Current Clinical Neurology

Series Editor

Daniel Tarsy
Beth Israel Deaconness Medical Center
Department of Neurology
Boston, MA
USA

Current Clinical Neurology offers a wide range of practical resources for clinical neurologists. Providing evidence-based titles covering the full range of neurologic disorders commonly presented in the clinical setting, the Current Clinical Neurology series covers such topics as multiple sclerosis, Parkinson's Disease and nonmotor dysfunction, seizures, Alzheimer's Disease, vascular dementia, sleep disorders, and many others. Series editor Daniel Tarsy, MD, is professor of neurology, Vice Chairman of the Department of Neurology, and Chief of the Movement Disorders division at Beth Israel Deaconness Hospital, Boston, Massachusetts.

More information about this series at http://www.springer.com/series/7630

Steven J. Frucht
Editor

Movement Disorder Emergencies

Diagnosis and Treatment

Third Edition

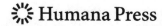 Humana Press

Editor
Steven J. Frucht
Department of Neurology
NYU Langone Health
New York, NY
USA

ISSN 1559-0585   ISSN 2524-4043   (electronic)
Current Clinical Neurology
ISBN 978-3-030-75900-1   ISBN 978-3-030-75898-1   (eBook)
https://doi.org/10.1007/978-3-030-75898-1

This Humana imprint is published by the registered company Springer Nature Switzerland AG
The registered company address is: Gewerbestrasse 11, 6330 Cham, Switzerland

For Rachel, Emma, Clare, and Lucy

Preface

Fifteen years have passed since the publication of the first edition of *Movement Disorder Emergencies*. In this time, what first seemed an unusual and esoteric topic has become mainstream. Teaching courses on movement disorder emergencies are a regular feature of the American Academy of Neurology and International Movement Disorders Congress' annual meetings, and the literature devoted to these rare but important topics has significantly grown.

In this third edition, all of the chapters have been revised and updated, and a number of new authors were added based on their expertise. We modified the organization of the chapters to better serve the practicing clinician, beginning with a practical approach to the patient, hyperacute emergencies, acute emergencies, emergencies of recognition (diagnostic pitfalls), and practical risks in the clinic (pitfalls in management). Key teaching points (shown with a key) and important lessons (shown with a lightning bolt) appear throughout each chapter. As before, videos are an indispensable resource, and the video segments accompanying 20 of the chapters have been expanded and are now available online. New chapters have been added, including discussion of the approach to the movement disorders patient in the emergency room and intensive care unit, neuro-ophthalmologic evaluation in movement disorders, posthypoxic myoclonus, X-linked adrenoleukodystrophy, and an unusual presentation of Wilson's disease.

We wish to thank Diane Lamsback for her enthusiasm, meticulous attention to detail, and indispensable effort in bringing this latest edition to fruition. We also thank the patients and their families who generously gave permission for publication of their videos. Finally, three young co-authors died tragically between the publication of the second edition and the present version. Dr. Jessica Panzer, Dr. Daniel Schneider, and Dr. John Lynch were highly skilled, compassionate clinicians whose contributions to patient care, education, and research will be sorely missed.

We dedicate this third edition to their memory.

New York, NY, USA   Steven J. Frucht

Series Editor Introduction

Welcome to the third edition of *Movement Disorders Emergencies. Diagnosis and Treatment* edited by Steven J. Frucht. The first and second editions were published by Springer in 2005 and 2013, respectively, and have been very well received. Both filled an important niche in the knowledge base of clinical neurologists who see most of their patients in the outpatient clinic or hospital emergency room.

The number of chapters has increased from 20 to 28 between the first two editions to 32 chapters in this new third edition. All previous chapters have been updated and revised, and important teaching points have been highlighted in many of the chapters. Patient videos continue to be available on the Springer website for nearly all of the chapters. New chapters by new authors which have been added in this volume include "Neuro-ophthalmologic Evaluation in Movement Disorders," "Movement Disorder Emergencies of the Upper Aerodigestive Tract," "Posthypoxic Myoclonus and its Management," "Tic Emergencies," "Coprolalia and Malignant Phonic Tics," "Startle Disorders," Functional Movement Disorders," "X-linked Adrenoleukodystrophy," and "Genetics and Genetic Counseling."

As previously emphasized by Dr. Frucht, emergencies have not only been defined in these volumes by the acute and serious nature of the disorders being described but also by the extreme rarity of many of these disorders which usually and even typically delays diagnosis and often regrettably results in a diagnosis of "psychogenic" or "functional" movement disorder born largely out of ignorance and lack of experience in the clinician asked to make a diagnosis in such cases. Once again, the neurologic community at all levels owes a large debt of gratitude to Dr. Frucht for his diligence in continuing to bring this topic to the attention of all of us.

Daniel Tarsy
Parkinson's Disease and Movement Disorders Center
Beth Israel Deaconess Medical Center, Harvard Medical School
Boston, MA, USA

Contents

Contributors

Umer Akbar, MD Department of Neurology, Brown University, Alpert Medical School Movement Disorders Program, Rhode Island Hospital, Providence, RI, USA

Boris Bentsianov, MD Department of Otolaryngology and Division of Laryngology, Voice and Swallowing Disorders, Downstate Medical Center, State University of New York, Brooklyn, NY, USA

Andrew Blitzer, MD, DDS Otolaryngology-Head and Neck Surgery, Columbia University College of Physicians and Surgeons, New York, NY, USA

Icahn School of Medicine at Mount Sinai, New York, NY, USA

New York Center for Voice and Swallowing Disorders, New York, NY, USA

Adam P. Burdick, MD Department of Neurosurgery, Scripps Clinic Medical Group, San Diego, CA, USA

Laura Buyan Dent, MD, PhD Department of Neurology, University of Wisconsin School of Medicine and Public Health, Madison, WI, USA

E. Cabrina Campbell, MD Department of Psychiatry, Corporal Michael J. Crescenz VA Medical Center and the University of Pennsylvania Perelman School of Medicine, Philadelphia, PA, USA

Stanley N. Caroff, MD Department of Psychiatry, Corporal Michael J. Crescenz VA Medical Center and the University of Pennsylvania Perelman School of Medicine, Philadelphia, PA, USA

Lesley F. Childs, MD Department of Otolaryngology – Head & Neck Surgery, UT Southwestern Medical Center, Dallas, TX, USA

Ajay E. Chitkara, MD ENT and Allergy Associates, LLP, Voice and Swallowing Disorders, Port Jefferson Station, NY, USA

Jenna Conway, MD Department of Neurology, New York University Grossman School of Medicine, New York, NY, USA

Blas Couto, MD, PhD Toronto Western Hospital, Morton and Gloria Shulman Movement Disorders Center and the Edmond J. Safra Program in Parkinson's Disease, Toronto, ON, Canada

Anthony Cultrara, MD Advanced ENT and Allergy, Voorhees, NJ, USA

Russell C. Dale, MBCHB, MSC, MRCPCH, PhD The Children's Hospital at Westmead, University of Sydney Specialty of Child & Adolescent Health, Westmead, NSW, Australia

Josep Dalmau, MD, PhD, ICREA Hospital Clinic, University Barcelona, Barcelona, Spain

University Pennsylvania, Philadelphia, PA, USA

Andrés De la Cerda, MD Department of Neuroscience, Clínica Dávila, Santiago, Chile

CETRAM, Santiago, Chile

Patrick S. Drummond, MD Department of Neurology, NYU Langone Health, New York, NY, USA

Stewart A. Factor, DO Movement Disorders Program, Vance Lanier Chair for Neurology, Emory University School of Medicine, Atlanta, GA, USA

Alfonso Fasano, MD, PhD Toronto Western Hospital, Movement Disorders Centre, Toronto, ON, Canada

Hubert H. Fernandez, MD Center for Neurological Restoration, Neurological Institute, Cleveland Clinic, Cleveland, OH, USA

Joseph H. Friedman, MD Butler Hospital, Providence, RI, USA

Steven J. Frucht, MD Department of Neurology, NYU Langone Health, New York, NY, USA

Yoshiaki Furukawa, MD, PhD Department of Neurology, Juntendo Tokyo Koto Geriatric Medical Center, Tokyo, Japan

Department of Neurology, Faculty of Medicine, Juntendo University, Tokyo, Japan

Philippe A. Salles, MD Department of Neuroscience, Clínica Dávila, Santiago, Chile CETRAM, Santiago, Chile

Center for Neurological Restoration, Neurological Institute, Cleveland Clinic, Cleveland, OH, USA

Christopher G. Goetz, MD Department of Neurological Sciences, Rush University Medical Center, Chicago, IL, USA

Jennifer G. Goldman, MD, MS Shirley Ryan AbilityLab, Northwestern University Feinberg School of Medicine, Chicago, IL, USA

Mark Forrest Gordon, MD Specialty Clinical Development, Teva Pharmaceuticals, West Chester, PA, USA

Mark Guttman, MD, FRCPC Centre for Movement Disorders, Toronto, ON, Canada

Peter Hedera, MD, PhD Department of Neurology, University of Louisville Medical Center, Louisville, KY, USA

Vanessa K. Hinson, MD, PhD Department of Neurology, Medical University of South Carolina, Charleston, SC, USA

Daniel E. Huddleston, MD Department of Neurology, Emory University School of Medicine, Atlanta, GA, USA

Tooru Inoue, MD, PhD Department of Neurosurgery, Fukuoka University Faculty of Medicine, Fukuoka, Japan

Prudencio Lozano-Iraguen, MD Department of Neuroscience, Clínica Dávila, Santiago, Chile

Eiji Isozaki, MD Department of Neurology, Tokyo Metropolitan Neurological Hospital, Fuchu, Tokyo, Japan

Joseph Jankovic, MD Parkinson's Disease Center and Movement Disorders Clinic, Department of Neurology, Baylor College of Medicine, Houston, TX, USA

Beomseok Jeon, MD, PhD Department of Neurology, Seoul National University College of Medicine, Seoul, South Korea

Laura A. Ketigian, BS New York Institute of Technology—College of Osteopathic Medicine, Old Westbury, NY, USA

Jong-Min Kim, MD, PhD Department of Neurology, Seoul National University College of Medicine, Seoul, South Korea

Stephen J. Kish, PhD Human Brain Laboratory, Centre for Addiction and Mental Health, University of Toronto, Toronto, ON, Canada

Anthony E. T. Lang, MD, FRCPC Toronto Western Hospital, Morton and Gloria Shulman Movement Disorders Center and the Edmond J. Safra Program in Parkinson's Disease, Toronto, ON, Canada

Adena N. Leder, DO, FAAN Adele Smithers Parkinson's Disease Treatment Center, New York Institute of Technology—College of Osteopathic Medicine, Old Westbury, NY, USA

Valentina Besa-Lehmann, MD Department of Neuroscience, Clínica Dávila, Santiago, Chile

CETRAM, Santiago, Chile

John Lynch, (Deceased), MD

Timothy Lynch, MB, BSc, FRCPI, FRCP Department of Neurology, Dublin Neurological Institute at the Mater Misericordiae University Hospital, Dublin, Ireland

Stephan C. Mann, MD, DLFAPA Private Practice, Harleysville, PA, USA

Inge A. Meijer, MD, PhD Department of Neurosciences, CHU Sainte Justine, Montreal, QC, Canada

Takashi Morishita, MD, PhD Department of Neurosurgery, Fukuoka University Faculty of Medicine, Fukuoka, Japan

Eoin Mulroy, MB, BCh, BAO Dublin Neurological Institute at the Mater Misericordiae University Hospital, Dublin, Ireland

Department of Clinical and Movement Neurosciences, UCL Queen Square Institute of Neurology, London, UK

Martha A. Nance, MD Struthers Parkinson's Center, Golden Valley, MN, USA

Jessica Panzer, (Deceased), MD, PhD

Roser Pons, MD First Department of Pediatrics, National and Kapodistrian University of Athens, Agia Sofia, Athens, Greece

Ronald B. Postuma, MD, MSc Department of Neurology, McGill University, Montreal General Hospital, Montreal, QC, Canada

Giulietta Maria Riboldi, MD Department of Neurology, NYU Langone Health, The Marlene and Paolo Fresco Institute for Parkinson's and Movement Disorders, New York, NY, USA

Scott Rickert, MD Division of Pediatric Otolaryngology, Department of Otolaryngology, Pediatrics, and Plastic Surgery, NYU Langone Health, New York, NY, USA

Janet C. Rucker, MD Department of Neurology, New York University Grossman School of Medicine, New York, NY, USA

Daniel Schneider, (Deceased), MD, MA Department of Neurology, Robert Wood Johnson Medical School, New Brunswick, NJ, USA

Meagan D. Seay, DO University of Utah Moran Eye Center, Salt Lake City, UT, USA

Kathleen M. Shannon, MD Department of Neurology, University of Wisconsin School of Medicine and Public Health, Madison, WI, USA

Christine M. Stahl, MD Department of Neurology, NYU Langone Health, New York, NY, USA

Christopher D. Stephen, MB ChB, MRCP (UK), MS Ataxia Center, Dystonia Center, Movement Disorders Unit, and Functional Neurological Disorder Research Program, Department of Neurology, Massachusetts General Hospital and Harvard Medical School, Boston, MA, USA

Thomas Stewart, FRACS (OHNS), MMed, MBBS, BMedSc New York Centre for Voice and Swallowing Disorders, New York, NY, USA

Kenneth A. Sullivan, PhD Department of Psychiatry, Corporal Michael J. Crescenz VA Medical Center and the University of Pennsylvania Perelman School of Medicine, Philadelphia, PA, USA

Pichet Termsarasab, MD Division of Neurology, Department of Medicine, Faculty of Medicine Ramathibodi Hospital, Bangkok, Thailand

Philip D. Thompson, MB, BS, PhD, FRACP The University of Adelaide, Adelaide, SA, Australia

Yuji Tomizawa, MD, PhD Department of Neurology, Juntendo Tokyo Koto Geriatric Medical Center, Juntendo University, Tokyo, Japan

Department of Neurology, Faculty of Medicine, Juntendo University, Tokyo, Japan

Ergun Y. Uc, MD Department of Neurology, Division of Movement Disorders and Parkinson's Foundation Center of Excellence, University of Iowa Carver College of Medicine, Iowa City, IA, USA

Carolina Pelayo-Varela, MD Department of Neuroscience, Clínica Dávila, Santiago, Chile

Christina L. Vaughan, MD, MHS Departments of Neurology and Medicine, University of Colorado, Anschutz Medical Center, Aurora, CO, USA

Valerie Voon, MD, PhD Department of Psychiatry, University of Cambridge, Addenbrooke's Hospital, Cambridge, UK

Daniel T. Williams, MD Department of Psychiatry, Columbia University Medical Center, New York, NY, USA

List of Videos

ing basic activities of daily living. Profound negative axial myoclonic jerks prevented him from standing even with two-person
assist. The next patient, a young woman who developed LAS after
an unrecognized esophageal intubation during a gynecologic surgery,
was incapacitated by medication-refractory myoclonus. She is shown
before and 20 minutes after ingestion of two glasses of wine, with
profound improvement in myoclonus and functional performance.
The final patient developed LAS after surviving a cardiopulmonary
arrest from spontaneous bilateral pneumothorax. Vocal myoclonus
prevented him from communicating, and myoclonus at rest and with
action left him completely functionally disabled. He is shown in
hospital before and 1 hour after ingestion of two grams of sodium
oxybate, with profound improvement in myoclonus.   201

Six patients with severe tic disorders are presented. An adult woman
with a 20-year history of tics had been under recent stress, and her
tics became severe enough for her to seek additional care. Whereas
her usual tics involved eye and neck movements, over 3 months their
severity increased to included flailing arm jerks and truncal movements that caused her to stumble and, in some instances, fall to the
ground. She became cautious about taking public transportation and
standing on train platforms because of fears she would stumble and
fall onto the train tracks. The second patient, an adult with a history
of over 40 years of tics, was concerned about muscle wasting and
numbness in one leg. He had an array of fluctuating tics that
included loud vocalizations, bruxism, and nasal and facial movements that waxed and waned. Over the last year, he developed leg
tics that involved knee banging and unusual rotational movements of
one leg. When he performed these leg tics, he had a tingling sensation in one leg that was uncomfortable but "strangely satisfying." On
examination, tics were observed, but also wasting of muscles
supplied by the sciatic nerve. Electromyography confirmed a sciatic
neuropathy at the level of the sciatic notch. The third patient had a
10-year history of GTS, and presented with a complaint of worsening leg and truncal tics. He had been started on pimozide 3 weeks
prior because of facial and neck tics. His family physician further
increased the pimozide because of his complaint of new leg movements and truncal rocking 1 week later. On examination by a
neurologist, multifocal motor tics affecting eyes, face, neck and
shoulder were present, as well as complex phonic tics. In addition,
marked rhythmic leg movements and rocking motions were accompanied by a subjective sense of inner restlessness and an inability to
sit still. When asked if the leg and truncal movements seemed
different than his familiar tics, he affirmed that they were. Whereas
he could suppress his eye, face and neck movements for several

minutes, he could not keep his legs or trunk still for even a few seconds. He was diagnosed with neuroleptic-induced akathisia. The fourth patient presented for evaluation of vocal tics (groaning tics) that were intrusive. Tetrabenazine was started with good control of these tics, and he was scheduled to return to school. However, anxiety surrounding his return to the classroom triggered a stress reaction, with involuntary movements that were flailing and distractible. The next patient, a young boy, presented with screaming vocal tics which were so loud that they could be heard four houses away at home; he was treated successfully with risperidone. The final patient developed continuous, unremitting tics with coprolalia, resistant to all available medications, even monitored sedation in the ICU. After an extensive review and discussion, he underwent implantation of bilateral GPi deep brain stimulators, with excellent response. . .   221

Video 13.1   Coprolalia and Malignant Phonic Tics

Five patients illustrate the significant challenge of malignant motor tics. The first patient, with "Gilles de la Tourette" syndrome (TS) exhibits loud vocalizations and screams that have markedly impaired his quality of life. His mother has only blinking tics. The second patient has severe TS and complex tics, one of which is manifested by a severe Valsalva maneuver and loud noise imitating "monsters." The third patient, an adult with TS and severe obsessive-compulsive disorder (OCD), had to stop working because of the loud screaming vocalizations. The fourth patient is a 46-year-old professor referred to our clinic with uncontrollable phonic tics such as bursts of screaming and obscene words. He developed phonic tics of coughing and wheezing, which was diagnosed as a "psychogenic motor disorder." He had other phonic tics of sniffing, sudden loud outbursts of laughing, and shouting of phrases such as "shut up" and "help." He also developed severe coprolalia. His motor tics presented in adulthood including facial grimacing, head jerking, and complex maneuvers of slapping his right upper extremity and knee. Because of the persistent and severe nature of his phonic tics, the patient resigned from lecturing at the university and transitioned to teaching classes on-line through internet-based learning. The last patient, a subject of the initial report of treatment of malignant coprolalia with botulinum toxin experienced initial onset of motor tics at age 2 years with facial grimacing, nose twitching, snorting, and sniffing. He also exhibited bulimic eating patterns, with a compulsion to vomit because it "felt good." He later developed severe coprolalia, frequently blurting words like "bitch," "mother fucker," and "asshole." He described an urge to have to make the movements and shout the obscenities. He reported that he was able to suppress his tics and vocalizations transiently, until he "let it all out" in the bathroom. His vocalizations resulted in several fights, social stigmatization and isolation from his peers, poor academic performance, depression and anxiety. The phonic tics and coprolalia were initially well controlled with pimozide, approx. 6 mg/day, and fluphenazine, approx. 5 mg/ day. However, his symptoms became very severe and a trial of BoNT type A (OnabotulinumtoxinA) injection, 30 U into the left vocal cord resulted in drastic improvement of his vocal symptoms. The patient received four treatment sessions over a period of 15 months. He reported a mean beneficial response of 2.3 at peak effect on a 0-4-point scale (0, no effect; 1, mild effect but no functional improvement; 2, moderate improvement but no change in functional disability; 3, moderate change in both severity and function; 4. marked improvement in both severity and function). A mean dose of 25 mouse U was injected, and mean duration of response was 20 weeks. He had no response (peak effect score 0) with a low dose of 20 U. However, he reported a mean peak effect score of 3.3 with dosages of 25-30 U. He noted that the BoNT injections markedly improved his quality of life, allowing him to socialize and secure employment. His phonic tics improved during young adulthood, and he is currently not taking any anti-tic medications.   233

Video 14.1   Hemiballism-Hemichorea

Four patients with hemiballism, three with nonketoic hyperglycemic chorea, and three with chorea storm are seen in this video segment. The first patient developed hemiballism secondary to left hemi-spheric cortical ischemia, demonstrated on MRI. The following patient developed left hemiballism from a right pontine hemorrhage. The next patient is shown in hospital after developing acute right hemiballism from a left midbrain hemorrhage. Ballistic movements were severe enough to cause bruising on his right arm and leg, requiring protective padding on his hospital bed. The next patient, a 55-year-old man, developed acute right hemiballism from a left subthalamic nucleus infarct, shown on imaging. The next patient presented to the emergency room with new, acute generalized chorea, and was found to have a blood sugar of 400. Her MRI revealed characteristic lesions of nonketotic hyperglycemic chorea. She also was treated with tetrabenazine, with good response. The following woman was admitted with new right hemiballism due to nonketoic hyperglycemia. In-hospital treatment with 1 mg of haloperidol substantially improved her involuntary movements. The final patient with nonketotic hyperglycemia is shown in hospital, with left hemiballism. Characteristic lesions are seen on CT and T1-weighted MRI images. The next patient, a 2-year-old girl, developed an encephalopathy of unknown etiology associated with severe generalized chorea (chorea storm). Chorea did not improve with any standard treatment including high dose neuroleptics, and

Part I

Practical Approach to the Patient with a Movement Disorder Emergency

Practical Approach to Management of the Movement Disorders Patient in the Hospital and Intensive Care Unit

1

Pichet Termsarasab

Patient Vignette

A 12-year-old boy with known DYT1 generalized dystonia presented to the emergency room with marked worsening of his dystonic symptoms over the last day. He initially presented with bilateral foot dystonia at the age of 5 years, which then spread upward becoming generalized within 1.5 years. He was managed with oral medications and an intrathecal baclofen pump, as his parents did not want to pursue deep brain stimulation. His dystonia had been under good control with trihexyphenidyl 12 mg/day, clonazepam 2 mg/day, and intrathecal baclofen. In the emergency room, severe generalized dystonia involving both arms, legs, and trunk was obvious, with temperature of 39.2 °C, blood pressure 154/95 mmHg, pulse 100/minute, respiratory rate 26/minute, and oxygen saturation 91% on room air. He was agitated and diaphoretic, and quickly diagnosed with dystonic storm. On arrival in the emergency room, his airway, breathing, and circulation were assessed, and he was given 2 liters of oxygen by nasal cannula which improved his oxygen saturation to 98%. Intravenous access was secured, and the basic labs including complete blood count, serum electrolytes, blood urea nitrogen, creatinine, creatine kinase (CK), urinalysis, as well as blood and urine cultures were collected. Intravenous fluids were promptly initiated, and an intensive care unit (ICU) consult was immediately called. He was given intravenous antipyretics without improvement in his temperature, and subsequently required a cooling blanket. Intravenous benztropine and lorazepam were given with only slight improvement in dystonia. Due to marked agitation and dystonia, continuous infusion of intravenous midazolam was started in the intensive care unit. The CK result returned at 853 units/liter. Urine myoglobin was negative. Aggressive IV fluid hydration was continued.

P. Termsarasab (✉)
Division of Neurology, Department of Medicine, Faculty of Medicine Ramathibodi Hospital, Bangkok, Thailand

© Springer Nature Switzerland AG 2022
S. J. Frucht (ed.), *Movement Disorder Emergencies*, Current Clinical Neurology,
https://doi.org/10.1007/978-3-030-75898-1_1

Further work-up with X-ray shunt series demonstrated breakage and kinking of the baclofen pump catheter, consistent with abrupt discontinuation of baclofen delivery. Treatment options, including repairing the pump or emergency deep brain stimulation, were discussed with his parents, and the decision was made to pursue the first. The patient was brought to the operating room, and intrathecal baclofen delivery was resumed. Dystonia and autonomic instability gradually improved in the ICU, and he returned back to his baseline over the next couple of days.

Discussion

This case demonstrates several important principles of management of movement disorder emergencies in the hospital and intensive care unit. Rapid decision-making, prompt and aggressive management, and identification of etiologies and/or precipitating factors should occur in parallel. Crucial steps in the management of movement disorder emergencies include activating intensive care unit expertise with close monitoring, management of temperature and autonomic instability, as well as symptomatic treatment when the precipitant of the emergency is identified.

Introduction

Patients with movement disorder emergencies may be encountered in the emergency room or intensive care unit, and are often critically ill. After initial evaluation, transfer to an intensive care unit is often required. Understanding the principles of management of movement disorder emergencies will help clinicians make appropriate clinical decisions and minimize risks of morbidity and mortality [1]. This chapter presents a practical approach to the management of patients with severe movement disorder emergencies in the hospital and intensive care unit (ICU).

Principles of the Management of the Patient in the Hospital and Intensive Care Unit

The management of the acutely ill movement disorder emergency patient requires a two-pronged approach. Stabilizing the patient is the first priority. While identification of etiologies and/or precipitating factors begins, symptomatic therapies should not be delayed. In short, diagnostic and therapeutic processes should occur in parallel, not sequentially.

     Acute management and identification of etiologies and/or precipitating factors should occur in parallel.

The framework for the management of movement disorder emergencies in the hospital and ICU is demonstrated in Fig. 1.1.

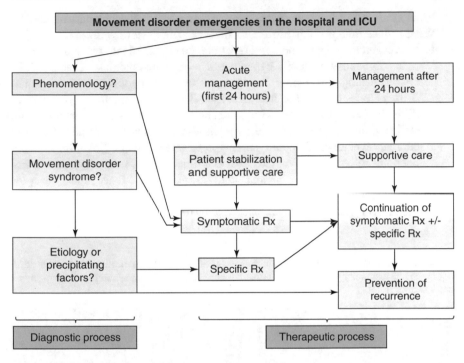

Fig. 1.1 An algorithm for the management of movement disorder emergencies in the hospital or intensive care unit. The diagnostic and therapeutic processes should occur in parallel. In clinical practice, these steps are usually performed simultaneously

Correct identification of the etiology of the movement disorder emergency begins with phenomenology. Movement disorder emergencies can be classified into two main categories, namely hypokinetic and hyperkinetic emergencies. Once the main phenomenology is identified, the next step is to identify the specific syndrome. For example, once parkinsonism along with rigidity is recognized, neuroleptic malignant syndrome can be identified. After the movement disorder emergency is correctly diagnosed, the etiologies and/or precipitating factors can be sought and appropriate therapies employed. Early and aggressive treatment is key. Treatment can be divided into acute management (<24 hours), and subacute management (>24 hours). In the first 24 hours, the main goals are patient stabilization and identification of etiologies and/or precipitating factors. After the first 24 hours, the management aims to provide supportive therapies and prevent recurrence.

Identification of Etiologies and/or Precipitating Factors

Three main questions should guide the clinician:

1. What is the predominant *phenomenology* in this patient?

2. What *syndrome* of the movement disorder emergencies does the patient have?
3. What is the *etiology* of this movement disorder emergency syndrome?
    1. Movement disorder phenomenologies can be classified into two main catego-
       ries: hypokinetic and hyperkinetic phenomenologies (Table 1.1).
       Distinguishing movements that are too slow (aka. hypokinetic movements)
       from the ones that are too fast (aka. hyperkinetic movements) is usually not
       difficult. Examples of hypokinetic phenomenologies include parkinsonism,
       stiffness, and catatonia. Acute hyperkinetic emergencies include dystonia,
       chorea, myoclonus, tics, and stereotypies, among others. Sometimes, acute
       phenomenologies may be mixed, for example, chorea, stereotypy, and dysto-
       nia may co-exist in a patient with anti-N-methyl-D-aspartate receptor
       (NMDAR) encephalitis [2]. Tremor is also considered a hyperkinetic phe-
       nomenology, but is rarely present in isolation.

Table 1.1 Three main diagnostic steps in movement disorder emergencies include identification of (1) the phenomenology, (2) movement disorder emergency syndromes, and (3) etiology and/or precipitating factor

1. Phenomenology	2. Syndrome	3. Etiology/Precipitating factor
Hypokinetic		
Parkinsonism	Neuroleptic malignant syndrome	Neuroleptics or other dopamine receptor blocking agents
	Parkinsonism-hyperpyrexia syndrome[1]	Abrupt discontinuation of levodopa
	Acute parkinsonism	CNS infection such as viral encephalitis, prion; drugs
Catatonia	Malignant catatonia	Underlying psychiatric disorders such as depression or schizophrenia
Stiffness	Acute severe exacerbation of spasms and rigidity/status spasticus in SPSD	Natural history of the diseases; can be triggered by intercurrent illness such as infection
Hyperkinetic		
Dystonia	Dystonic storm	Infection, abrupt discontinuation of anti-dystonic treatment such as baclofen or anticholinergics
	Acute dystonic reaction	Neuroleptics or other dopamine receptor blocking agents
Myoclonus + tremor (also with rigidity)	Serotonin syndrome[2]	Serotonergic agents (dose-dependent)
Chorea	Choreic storm	Underlying choreic disorders; can be triggered by intercurrent illness such as infection
Myoclonus	Myoclonic status	Underlying myoclonic disorders such as posthypoxic myoclonus, not responsive to medical treatment
Tic	Tic status	Exacerbation of an underlying tic disorder

CNS central nervous system, *SPSD* stiff-person spectrum disorders
[a]Clinical features identical to neuroleptic malignant syndrome
[b]Some may classify serotonin syndrome as a hypokinetic emergency due to prominent rigidity

2. Once the movement disorder phenomenology is identified, the next step is to determine the movement disorder emergency syndrome. To identify the syndrome, clinicians must consider phenomenology, along with additional information including time course, level of consciousness, fever, and autonomic features. The features of selected movement disorder emergency syndromes are outlined in Table 1.2.

   Hypokinetic movement disorder syndromes include parkinsonism-hyperpyrexia syndrome, neuroleptic malignant syndrome, serotonin syndrome, acute parkinsonism due to other causes, malignant catatonia, and acute severe exacerbation of spasms and rigidity in stiff-person spectrum disorders [3]. Examples of the syndromes related to hyperkinetic movement disorder emergencies include dystonic storm (aka. status dystonicus), choreic storm, myoclonic status, and tic status, among others. In addition, some syndromes are encountered in patients with known underlying movement disorders. Examples include severe stridor or respiratory compromise due to vocal abductor paresis in multiple system atrophy [4], psychosis in Parkinson's disease, and cervical myelopathy in patients with severe cervical tics [5].

3. After the correct syndrome is identified, precipitating factors should be sought (see Table 1.1), and specific treatments employed. For example,

Table 1.2 Clinical features of selected movement disorder emergency syndromes in the hospital and intensive care unit including the main phenomenology, co-existing features, fever, other autonomic features, and mental status

MD emergency syndrome	Main phenomenology	Co-existing features	Fever	Other autonomic features	Altered mental status
Neuroleptic malignant syndrome[a]	Parkinsonism including rigidity		++	++	++
Serotonin syndrome	Myoclonus, shivering-like movements	Rigidity, hyperreflexia	+	++	++
Malignant catatonia	Catatonia		+	+	++
Acute severe exacerbation of spasms and rigidity/ status spasticus in SPSD	Stiffness, muscle spasms, and rigidity		+	++	+/++
Acute dystonic reaction	Dystonia, typically retrocollis and lower cranial dystonia	Can co-occur with oculogyric crisis	+/−	+/−	−
Dystonic storm	Dystonia		+	+	−
Choreic storm	Chorea		+/−	+/−	−
Myoclonic status	Myoclonus		+	+	−
Tic status	Tic		−	−	−

"+" indicates presence of these features; "++" indicates higher association and/or severity; "−" indicates lack of these features

SPSD stiff-person spectrum disorder

[a]Parkinsonism-hyperpyrexia syndrome is also included in this category

once neuroleptic malignant syndrome is identified, dopamine receptor blocking agents should be immediately discontinued. Symptoms reminiscent of neuroleptic malignant syndrome in a patient with Parkinson's disease are termed the parkinsonism-hyperpyrexia syndrome [6, 7]. Levodopa withdrawal is often a trigger, and specific treatment employs delivery of levodopa or other dopaminergic agents. In hyperkinetic storms such as dystonic storm, precipitating factors include intercurrent illness or infection, or baclofen withdrawal due to malfunction of intrathecal baclofen pump (as in our patient) [8]. Once the precipitating factor is addressed, appropriate specific treatments (antibiotics and resuming baclofen delivery) can be provided. In contrast, if a patient develops acute dystonia in the cervical (retrocollis) or lower cranial regions, a different syndrome may be recognized: an acute dystonic reaction, usually due to a D2 receptor blocker. Discontinuation of the offending agent and institution of parenteral diphenhydramine or biperiden may be life-saving.

⊙━━━▪   Treatment of movement disorder emergencies begins with phenomenology: to establish whether it is a hyperkinetic or hypokinetic syndrome.

Principles of Management

Table 1.3 demonstrates principles of management in the acute and subacute periods.

Table 1.3 Principles of management of movement disorder emergencies in the hospital and intensive care unit

1. Acute management in the first 24 hours
Maintain ABC (Airway, Breathing and Circulation)
Early ICU transfer: Be aggressive and proactive
Secure IV access
Aggressive IV fluid hydration
Temperature reduction measures, e.g., acetaminophen or cooling blanket if >40 °C
Treatment of autonomic instability such as hypertension, tachycardia
Assess and consider needs for ventilatory support
Close monitoring of vital signs and other parameters such as urine output
Obtain necessary lab tests, e.g., CBC, electrolytes, BUN, Cr, CK, UA, ABG, infectious work-up, but these should not delay other steps
Symptomatic therapies of movement disorders
Selection is based on the phenomenology and movement disorder emergency syndromes (see Table 1.1)
IV sedatives/anesthetics, if needed, e.g., benzodiazepines, propofol, barbiturates
Specific therapies: Address and treat underlying etiology and precipitating factors
2. Management after 24 hours
Continue supportive care and symptomatic therapies
Prevent recurrence or relapses

ABG arterial blood gas, *BUN* blood urea nitrogen, *CBC* complete blood count, *CK* creatine kinase, *Cr* creatinine, *ICU* intensive care unit, *IV* intravenous, *UA* urinalysis

Acute Management (<24 Hours)

The primary goal in the first 24 hours is to reduce morbidity and mortality. Early, prompt and aggressive intervention is key. It is always better to err on the side of action and to transfer a patient to the ICU before they decompensate with respiratory embarrassment or cardiovascular collapse.

Prompt, aggressive management in the acute phase is key.

Intravenous (IV) access should be secured, preferably with at least two lines for IV fluid and IV drug administration. Aggressive IV fluid hydration helps address hypotension and myoglobinuria, (e.g., neuroleptic malignant syndrome, dystonic storm) [9, 10]. IV fluid hydration also has an important role in hyperkinetic emergencies such as dystonic or choreic storm where metabolic derangements can lead to massive fluid loss and "third spacing" of interstitial fluid. Fever, dehydration, and hypotension increase morbidity [11]. Temperature reduction includes pharmacological treatment such as intravenous antipyretics (acetaminophen or non-steroidal anti-inflammatory agents). Physical methods such as cooling blankets may also be used. If the temperature is very high (e.g., greater than 40 °C) or refractory to the initial temperature management, more aggressive measures such as intravascular cooling catheters should be considered [11, 12]. In this case, continuous core temperature monitoring (e.g., by using an esophageal probe) is required during the maintenance of normothermia.

Autonomic instability such as hyperthermia, labile blood pressure, tachycardia, and diaphoresis is common in neuroleptic malignant syndrome, serotonin syndrome, and dystonic storm. Blood pressure should be closely monitored, and interventions such as IV antihypertensive agents or vasopressors should be initiated promptly. Patients with labile blood pressure may benefit from continuous blood pressure monitoring with an arterial line. Early detection of respiratory compromise by checking an arterial blood gas helps to identify respiratory failure before a crisis. Intubation in patients with severe rigidity or muscle spasms may require IV sedatives or neuromuscular blocking agents. Typically, blood samples are collected during the process of securing an IV access, including complete blood count, serum electrolytes, creatine kinase (CK), blood urea nitrogen, creatinine, urinalysis, among others. A septic work-up should always be performed, especially when there is fever. CK is often elevated in neuroleptic malignant syndrome, serotonin syndrome, or any other movement disorder emergencies that result in rhabdomyolysis. Urine myoglobin can be considered when there is rhabdomyolysis or red-colored urine but absence of erythrocytes. Aggressive IV fluid hydration is required in these patients to prevent renal failure in the setting of myoglobinuria. Urine output, renal function, and serum CK should be monitored. Metabolic acidosis due to lactic acidosis and rhabdomyolysis can result in hyperkalemia which can potentially lead to cardiac arrhythmias and sudden cardiac arrest.

The phenomenology of movement disorder emergencies helps guide symptomatic therapies (Table 1.4). For example, in dystonic emergencies such as dystonic storm, intravenous anticholinergics and/or benzodiazepines should be employed [8]. Parenteral baclofen is available only for an intrathecal route, and intrathecal baclofen should *not* be injected intravenously. Severe muscle rigidity or spasms (such as in neuroleptic malignant syndrome or status spasticus in stiff-person spectrum disorders) or excessive movements in various hyperkinetic emergencies may result in rhabdomyolysis, increased energy consumption, and metabolic acidosis. In these circumstances, sedation with intravenous anesthetic agents such as benzodiazepines or propofol should be considered. Medications should be administered parenterally by intravenous route, not orally or via a nasogastric tube. Rapidly acting medications are usually preferred, as gastrointestinal motility and absorption may not be reliable in critically ill patients [13]. Pharmacological therapies commonly

Table 1.4 Symptomatic and specific therapies in some selected movement disorder emergency syndromes

Movement disorder emergency syndrome	Symptomatic Rx	Specific Rx
Neuroleptic malignant syndrome	Dopamine agonists, e.g., bromocriptine; Dantrolene	Discontinue neuroleptics; avoid restarting at least in the next 2 weeks
Serotonin syndrome	Cyproheptadine, propranolol	Discontinue serotonergic agents
Malignant catatonia	BZDs such as lorazepam	Treat underlying psychiatric disorders; consider electroconvulsive therapy (ECT)
Acute severe exacerbation of spasms and rigidity/status spasticus in SPSD	BZDs, baclofen, anesthetic agents	Treat precipitating factors such as infection
Acute dystonic reaction	IV anticholinergics or antihistamines, BZDs may be an alternative	Discontinue neuroleptics
Dystonic storm	BZDs, baclofen, anticholinergics, sedative/anesthetic agents; DBS can be considered in DYT1, DYT6, and tardive dystonia	Treat underlying precipitating factors; resume baclofen in case of baclofen withdraw
Choreic storm	High-potency neuroleptics, tetrabenazine, sedative/anesthetic agents	Treat underlying etiologies of chorea such as blood sugar control in non-ketotic hyperglycemia
Myoclonic status	Valproate, levetiracetam, BZDs; DBS can be considered in posthypoxic myoclonus	Treat underlying precipitating factors, if any
Tic status	High potency neuroleptics, tetrabenazine, BZD, clonidine	Treat underlying precipitating factors, if any

BZD benzodiazepine, *SPSD* stiff-person spectrum disorders used in the hospital and ICU for movement disorder emergencies are demonstrated in Table 1.5.

Surgical intervention plays an important role in some movement disorder emergencies. For example, deep brain stimulation (DBS) of bilateral globus pallidi (GPi) in patients with dystonic storm may be life-saving, especially in DYT1 dystonia [8, 14]. The modern approach is to consider DBS in the first 24 hours after patients are stabilized, as DBS can rapidly terminate storm.

Identification of etiologies and/or precipitating factors impacts appropriate selection of specific therapies. For example, if anti-NMDAR encephalitis is identified in a patient with severe stereotypy, chorea, and altered mental status, prompt initiation of immunotherapies including intravenous methylprednisolone and/or intravenous immunoglobulin will often lead to a good outcome. In neuroleptic

Table 1.5 Pharmacologic therapies commonly used for movement disorder emergencies in the hospital and intensive care unit

Medication	Route[a]	Dosage	Dosing interval	Note
Bromocriptine	PO/ NG	2.5–5 mg/dose	q 8 h	If not available, other DAs can be considered as an alternative
Dantrolene	IV	1–2.5 mg/kg/dose	q 6 h	
Cyproheptadine	PO/ NG	2–12 mg/dose	q 2 h	Start with 12 mg, followed by 2 mg q 2 h
Benztropine	IV/IM	1–2 mg/dose	Single dose	
Diphenhydramine	IV	25–50 mg/dose	Single dose	
Baclofen	PO/ NG	15–120 mg/d	TID	Intrathecal form should *not* be injected intravenously
Lorazepam[b]	IV/IM	1–4 mg/dose	q 5 min to 4–6 h	Dosing interval depends on indications[c]
Diazepam[b]	IV/IM	5–10 mg/dose	q 8 min to 8 h	Dosing interval depends on indications[c]
Midazolam[b]	IV	Initiation 0.01–0.05 mg/ kg; maintenance 0.02–0.1 mg/kg/h	Continuous infusion	
Propofol	IV	Initiation 0.3 mg/kg/h; maintenance 0.3–3 mg/ kg/h	Continuous infusion	
Pentobarbital	IV	Loading 1 mg/kg, then 1–3 mg/kg/h (maximum 5 mg/kg/h)	Continuous infusion	

d day, *DA* dopamine agonists, *h* hour, *IM* intramuscular, *IV* intravenous, *kg* kilogram, *mcg* microgram, *mg* milligram, *min* minute, *NG* via nasogastric tube, *PO* per oral, *q* every
[a]When there are multiple options for parenteral administration, an intravenous route is preferred in movement disorder emergencies
[b]These medications are benzodiazepines
[c]Lorazepam or diazepam can be given every 8–10 minutes in serotonin syndrome. In neuroleptic malignant syndrome, it can be given every 8 hours

malignant syndrome or serotonin syndrome, removal of offending agents is a crucial step in termination of these movement disorder emergencies. In neuroleptic malignant syndrome, neuroleptics should be avoided for at least 2 weeks, and when rechallenged, low dosage, gradual titration, and low-potency neuroleptics are preferred [15, 16]. In serotonin syndrome, the washout period of previously offending agents depends on the half-life of serotonergic medications. In dystonic storm, precipitating factors such as infection or abrupt discontinuation of anti-dystonic medications including baclofen or anticholinergics should be addressed promptly [8, 17, 18].

Management After the First 24 Hours

Management after the first 24 hours aims to provide supportive care and symptomatic treatment, as well as prevent recurrence. This process may take 2–4 weeks until the movement disorder emergency completely resolves. Some patients may require prolonged admission to the ICU due to difficult ventilator weaning or complicated infections such as pneumonia or urinary tract infections. Prevention of recurrence is also of importance. IV medications can be switched to an oral route during the maintenance phase. Early discontinuation of symptomatic therapies without maintenance can lead to recurrence of movement disorder emergencies. For example, in patients with acute dystonic reactions, after termination of the reaction with IV anticholinergics, oral anticholinergics should be continued for at least a week to prevent recurrence [19]. Continuation of specific therapies depends on the underlying etiology. For example, in cases of infection as a trigger, some patients may require a prolonged course of antibiotics. Rechallenging of medications such as antipsychotics or serotonergic medications requires special caution.

Table 1.6 demonstrates pearls and pitfalls in management of movement disorder

Table 1.6 Pearls and pitfalls in the management of movement disorder emergencies in the hospital and intensive care unit

Be aggressive, intervene early. Do not exercise a "wait-and-see" approach.
Consider early ICU admission.
General ICU care including vital sign monitoring, IV fluid hydration, temperature reduction measures is paramount.
Aggressive IV fluid hydration to prevent renal failure, especially when at risk for rhabdomyolysis and myoglobinuria.
Close monitoring is required.
An IV route of medication administration is preferred in the first 24 hours.
Maintain with oral symptomatic medication(s) after acute treatment with IV medications; early discontinuation of symptomatic therapies may lead to recurrence.
Be cautious about movement disorder emergency mimics such as pseudodystonic emergencies and sepsis (mimicking neuroleptic malignant syndrome or malignant hyperthermia).

ICU intensive care unit, *IV* intravenous

emergencies in the hospital and ICU.

Conclusion

Management of most movement disorder emergencies begins with diagnosis at the bedside. Clinical acumen helps determine the nature of the problem (hypokinetic or hyperkinetic), allowing disease-specific interventions to begin while patients are stabilized.

References

1. Poston KL, Frucht SJ. Movement disorder emergencies. J Neurol. 2008;255(Suppl 4):2–13. https://doi.org/10.1007/s00415-008-4002-9.
2. Varley JA, Webb AJS, Balint B, Fung VSC, Scthi KD, Tijssen MAJ, et al. The movement disorder associated with NMDAR antibody encephalitis is complex and characteristic: an expert video-rating study. J Neurol Neurosurg Psychiatry. 2019;90(6):724–6. https://doi.org/10.1136/jnnp-2018-318584.
3. Termsarasab P, Thammongkolchai T, Katirji B. Emergencies in stiff-person spectrum disorders. In: Stiff-person syndrome and related disorders. Cham: Springer; 2020.
4. Blumin JH, Berke GS. Bilateral vocal fold paresis and multiple system atrophy. Arch Otolaryngol Head Neck Surg. 2002;128(12):1404–7. https://doi.org/10.1001/archotol.128.12.1404.
5. Dobbs M, Berger JR. Cervical myelopathy secondary to violent tics of Tourette's syndrome. Neurology. 2003;60(11):1862–3. https://doi.org/10.1212/01.wnl.0000064285.98285.cf.
6. Friedman JH, Feinberg SS, Feldman RG. A neuroleptic malignantlike syndrome due to levodopa therapy withdrawal. JAMA. 1985;254(19):2792–5. https://doi.org/10.1001/jama.1985.03360190098033.
7. Granner MA, Wooten GF. Neuroleptic malignant syndrome or parkinsonism hyperpyrexia syndrome. Semin Neurol. 1991;11(3):228–35. https://doi.org/10.1055/s-2008-1041226.
8. Termsarasab P, Frucht SJ. Dystonic storm: a practical clinical and video review. J Clin Mov Disord. 2017;4:10. https://doi.org/10.1186/s40734-017-0057-z.
9. Fink RA. Myoglobinuria in neuroleptic malignant syndrome. Arch Intern Med. 1985;145(9):1736. https://doi.org/10.1001/archinte.1985.00360090212035.
10. Bertorini TE. Myoglobinuria, malignant hyperthermia, neuroleptic malignant syndrome and serotonin syndrome. Neurol Clin. 1997;15(3):649–71. https://doi.org/10.1016/s0733-8619(05)70338-8.
11. Faulds M, Meekings T. Temperature management in critically ill patients. Contin Educ Anaesth Crit Care Pain. 2013;13(3):75–9. https://doi.org/10.1093/bjaceaccp/mks063.
12. Lopez GA. Temperature Management in the Neurointensive Care Unit. Curr Treat Options Neurol. 2016;18(3):12. https://doi.org/10.1007/s11940-016-0393-6.
13. Vazquez-Sandoval A, Ghamande S, Surani S. Critically ill patients and gut motility: are we addressing it? World J Gastrointest Pharmacol Ther. 2017;8(3):174–9. https://doi.org/10.4292/wjgpt.v8.i3.174.
14. Ben-Haim S, Flatow V, Cheung T, Cho C, Tagliati M, Alterman RL. Deep brain stimulation for status dystonicus: a case series and review of the literature. Stereotact Funct Neurosurg. 2016;94(4):207–15. https://doi.org/10.1159/000446191.
15. Strawn JR, Keck PE Jr, Caroff SN. Neuroleptic malignant syndrome. Am J Psychiatry. 2007;164(6):870–6. https://doi.org/10.1176/ajp.2007.164.6.870.
16. Sarkar S, Gupta N. Drug information update. Atypical antipsychotics and neuroleptic malignant syndrome: nuances and pragmatics of the association. BJPsych Bull. 2017;41(4):211–6. https://doi.org/10.1192/pb.bp.116.053736.

17. Allen NM, Lin JP, Lynch T, King MD. Status dystonicus: a practice guide. Dev Med Child Neurol. 2014;56(2):105–12. https://doi.org/10.1111/dmcn.12339.
18. Mariotti P, Fasano A, Contarino MF, Della Marca G, Piastra M, Genovese O, et al. Management of status dystonicus: our experience and review of the literature. Mov Disord. 2007;22(7):963–8. https://doi.org/10.1002/mds.21471.
19. Frucht SJ. Treatment of movement disorder emergencies. Neurotherapeutics. 2014;11(1):208–12. https://doi.org/10.1007/s13311-013-0240-3.

Neuro-Ophthalmologic Emergencies in Movement Disorders

2

Jenna Conway, Meagan D. Seay, and Janet C. Rucker

Abbreviations

ACTH	Adrenocorticotropic hormone
CJD	Creutzfeldt-Jakob disease
CNS	Central nervous system
CSF	Cerebrospinal fluid
DBN	Downbeat nystagmus
EEG	Electroencephalogram
GABAA	γ-Aminobutyric acid A
GAD	Glutamic acid decarboxylase
INC	Interstitial nucleus of Cajal
IV	Intravenous
IVIG	Intravenous immunoglobulin
MRI	Magnetic resonance imaging
NMDA	N-methyl-D-aspartate
OKN	Optokinetic nystagmus
PAS	Periodic acid-Schiff
PCA	Posterior cerebral arteries

Supplementary Information The online version of this chapter (https://doi.org/10.1007/978-3-030-75898-1_2) contains supplementary material, which is available to authorized users.

J. Conway · J. C. Rucker (✉)
Department of Neurology, New York University Grossman School of Medicine, New York, NY, USA
e-mail: Janet.Rucker@nyulangone.org

M. D. Seay
University of Utah Moran Eye Center, Salt Lake City, UT, USA

PCR	Polymerase chain reaction
PERM	Progressive encephalomyelitis with rigidity and myoclonus
PET-CT	Positron emission tomography-computed tomography
PPRF	Paramedian pontine reticular formation
PSP	Progressive supranuclear palsy
RIMLF	Rostral interstitial medial longitudinal fasciculus
UBN	Upbeat nystagmus
VOR	Vestibulo-ocular reflexes

Patient Vignettes

Patient 1

A 42-year-old man with no past medical history presented to the emergency department with acute-onset dizziness, shakiness, and oscillopsia. Examination revealed opsoclonus, head titubation, and truncal myoclonus. Brain magnetic resonance imaging (MRI) with contrast, cerebrospinal fluid (CSF) analysis, paraneoplastic antibody panel, and co-registered body positron emission tomography-computed tomography (PET-CT) scan were unremarkable. Infectious and immune serologies were unremarkable. He was treated empirically with intravenous immunoglobulin (IVIG) and gradually recovered fully over 3 months. The working diagnosis was para-infectious brainstem encephalitis, although no specific infectious agent was identified.

Patient 2

A 59-year-old woman presented to the emergency department with acute-onset vertical oscillopsia and double vision. She denied other neurological symptoms, though her family reported mild confusion. Medical history included diabetes and hypertension. She denied tobacco use, but reported daily alcohol intake. On examination, she was oriented to person and place, but not to year. Eye movement examination revealed incomplete bilateral abduction and adduction and upbeat nystagmus. Gait was narrow-based and steady, but she had mild difficulty with tandem gait. MRI revealed increased T2 signal around the third ventricle in bilateral thalami. She was diagnosed with Wernicke's encephalopathy and treated with intravenous (IV) thiamine.

Introduction

Eye movement abnormalities that occur in emergent settings in movement disorders include acute/subacute onset supranuclear saccadic gaze palsies, ocular flutter and opsoclonus, various types of nystagmus, and oculogyric crisis. In this chapter, we review and discuss each of these eye movement disorders.

Acute/Subacute-Onset Supranuclear Saccadic Gaze Palsies

Description

Failure of brainstem supranuclear saccadic burst neurons results in a brainstem-mediated supranuclear saccadic gaze palsy with slowing of saccades horizontally and/or vertically. The slowing of saccades may or may not be accompanied by range of motion limitation of eye movements.

Mechanism

Supranuclear saccadic gaze palsies may occur with pathology involving the pons or midbrain. Saccadic excitatory burst neurons that control horizontal saccades are located in the pons in the paramedian pontine reticular formation (PPRF) just rostral to the sixth nerve nucleus [1]. The rostral interstitial medial longitudinal fasciculus (RIMLF) in the mesencephalic reticular formation in the midbrain houses saccadic excitatory burst neurons that control vertical and torsional saccades [2], though a few are also located in the interstitial nucleus of Cajal (INC) [3, 4].

Clinical Evaluation

Detection of a saccadic gaze palsy on exam requires assessment of the static range of ocular motility and dynamic eye movements. Assessment of the following eye movement types should be performed both horizontally and vertically: saccades, smooth pursuit, vestibulo-ocular reflexes (VOR), and optokinetic nystagmus (OKN). Saccades are tested by having the patient make rapid jumps with their eyes between two stationary visual targets, while assessing timing of initiation, speed, accuracy, and trajectory. Regarding saccade speed, a general "rule-of-thumb" is that the examiner should not be able to see the eye move through the full trajectory of motion, but rather should see it start and then land on target. If the eye can follow the full trajectory of the saccade, then it is too slow. Smooth pursuit is evaluated by having the patient follow a slowly moving target, while observing for corrective saccades. VOR is tested by passive head movement, while the patient fixates on a visual target, noting the range of eye movements and the smoothness of the movement. OKN is examined by moving a striped drum or tape in front of the patient, while observing for slow tracking movements of the eyes and corrective saccadic quick phases.

    ⊶   Saccades should not be visible throughout their trajectory: "if you can see the entire saccadic movement, it is too slow."

Supranuclear saccadic gaze palsies produce slowing of horizontal and/or vertical saccades with or without limitation of range of motion. Pontine lesions involving the PPRF cause horizontal gaze palsy, and midbrain lesions involving the

RIMLF produce vertical gaze palsy. When range limitations occur, they are typically worse with saccades than with smooth pursuit testing. They can be overcome by VOR, which establishes them as supranuclear. Saccadic gaze palsies cause loss of OKN quick phases with slow tonic deviation of the eyes in the direction of stimulus motion. Loss of OKN quick phases is often an early sign of a developing supranuclear gaze palsy. With instantaneous catastrophic lesions such as stroke, the above patterns may not be seen acutely and all eye movement types may be affected. Saccade slowing in isolation may also be evidence of a saccadic gaze palsy, even with full eye movement range. Isolated mild impairment of eye elevation is not sufficient to diagnose a saccadic gaze palsy, as this may be seen in healthy elderly individuals secondary to mechanical orbital changes [5]. Some patients with selective slowing of horizontal or vertical saccades will demonstrate a curved trajectory with saccade testing, such as "round-the-house" saccades seen in vertical saccadic gaze palsies [6].

Etiologies

Chronic saccadic gaze palsies occur in neurodegenerative disorders (e.g., progressive supranuclear palsy [PSP]) and metabolic/inherited conditions (e.g., spinocerebellar ataxia), however we will focus on acute/subacute saccadic gaze palsies of vascular, neoplastic/paraneoplastic, infectious, and inflammatory origin [7] (Table 2.1).

Stroke is a common cause of acute saccadic gaze palsy. Acute-onset vertical saccadic gaze palsy is usually due to midbrain infarction. "Top of the basilar" strokes can cause vertical saccadic gaze palsy in the distribution of the paramedian-penetrating arteries originating from the proximal posterior cerebral arteries (PCA) at the basilar bifurcation. The RIMLF in the midbrain is supplied by the posterior thalamo-subthalamic paramedian artery. In 20% of the population, an anatomic variant in the form of a single perforating artery (of Percheron) supplies both RIMLFs, making bilateral lesions possible from a single vessel infarct. Radiographically, the lesions may take on a "butterfly" shape in the coronal plane [8, 9]. Saccadic gaze palsies can also result from a unilateral midbrain infarct [10]. Midbrain strokes causing isolated supranuclear vertical gaze palsies usually result from vertebrobasilar atherosclerosis, although they may also be due to emboli from the proximal PCA to the basilar bifurcation [11]. Another vascular cause of vertical saccadic gaze palsy is thalamic hemorrhage with caudal extension to the midbrain or resultant hydrocephalus from intraventricular extension causing a dorsal midbrain syndrome [12]. Acute-onset horizontal saccadic gaze palsy usually occurs in pontine infarction involving the PPRF [13].

Neoplasms causing midbrain compression can present with a subacute saccadic gaze palsy. Specifically, tumors involving the pineal gland, including pineal germinoma or teratoma, pineocytoma, pineoblastoma, glioma, or metastases, can lead to the dorsal midbrain syndrome with upgaze palsy, eyelid retraction, pupillary light-near dissociation, and convergence-retraction nystagmus. Pineal lesions can rarely mimic PSP in older patients [14].

Table 2.1 Supranuclear saccadic gaze palsies[a]

Saccadic gaze palsy subtype	Emergent etiologies	Subacute/chronic etiologies

Vertical	Vascular
	  Midbrain infarction
	Neoplastic
	  Dorsal midbrain syndrome due to compressive lesion or hydrocephalus
		Neurodegenerative disorders:
		  PSP
		  CBD (rarely)
		  HD
		  LBD (rarely)
		Metabolic and genetic:
		  Niemann-Pick type C
		Paraneoplastic/autoimmune
		  Anti Ma1 and Ma2/GAD/glycine receptor/IgLON5
		Demyelinating
		Infectious:
		  Whipple's disease
		  Chronic dengue encephalitis
		  Prion (CJD)

Horizontal	Vascular
	  Pontine infarction
	Neoplastic
	  Pontine glioma
		Neurodegenerative disorders:
		  PSP (late)
		Metabolic and genetic:
		  Gaucher
		  Spinocerebellar ataxia type 2
		Paraneoplastic/autoimmune
		  Anti Ma1 and Ma2/GAD/glycine receptor/IgLON5
		Demyelinating

PSP progressive supranuclear palsy, *CBD* corticobasal degeneration, *HD* Huntington's disease, *LBD* Lewy body dementia, *CJD* Creutzfeldt-Jakob disease
[a]Common and representative causes, not comprehensive

A well-recognized infectious cause of saccadic gaze palsy is Whipple's disease, a chronic infection caused by the gram-positive bacillus Tropheryma whipplei. The pathogen has a predilection for the periaqueductal gray matter, hypothalamus, hippocampus, basal ganglia, cerebellum, and cerebral cortex [15]. In approximately one-third of patients with central nervous system (CNS) involvement, supranuclear vertical saccadic gaze palsy (either upgaze or downgaze) may occur [16]. When dementia and gait disturbance occur with vertical supranuclear gaze palsy, Whipple's disease may mimic PSP. In some patients, the vertical saccadic gaze palsy may progress to complete ophthalmoplegia [17]. While not consistently present, oculo-masticatory myorhythmia is considered pathognomonic and comprises pendular convergent-divergent nystagmus with concurrent masticatory muscle contractions [15]. Other neurologic findings may include cerebellar ataxia, tremor, postural instability, dystonia, myoclonus, cognitive deficits, psychiatric symptoms, delirium, seizures, and signs of hypothalamic involvement (e.g., syndrome of inappropriate antidiuretic hormone secretion, insomnia, hypersomnia, and hyperphagia) [16]. Systemic features of Whipple's disease, which may be absent in CNS Whipple's disease, include gastrointestinal symptoms (e.g., malabsorption, abdominal pain, diarrhea), weight loss, fever, and polyarthralgia [16]. While MRI and CSF analysis may be normal, they can also reveal midbrain, hypothalamic, and temporal lobe hyperintensities and CSF pleocytosis with elevated protein [18]. Diagnosis is made by small bowel biopsy and polymerase chain reaction (PCR) testing [19]. While staining for periodic acid-Schiff (PAS)-positivity in macrophages can also be used, it is not as sensitive or specific [11]. Treatment of Whipple's disease requires long-term antibiotics such as trimethoprim-sulfamethoxazole or ceftriaxone [20]. Prion disease, such as Creutzfeldt–Jakob disease (CJD), can also mimic PSP with early falls and vertical saccadic gaze palsy, although the disease course is typically more rapid [21, 22]. MRI clues include basal ganglia T2-hyperintensities and cortical ribboning on diffusion-weighted imaging.

Paraneoplastic, autoimmune, and inflammatory processes can also present with saccadic gaze palsy. Both supranuclear and nuclear ophthalmoparesis can be a manifestation of paraneoplastic/autoimmune brainstem encephalitis. Various antibodies have been associated, such as anti-Ma [23], anti-glutamic acid decarboxylase (GAD) [24–26], anti-GlyR [27], and anti-IgLON5 [28] antibodies. Anti-Ma antibodies are commonly found in testicular cancer and cause limbic encephalitis and/or brainstem dysfunction with various ocular motor deficits including saccadic gaze palsy, opsoclonus, ocular flutter, oculogyric crisis, nystagmus (horizontal, horizontal-torsional, and downbeat), and skew deviation [23]. GAD antibodies are associated with many eye movement abnormalities including nystagmus (downbeat and periodic alternating nystagmus), ocular flutter and opsoclonus, and ophthalmoplegia with or without stiff person syndrome or cerebellar dysfunction [24–26]. Anti-GlyR antibodies are associated with progressive encephalomyelitis with rigidity and myoclonus (PERM), characterized by brainstem, spinal cord, and autonomic involvement, and may also involve saccadic gaze palsy [27]. Anti-IgLON5 antibodies are associated with cell surface antibody-associated neurodegeneration [28] and may present with vertical or horizontal saccadic gaze palsy. Parkinsonism tends to be absent with Ig-LON5 antibodies [29]. Immunosuppression is the treatment of choice for paraneoplastic, autoimmune, and inflammatory causes of saccadic gaze palsies, as well as treatment of any underlying tumor.

⚷ Supranuclear saccadic gaze palsies present with slowing of saccades with or without range of motion limitation. It is important to rule out acute/subacute causes including vascular, neoplastic/paraneoplastic, infectious, and inflammatory etiologies.

Ocular Flutter and Opsoclonus

Description

Ocular flutter and opsoclonus, also called "saccadomania," are erratic bursts of rapid high frequency saccades that have no intersaccadic interval and that oscillate about the visual midline. Specifically, ocular flutter comprises saccades that occur only in the horizontal plane (not vertical or torsional). In contrast, opsoclonus has conjugate multidirectional saccades occurring in all trajectories (horizontal, vertical, and torsional). These eye movement abnormalities may be associated with eye blinking, facial twitching, myoclonus, and ataxia ("dancing eyes and feet") [30]. As with all saccadic intrusions, opsoclonus and ocular flutter are often not continuous, but occur sporadically and are typically provoked by gaze shifting.

Mechanism

Ocular flutter and opsoclonus may occur with pathology involving the pons (where saccadic burst neurons that control horizontal saccades are located) or the cerebellum (from malfunctioning of the vermis Purkinje cells leading to disinhibition of the cerebellar fastigial nucleus) [31, 32]. There is evidence for increased γ-aminobutyric acid A (GABA-A) receptor sensitivity in a circuit involving the cerebellum, inferior olives, and brainstem saccadic premotor burst neurons [33]. Further, the saccadic burst neurons are inherently prone to oscillating due to synaptic feedback loops and their post-inhibitory rebound properties [34].

Clinical Evaluation

Patients with ocular flutter or opsoclonus will typically present with oscillopsia, a subjective sense of motion in visual space. While flutter and opsoclonus are usually large enough to be seen on clinical examination, they can also be small in amplitude requiring ophthalmoscopy or quantified eye movement recordings to capture. As such, any patient with new-onset oscillopsia that is unexplained on examination should be assessed for small oscillations with further testing.

Etiologies

Ocular flutter and opsoclonus are most commonly seen in two clinical settings: parainfectious brainstem encephalitis or paraneoplastic/autoimmune disease (Table 2.2). Various antibodies have been associated including Hu (ANNA1) [35], Ri (ANNA2) [36], Yo (anti-Purkinje cell) [37], Ma, amphiphysin, P/Q-type calcium channel [38], N-methyl-D-aspartate (NMDA) receptor [39, 40], GABA-B [41], glycine [42], glutamate receptors [43], GAD [26], and GQ1b [44]. Tumors associated with these eye movement abnormalities include small-cell lung (e.g., anti-Hu antibodies), breast (e.g., anti-Ri antibodies), and gynecologic malignancies. Older age and encephalopathy are more commonly seen in paraneoplastic compared to parainfectious opsoclonus [42]. Para-infectious brainstem encephalitis is often accompanied by truncal myoclonus, ataxia, and emotional lability. Infectious pathogens include enterovirus [45], West Nile virus [46], Lyme disease [47], mumps [48], HIV [49], malaria [50], dengue [51], Zika virus [52], and SARS-CoV-2 [personal communication]. Ocular flutter and opsoclonus have also been reported secondary to

Table 2.2 Characteristics and potential etiologies of ocular flutter and opsoclonus[a]

	Characteristic eye movement	Etiologies
Ocular flutter	Back-to-back, conjugate, horizontal saccades with no intersaccadic interval	Idiopathic Para-infectious

Opsoclonus	Back-to-back, conjugate, horizontal, vertical and torsional saccades with no intersaccadic interval	HIV
		Enterovirus
		Mumps
		Zika virus
		Cytomegalovirus
		SARS-CoV-2
		Paraneoplastic
		  Neuroblastoma (children)
		  Small cell lung cancer
		  Breast and ovarian cancer
		Toxic/metabolic states
		  Cocaine, PCP
		  Phenytoin, lithium,
		    amitriptyline, venlafaxine
		  Inborn errors of metabolism
		  Celiac disease
		Demyelinating syndromes
		  Multiple sclerosis
		  NMOSD
		  MOG IgG

NMOSD neuromyelitis optica spectrum disorder, *MOG IgG* myelin oligodendrocyte glycoprotein immunoglobulin, *PCP* Phencyclidine
[a]Common and representative causes, not comprehensive

traumatic brain injury, including in concussion [53–55]. Finally, opsoclonus and flutter may also be drug induced (e.g., amitriptyline, lithium, phenytoin, cocaine, and organophosphates) [56–58]. Regarding disease course, para-infectious opsoclonus typically slowly improves, while paraneoplastic opsoclonus often depends on treatment of the underlying tumor [42]. Both para-infectious and paraneoplastic opsoclonus have been anecdotally reported to improve with clonazepam, topiramate, gabapentin, corticosteroids, and other immunosuppressive agents such as IVIG or plasmapheresis [59].

Ocular flutter and opsoclonus are erratic bursts of high frequency and velocity back-to-back saccades that oscillate about the midline with no intersaccadic interval. Ocular flutter and opsoclonus are typically due to either infectious/para-infectious brainstem encephalitis or paraneoplastic/autoimmune disease.

In children with opsoclonus (and ocular flutter), more than 50% have an underlying neuroblastoma requiring a careful search [56, 60, 61]. The eye movement abnormality may present prior to identification of the underlying tumor. Compared to those without opsoclonus, children with both neuroblastoma and opsoclonus tend to have a more favorable prognosis, which may be due to immune surveillance, earlier tumor detection, and/or favorable tumor biology. Opsoclonus-myoclonus may respond to tumor removal and adrenocorticotropic hormone (ACTH) or corticosteroids, sometimes in combination with immunomodulatory therapy (e.g., IVIG, plasmapheresis, azathioprine, or rituximab) [62]. The response to these therapies suggests an underlying autoimmune mechanism of opsoclonus associated with neuroblastoma. Relapses and corticosteroid dependence are common in opsoclonus associated with neuroblastoma. Many children have permanent neurologic abnormalities including ataxia and cognitive issues, the latter of which may be related to a cerebellar cognitive affective syndrome [63]. Cerebellar atrophy of the vermis, cerebellar hemispheres, and flocculonodular lobes may be seen, with the degree of atrophy correlating with neurologic outcome [64]. Other forms of opsoclonus can also occur in children, such as opsoclonus associated with severe visual disturbances, para-infectious cerebellitis, and encephalitis [56]. Similar to paraneoplastic opsoclonus myoclonus, the para-infectious type may require ACTH or corticosteroids; however, the prognosis is usually better [11]. Any child with opsoclonus requires a brain MRI and CSF examination, in addition to a neuroblastoma screen.

Given that some individuals are capable of generating these large-amplitude eye movements [65], it can be difficult to differentiate pathologic ocular flutter and opsoclonus from voluntary eye movements. A mimic of ocular flutter is called voluntary nystagmus, though it is flutter-like and not a true nystagmus. This eye movement can be performed voluntarily by some individuals, usually with convergence of the eyes and other features of the near vision response (e.g., pupillary constriction). Voluntary nystagmus cannot usually be sustained for an extended period of time.

Nystagmus

Nystagmus is a rhythmic biphasic oscillation of the eyes, initiated by a slow drift of the eyes. In jerk nystagmus, the slow drifts are followed by fast phases in the opposite direction, for which the jerk nystagmus is named (i.e., nystagmus with slow drifts downward followed by fast phases upward is called upbeat nystagmus). When the slow drifts in one direction are followed by slow drifts in the opposite direction, the nystagmus is pendular. Nystagmus may be physiological in response to environmental stimuli (e.g., OKN), congenital, or acquired (Table 2.3) and exists in many forms with highly variable etiologies and treatments. Comprehensive coverage of nystagmus is beyond the scope of this chapter and can be found elsewhere [66, 67]. Here, a few acute to subacute causes of nystagmus are highlighted.

Downbeat Nystagmus

Description
Downbeat nystagmus (DBN) is jerk nystagmus with slow upward drifts followed by downward corrective fast phases. It typically increases in amplitude and frequency in downward-lateral gaze. On examination, DBN may be accompanied by impaired downward smooth pursuit and other eye movement abnormalities reflecting cerebellar disease, such as an alternating skew deviation on lateral gaze (i.e., right hypertropia in right gaze and left hypertropia in left gaze) [68]. Patients may or may not experience vertical oscillopsia with DBN.

Table 2.3 Acute and subacute/chronic etiologies of nystagmus subtypes[a]

Nystagmus Type	Acute etiologies	Subacute/chronic etiologies

Downbeat	Cervicomedullary junction lesions:
	  Tumor
	  Stroke
	Wernicke encephalopathy
		Cervicomedullary junction lesions:
		  Chiari malformation
		  Demyelination
		  Syringomyelia
		Paraneoplastic disorders:
		  Anti-GAD/Hu/Yo/Ma1/Ma2/VGCC
		Degenerative disorders:
		  Olivopontocerebellar atrophy
		  Friedreich's ataxia
		  Spinocerebellar ataxia
		Toxic and metabolic:
		  Lithium, amiodarone, anti-convulsants
		  B12, magnesium deficiency

Upbeat	Wernicke encephalopathy
	Medullary or midbrain lesions:
	  Stroke
		Paraneoplastic disorders:
		  Anti-Hu
		Medullary or midbrain lesions:
		  Demyelination

Gaze evoked	Wernicke encephalopathy	Drug toxicities:
		  Anti-convulsants
		  Alcohol
		  Sedatives
		Chiari I malformation

Acquired pendular		Oculopalatal myoclonus:
		  Few months following brainstem stroke;
		  cavernous malformation
		Convergence-divergence pattern:
		  Whipple disease
		Demyelination
		Pelizaeus-Merzbacher disease
		Toluene abuse (glue sniffing)

Convergence-retraction	Dorsal midbrain syndrome
	  Stroke
	  Tumor
	  Hydrocephalus
		Dorsal midbrain syndrome
		  Demyelination

GAD glutamic acid decarboxylase, *VGCC* voltage gated calcium channel
[a]Common and representative causes, not comprehensive

Etiologies

DBN is most commonly due to cerebellar dysfunction, with lesions involving the cervicomedullary junction or vestibulocerebellum (flocculus, paraflocculus, nodulus, and uvula). It has also occasionally been reported with brainstem lesions involving the paramedian medullary or pontomedullary region, which may relate to damage involving paramedian tract cell groups, or damage to the pontine portion of the medial longitudinal fasciculus [69–71].

Acute or subacute onset DBN can occur from cerebellar ischemia or paraneoplastic cerebellar degeneration (e.g., Yo or Hu antibodies with underlying malignancy or GAD antibodies associated with stiff person syndrome and cerebellar syndrome) [72]. It may also be seen in toxic-metabolic conditions (e.g., hypomagnesemia [73], thiamine deficiency following the acute phase [74] or B12 deficiency [75]) and drug-induced states (e.g., carbamazepine [76], lithium [77], alcohol [78], opioids [79]). More chronic etiologies include craniocervical abnormalities (e.g., Chiari I malformations [80]), degenerative diseases (e.g., spinocerebellar degenerations [80]), neoplasms (e.g., foramen magnum mass lesions [80]), infectious diseases (e.g., West Nile virus encephalomyelitis [81]), and congenital disorders [82]. Despite standard MRI of the cervicomedullary junction, no cause is found in 30–40% of acquired DBN [83].

O———⚷   Vertical nystagmus suggests a central etiology, requiring a thorough workup. Downbeat nystagmus may occur acutely/subacutely from ischemic and paraneoplastic cerebellar disorders. Upbeat nystagmus occurs in Wernicke's encephalopathy and brainstem stroke.

Mechanism
The mechanism of DBN is most often considered to be due to up-down asymmetries in the brainstem–cerebellar network that normally stabilizes vertical gaze [84]. Three main hypotheses exist regarding the mechanism of DBN: (1) a tone imbalance in the central connections of the semicircular canals or otolithic system that control eye movements [85], (2) asymmetric vertical smooth pursuit [68], and (3) abnormalities in the brainstem-cerebellar connections that control vertical gaze holding (i.e., neural integrator) [86]. For instance, efferent cerebellar Purkinje cells of the flocculus inhibit upward eye movements via vestibular nuclei connections [87], and thus reduced inhibition from a cerebellar lesion results in slow upward drifts and corrective downward fast phases.

Treatment
Treatment options for downbeat nystagmus are based on identifying and treating the underlying etiology, if possible. However, certain medications may reduce downbeat nystagmus such as potassium channel blockers including 3,4-diaminopyridine and 4-aminopyridine (4-AP), the latter of which is preferred as it more readily crosses the blood-brain barrier [88–92]. These medications increase the excitability of cerebellar Purkinje cells and therefore may restore normal inhibitory influence of the cerebellum upon the anterior semicircular canal pathways [90]. Other medications that can be tried include clonazepam, chlorzoxazone, baclofen, or gabapentin [93–95]. Some patients may also respond to prism therapy to induce convergence or deflect the perceived image upward [96].

Upbeat Nystagmus

Description
Upbeat nystagmus (UBN) is jerk nystagmus with slow downward phases followed by upward corrective fast phases. Nystagmus amplitude and frequency often increase with upward gaze. It is typically associated with impaired upward smooth pursuit.

Etiologies

UBN typically arises from lesions in the medulla and, less often, the midbrain. It is commonly seen in Wernicke's encephalopathy from thiamine deficiency, in which it is associated with horizontal gaze deficits and sometimes with accompanying gaze-evoked nystagmus [66]. Recent evidence suggests that UBN in Wernicke's encephalopathy may convert to DBN during convergence in the acute phase of the condition, and eventually may convert to persistent DBN in the chronic phase [74]. Other causes of UBN include demyelinating disease, brainstem stroke (typically medullary), cerebellar degeneration, and tumors.

Mechanism

The mechanism of UBN may be disruption of structures mediating upward eye movements such as the superior cerebellar peduncle (brachium conjunctivum) that contains connections from the vestibular to ocular motor nuclei via anterior semicircular canal pathways [97]. It may also result from asymmetry in which posterior semicircular canal pathways are hyperactive causing a downward bias and upbeat nystagmus [98]. Medullary lesions causing UBN typically involve the caudal medullary perihypoglossal nuclei [99, 100].

Treatment

UBN usually resolves within weeks, but since it can be quite symptomatic, treatment options are similar to those used for DBN and include 4-AP, baclofen, or clonazepam [101, 102].

Oculogyric Crisis

Description

Oculogyric crisis is an acute dystonic reaction of extraocular muscles with a conjugate, typically upward, deviation of the eyes lasting seconds to hours [103]. Oculogyric crises are often associated with other dystonic or dyskinetic movements, such as tongue protrusion, lip smacking, blepharospasm, choreoathetosis, anterocollis, and retrocollis [104].

Etiologies

Initially described in postencephalitic parkinsonism, oculogyric crises today are seen in acute or tardive extrapyramidal reactions to neuroleptics [105] (Table 2.4). First-generation neuroleptics are frequently implicated, but oculogyric crises can also occur with newer neuroleptics (quetiapine [106], olanzapine [107], ziprasidone [108], and aripiprazole [109]). Other medications can also induce oculogyric crises, such as carbamazepine [110], lamotrigine [111], lithium [112], metoclopramide [113], cefixime [114], gabapentin [115], tetrabenazine [116], and cetirizine [117].

Oculogyric crises have also been associated with numerous other neurologic disorders, such as various movement disorders (Parkinson's disease [118], familial Parkinson-dementia syndrome [119], dopa-responsive dystonia [120], parkinsonism with basal ganglia calcifications or Fahr's disease [121]), infectious diseases (neurosyphilis, acute herpetic brainstem encephalitis [122]), inflammatory disorders (multiple sclerosis, paraneoplastic disease [123]), vascular disease (striatocapsular infarction [124]), metabolic/genetic conditions (ataxia-telangiectasia [125], Rett's syndrome [126], Wilson's disease [127]), and other neurologic disorders (cerebellar disease, trauma [128], cystic glioma of the third ventricle [129], midbrain lesions [130]). In a patient with oculogyric crisis, seizures should be ruled out with an electroencephalogram (EEG).

👌━━📌 Oculogyric crisis is an acute dystonic reaction of ocular muscles with a conjugate deviation of the eyes, typically upward and lateral. Oculogyric crises are most commonly acute or tardive reactions to neuroleptics, though other etiologies exist.

Mechanism

The underlying mechanism of oculogyric crisis is unclear and various hypotheses have been proposed [11]. In postencephalitic patients, it was proposed that oculogyric crises result from a release of supranuclear control of the ocular motor centers as a result of injury to the corpus striatum or subthalamic nucleus [131]. It has also been hypothesized that oculogyric crises result from abnormal VOR due to brainstem lesions involving the vestibular pathways [132]. Given the response to anticholinergic agents, it has also been thought to result from a defect in mesencephalic vertical gaze-holding mechanisms that are dependent on balanced cholinergic and dopaminergic systems [133]. Lastly, a limbic-motor disorder has been hypothesized to explain oculogyric crises [128].

Table 2.4 Description, etiologies, and treatments of oculogyric crisis

Characteristics	Etiologies	Treatment
Sustained, upward deviation of eyes lasting seconds to hours Ranges from mild and brief to severe, prolonged, and painful May have neck flexion, jaw opening, blepharospasm, and autonomic symptoms Psychiatric symptoms may be present	Drug induced: Typical and atypical neuroleptics Antiemetics Antidepressants Anticonvulsants Disorders of dopamine metabolism Hereditary and sporadic movement disorders Brain lesions: Dorsal midbrain Substantia nigra Basal ganglia Posterior third ventricle	Remove or reduce the dose of the offending agent Anticholinergics: Benztropine Biperiden Antihistamines: Diphenhydramine L-dopa may be beneficial in patients with parkinsonism

Treatment

Treating the underlying condition is important and removal of the offending drug is critical if the oculogyric crisis is drug-induced. Oculogyric crises that are severe/painful can be treated acutely with IV or intramuscular (IM) benztropine or diphenhydramine [128]. If unsuccessful, IV/IM benzodiazepines (e.g., lorazepam or diazepam) can be tried [128]. In some patients, short-term treatment with oral benztropine or trihexyphenidyl following the acute episode may be needed [128].

Conclusion

Eye movement abnormalities that may be due to urgent or emergent etiologies in movement disorders include acute/subacute onset supranuclear saccadic gaze palsies, ocular flutter and opsoclonus, various types of nystagmus, and oculogyric crisis. Given the varying etiologies and thus treatments, it is important for the clinician to be aware of these eye movement abnormalities.

References

 1. Horn AK, Büttner-Ennever JA, Suzuki Y, Henn V. Histological identification of premotor neurons for horizontal saccades in monkey and man by parvalbumin immunostaining. J Comp Neurol. 1995;359(2):350–63.
 2. Horn AK, Büttner-Ennever JA. Premotor neurons for vertical eye movements in the rostral mesencephalon of monkey and human: histologic identification by parvalbumin immunostaining. J Comp Neurol. 1998;392(4):413–27.
 3. Moschovakis A, Scudder C, Highstein S. Structure of the primate oculomotor burst generator. I. Medium-lead burst neurons with upward on-directions. J Neurophysiol. 1991;65(2):203–17.
 4. Moschovakis A, Scudder C, Highstein S, Warren J. Structure of the primate oculomotor burst generator. II. Medium-lead burst neurons with downward on-directions. J Neurophysiol. 1991;65(2):218–29.
 5. Clark RA, Demer JL. Effect of aging on human rectus extraocular muscle paths demonstrated by magnetic resonance imaging. Am J Ophthalmol. 2002;134(6):872–8.
 6. Quinn N. The "round the houses" sign in progressive supranuclear palsy. Ann Neurol. 1996;40(6):951.
 7. Lloyd-Smith Sequeira A, Rizzo J-R, Rucker JC. Clinical approach to supranuclear brainstem saccadic gaze palsies. Front Neurol. 2017;8:429.
 8. Percheron G. The anatomy of the arterial supply of the human thalamus and its use for the interpretation of the thalamic vascular pathology. Z Neurol. 1973;205(1):1–13.
 9. Matheus MG, Castillo M. Imaging of acute bilateral paramedian thalamic and mesencephalic infarcts. Am J Neuroradiol. 2003;24(10):2005–8.
10. Ranalli PJ, Sharpe JA, Fletcher WA. Palsy of upward and downward saccadic, pursuit, and vestibular movements with a unilateral midbrain lesion: pathophysiologic correlations. Neurology. 1988;38(1):114–22.
11. Liu GT, Volpe NJ, Galetta SL. Liu, Volpe, and Galetta's neuro-ophthalmology E-book: diagnosis and management. Philadelphia: Elsevier Health Sciences; 2018.
12. Chung C-S, Caplan LR, Han W, Pessin MS, Lee K-H, Kim J-M. Thalamic haemorrhage. Brain. 1996;119(6):1873–86.

13. Kataoka S, Hori A, Shirakawa T, Hirose G. Paramedian pontine infarction: neurological/ topographical correlation. Stroke. 1997;28(4):809–15.
14. Siderowf AD, Galetta SL, Hurtig HI, Liu GT. Posey and Spiller and progressive supranuclear palsy: an incorrect attribution. Move Disord. 1998;13(1):170–4.
15. Simpson DA, Wishnow R, Gargulinski RB, Pawlak AM. Oculofacial-skeletal myorhythmia in central nervous system Whipple's disease: additional case and review of the literature. Move Disord. 1995;10(2):195–200.
16. Louis E, Lynch T, Kaufmann P, Fahn S, Odel J. Diagnostic guidelines in central nervous system Whipple's disease. Ann Neurol. 1996;40(4):561–8.
17. Compain C, Sacre K, Puéchal X, Klein I, Vital-Durand D, Houeto J-L, et al. Central nervous system involvement in Whipple disease: clinical study of 18 patients and long-term follow-up. Medicine. 2013;92(6):324.
18. Verhagena W, Huygen P, Dalman J, Schuurmans M. Whipple's disease and the central nervous system a case report and a review of the literature. Clin Neurol Neurosurg. 1996;98(4):299–304.
19. Ramzan NN, Loftus E, Burgart LJ, Rooney M, Batts KP, Wiesner RH, et al. Diagnosis and monitoring of Whipple disease by polymerase chain reaction. Ann Intern Med. 1997;126(7):520–7.
20. Fenollar F, Puéchal X, Raoult D. Whipple's disease. N Engl J Med. 2007;356(1):55–66.
21. Prasad S, Ko MW, Lee EB, Gonatas NK, Stern MB, Galetta S. Supranuclear vertical gaze abnormalities in sporadic Creutzfeldt–Jakob disease. J Neurol Sci. 2007;253(1–2):69–72.
22. Rowe DB, Lewis V, Needham M, Rodriguez M, Boyd A, McLean C, et al. Novel prion protein gene mutation presenting with subacute PSP-like syndrome. Neurology. 2007;68(11):868–70.
23. Dalmau J, Graus F, Villarejo A, Posner JB, Blumenthal D, Thiessen B, et al. Clinical analysis of anti-Ma2-associated encephalitis. Brain. 2004;127(8):1831–44.
24. Tilikete C, Vighetto A, Trouillas P, Honnorat J. Potential role of anti-GAD antibodies in abnormal eye movements. Ann N Y Acad Sci. 2005;1039(1):446–54.
25. Markakis I, Alexiou E, Xifaras M, Gekas G, Rombos A. Opsoclonus–myoclonus–ataxia syndrome with autoantibodies to glutamic acid decarboxylase. Clin Neurol Neurosurg. 2008;110(6):619–21.
26. Dubbioso R, Marcelli V, Manganelli F, Iodice R, Esposito M, Santoro L. Anti-GAD antibody ocular flutter: expanding the spectrum of autoimmune ocular motor disorders. J Neurol. 2013;260(10):2675–7.
27. Peeters E, Vanacker P, Woodhall M, Vincent A, Schrooten M. Supranuclear gaze palsy in glycine receptor antibody-positive progressive encephalomyelitis with rigidity and myoclonus. Move Disord. 2012;27(14):1830–2.
28. Dale RC, Ramanathan S. Cell surface antibody–associated neurodegeneration: the case of anti-IgLON5 antibodies. Neurology. 2017;88(18):1688–90.
29. Gaig C, Graus F, Compta Y, Högl B, Bataller L, Brüggemann N, et al. Clinical manifestations of the anti-IgLON5 disease. Neurology. 2017;88(18):1736–43.
30. Imtiaz KE, Vora J. Dancing eyes-dancing feet. Lancet. 1999;354(9176):390.
31. Schon F, Hodgson TL, Mort D, Kennard C. Ocular flutter associated with a localized lesion in the paramedian pontine reticular formation. Ann Neurol. 2001;50(3):413–6.
32. Helmchen C, Rambold H, Sprenger A, Erdmann C, Binkofski F. Cerebellar activation in opsoclonus: an fMRI study. Neurology. 2003;61(3):412–5.
33. Optican LM, Pretegiani E. A GABAergic dysfunction in the olivary–cerebellar–brainstem network may cause eye oscillations and body tremor. II Model simulations of saccadic eye oscillations. Front Neurol. 2017;8:372.
34. Shaikh AG, Ramat S, Optican LM, Miura K, Leigh RJ, Zee DS. Saccadic burst cell membrane dysfunction is responsible for saccadic oscillations. J Neuroophthalmol. 2008;28(4):329.
35. Fisher PG, Wechsler DS, Singer HS. Anti-Hu antibody in a neuroblastoma-associated paraneoplastic syndrome. Pediatr Neurol. 1994;10(4):309–12.

36. Luque FA, Furneaux HM, Ferziger R, Rosenblum MK, Wray SH, Schold SC Jr, et al. Anti-Ri: an antibody associated with paraneoplastic opsoclonus and breast cancer. Ann Neurol. 1991;29(3):241–51.

37. Connolly AM, Pestronk A, Mehta S, Pranzatelli MR, Noetzel MJ. Serum autoantibodies in childhood opsoclonus-myoclonus syndrome: an analysis of antigenic targets in neural tissues. J Pediatr. 1997;130(6):878–84.

38. Josephson CB, Grant I, Benstead T. Opsoclonus-myoclonus with multiple paraneoplastic syndromes and VGCC antibodies. Can J Neurol Sci. 2009;36(4):512–4.

39. Urriola NX, Helou J, Maamary J, Pogson J, Lee F, Parratt K, et al. NMDA receptor antibody in teratoma-related opsoclonus-myoclonus syndrome. J Clin Neurosci. 2018;58:203–4.

40. Player B, Harmelink M, Bordini B, Weisgerber M, Girolami M, Croix M. Pediatric opsoclonus-myoclonus-ataxia syndrome associated with anti-N-methyl-D-aspartate receptor encephalitis. Pediatr Neurol. 2015;53(5):456–8.

41. DeFelipe-Mimbrera A, Masjuan J, Corral Í, Villar LM, Graus F, García-Barragán N. Opsoclonus–myoclonus syndrome and limbic encephalitis associated with GABAB receptor antibodies in CSF. J Neuroimmunol. 2014;272(1–2):91–3.

42. Armangué T, Sabater L, Torres-Vega E, Martínez-Hernández E, Ariño H, Petit-Pedrol M, et al. Clinical and immunological features of opsoclonus-myoclonus syndrome in the era of neuronal cell surface antibodies. JAMA Neurol. 2016;73(4):417–24.

43. Kambe T, Takahashi Y, Furukawa Y. A mild form of adult-onset opsoclonus-myoclonus syndrome associated with antiglutamate receptor antibodies. JAMA Neurol. 2013;70(5):654–5.

44. Zaro-Weber O, Galldiks N, Dohmen C, Fink GR, Nowak DA. Ocular flutter, generalized myoclonus, and trunk ataxia associated with anti-GQ1b antibodies. Arch Neurol. 2008;65(5):659–61.

45. Wiest G, Safoschnik G, Schnaberth G, Mueller C. Ocular flutter and truncal ataxia may be associated with enterovirus infection. J Neurol. 1997;244(5):288–92.

46. Khosla JS, Edelman MJ, Kennedy N, Reich SG. West Nile virus presenting as opsoclonus-myoclonus cerebellar ataxia. Neurology. 2005;64(6):1095.

47. Gyllenborg J, Milea D. Ocular flutter as the first manifestation of Lyme disease. Neurology. 2009;72(3):291.

48. Ichiba N, Miyake Y, Sato K, Oda M, Kimoto H. Mumps-induced opsoclonus-myoclonus and ataxia. Pediatr Neurol. 1988;4(4):224–7.

49. Guedes BF, Vieira Filho MA, Listik C, Carra RB, Pereira CB, da Silva ER, et al. HIV-associated opsoclonus-myoclonus-ataxia syndrome: early infection, immune reconstitution syndrome or secondary to other diseases? Case report and literature review. J Neurovirol. 2018;24(1):123–7.

50. Poungvarin N, Praditsuwan R. Opsoclonus in malaria: the first report in the literature. J Med Assoc Thai = Chotmaihet Thangphaet. 1990;73(8):462–6.

51. Mahale RR, Mehta A, Buddaraju K, Srinivasa R. Parainfectious ocular flutter and truncal ataxia in association with dengue fever. J Pediatr Neurosci. 2017;12(1):91.

52. Karam E, Giraldo J, Rodriguez F, Hernandez-Pereira CE, Rodriguez-Morales AJ, Blohm GM, et al. Ocular flutter following Zika virus infection. J Neurovirol. 2017;23(6):932–4.

53. Turazzi S, Alexandre A, Bricolo A, Rizzuto N. Opsoclonus and palatal myoclonus during prolonged post-traumatic coma. Eur Neurol. 1977;15(5):257–63.

54. Digre KB. Opsoclonus in adults: report of three cases and review of the literature. Arch Neurol. 1986;43(11):1165–75.

55. Rizzo J-R, Hudson TE, Sequeira AJ, Dai W, Chaudhry Y, Martone J, et al. Eye position-dependent opsoclonus in mild traumatic brain injury. Prog Brain Res. 2019;249:65–78.

56. Pranzatelli MR. The neurobiology of the opsoclonus-myoclonus syndrome. Clin Neuropharmacol. 1992;15(3):186–228.

57. Liang TW, Balcer L, Solomon D, Messe S, Galetta S. Supranuclear gaze palsy and opsoclonus after Diazinon poisoning. J Neurol Neurosurg Psychiatry. 2003;74(5):677–9.

58. Au WJ, Keltner WJ. Opsoclonus with amitriptyline overdose. Ann Neurol. 1979;6(1):87.

59. Klaas JP, Ahlskog JE, Pittock SJ, Matsumoto JY, Aksamit AJ, Bartleson J, et al. Adult-onset opsoclonus-myoclonus syndrome. Arch Neurol. 2012;69(12):1598–607.
60. Moe PG, Nellhaus G. Infantile polymyoclonia-opsoclonus syndrome and neural crest tumors. Neurology. 1970;20(8):756.
61. Rudnick E, Khakoo Y, Antunes NL, Seeger RC, Brodeur GM, Shimada H, et al. Opsoclonus-myoclonus-ataxia syndrome in neuroblastoma: clinical outcome and antineuronal antibodies—a report from the children's cancer group study. Med Pediatr Oncol. 2001;36(6):612–22.
62. Tate ED, Pranzatelli MR, Verhulst SJ, Markwell SJ, Franz DN, Graf WD, et al. Active comparator-controlled, rater-blinded study of corticotropin-based immunotherapies for opsoclonus-myoclonus syndrome. J Child Neurol. 2012;27(7):875–84.
63. De Grandis E, Parodi S, Conte M, Angelini P, Battaglia F, Gandolfo C, et al. Long-term follow-up of neuroblastoma-associated opsoclonus-myoclonus-ataxia syndrome. Neuropediatrics. 2009;40(03):103–11.
64. Anand G, Bridge H, Rackstraw P, Chekroud AM, Yong J, Stagg CJ, et al. Cerebellar and cortical abnormalities in paediatric opsoclonus-myoclonus syndrome. Dev Med Child Neurol. 2015;57(3):265–72.
65. Yee RD, Spiegel PH, Yamada T, Abel LA, Suzuki DA, Zee DS. Voluntary saccadic oscillations, resembling ocular flutter and opsoclonus. J Neuroophthalmol. 1994;14(2):95–101.
66. Rucker JC. Nystagmus and saccadic intrusions. CONTINUUM: Lifelong Learn Neurol. 2019;25(5):1376–400.
67. Leigh RJ, Zee DS. The neurology of eye movements. New York: Oxford University Press; 2015.
68. Zee DS, Friendlich AR, Robinson DA. The mechanism of downbeat nystagmus. Arch Neurol. 1974;30(3):227–37.
69. Wagner J, Lehnen N, Glasauer S, Rettinger N, Büttner U, Brandt T, et al. Downbeat nystagmus caused by a paramedian ponto-medullary lesion. J Neurol. 2009;256(9):1572–4.
70. Nakamagoe K, Shimizu K, Koganezawa T, Tamaoka A. Downbeat nystagmus due to a paramedian medullary lesion. J Clin Neurosci. 2012;19(11):1597–9.
71. Nakamagoe K, Fujizuka N, Koganezawa T, Yamaguchi T, Tamaoka A. Downbeat nystagmus associated with damage to the medial longitudinal fasciculus of the pons: a vestibular balance control mechanism via the lower brainstem paramedian tract neurons. J Neurol Sci. 2013;328(1–2):98–101.
72. Ances BM, Dalmau JO, Tsai J, Hasbani MJ, Galetta SL. Downbeating nystagmus and muscle spasms in a patient with glutamic-acid decarboxylase antibodies. Am J Ophthalmol. 2005;140(1):142–4.
73. Saul RF, Selhorst JB. Downbeat nystagmus with magnesium depletion. Arch Neurol. 1981;38(10):650–2.
74. Kattah JC, Tehrani AS, du Lac S, Newman-Toker DE, Zee DS. Conversion of upbeat to downbeat nystagmus in Wernicke encephalopathy. Neurology. 2018;91(17):790–6.
75. Mayfrank L, Thoden U. Downbeat nystagmus indicates cerebellar or brain-stem lesions in vitamin B 12 deficiency. J Neurol. 1986;233(3):145–8.
76. Chrousos GA, Cowdry R, Schuelein M, Abdul-Rahim AS, Matsuo V, Currie JN. Two cases of downbeat nystagmus and oscillopsia associated with carbamazepine. Am J Ophthalmol. 1987;103(2):221–4.
77. Lessell I, Halmagyi GM, Curthoys IS, Lessell S, Hoyt WF. Lithium-induced downbeat nystagmus. Am J Ophthalmol. 1989;107(6):664–70.
78. Zasorin N, Baloh RW. Downbeat nystagmus with alcoholic cerebellar degeneration. Arch Neurol. 1984;41(12):1301–2.
79. Kaut O, Kornblum C. Transient downbeat nystagmus after intravenous administration of the opioid piritramide. J Neuro-ophthalmol. 2010;30(2):164.
80. Halmagyi GM, Rudge P, Gresty MA, Sanders MD. Downbeating nystagmus: a review of 62 cases. Arch Neurol. 1983;40(13):777–84.
81. Prasad S, Brown MJ, Galetta SL. Transient downbeat nystagmus from West Nile virus encephalomyelitis. Neurology. 2006;66(10):1599–600.

82. Brodsky MC. Congenital downbeat nystagmus. J Pediatr Ophthalmol Strabismus. 1996;33(3):191–3.
83. Bronstein A, Miller D, Rudge P, Kendall B. Down beating nystagmus: magnetic resonance imaging and neuro-otological findings. J Neurol Sci. 1987;81(2–3):173–84.
84. Halmagyi GM, Leigh RJ. Upbeat about downbeat nystagmus. Neurology. 2004;63:606–7.
85. Baloh RW, Spooner JW. Downbeat nystagmus: a type of central vestibular nystagmus. Neurology. 1981;31(3):304.
86. Glasauer S, Hoshi M, Kempermann U, Eggert T, Buttner U. Three-dimensional eye position and slow phase velocity in humans with downbeat nystagmus. J Neurophysiol. 2003;89(1):338–54.
87. Ito M, Nisimaru N, Yamamoto M. Specific patterns of neuronal connexions involved in the control of the rabbit's vestibulo-ocular reflexes by the cerebellar flocculus. J Physiol. 1977;265(3):833–54.
88. Strupp M, Schüler O, Krafczyk S, Jahn K, Schautzer F, Büttner U, et al. Treatment of downbeat nystagmus with 3, 4-diaminopyridine: a placebo-controlled study. Neurology. 2003;61(2):165–70.
89. Kalla R, Glasauer S, Schautzer F, Lehnen N, Büttner U, Strupp M, et al. 4-aminopyridine improves downbeat nystagmus, smooth pursuit, and VOR gain. Neurology. 2004;62(7):1228–9.
90. Kalla R, Glasauer S, Büttner U, Brandt T, Strupp M. 4-aminopyridine restores vertical and horizontal neural integrator function in downbeat nystagmus. Brain. 2007;130(9):2441–51.
91. Claassen J, Spiegel R, Kalla R, Faldon M, Kennard C, Danchaivijitr C, et al. A randomised double-blind, cross-over trial of 4-aminopyridine for downbeat nystagmus—effects on slowphase eye velocity, postural stability, locomotion and symptoms. J Neurol Neurosurg Psychiatry. 2013;84(12):1392–9.
92. Kalla R, Spiegel R, Claassen J, Bardins S, Hahn A, Schneider E, et al. Comparison of 10-mg doses of 4-aminopyridine and 3, 4-diaminopyridine for the treatment of downbeat nystagmus. J Neuroophthalmol. 2011;31(4):320–5.
93. Young YH, Huang TW. Role of clonazepam in the treatment of idiopathic downbeat nystagmus. Laryngoscope. 2001;111(8):1490–3.
94. Averbuch-Heller L, Tusa R, Fuhry L, Rottach K, Ganser G, Heide W, et al. A double-blind controlled study of gabapentin and baclofen as treatment for acquired nystagmus. Ann Neurol. 1997;41(6):818–25.
95. Feil K, Claaßen J, Bardins S, Teufel J, Krafczyk S, Schneider E, et al. Effect of chlorzoxazone in patients with downbeat nystagmus: a pilot trial. Neurology. 2013;81(13):1152–8.
96. Carlow TJ. Medical treatment of nystagmus and ocular motor disorders. Int Ophthalmol Clin. 1986;26(4):251–64.
97. Nakada T, Remler MP. Primary position upbeat nystagmus. Another central vestibular nystagmus? J Clin Neuroophthalmol. 1981;1(3):185–9.
98. Gresty MA, Bronstein AM, Brookes GB, Rudge P. Primary position upbeating nystagmus associated with middle ear disease. Neuro-Ophthalmology. 1988;8(6):321–8.
99. Büttner-Ennever J, Horn A. Pathways from cell groups of the paramedian tracts to the floccular region a. Ann N Y Acad Sci. 1996;781(1):532–40.
100. Saito T, Aizawa H, Sawada J, Katayama T, Hasebe N. Lesion of the nucleus intercalatus in primary position upbeat nystagmus. Arch Neurol. 2010;67(11):1403–4.
101. Glasauer S, Kalla R, Büttner U, Strupp M, Brandt T. 4-aminopyridine restores visual ocular motor function in upbeat nystagmus. J Neurol Neurosurg Psychiatry. 2005;76(3):451–3.
102. Strupp M, Kremmyda O, Brandt T, editors. Pharmacotherapy of vestibular disorders and nystagmus. Semin Neurol. 2013;33(3):286–96.
103. Fahn S. Classification and investigation of dystonia. Move Disord. 1987;2:332–58.
104. FitzGerald PM, Jankovic J. Tardive oculogyric crises. Neurology. 1989;39(11):1434.
105. Nasrallah HA, Pappas NJ, Crowe RR. Oculogyric dystonia in tardive dyskinesia. Am J Psychiatry. 1980;137(7):850–1.

106. Ghosh S, Dhrubajyoti B, Bhattacharya A, Roy D, Saddichha S. Tardive oculogyric crisis associated with quetiapine use. J Clin Psychopharmacol. 2013;33(2):266.
107. Praharaj SK, Jana AK, Sarkar S, Sinha VK. Olanzapine-induced tardive oculogyric crisis. J Clin Psychopharmacol. 2009;29(6):604–6.
108. de Mattos Viana B, Prais HAC, Camargos ST, Cardoso FEC. Ziprasidone-related oculogyric crisis in an adult. Clin Neurol Neurosurg. 2009;111(10):883–5.
109. Bhachech JT. Aripiprazole-induced oculogyric crisis (acute dystonia). J Pharmacol Pharmacother. 2012;3(3):279.
110. Berchou RC, Rodin EA. Carbamazepine-Induced oculogyric crisis. Arch Neurol. 1979;36(8):522–3.
111. Veerapandiyan A, Gallentine WB, Winchester SA, Baker J, Kansagra SM, Mikati MA. Oculogyric crises secondary to lamotrigine overdosage. Epilepsia. 2011;52(3):e4–6.
112. Sandyk R. Oculogyric crisis induced by lithium carbonate. Eur Neurol. 1984;23(2):92–4.
113. Koban Y, Ekinci M, Cagatay HH, Yazar Z. Oculogyric crisis in a patient taking metoclo pramide. Clin Ophthalmol (Auckland, NZ). 2014;8:567.
114. Bayram E, Bayram MT, Hiz S, Turkmen M. Cefixime-induced oculogyric crisis. Pediatr Emerg Care. 2012;28(1):55–6.
115. Reeves AL, So EL, Sharbrough FW, Krahn LE. Movement disorders associated with the use of gabapentin. Epilepsia. 1996;37(10):988–90.
116. Burke RE, Reches A, Traub MM, Ilson J, Swash M, Fahn S. Tetrabenazine induces acute dystonic reactions. Ann Neurol. 1985;17(2):200–2.
117. Fraunfelder FW, Fraunfelder FT. Oculogyric crisis in patients taking cetirizine. Am J Ophthalmol. 2004;137(2):355–7.
118. Smith JL, editor. Ocular signs of parkinsonism. J Neurosurg. 1966;24:284–5.
119. Mata M, Dorovini-Zis K, Wilson M, Young AB. New form of familial Parkinson-dementia syndrome: clinical and pathologic findings. Neurology. 1983;33(11):1439.
120. Lamberti P, de Mari M, Iliceto G, Caldarola M, Serlenga L. Effect of l-dopa on oculogyric crises in a case of dopa-responsive dystonia. Move Disord. 1993;8(2):236–7.
121. Kis B, Hedrich K, Kann M, Schwinger E, Kömpf D, Klein C, et al. Oculogyric dystonic states in early-onset parkinsonism with basal ganglia calcifications. Neurology. 2005;65(5):761.
122. Matsumura K, Sakuta M. Oculogyric crisis in acute herpetic brainstem encephalitis. J Neurol Neurosurg Psychiatry. 1987;50(3):365.
123. Bennett J, Galetta SL, Frohman L, Mourelatos Z, Gultekin S, Dalmau J, et al. Neuro-ophthalmologic manifestations of a paraneoplastic syndrome and testicular carcinoma. Neurology. 1999;52(4):864.
124. Liu GT, Carrazana EJ, Macklis JD, Mikati MA. Delayed oculogyric crises associated with striatocapsular infarction. J Clin Neuroophthalmol. 1991;11(3):198–201.
125. Urra D, Campos J, Ruiz P. Movement disorders in ataxia-telangiectasia: review of six patients: PP474. Neurology. 1989;39(3).
126. FitzGerald P, Jankovic J, Glaze D, Schultz R, Percy A. Extrapyramidal involvement in Rett's syndrome. Neurology. 1990;40(2):293.
127. Lee M, Kim Y, Lyoo C. Oculogyric crisis as an initial manifestation of Wilson's disease. Neurology. 1999;52(8):1714.
128. Joseph AB, Young RR. Movement disorders in neurology and neuropsychiatry. Hoboken: Blackwell Scientific Publications; 1992.
129. Heimburger RF. Positional oculogyric crises: case report. J Neurosurg. 1988;69(6):951–3.
130. Della Marca G, Frisullo G, Vollono C, Dittoni S, Losurdo A, Testani E, et al. Oculogyric crisis in a midbrain lesion. Arch Neurol. 2011;68(3):390–1.
131. McCowan P, Cook L. Oculogyric crises in chronic epidemic encephalitis. Brain. 1928;51(3):285–309.
132. Onuaguluchi G. Crises in post-encephalitic parkinsonism. Brain. 1961;84(3):395–414.
133. Leigh RJ, Foley JM, Remler BF, Civil RH. Oculogyric crisis: a syndrome of thought disorder and ocular deviation. Ann Neurol. 1987;22(1):13–7.

Movement Disorder Emergencies of the Upper Aerodigestive Tract

3

Thomas Stewart, Lesley F. Childs, Scott Rickert,
Boris Bentsianov, Ajay E. Chitkara, Anthony Cultrara,
and Andrew Blitzer

Patient Vignette

A 52-year-old man was transferred to the emergency room of a major hospital from a referral facility because of recent slurred speech. He had been admitted to the referral facility the week before for treatment of alcohol abuse. Upon his arrival in the emergency room, the neurology resident was called to evaluate the patient after a normal computed tomography scan was obtained. Examination revealed normal comprehension and expression, slurring of speech, and an inability to fully open his

T. Stewart
New York Centre for Voice and Swallowing Disorders, New York, NY, USA

L. F. Childs
Department of Otolaryngology – Head & Neck Surgery, UT Southwestern Medical Center, Dallas, TX, USA

S. Rickert
Division of Pediatric Otolaryngology, Department of Otolaryngology, Pediatrics, and Plastic Surgery, NYU Langone Health, New York, NY, USA

B. Bentsianov
Department of Otolaryngology and Division of Laryngology, Voice and Swallowing Disorders, Downstate Medical Center, State University of New York, Brooklyn, NY, USA

A. E. Chitkara
ENT and Allergy Associates, LLP, Voice and Swallowing Disorders, Port Jefferson Station, NY, USA

A. Cultrara
Advanced ENT and Allergy, Voorhees, NJ, USA

A. Blitzer (✉)
Otolaryngology-Head and Neck Surgery, Columbia University College of Physicians and Surgeons, New York, NY, USA

Icahn School of Medicine at Mount Sinai, New York, NY, USA

New York Center for Voice and Swallowing Disorders, New York, NY, USA

© Springer Nature Switzerland AG 2022
S. J. Frucht (ed.), *Movement Disorder Emergencies*, Current Clinical Neurology,
https://doi.org/10.1007/978-3-030-75898-1_3

jaw and protrude his tongue. There were no defects in visual field perception, power, or sensation. Review of the medical record from the referring institution revealed that the patient had been started on 5 mg of haloperidol four times daily on his admission to the referral facility as part of his treatment for alcohol abuse—he was unaware he was receiving the medication. An acute dystonic reaction was diagnosed, and 25 mg of intravenous diphenhydramine was administered, with resolution of the dysarthria and jaw restriction within 90s of infusion. He was maintained on oral diphenhydramine (25 mg twice daily) for 1 week after discharge.

Introduction

Respiratory emergencies secondary to movement disorders are a rare but potentially life-threatening phenomenon. The clinician treating this patient population should be aware of the differential diagnosis and proper treatment to prevent adverse outcomes. The primary goal of intervention is to ensure a secure airway and to prevent respiratory embarrassment. Breathing disturbances of the larynx may be caused by primary movement disorders or may be iatrogenically induced, for example secondary to neuroleptic agents. In general, movement disorders of the upper aerodigestive tract lead to gradual respiratory compromise by diminishing the ability of the larynx to protect the lungs from aspiration. In this section, we will focus on movement disorders that produce acute airway obstruction as a result of mechanical blockage by glottic dysfunction. Laryngeal anatomy and physiology, history and physical exam, differential diagnosis, and treatment of airway emergencies will also be discussed.

     Securing the airway and preventing respiratory embarrassment is the primary goal of intervention.

Acute Airway Assessment and Management

The management of any patient with potential airway compromise starts with a rapid and accurate assessment of the severity and urgency of the clinical problem. Airway management can usually be classified as emergent, urgent, or chronic. An accurate history, patient assessment, and physical examination will help categorize various patients, allowing potentially life-saving measures to be executed appropriately.

Basic history with respect to the airway includes several key items. While dyspnea or shortness of breath is often the focus, this symptom may occur late in the course of events and herald a true airway emergency. More subtle findings occur earlier and are critical to recognize. Stridor or "noisy breathing" suggests a disturbance of the normal laminar airflow pattern. Inspiratory stridor usually implies a laryngeal or supraglottic obstruction, with isolated expiratory stridor suggesting an intrathoracic or tracheobronchial obstruction. A biphasic stridor classically implies a subglottic origin for the stridor. Dysphonia, or hoarseness, is an important early finding. Questions about onset (acute vs. chronic), duration (continuous vs. episodic), and quality (harsh, raspy, breaks, breathy, fatigable) give important information about airway stability.

The physical examination of the upper airway depends on accurate interpretation of findings on flexible fiberoptic laryngoscopy. Neurologic conditions present a particular challenge because there is often no anatomic distortion of laryngeal anatomy. Instead, they often manifest as complex functional disturbances requiring an experienced, trained observer. Failure of bilateral vocal fold abduction may warrant emergency intervention, cricothyroidotomy, or tracheotomy. The specific history and physical findings of each of the neurologic emergencies of the airway, including adductor breathing dystonia, Shy Drager syndrome, and iatrogenic-related emergencies, will be discussed below.

Many neurologic airway emergencies will respond to medical intervention including high flow humidified oxygen, intravenous infusion of steroids, and continuous pulse oximetry monitoring (preferably in a critical care unit). These measures help stabilize the situation; either completely avoiding the need for definitive airway management or at least allowing staff trained in advanced airway management to arrive for assistance with care. Caution should be taken prior to attempted intubation in this patient group, as bilateral true vocal fold adduction may leave the vocal folds in a median or paramedian position making endotracheal intubation potentially challenging. Repeated attempts can further aggravate the situation by traumatizing the larynx and true vocal folds, causing bleeding and edema in an already compromised airway. Fiberoptic-guided intubation performed in a controlled operating room setting, with back-up surgical airway assistance is far superior if time allows. Should this option not be available, or the situation too acute, cricothyroidotomy by incision into the cricothyroid membrane and insertion of a small endotracheal tube (e.g., #5.0 or #5.5) can be performed. This should be followed by conversion to tracheotomy as early as possible to prevent injury to the subglottis and potential further injury to the larynx and vocal folds.

Breathing Disturbances from Primary Disorders

Spasmodic Dysphonia

Dystonia is defined as involuntary sustained muscle contractions frequently causing twisting and repetitive movements or abnormal postures that may be sustained or intermittent. Spasmodic dysphonia (SD) is a clinical term used to describe focal laryngeal dystonia. The vocal apparatus usually functions normally during respiration, and laryngeal dystonia is triggered by speech. Most SD is idiopathic; however, it may occur secondary to neurological disorders (Wilson's disease, parkinsonism,

Huntington's disease, ceroid lipofuscinosis), environmental factors (posttraumatic, postinfectious, vascular, neoplastic, toxic) and even psychogenic [1]. SD is generally categorized into an adductor (AdSD) form, abductor (AbSD) form, or mixed type.

In AbSD, inappropriate contraction of the posterior cricoarytenoid muscles (the sole laryngeal abductors) results in hyper-abduction of the vocal folds. The voice quality is breathy and aphonic breaks occur during connected speech. In AdSD, inappropriate hyper-adduction of the laryngeal adductors (primarily the thyroarytenoids) results in a choked, strained voice quality with breaks in phonation. Laryngeal dystonias are task-specific (i.e., they occur only during speaking) and generally do not interfere with normal breathing, therefore respiratory compromise is not seen. Some studies have suggested that the sensation of dyspnea experienced by patients with laryngeal dystonia may be exacerbated by desynchronized contractions of the diaphragm [2]. The primary treatment of SD is with botulinum toxin injections to partially chemically denervate the specific laryngeal muscles responsible for the abnormal movements.

Adductor Laryngeal Breathing Dystonia

As mentioned earlier, focal laryngeal dystonias usually do not interfere with respiration; however, patients with adductor laryngeal breathing dystonia present with adductor spasms, which occur selectively during inspiration. This usually presents as stridor of unknown etiology. Gerhardt first described this disorder, attributing it to paralysis of the abductor muscles. In 1992, Marion [3] studied three patients with Gerhardt's syndrome with laryngeal electromyography to show that adductor muscles were hyperactive. No weakness or denervation of the abductors was present, suggesting that the syndrome occurred as the result of AdSD. In 1994, our group reported seven patients with stridor and paradoxical movement of the vocal folds [4]. They had normal abduction on coughing and laughing, but during inspiration they had closure of the vocal folds increasing airway resistance and producing stridor. Hyperactive adductor muscles were demonstrated on EMG, while normal activity was seen in the abductor muscles. None of these patients desaturated on pulse oximetry and none required tracheostomy or ventilatory assistance. Stridor disappeared during sleep, typical of dystonia, and reappeared on awakening. All of the patients improved with injections of botulinum toxin to weaken the adductor muscles. Adductor breathing dystonia has also been reported in association with Lubag syndrome [5] (X-linked dystonia-parkinsonism), with multiple system atrophy (MSA) [6], with progressive supranuclear palsy [7] (both atypical parkinsonian syndromes) and as a complication of chimeric-antigen receptor T-cell immunotherapy (CAR-T) [8].

Multiple System Atrophy: Abductor Weakness

MSA is a progressive degenerative neurological disorder affecting multiple systems, characterized clinically by a variety of parkinsonian, cerebellar, and autonomic signs and symptoms. MSA is categorized into MSA-P (predominant parkinsonism) and MSA-C (predominant cerebellar) [9], with three levels of diagnostic certainty: possible, probable, and definite. Stridor is an additional feature of possible MSA-P or MSA-C; this partial airway obstruction is secondary to progressive vocal fold dysfunction, typically presenting as stridor that occurs first in sleep. With the limitation of a frequently delayed diagnosis, stridor within 3 years of motor or autonomic symptoms may shorten overall survival [10]. Nocturnal stridor signifies a poor prognosis, with an increased risk of sudden death [11, 12]. Deguchi studied the relationship between urine storage dysfunction, abductor paralysis, and central sleep apnea in these patients, noting that a deterioration of urine storage function might serve as a useful predictor of a parallel patient decline from abductor paralysis and central sleep apnea [13].

Stridor, particularly daytime stridor, increases the risk of sudden death. A complaint or history of stridor should prompt urgent referral to an experienced otolaryngologist.

Vocal fold paresis and paralysis have been documented; however, the etiology of the vocal fold dysfunction is still elusive. Some authors have postulated that there is progressive weakness of the laryngeal abductors, while others suggest a dyskinesia or dystonia of the adductors leading to paradoxical vocal fold movement. Yoshihara noted a variety of stages of neurogenic degeneration of the muscle fibers and neuromuscular junctions of the posterior cricoarytenoid muscle, corresponding with abductor immobility in a patient with MSA [14]. Some authors have demonstrated adductor hyperfunctioning by laryngeal electromyography in patients with MSA, which responded to botulinum toxin injection to the thyroarytenoid muscles [6]. Flexible endoscopic evaluation usually reveals vocal fold adduction during inspiration. Earlier in the disease process, continuous positive airway pressure therapy has been proposed as a treatment for MSA-associated stridor, which often leads to excessive daytime sleepiness in these patients. CPAP can also serve as a tool for uncovering the possibility of central apnea in this population [15–17]. As the laryngeal dysfunction progresses, patients may require tracheotomy to protect the airway.

There is no cure for MSA and life expectancy is generally 7–10 years after diagnosis; medical treatment is symptomatic. Surgical intervention may be necessary to provide alternatives for nutritional support secondary to dysphagia and/or tracheotomy to secure the dysfunctional airway.

Iatrogenic Causes of Breathing Disturbances

Spasmodic Dysphonia: Airway Obstruction Secondary to Botulinum Toxin Treatment

The treatment of SD entails manipulation of the larynx in order to deliver botulinum toxin to the appropriate laryngeal muscles. Airway compromise may occur iatrogenically as the result of laryngospasm, excessive volume injection, or paralysis of the laryngeal abductors bilaterally. Laryngospasm is a sudden, sustained adduction of the vocal folds resulting in occlusion of the airway. This reflex is mediated via the vagus nerve and usually occurs in response to irritation of the vocal folds. It is thought to be a protective response that prevents irritants from reaching the lower airway. The treatment of AdSD requires botulinum toxin injection under EMG guidance into the thyroarytenoid muscles. The needle is advanced through the cricothyroid membrane into the body of the thyroarytenoid muscle, remaining extramucosally and preventing breach of the needle into the airway throughout the procedure. In some individuals, the needle may stimulate laryngospasm resulting in acute airway obstruction. Initial treatment requires the patient to remain calm and to inhale nasally ("sniffing" maneuver) until the spasm breaks: this technique is usually successful. Failure of the spasm to break with conservative measures may require securing the airway via intubation, cricothyroidotomy, or tracheotomy. In the operating room, laryngospasm may be arrested with positive pressure ventilation, or with paralytic agents followed by endotracheal intubation. Injection of excessive volume into the vocal folds may lead to dyspnea and subsequent mechanical obstruction of the glottic inlet. In our practice the senior author tries to limit the injection to 0.1 mL per vocal fold to avoid stridor and/or glottic obstruction.

The treatment of AbSD requires botulinum toxin injection under EMG guidance into the posterior cricoarytenoid muscles. Because these are the only intrinsic laryngeal muscles responsible for abducting the vocal folds, bilateral paralysis can result in acute laryngeal obstruction. To prevent this from occurring, we usually inject only one side per clinical visit. Approximately 2 weeks later, after the peak effect of the botulinum toxin has passed, flexible nasolaryngoscopy is performed to evaluate the abductor capability of the injected vocal fold. If there is satisfactory motion of the treated vocal fold, the contralateral posterior cricoarytenoid muscle is treated. Precise unilateral injection is mandatory to prevent inadvertent bilateral posterior cricoarytenoid muscle paralysis by direct injection or local diffusion.

There are no antidotes for mechanical obstruction of the larynx caused by overzealous injection of the vocal folds or inadvertent bilateral paralysis of the laryngeal abductors. Treatment is guided by the severity of the obstruction and may include intubation and/or procurement of a surgical airway.

Drug-Induced Tardive Dystonia

Typical neuroleptics and antipsychotics may trigger tardive dyskinesia or tardive dystonia, which can cause acute respiratory compromise if the larynx is involved. The extra-pyramidal side effects of neuroleptic and antipsychotic medications have been extensively reviewed in the literature [18–20]. We will focus on tardive dystonia, as laryngeal involvement may precipitate acute respiratory embarrassment and sudden death if not properly diagnosed and treated. Tardive dyskinesia typically presents as involuntary choreic movements of oral, buccal and lingual areas, whereas tardive dystonia produces involuntary spasmodic movements of the head, neck, tongue, and mouth. When the dystonia involves the laryngeal musculature, respiratory compromise may ensue as a result of vocal fold spasms. The diagnosis of tardive dystonia of the larynx should always be suspected in patients with a history of neuroleptic use. Patients may present with acute stridor without obvious precipitating cause. The diagnosis is based on history and clinical examination including endoscopy to rule out other causes of airway obstruction [21]. Primary medical management of tardive dystonia is with anticholinergics such as diphenhydramine, which should be administered parenterally in the acute setting. Once the patient is stabilized, pharmaceutical treatment should be continued orally as an outpatient for 3–5 days. Patients with laryngeal dystonia may require resuscitative treatment, that is, supplemental oxygen therapy, intubation, or a surgical airway while diagnosis and treatment are provided [22]. Fortunately, tardive dystonias respond promptly when properly diagnosed and treated.

Parkinson's Disease: Airway Compromise Related to Deep Brain Stimulator

Deep brain stimulation therapy is a now well-established intervention for the treatment of Parkinson's disease, particularly for motor symptoms refractory to medical therapy [23]. The development of bilateral vocal fold immobility following the placement of subthalamic electrodes has been reported, requiring placement of a temporary or permanent tracheotomy [24, 25]. While this is an uncommon complication, awareness of this association is important for the treating physician both for prior informed consent for the patient and for subsequent perioperative care.

Swallowing Emergencies

Deglutition is a complex act of the laryngopharynx, requiring the successful passage of a food bolus into the upper esophagus and simultaneous protection of the laryngotracheal airway. This act relies upon the complex interrelationship of neuromuscular coordination of the oral cavity, oropharynx, hypopharynx, and larynx. Breakdown in the neuromuscular coordination of deglutition causes dysphagia (difficulty swallowing) or aspiration (food bolus passing into the airway distal to the level of the true vocal folds). Emergencies of swallowing can be categorized into those related to dysmotility and those related to aspiration; in the first, the patient is unable to maintain nutritional sustenance via oral intake, and in the second, the patient is unsafe to maintain an oral diet due to airway protection. These emergencies of swallowing rarely require immediate attention but often benefit from urgent intervention to allow adequate nutritional intake and to prevent aspiration pneumonia.

Swallowing Assessment

The swallowing assessment should include a history of the type and quantity of foods tolerated, weight loss or gain, and a history of coughing or choking. The clinical exam should include a comprehensive head and neck examination including cranial nerve examination and flexible nasoendoscopy of the pharynx and larynx. In addition to structural and functional assessment of the larynx, the specific act of deglutition should be witnessed endoscopically.

Objective methods of evaluating swallowing function include modified barium swallow and fiberoptic endoscopic evaluation of swallowing (FEES). The modified barium swallow (MBS) [26] involves videofluoroscopic evaluation in both anteroposterior and lateral views of swallowing while the patient is given barium coated foods of different consistencies (thin and thick liquid, puree, and solid). The examiner assesses for dysfunction in either structural or mechanical dysmotility during swallowing in the oral, pharyngeal and upper esophageal phases. In order to evaluate the entire esophagus, a barium esophagram is performed which involves the patient swallowing liquid barium. Views are taken before, during and after the barium is administered. If a difficulty is identified, feeding position and strategy can be tested using the barium to evaluate the efficacy of the compensatory maneuvers. FEES allows direct visualization of swallowing with a flexible laryngoscope in place during deglutition [27, 28]. The patient is offered food boluses of different consistencies with the addition of food coloring. The swallow is observed through the flexible videolaryngoscope. Many aspects of the swallow can be assessed in this manner except during velopharyngeal closure when the view is transiently obstructed. FEES can be performed at the bedside or in the office. MBS and FEES, when performed by experienced examiners, have similar specificity and sensitivity [29].

Laryngeal sensory testing is a method of evaluating the afferents of the laryngopharynx [28]. This is done at the same time as the FEES and evaluates the laryngeal adductor reflex. When present, the reflex implies that sensory input to the larynx is intact. A calibrated air puff stimulus is applied to the aryepiglottic fold mucosa while watching for the adductor reflex. Sensory deficits have been shown to contribute to aspiration [30]; however, the role of sensation in dysphagia associated with movement disorders requires further investigation.

Esophageal function can also be evaluated with manometry. This technique measures the sequential muscular function of the esophagus and can thus confirm dysmotility disorders of the esophagus [31]. This technique may be combined with videofluoroscopy, which adds information regarding bolus location [32].

Treatment of Swallowing Disorders

The treatment of dysphagia begins with behavior modification and speech and swallowing therapy. This entails both positional and functional maneuvers to improve swallowing efficiency and prevent aspiration of the food bolus into the trachea. In severe cases, oral feeding may be inadequate for nutritional sustenance, and tube feeding is required for supplementation. Early intervention is crucial to maintain adequate caloric needs. Nasogastric tube feeding is appropriate for initiating enteral feeds. Percutaneous endoscopic gastrostomy (PEG) or open gastrostomies are long-term, reversible means of maintaining enteral feeding in patients with debilitating dysphagia. In some cases, treating the underlying movement disorder may improve the symptoms of dysphagia.

Aspiration of a food or liquid bolus can result in aspiration pneumonia, which is associated with significant morbidity in patients with degenerative movement disorders. Behavioral modifications through speech and swallowing therapy are first implemented. If vocal fold immobility is contributing to aspiration, then medialization laryngoplasty may help the patient to swallow safely [33]. Gastric tube feeding bypasses the upper aerodigestive tract and may decrease the frequency of aspiration. Tube feeding, however, does not prevent the aspiration of oral secretions, and patients may develop aspiration pneumonia even with a PEG. Patients who continue to aspirate oral secretions despite the presence of a gastric feeding tube may benefit from surgical airway protection. This includes glottic closure, epiglottic closure, laryngotracheal separation, and total laryngectomy [34, 35]. Tracheotomy does not prevent aspiration, and it may actually increase the risk of aspiration. This is due to the tethering effect of the trachea, which may inhibit laryngeal elevation, along with the inability to create adequate subglottic pressure during the swallow. Tracheotomy, however, does improve pulmonary toilet.

Specific Disorders Related to Swallowing Emergencies

Oromandibulolingual Dystonia

Oromandibulolingual dystonia [36, 37] (OMD) is a form of focal dystonia involving the masticatory, lower facial and tongue musculature, producing spasms and often jaw deviation. In the early sixteenth century, Brueghel often painted faces with open mouths and contracted facial muscles, perhaps due to OMD [38]. In 1899, Gowers [39] described conditions producing tonic and clonic jaw contractions. The differential diagnosis of tonic jaw spasms includes dystonia, tetanus, trauma, hysteria, brainstem lesions, and hypothermia. Just after the turn of the century, Meige [40] reported a syndrome of spasms of the eyelids in addition to contractions of the pharyngeal, jaw, and tongue muscles. These spasms were often provoked by voluntary action (talking and/or eating) and lessened by humming, singing, yawning, or voluntarily opening the mouth. Some patients with Meige's syndrome developed other signs of dystonia, including torticollis, spasmodic dysphonia, or writer's cramp. In 1976, Marsden [41] realized that blepharospasm and oromandibular dystonia were both forms of adult-onset focal dystonia, a view supported by others [42–52]. In the most severe cases of OMD, dysphagia and/or airway obstruction can occur. One such case was published in a patient who sustained hypoxic brain injury, presenting several years later with intermittent respiratory distress requiring tracheostomy [53].

The etiology and differential diagnosis of OMD are similar to other forms of focal dystonia [54]. Misdiagnosis is common. Sustained or repetitive muscle contractions associated with bruxism typically occur in sleep and OMD disappears in sleep. Many patients are initially diagnosed as having temporomandibular disorders (TMD) and are treated with a variety of appliances [55]. Dental appliances may be useful, as sensory tricks help orofacial dyskinesias and OMD. On the basis of clinical exam, patients can be classified as having predominantly jaw-closing, jaw-opening, or jaw-deviation dystonia. Drug therapy is the mainstay of treatment; anticholinergics, benzodiazepines, and baclofen have proven to be most effective [56, 57]. We and others have reported success in managing OMD with local injections of botulinum toxin [58, 59]. There have been reports of successful management of the jaw spasms using anesthetics and alcohol, suggesting an important role for modulating afferents in OMD [60].

Side effects and complications of botulinum toxin injection of OMD are uncommon. In our initial report, there were 14 instances of dysphagia, mostly of the jaw-opening dystonia variety, where the anterior digastric muscles were injected. This injection can cause weakness of the suprahyoid muscle causing poor elevation of the larynx on swallowing and also changing the effectiveness of the tongue base on swallowing. One patient had severe dysphagia requiring a change of diet. One patient with jaw-closing dystonia had marked weakness of jaw closing and required an elastic bandage wrapped around his jaw to assist with chewing. Injection of the external pterygoid muscles occasionally caused rhinolalia or nasal regurgitation when drinking liquids. One patient with severe jaw-opening dystonia was treated too aggressively and developed antibodies to botulinum toxin type A [61]. We initially treated a number of patients with severe lingual dystonia that caused posturing of the tongue or even prevented jaw closing. However, this approach converts a hyperfunctional tongue to a hypofunctional tongue. In most cases, we found the disability from the treatment worse than the disease. We recommend not treating the tongue, particularly the tongue base, since this worsens both speech and swallowing. In our initial series, six patients experienced such severe dysphagia that they required a temporary nasogastric tube for enteral feeding for 3–8 weeks. Two patients with severe lingual dystonia (tongue remained postured out of their mouths most of the time) were treated successfully because they already had a tracheostomy and a gastrostomy tube. In these cases, a hypofunctional tongue was a clinical improvement [62, 63]. Some authors report benefits with low dose injections of lingual musculature [64]. Lyons recently reported on deep brain stimulation as an effective and safe treatment for patients with medically refractory Meige's syndrome [65].

Multiple System Atrophy

The main laryngopharyngeal deficit in patients with MSA is vocal fold immobility, which may be related to abductor paresis [6]. Persistent activity of the cricopharyngeus muscle during swallowing has also been noted in EMG studies [6]. Clinically, patients with advanced stages of MSA are more likely to have vocal fold immobility. This, along with dysfunction of the cricopharyngeus muscle, contributes to dysphagia. There is an increase in bolus stasis at the level of the piriform sinuses and the cricopharyngeus [66]. The presence of vocal fold immobility has been associated with increased risk of aspiration in patients with MSA, and therefore increased risk of aspiration pneumonia [66]. Patients with laryngopharyngeal deficits related to MSA often require a tracheotomy to maintain the airway as the disease advances. At this point, there is often the need for gastric tube feeding to maintain adequate nutrition in these patients.

Multiple Sclerosis

Dysphagia is a secondary symptom of multiple sclerosis (MS), and a leading cause of morbidity and mortality in patients with MS [67]. Difficulty swallowing can lead to dehydration, malnutrition, and aspiration pneumonia. Dysphagia may be present in up to 43% of patients with MS, and the severity of the disease does not correlate with the degree of dysphagia. Dysphagia is caused by dysmotility at the level of the pharyngeal constrictors. This can result in penetration of the food bolus into the laryngeal vestibule. Slowing of the laryngopharyngeal phase of swallowing results in pharyngeal dysmotility [67]. Since there is no specific correlation between the disease state and the degree of dysphagia in MS, any complaint of swallowing dysfunction should be evaluated and treated regardless of the patient's overall disability. Speech and swallowing therapy may be beneficial to help compensate for the laryngopharyngeal dysfunction [68]. Patients at risk for aspiration or who are unable to maintain oral intake may require tube feeding for maintenance of nutrition.

Amyotrophic Lateral Sclerosis

Dysphagia in amyotrophic lateral sclerosis (ALS) usually manifests several months after the onset of the disease [69]. Dysphagia in these patients may progress to aspiration pneumonia, poor nutrition, and dehydration. Dysphagia in ALS is related to dysfunction at various phases of swallowing. There is generalized weakness of the perioral, submental, suprahyoid muscles, and the tongue. This affects the oral preparatory and oral phases of swallowing and can result in difficulty controlling liquids and purees [69]. There is a delay in triggering the pharyngeal phase of swallowing in patients with early, moderate dysphagia. In addition, there is a delay in laryngeal elevation in ALS patients with dysphagia. These patients also exhibit decreased tonic pause duration of the cricopharyngcus muscle during associated swallowing and laryngeal elevation, resulting in shorter periods of upper esophageal sphincter opening [70]. ALS patients with dysphagia have weakness of laryngeal and respiratory muscles. They also exhibit brisk mandibular and gag reflexes. In advanced stages, patients can lose all voluntary control of the swallow resulting in a spontaneous reflex swallow [70]. Using a mouse model, Lever suggested that pharyngeal dysphagia in ALS may be attributed to both motor and sensory pathologies [71].

⚡ Bulbar-onset ALS may present to the otolaryngologist first, mimicking adductor spasmodic dysphonia. Care must be taken to avoid injecting botulinum toxin unless the features of spasmodic dysphonia are clear.

Speech and swallowing therapy may provide compensatory techniques for early and moderate dysphagia. As the disease progresses and dysphagia becomes debilitating, gastric tube feedings are required. Spataro showed that PEG placement improves survival in dysphagic ALS patients, with few side effects [72]. Some patients with severe aspiration of secretions may benefit from surgical airway protection via glottal closure, laryngotracheal separation, or total laryngectomy.

Parkinson's Disease

Swallowing dysfunction is present in 30–52% of patients with Parkinson's disease (PD); in fact, gastrointestinal symptoms (including dysphagia) are among the most common nonmotor manifestations of PD [73–75]. Dysphagia and aspiration in the setting of respiratory insufficiency are a major cause of death in patients with PD [76]. In patients with PD, there is a positive correlation between dysphagia and both disease duration and severity [77]. Potulska [73] compared swallowing function in PD patients with normal subjects using EMG and pharyngoesophageal scintigraphy. PD patients exhibited either subclinical dysphagia or overt dysphagia. Overall pharyngeal transit times, laryngeal movement times, and esophageal transit times were prolonged in PD patients with overt dysphagia. As the dysphagia progressed, the pharyngeal phase of swallowing became more disrupted. Also, the dysphagia limit (maximum bolus volume safely swallowed) was significantly less in patients with overt dysphagia compared to patients with subclinical dysphagia [73]. EMG studies showed prolonged triggering of the swallowing reflex and prolonged duration of the pharyngeal reflex time without disturbance in the function of the cricopharyngeus muscle [70]. In the early stages of PD, patients have been shown to have manometric abnormalities even before clinical manifestations of dysphagia [78]. In a meta-analysis performed by Menezes and Melo, levodopa intake was shown not to be associated with an improvement in swallowing function in patients with Parkinson's disease [79]. PD patients with dysphagia may benefit from speech and swallowing therapy to compensate for the impaired swallowing mechanism. Expiratory muscle strength training may improve swallow safety [80]. If the dysphagia progresses such that oral nutrition is either inadequate or unsafe, then tube feeding should be implemented.

Huntington's Disease

Huntington's disease (HD) is a neurodegenerative disorder of the basal ganglia resulting in choreic movements, dementia, and neuropsychiatric features. These patients have impaired motor control of nearly all voluntary muscles, with many patients suffering from dysphagia [81]. In a review of the Nationwide Inpatient Sample database from 1996 to 2002, the most common HD-associated reason for hospital admission was pneumonia, of which aspiration pneumonia represented 22% of cases [82]. Death occurs within 20 years in most patients and is often due to aspiration pneumonia. HD-related dysphagia is classified as hyperkinetic or bradykinetic [83]. The hyperkinetic variant is more prevalent of the two. This type is associated with uncoordinated, hyperactive movements of the tongue, mandible, and soft palate. There is also reduced activity of the suprahyoid, cricopharyngeus, and extrinsic muscles of the larynx [83]. In addition, there are abrupt swallowing and involuntary respiratory maneuvers associated with the hyperkinetic variant [84]. Tachyphagia, or rapid swallowing maneuvers, is a unique characteristic of HD-related dysphagia. The bradykinetic variant of HD manifests with reduced motor function, range of motion, and coordination of the lips, mandible, tongue, and extrinsic laryngeal musculature [83]. Lingual sensory deficits may be present in both hyperkinetic and bradykinetic variants of HD. Kagel and Leopold [83] reviewed patients with HD over a 16-year period and found 28 of 29 patients had severe oral phase dysphagia by videofluoroscopic swallowing study, 17 of 29 patients had severe pharyngeal phase dysphagia, yet only 2 of 29 patients penetrated or aspirated. It should be noted that these swallow studies were performed with the patients in specially designed chairs to facilitate safe swallowing via postural fixation and spinal extension. Over one half of the patients studied exhibited uncoordinated and asynchronous vocal fold function. This laryngeal chorea resulted in almost one-third of the patients with a potentially unprotected tracheal airway [83].

Treatment of swallowing dysfunction in HD patients should begin with speech therapy and dietary modifications. This technique is limited by each patient's cognitive decline and ability to cooperate. Other techniques to optimize safe swallowing include specially designed chairs and prostheses, which limit some of the choreic activity and increase the efficiency of swallowing. When the disease progresses to unsafe swallowing, gastric tube feeding is recommended.

Palatal Myoclonus

Palatal myoclonus is a form of focal myoclonus, which manifests as repetitive contractions of the soft palate and uvula. It may affect only one side, although bilateral symmetric involvement is more common. Continuous, synchronous contractions of the uvula and soft palate occur at a frequency of 100–150 beats per minute [85]. The myoclonic activity persists during sleep. There may be associated focal myoclonic involvement of the larynx, extraocular muscles, neck, diaphragm, tongue, and face [85]. Palatal myoclonus is classified as symptomatic or essential. Symptomatic myoclonus occurs secondary to an underlying central nervous system disturbance, most commonly a brainstem stroke [86]. Other causes of symptomatic myoclonus include trauma, brainstem tumors or lesions, multiple sclerosis, encephalitis, progressive bulbar palsy, syringobulbia, obstructive hydrocephalus, and infectious causes (syphilis, malaria) [85–87]. There may be a latency period between the brainstem insult and onset of myoclonus of 3 weeks to 3 years [85]. Essential myoclonus, which is much less common, has no identifiable etiology [87]. The essential variant is associated with earlier onset (30–40 years), equal incidence in men and women, and often presents with the sole complaint of ear clicking. Symptomatic palatal myoclonus usually occurs in older males with less frequent subjective complaints [86]. There are occasional reports of palatal myoclonus contributing to dysphagia, dysarthria, and aspiration [87].

Treatment regimens for palatal myoclonus may include medical therapy with or without speech and swallowing therapy. Unfortunately, palatal myoclonus is often refractory to systemic medications. Occasionally successful medications include anticholinergics and clonazepam. Botulinum toxin has been used for treatment with successful results as well [85]. Swallowing therapy can also benefit patients with significant dysphagia and aspiration related to the palatal myoclonus. Behavioral techniques such as the supraglottic swallow can allow safe oral feeding [87].

Conclusion

Movement disorder emergencies of the aerodigestive tract are dramatic and often life threatening. With appropriate, timely evaluation and intervention, most patients can be effectively managed and major morbidity avoided.

References

1. Brin MF, Fahn S, Blitzer A, Ramig LO, Stewart C. Movement disorders of the larynx. In: Blitzer A, Brin MF, Sasaki CT, Fahn S, Harris KS, editors. Neurologic disorders of the larynx. New York: Thieme Medical Publishers Inc.; 1992. p. 248–78.
2. Braun N, Abd A, Baer J, Blitzer A, Stewart C, Brin M. Dyspnea in dystonia; a functional evaluation. Chest. 1995;107:1309–16.
3. Marion MH, Klap P, Perrin A, Cohen M. Stridor and focal laryngeal dystonia. Lancet. 1992;339:815.

4. Grillone GA, Blitzer A, Brin MF, Annino DJ Jr, Saint-Hilaire MH. Treatment of adductor laryngeal breathing dystonia with botulinum toxin type A. Laryngoscope. 1994;104:30–2.
5. Lew MF, Shindo M, Moscowitz CB, Wilhemsen KC, Fahn S, Waters CH. Adductor laryngeal breathing dystonia in a patient with lubag (X-linked dystonia-Parkinsonism syndrome). Mov Disord. 1994;9:318–20.
6. Merlo IM, Occhini A, Pacchetti C, Alfonsi E. Not paralysis, but dystonia causes stridor in multiple system atrophy. Neurology. 2002;58:649–52.
7. Panegyres PK, Hillman D, Dunne JW. Laryngeal dystonia causing upper airway obstruction in progressive supranuclear palsy. J Clin Neurosci. 2007;14:380–1.
8. Lee DD, Lin Y, Galati LT, Shapshay SM. Head and neck dystonia following chimeric-antigen receptor T-cell immunotherapy: a case report. Laryngoscope. 2020;130(12):E863–4.
9. Gilman S, Wenning GK, Low PA, Brooks DJ, Mathias CJ, Trojanowski JQ, et al. Second consensus statement on the diagnosis of multiple system atrophy. Neurology. 2008;71:670–6.
10. Giannini G, Calandra-Buonaura G, Mastrolilli F, Righini M, Bacchi-Reggiani ML, Cecere A, et al. Early stridor onset and stridor treatment predict survival in 136 patients with MSA. Neurology. 2016;87:1375–83.
11. Cortelli P, Calandra-Buonaura G, Benarroch EE, Giannini G, Iranzo A, Low PA, Martinelli P, et al. Stridor in multiple system atrophy: consensus statement on diagnosis, prognosis, and treatment. Neurology. 2019;93(14):630–9.
12. Tousi B. Movement disorder emergencies in the elderly: recognizing and treating an often-iatrogenic problem. Cleve Clin J Med. 2008;75:449–57.
13. Deguchi K, Ikeda K, Goto R, Tsukaguchi M, Urai Y, Kurokohchi K, et al. The close relationship between life-threatening breathing disorders and urine storage dysfunction in multiple system atrophy. J Neurol. 2010;257(8):1287–92.
14. Yoshihara T, Yamamura Y, Kaneko F, Abo N, Nomoto M. Neuromuscular junctions of the posterior cricoarytenoid muscle in multiple system atrophy: a case study. Acta Otolaryngol Suppl. 2009;562:115–9.
15. Kuzniar TJ, Morgenthaler TI, Prakash UB, Pallanch JF, Silber MH, Tippmann-Peikert M. Effects of continuous positive airway pressure on stridor in multiple system atrophy-sleep laryngoscopy. J Clin Sleep Med. 2009;15:65–7.
16. Suzuki M, Saigusa H, Shibasaki K, Kodera K. Multiple system atrophy manifesting as complex sleep-disordered breathing. Auris Nasus Larynx. 2010;37:110–3.
17. Moreno-Lopez C, Santamaria J, Salamero M, Del Sorbo F, Albanese A, Pellecchia MT, et al. Excessive daytime sleepiness in multiple system atrophy (SLEEMSA study). Arch Neurol. 2011;68:223–30.
18. Wirshing WC. Movement disorders associated with neuroleptic treatment. J Clin Psychiatry. 2001;21:15–8.
19. Glazer WM. Extrapyramidal side effects, tardive dyskinesia, and the concept of atypicality. J Clin Psychiatry. 2000;61:16–21.
20. Marsden CD, Jenner P. The pathophysiology of extrapyramidal side effects of neuroleptic drugs. Psychol Med. 1980;10:55–72.
21. Rowley H, Lynch T, Keogh I, Russell J. Tardive dystonia of the larynx in a quadriplegic patient: an unusual cause of stridor. J Laryngol Otol. 2001;115:918–9.
22. Fines RE, Brady WJ Jr, Martin ML. Acute laryngeal dystonia related to neuroleptic agents. Am J Emerg Med. 1999;17:319–20.
23. National Collaborating Centre for Chronic Conditions. Parkinson's disease: national clinical guideline for diagnosis and management in primary and secondary care. London: Royal College of Physicians; 2006.
24. Arocho-Quinones EV, Hammer MJ, Bock JM, Pahapill PA. Effects of deep brain stimulation on vocal fold immobility in Parkinson's disease. Surg Neurol Int. 2017;8:22.
25. Wang M, Saasouh W, Botsford T, Keebler A, Zura A, Benninger MS, et al. Postoperative stridor and acute respiratory failure after Parkinson disease deep brain stimulator placement: case report and review of literature. World Neurosurg. 2018;111:22–5.
26. Logemann J. Manual for the videoflouroscopic study of swallowing. Proed: Austin; 1993.

27. Bastien RW. Videoendoscopic evaluation of patients with dysphagia: an adjunct to the modified barium swallow. Otolaryngol Head Neck Surg. 1991;104:339–50.
28. Aviv JE, Kin T, Sacco RL, Kaplan S, Goodhart K, Diamond B, et al. FEESST: a new bedside endoscopic test of the motor and sensory components of swallowing. Ann Otol Rhinol Laryngol. 1998;107:378–87.
29. Aviv JE. Prospective randomized outcome study of endoscopy versus modified barium swallow in patients with dysphagia. Laryngoscope. 2000;110:563–74.
30. Setzen M, Cohen MA, Mattucci KF, Perlman PW, Ditkoff MK. Laryngopharyngeal sensory deficits as a predictor of aspiration. Otolaryngol Head Neck Surg. 2001;124:622–4.
31. McConnel FMS. Analysis of pressure generation and bolus transit during pharyngeal swallowing. Laryngoscope. 1988;98:71–8.
32. McConnel FMS, Cevenko D, Mendelsohn MS. Manofluorographic analysis of swallowing. Otolaryngol Clin N Am. 1988;21:625–35.
33. Flint PW, Purcell LL, Cummings CW. Pathophysiology and indications for medialization thy- roplasty in patients with dysphagia and aspiration. Otolaryngol Head Neck Surg. 1997;16:349–54.
34. Strome SE. Aspiration. In: Gates G, editor. Current therapy in otolaryngology head and neck surgery. 6th ed. St. Louis: Mosby; 1998. p. 453–6.
35. Wisdom G, Krespi YP, Blitzer A. Surgical therapy for chronic aspiration. Oper Tech Otolaryngol Head Neck Surg. 1997;8:199–208.
36. Brin MF, Blitzer A, Herman S, Stewart C. Oromandibular dystonia: treatment of 96 patients with botulinum toxin type A. In: Jankovic J, Hallett M, editors. Therapy with botulinum toxin. New York: Marcel Dekker, Inc.; 1994. p. 429–35.
37. Brin MF, Danisi F, Blitzer A. Blepharospasm, oromandibular dystonia, Meige's syndrome and hemifacial spasm. In: Moore P, editor. Handbook of botulinum toxin treatment. 2nd ed. London: Blackwell Science; 2003. p. 119–41.
38. Parkes D, Schachter M. Meige, Breughel, or Blake. Neurology. 1981;31:498.
39. Gowers WR. Manual of diseases of the nervous system. 3rd ed. London: Churchill; 1899. p. 200.
40. Meige H. Les convusions de la face: une forme clinique de la convulsions faciales, bilateral et mediane. Rev Neurol (Paris). 1910;21:437–43.
41. Marsden CD. Blepharospasm-oromandibular dystonia syndrome (Brueghal's syndrome). A variant of adult-onset torsion dystonia? J Neurol Neurosurg Psychiatry. 1976;39:1204–9.
42. Thompson PD, Obeso JA, Delgato G, Gallego J, Marsden CD. Focal dystonia of the jaw and the differential diagnosis of unilateral jaw and masticatory spasm. J Neurol Neurosurg Psychiatry. 1986;49:651–6.
43. Jankovic J. Blepharospasm and oromandibular-laryngeal-cervical dystonia: a controlled trial of botulinum A toxin therapy. Adv Neurol. 1988;50:583–91.
44. Tolosa E, Marti MJ. Blepharospasm-oromandibular dystonia (Meige's syndrome): clinical aspects. Adv Neurol. 1988;49:73–84.
45. Tolosa E, Kulisevsky J, Fahn S. Meige syndrome: primary and secondary forms. Adv Neurol. 1988;50:509–15.
46. Tolosa ES. Clinical features of Meige's disease (idiopathic orofacial dystonia). A report of 17 cases. Arch Neurol. 1981;38:147–51.
47. Jankovic J, Ford J. Blepharospasm and orofacial-cervical dystonia: clinical and pharmacological findings in 100 patients. Ann Neurol. 1983;13:402–11.
48. Berardelli A, Rothwell J, Day B, Marsden CD. Pathophysiology of blepharospasm and oromandibular dystonia. Brain. 1985;108:593–608.
49. Nutt JG, Hammerstad JP. Blepharospasm and oromandibualr dystonia (Meige's syndrome) in sisters. Ann Neurol. 1981;9:189–91.
50. Marsden CD. Problems of adult-onset idiopathic torsion dystonia and other isolated dyskinesias in adult life. Adv Neurol. 1976;14:259–76.
51. Defazio G, Lamberti P, Lepore V, Livrea P, Ferrari E. Facial dystonia: clinical features, prognosis, and pharmacology in 31 patients. Ital J Neurol Sci. 1989;10:553–60.

52. Jordan DR, Patrinely JR, Anderson RL, Thiese SM. Essential blepharospasm and related dystonias. Surv Ophthalmol. 1989;34:123–32.
53. Kirton CA, Riopelle RJ. Meige syndrome secondary to basal ganglia injury: a potential cause of acute respiratory distress. Can J Neurol Sci. 2001;28:167–73.
54. Brin MF. Advances in dystonia: genetics and treatment with botulinum toxin. In: Smith B, Adelman G, editors. Neuroscience year, supplement to the encyclopedia of neuroscience. Boston: Birkhauser; 1992. p. 56–8.
55. Blitzer A, Brin MF, Greene PE, Fahn S. Botulinum toxin injection for the treatment of oromandibular dystonia. Ann Otol Rhinol Laryngol. 1989;98:93–7.
56. Greene P, Shale H, Fahn S. Analysis of open-label trial in torsion dystonia using high dosages of anticholinergics and other drugs. Mov Disord. 1988;3:46–60.
57. Gollomp SM, Fahn S, Burke RE, Reches A, Ilson J. Therapeutic trials in Meige syndrome. Adv Neurol. 1983;37:207–13.
58. Tan EK, Jankovic J. Botulinum toxin A in patients with oromandibular dystonia: long-term follow-up. Neurology. 1999;53:2102–7.
59. Charous SJ, Comella CL, Fan W. Jaw-opening dystonia: quality of life after botulinum toxin injections. Ear Nose Throat J. 2011;90:E9.
60. Yoshida K, Kaji R, Shibasaki H, Iizuka T. Factors influencing the therapeutic effect of muscle afferent block for oromandibular dystonia and dyskinesia: implications for their distinct pathophysiology. Int J Oral Maxillofac Surg. 2002;31:499–505.
61. Adler CH, Factor SA, Brin MF, Sethi KD. Secondary nonresponsiveness to botulinum toxin A in patients with oromandibular dystonia. Mov Disord. 2002;17:158–61.
62. Brin MF, Blitzer A, Greene PE, Fahn S. Botulinum toxin therapy for the treatment of oromandibulolingual dystonia (OMD). Neurology. 1988;38(Suppl 1):294.
63. Blitzer A, Brin MF, Fahn S. Botulinum toxin injections for lingual dystonia. Laryngoscope. 1991;101:799.
64. Charles PD, Davis TL, Shannon KM, Hook MA, Warner JS. Tongue protrusion dystonia: treatment with botulinum toxin. South Med J. 1997;90:522–5.
65. Lyons MK, Birch BD, Hillman RA, Boucher OK, Evidente VG. Long-term follow-up of deep brain stimulation for Meige syndrome. Neurosurg Focus. 2010;29(2):E5.
66. Higo R, Tayama N, Watanabe T, Nitou T, Takeuchi S. Vocal fold motion impairment in patients with multiple system atrophy: evaluation of its relationship with swallowing function. J Neurol Neurosurg Psychiatry. 2003;74:982–4.
67. Abraham SS, Yun PT. Laryngopharyngeal dysmotility in multiple sclerosis. Dysphagia. 2002;16:69–74.
68. Prosiegel M, Schelling A, Wagner-Sonntag E. Dysphagia and multiple sclerosis. Int MS J. 2004;11(1):22–31.
69. Eretkin C, Aydogdu I, Yuceyar N, Kiylioglu N, Tarlaci S, Uludag B. Pathophysiological mechanisms of oropharyngeal dysphagia in amyotrophic lateral sclerosis. Brain. 2000;123:125–40.
70. Eretkin C, Tarlaci S, Aydogdu I, Kiylioglu N, Yuceyar N, Turman AB, et al. Electrophysiological evaluation of pharyngeal phase of swallowing in patients with Parkinson's disease. Mov Disord. 2002;17(5):942–9.
71. Lever TE, Simon E, Cox KT, Capra NF, O'Brien KF, Hough MS, et al. A mouse model of pharyngeal dysphagia in amyotrophic lateral sclerosis. Dysphagia. 2010;25:112–26.
72. Spataro R, Ficano L, Piccoli F, La Bella V. Percutaneous endoscopic gastrostomy in amyothrophic lateral sclerosis: effect on survival. J Neurol Sci. 2011;15:44–8.
73. Potulska A, Friedman A, Krolicki L, Spychala A. Swallowing disorders in Parkinson's disease. Parkinsonism Relat Disord. 2003;9:349–53.
74. Cloud LJ, Greene JG. Gastrointestinal features of Parkinson's disease. Curr Neurol Neurosci Rep. 2011;11(4):379–84.
75. Pfeiffer RF. Gastrointestinal dysfunction in Parkinson's disease. Parkinsonism Relat Disord. 2011;17:10–5.
76. Fuh JL, Lee RC, Wang SJ, Lin CH, Wang PN, Chiang JH, et al. Swallowing difficulty in Parkinson's disease. Clin Neurol Neurosurg. 1997;99:106–12.

77. Edwards LL, Quigley EM, Pfeiffer RF. Gastrointestinal dysfunction in Parkinson's disease: frequency and pathophysiology. Neurology. 1992;42:726–32.
78. Sung HY, Kim JS, Lee KS, Kim YI, Song IU, Chung SW, et al. The prevalence and patterns of pharyngoesophageal dysmotility in patients with early stage Parkinson's disease. Mov Disord. 2010;25:2361–8.
79. Menezes C, Melo A. Does levodopa improve swallowing dysfunction in Parkinson's disease patients? J Clin Pharm Ther. 2009;34:673–6.
80. Troche MS, Okun MS, Rosenbek JC, Musson N, Fernandez HH, Rodriguez R, et al. Aspiration and swallowing in Parkinson disease and rehabilitation with EMST: a randomized trial. Neurology. 2010;75:1912–9.
81. Heemskerk AW, Roos RA. Dysphagia in Huntington's disease: a review. Dysphagia. 2011;26:62–6.
82. Dubinsky RM. No going home for hospitalized Huntington's disease patients. Mov Disord. 2005;20:1316–22.
83. Kagel MC, Leopold NA. Dysphagia in Huntington's disease: a 16-year retrospective. Dysphagia. 1992;7:106–14.
84. Hamakawa S, Koda C, Umeno H, Yoshida Y, Nakashima T, Asaoka K, et al. Oropharyngeal dysphagia in a case of Huntington's disease. Auris Nasus Larynx. 2004;31:171–6.
85. Pappert E, Goetz C. Myoclonus. In: Kurlan R, editor. Treatment of movement disorders. Philadelphia: JB Lippincott; 1995. p. 247–336.
86. Rivest J. Myoclonus. Can J Neurol Sci. 2003;30:S53–8.
87. Drysdale AJ, Ansell J, Adeley J. Palato-pharyngo-laryngeal myoclonus: an unusual cause of dysphagia and dysarthria. J Laryngol Otol. 1993;107:746–7.

Part II

Hyperacute Movement Disorder Emergencies

Acute Parkinsonism

4

Umer Akbar, Hubert H. Fernandez,
and Joseph H. Friedman

Patient Vignettes

Patient 1

A 75-year-old woman with a history of bipolar disease dating back to her twenties was admitted to the hospital after falling and breaking her hip while walking her dog. She had been living alone. She underwent a total hip replacement without incident, and remained at her mental and physical baseline postoperatively in the recovery room and postsurgical floor. Two days after surgery she suddenly became mute, stiff, and unresponsive. In addition to her usual regimen of lithium 600 mg, fluoxetine 20 mg, and trifluoperazine 4 mg daily, she had received a total of five doses of meperidine 50 mg/bolus intravenously for pain control. She kept her eyes open and responded to visual threat and deep pain but not voice. She was akinetic, and tone was markedly increased. When her arms were passively elevated, she very slowly lowered them. Deep tendon reflexes were normal. Vital signs, laboratory tests

Supplementary Information The online version of this chapter (https://doi.org/10.1007/978-3-030-75898-1_4) contains supplementary material, which is available to authorized users.

U. Akbar (✉)
Department of Neurology, Brown University, Alpert Medical School Movement Disorders Program, Rhode Island Hospital, Providence, RI, USA
e-mail: umer_akbar@brown.edu

H. H. Fernandez
Center for Neurological Restoration, Neurological Institute, Cleveland Clinic, Cleveland, OH, USA

J. H. Friedman
Butler Hospital, Providence, RI, USA

© Springer Nature Switzerland AG 2022
S. J. Frucht (ed.), *Movement Disorder Emergencies*, Current Clinical Neurology,
https://doi.org/10.1007/978-3-030-75898-1_4

including lithium levels, and a head computerized tomography (CT) were unremarkable. She remained in this state for 3 days before a movement disorder consultation was requested.

Patient 2

A 15-year-old girl developed a 4-day febrile illness accompanied by a diffuse erythematous maculopapular rash, conjunctivitis, and headache. On the fifth day as her fever and rash resolved she became increasingly drowsy and difficult to arouse. When awake she followed commands very slowly. Her visual fields and eye movements were normal and no ptosis was noted. Her face was expressionless and her mouth was held partly open. She was diffusely rigid with a mild intermittent resting tremor in the left hand; no other adventitious movements were seen. Deep tendon reflexes were normal and plantar responses were equivocal. The remainder of her neurologic examination was unremarkable. Medical and family history was non-contributory.

Immunizations were up to date apart from measles. Her peripheral white blood cell count was 14.0×10^9/L with 45% neutrophils and 48% lymphocytes. Cerebrospinal fluid (CSF) analysis showed 20 white blood cells per millimeter (all lymphocytes), no red blood cells, and normal protein and glucose. Serum measles antibody titer (by complement fixation) 10 days after the rash was 1:160; 3 weeks later, the titer was 1:80. Electroencephalogram (EEG) and computerized tomography (CT) of the head were unremarkable. She was started on carbidopa/levodopa 25/100 mg at 1/2 tablets three times per day with significant improvement in her symptoms. Over the next 3 months, tremor, bradykinesia, and rigidity slowly resolved.

Introduction

There is no universally accepted definition of "acute parkinsonism." We use the term to define a bradykinetic-rigid syndrome developing over minutes to a few weeks. It may be difficult to recognize bradykinetic rigid syndromes early on, especially in patients who are systemically ill. Secondary parkinsonism, defined as an identifiable non-degenerative disorder, often occurs following exposure to medications that block dopamine D2 receptors [1]. In primary parkinsonism [2] the date of symptom onset is usually hard to pinpoint. In contrast, most secondary forms of parkinsonism including drug-induced forms evolve over weeks or even hours.

The major causes of acute parkinsonism are listed in Table 4.1. Parkinsonism may be a relatively minor aspect of a life-threatening disorder, or it may be the presenting and most obvious feature. In the latter, patients and families often note the symptoms only when the patient is brought to medical attention after a fall or a spell of incontinence. With diligent questioning, one can usually determine that the process began earlier than originally reported.

Table 4.1 Etiologies for acute parkinsonism	Infectious
	Post-infectious
	Autoimmune/paraneoplastic
	Systemic lupus erythematosus
	LGI1 antibodies
	IgLON5 antibodies
	Dopamine 2 receptor antibodies
	Ma2 antibodies
	Ri antibodies
	Medication
	"Typical" side effects of anti-dopamine drugs
	Idiosyncratic effects
	Neuroleptic malignant syndrome
	Scrotonin syndrome
	Chemotherapeutic drugs
	Toxic
	Carbon monoxide
	Cadmium
	MPTP
	Ethanol withdrawal
	Ethylene oxide
	Methanol
	Disulfiram
	Bone marrow transplantation
	Organophosphate exposure
	Structural
	Stroke
	Subdural hematoma
	Central and extra pontine myelinolysis
	Tumor
	Hydrocephalus
	Psychiatric
	Catatonia
	Conversion
	Obsessive-compulsive disorder (obsessional slowness)
	Malingering

Acute parkinsonism in primary psychiatric disorders occurs in two settings, catatonia, and conversion disorder. While parkinsonism may accompany severe depression [3] (particularly in the elderly) as well as severe obsessive-compulsive disorder [4], the onset is not usually acute.

Noninfectious Acute Parkinsonism

Structural Lesions

Normal pressure hydrocephalus often mimics parkinsonism, but the onset is insidious. In contrast, obstructive hydrocephalus is a well-known cause of acute parkinsonism [5]. Acute parkinsonism may occur in both adults and children, either due to shunt obstruction or at presentation. Obstructive hydrocephalus following meningitis or subarachnoid hemorrhage may also cause parkinsonism. One 16-year-old patient had parkinsonism noted on awakening from repair of a shunt malfunction; the shunt was blocked, although hydrocephalus was not present. Another case developed immediately after shunt revision. One developed acutely 1 year after shunting [6]. Some cases of obstructive parkinsonism are responsive to levodopa.

Acute development of hydrocephalus in patients with aqueductal stenosis can present with levodopa-responsive parkinsonism.

Vascular parkinsonism, previously called atherosclerotic parkinsonism, usually results from tiny lacunes in the basal ganglia compounded by microvascular white matter disease [7]. This is generally insidious in onset and slowly progressive, although sudden worsening may occur with new strokes. Acute parkinsonism following a single stroke is rare [8–16]. Kim described six patients who developed hemi-parkinsonism, three with rest tremor and cogwheeling rigidity [11]. Tremor and other signs of parkinsonism developed after weakness improved. Imaging studies revealed large infarcts involving the supplementary motor area or cingulate gyrus. Other frontal strokes have also caused acute parkinsonism [12, 13]. As one might expect, strokes in the substantia nigra (SN) may cause parkinsonism [8–10], but these are exceedingly rare. Interestingly, strokes in the lenticular nuclei do not cause parkinsonism [14]. Acute hemorrhage is a less common cause of acute parkinsonism [15].

Toxic/Metabolic

A number of poisons may induce parkinsonism. In some, like manganese, symptoms develop subacutely [17] or over long periods of time [18]. Parkinsonism may follow recovery from coma caused by carbon monoxide poisoning [19–21]. Carbon monoxide poisoning is a persistent problem in some countries, notably Korea where faulty oil burning heaters are used. The globus pallidus is typically involved, but data suggest that white matter deterioration must also be present for parkinsonism to develop. Cadmium [22] and ethylene oxide [23], disulfiram (used to prevent alcoholics from imbibing) [24], and cyanide poisoning are other uncommon causes [25, 26].

MPTP has a special place in the history of movement disorders [27]. After its identification by Langston and colleagues as the source of a mini-epidemic of severe, acute parkinsonism in IV drug abusers in the San Francisco Bay area, it was developed as a tool for research in Parkinson's disease (PD). The drug is taken up by glial cells and converted to MPP+, which is secreted and taken up by dopaminergic cells in the pars compacta of the substantia nigra. MPTP was the first systemically administered drug to selectively target these cells, and because it has a similar effect in other primates, it has been widely used to create animal models of PD. These models are superb for testing symptomatic treatments for motor dysfunction. The onset of parkinsonism occurs after the first few doses.

Acute parkinsonism is a rare complication of insect stings [28–30]. Acute parkinsonism developed within 3 days of a wasp sting [28] associated with pallidal necrosis, followed by acute deterioration 6 months later with degeneration of the nigrostriatal pathway. Bee stings have not been implicated. Parkinsonism due to alcohol withdrawal has been reported rarely [31–34]. A follow-up of some of these patients one or more years later proved that this withdrawal phenomenon was not a premature unmasking of subclinical PD. Parkinsonism occurred early in withdrawal, and sometimes resolved within a week [31]. The mechanism is postulated to be a metabolic effect of ethanol on striatal dopamine or dopamine receptors. Twelve days after overly rapid correction of hyponatremia, a 66-year-old woman became confused and developed parkinsonism. MRI revealed central pontine myelinolysis. She was responsive to very low doses of levodopa, and her parkinsonism gradually resolved [35]. Another similar case was also accompanied by pyramidal features [36]. Parkinsonism is however not a typical feature of central pontine myelinolysis [37]. Hypoxic insult to the basal ganglia may cause parkinsonism or dystonia [38–40]. This is uncommon and typically occurs after a major brain insult. The syndrome has occurred in children [39] as well as adults, and damage to the lenticular nuclei is clearly visible on magnetic resonance imaging (MRI). Onset is usually delayed, but symptoms may develop rapidly.

Neuroleptic malignant syndrome (NMS) is variably defined, but generally requires the presence of fever, altered mental status, and rigidity [41–43]. Many patients have extreme elevations of creatine phosphokinase (CPK) due to rhabdomyolysis, but this is not required for diagnosis. Elevations in the CPK to the 1000–2000 range are sometimes seen in otherwise normal, treated psychotic patients, even in the absence of signs or symptoms of muscle or tone abnormalities. It is critically important to exclude infection in patients presenting with fever, alteration in mental status, or CPK elevation. Infections frequently cause exacerbations of neurological syndromes, including parkinsonism, and both infection and NMS may occur in the same patient. NMS may begin at any point once a patient is treated with neuroleptics, but it usually occurs relatively shortly after initiation of the offending drug or after a dose increase. While there is general agreement that the newer atypical neuroleptics are less likely to cause NMS, there is as yet little data to support this.

The onset of NMS may be fulminant, progressing to coma over hours, but it usually develops over days. Patients develop fever, stiffness, and mental impairment with delirium and obtundation. The impaired mental state may initially be overlooked. Rigidity may be so severe that the limbs cannot be moved, and the stiffness may be fairly fixed. In some, muscle contractions may mimic a tonic seizure. Management of NMS requires excluding infection, identifying and discontinuing the offending drug, close monitoring of autonomic and respiratory parameters, and treatment with dopaminergic replacement (either levodopa or dopamine agonists).

⚷ The management of neuroleptic malignant syndrome begins with a high index of suspicion for the disorder.

Dopamine D2 receptor blocking drugs routinely cause parkinsonism [1]. This may also occur with lithium or valproic acid. The syndrome usually develops over the course of weeks, but may occasionally develop over 24 h [44]. In patients who have a primary parkinsonian syndrome, a low-potency neuroleptic or even an atypical antipsychotic can induce acute parkinsonism. This is not uncommon when a patient with PD is treated with an anti-emetic such as prochlorperazine or metoclopramide.

◢◤   Use of typical or atypical neuroleptics (with the exception of quetiapine, pimavanserin, or clozapine) in PD patients is contraindicated.

A handful of children who underwent bone marrow transplantation (BMT) and chemotherapy developed an acute parkinsonian syndrome, sometimes evolving over hours, 2–3 months after transplant [45, 46]. In addition to parkinsonism, cognitive and mental changes also occurred. No particular medication could be implicated, and one patient had an autologous transplant eliminating the possibility of a graft versus host reaction. MRI revealed demyelination, and brain biopsies revealed regions of variably active inflammatory demyelinating lesions. Severe and persistent neurologic sequelae were common. Several reports in the literature describe an acute parkinsonian syndrome occurring with a variety of chemotherapeutic agents [47] and with cyclosporin [48]. Some of these patients responded very well to levodopa, and parkinsonism was not permanent. In a case series of five subjects who were briefly exposed to organophosphate pesticide and developed acute parkinsonism, four recovered completely without treatment (one was lost to follow-up) [49].

Autoimmune/Paraneoplastic

Autoimmune pathology has been demonstrated to be associated with the development of acute parkinsonism. For example, a handful of teenagers with systemic lupus involving the nervous system developed acute parkinsonism in the setting of active central nervous system (CNS) involvement [49, 50]. Chorea, however, is a more common movement disorder associated both with systemic lupus and lupus anticoagulant antibody. Recently, parkinsonism has been reported in a growing number of immunologic processes. Several antibodies have been reported, including Ma2, Ri, IgLON5, and LGI1. Some—but not all—of these antibodies are linked to neoplasms. Paraneoplastic syndromes are a rare cause of movement disorders, including parkinsonism. The most common associated cancers found are small cell lung cancer, breast, gynecological, testicular, lymphoma, and thymoma. Identifying and treating the underlying cancer is critical. If cancer is not identified, immunotherapy is the mainstay of treatment.

Psychiatric

Catatonia is an important diagnostic possibility to consider in the setting of acute parkinsonism [51–53]. Catatonia should be strongly considered in any patient with acute-onset akinesia without an obvious cause such as toxin exposure, hypoxic ischemia, CNS infection, or hydrocephalus. Concurrent use of neuroleptic drugs that may cause parkinsonism may complicate the diagnosis. Although for many decades catatonia was considered a variant of schizophrenia, DSM criteria have been revised to recognize it as a manifestation of manic-depressive disorder as well. It is actually more common in the affective disorders. The patient may have experienced previous spells that may not have been recognized, or resolved over long periods of time. Catatonia may punctuate a manic spell or follow a bout of catatonic excitement. A catatonic, unlike someone with parkinsonism, will not attempt to move. He or she will not appear to be uncomfortable or become hungry. All studies will be normal and an EEG, if the eyes are closed, will be normal. Most physicians incorrectly think of catalepsy as the defining characteristic of catatonia. Not all patients have waxy flexibility or maintain postures that are externally imposed. The hallmark features of catatonia are negativism, a refusal to cooperate generally manifested as mutism or minimal interaction, and lack of movement. Patients may be stiff, or in contrast exhibit "mit-gehen," in which they move with the imposed movement, "helping" the movement. Thus, one sees a patient who is not moving but may not be in the typical flexed posture of parkinsonism. There is no tremor, and, despite an alert status, little interaction with the environment. Patients will not follow commands and may not respond to pain. Since the patient may keep his or her eyes closed, coma and encephalopathy must be excluded. However, if the eyes are closed and the patient is stiff, unresponsive to deep pain, the possibility of coma needs to be considered. If a patient is catatonic, there may be no response to deep pain but cranial nerve reflexes will remain intact. It is unlikely that a catatonic will respond to suggestion, but it is certainly worth trying. "If he is truly comatose/unable to move/stiff/etc., then he will keep his hand above his face when I drop it." If the patient is simply severely parkinsonian from neuroleptics, then he or she should be able to comply with some requests, such as moving the eyes and raising a finger.

Psychogenic or functional parkinsonism is not common but should always be considered, especially in young patients. In studies of new referrals to movement disorder specialists, about 2–5% have presumed functional diagnoses [54]. Acute-onset parkinsonism without a demonstrable cause is not likely organic. The behavioral causes are catatonia, conversion, and malingering. Conversion disorder is a type of somatoform disorder in which patients express mental stress as physical disability [55]. It usually begins abruptly, helping to distinguish it from organic disorders [56, 57]. In idiopathic PD, tremor tends to vary throughout the day, often becoming prominent in time of stress and disappearing during periods of relaxation.

These variations usually occur over minutes, whereas in conversion the symptoms tend to resolve for hours or even days at a time. Factors that typically worsen tremor in PD—cold, heavylifting, excitement—do not necessarily affect conversion tremor. On examination, signs of conversion resolve with distraction and vary in frequency, while PD is usually invariant in frequency. The slowness of conversion disorders has a more deliberate character, especially during handwriting. Balance impairment is usually not present. The presence of a "belle indifference" attitude is often but not always present in conversion. Some patients with bona fide PD will mask their concern, either because they do not understand the implications of the diagnosis or are in denial. Often patients with conversion have a background in medicine, such as nursing, medical secretary, a lab technician, or have experience with the disorder from a relative. The single most common stressor in women with conversion is a history of childhood sexual or physical abuse.

Infectious Parkinsonism

Classification and Clinical Features

Since von Economo first described acute parkinsonism, similar illnesses have been reported with a myriad of infectious agents. In this section, we have divided the infectious causes of parkinsonism into seven categories (Table 4.2).

Von Economo's disease (ED), also called encephalitis lethargica, was probably seen prior to his initial description of 13 cases with the onset between February and April 1917 in Vienna [58]. Urechia [59] probably described the first recorded credible case series of ED with the onset in April and May 1915 in Bucharest. Somewhat later (1915 or 1916), cases were described in the French army [60, 61]. A massive encephalitis outbreak affecting 65,000 Chinese in the province of Yunnanfu caused devastation from 1917 to 1927 [53, 62]. By 1919, cases had been reported throughout the world. The peak incidence in the United States was in 1923 with about 2000 reported deaths. No major outbreaks of epidemic encephalitis occurred after 1926, and by 1935 the disease had virtually disappeared.

Von Economo was the first to recognize and classify three distinct forms of the acute illness, which he called "encephalitis lethargica." He described the *somnolent-ophthalmoplegic form*: a "prodromal phenomena consisting of general discomfort, shivering, headache and slight pharyngitis. The temperature is generally only a little

Table 4.2 Classification of infectious causes of parkinsonism

A. Von Economo's disease (ED)/encephalitis lethargica
B. Post-encephalitic parkinsonism (PEP) of von Economo
C. Sporadic, post-pandemic ED-like and PEP-like cases
D. Parkinsonism associated with known viral encephalitis
Parkinsonism associated with nonviral encephalitis
Parkinsonism associated with non-encephalitic infectious
Postvaccine parkinsonism

raised. Within the next few days, somnolence begins to predominate. The patients, when left to themselves, fall asleep in the act of sitting and standing, and even while walking, or during meals with food in the mouth. If aroused, they wake up quickly and completely, are oriented and fully conscious, but soon drop back to sleep. Sleepiness in this form may last for weeks or even months but frequently deepens to a state of most intense stupor. Generally, during the first days of illness cranial nerve palsies appear. Ptosis is one of the first and most frequent symptoms. Rarely observed are supranuclear paralyses, paresis of convergence, nystagmus, optic neuritis, papilledema, pupillary disturbances and even Argyll Robertson's sign" [63]. In the *hyperkinetic form*, "chorea and hemichorea as well as myoclonic twitches were observed which may degenerate into wild jactations. On the other hand, it may find its mental expression in a general, curious restlessness of an anxious or hypomanic type. In most of these cases, there is a very distinct sleep disturbance and generally the condition is one of troublesome sleeplessness" [63]. Von Economo termed the least frequent form *amyostatic-akinetic*. He described it as "a rigidity, without a real palsy and without symptoms arising from the pyramidal tract. This form of encephalitis lethargica is particularly common in the chronic cases, dominating the clinical picture of parkinsonism. I reserve the name 'parkinsonism,' though symptomatically identical with the amyostatic-akinetic form, rather for the chronic cases. To look at these patients one would suppose them to be in a state of profound secondary dementia. Emotions are scarcely noticeable in the face, but they are mentally intact" [63].

ED was a serious, often lethal disease. "The prognosis of clinically well-documented cases of encephalitis lethargica is 40% mortality, 14% complete recovery, 26% recovery with defect, but able to work, and 20% chronic invalidity" [63]. It is estimated that more than 60% of ED patients who survived developed postencephalitic parkinsonism (PEP). The sequelae occurred more often in adults than in children. The latency period was less than 5 years in 50% of cases and less than 10 years in 85% [64]. The average age of the onset of PEP was approximately 27 years. Resting tremor was the presenting symptom in two-thirds of cases while akinetic-rigid features occurred alone in about one-third [65]. Symptoms were occasionally unilateral and often asymmetrical [66]. Other neurological abnormalities besides parkinsonism were present in most patients. One of the most notable features was the presence of oculogyric crises: "they consist of tonic visual convulsions, occurring in fits and generally lasting only a few minutes, during which the patients as a rule look upwards and sideways" [63]. Other features included dystonia (such as blepharospasm, torticollis, cranial, and torsional dystonia), myoclonus (focal or generalized), facial and respiratory tics, choreoathetosis, obsessive-compulsive behavior, pyramidal signs [66, 67], supranuclear gaze palsy, and eyelid apraxia [68]. One study assessing the accuracy of the diagnosis of PEP in pathologically proven cases showed a high reliability and sensitivity in diagnosis. The best predictors for the diagnosis included the onset below middle age, symptoms lasting more than 10 years, and oculogyric crisis [69]. Recent work has suggested that the relationship between ED and PEP is less clear [70].

The course of PEP is unclear. Duvoisin and Yahr [64] followed 49 patients with probable PEP and observed a stable course or very slow deterioration. On the other hand, Duncan [71] who studied 136 PEP inpatients in London was impressed with the progressive nature of parkinsonian disabilities. Calne and Lees [72] and Viereggel [73] both reported deterioration in motor function, generally late in life. The relatively uniform nature of the deterioration exceeded changes in motor function seen in normal elderly subjects and occurred without comparable age-related changes in intellect. In one report, the mean survival from the onset of symptoms was 23.2 years with the mean age at death of 74.3 years [65]. While there appears to be general agreement that ED and PEP share a viral etiology, no causative agent was ever identified. Its occurrence around the time of the influenza pandemic of 1918 and 1919 has led some to link ED/PEP to the influenza pandemic [74]. However, von Economo himself rejected this hypothesis on several grounds: (1) ED appeared prior to the influenza pandemic; (2) ED/PEP was not contagious, whereas influenza was highly so; (3) their clinical presentations were different; and (4) the pathology was different with typical midbrain lesions in ED/PEP contrasting with diffuse brain congestion in cases of post-influenzal encephalopathy [63]. Since the influenza pandemic affected at least 500 million persons [75] or over one-fourth of the world's population at that time, it is very possible that many individuals with ED may coincidentally also have had influenza [76]. Modern studies using immunocytochemistry and immunofluorescence to detect in situ antigens failed to consistently isolate influenza or any other virus in the remaining brain or CSF samples of neuropathologically confirmed ED and PEP [76–80]. Similarly, the search for autoantibodies did not support an autoimmune mechanism in PEP [81]. Finally, studies on genetic susceptibility of ED/PEP have been inconclusive. While Elizan [82] saw a highly significant increase in the frequency of HLA-B14 antigen in PEP cases, Lees [83] could not confirm this in their samples.

ED cases considered to be associated with the 1917–1927 pandemic occurred until the early 1930s, after which the disease disappeared. Thus, assuming up to a 20-year latency, no PEP cases would be expected to appear after the middle 1950s. Several sporadic ED-like and PEP-like cases, unrelated to the pandemic, have been reported with onset after 1959 [84–91]. Other than one report of positive influenza A antibody titer (1:>160) [90] and another report of CSF cultures yielding coxsackie B4 enterovirus [91], attempts to identify the viral agent in ED-like cases have failed. Nonetheless, the clinical presentation, laboratory studies, imaging, and pathological findings are reminiscent, if not identical, to ED/PEP. To distinguish these cases from parkinsonism associated with viral encephalitides, Howard and Lees [88] proposed major criteria for the diagnosis of ED. The illness should comprise an acute or subacute encephalitic illness with at least three out of the following seven features: (1) signs of basal ganglia involvement; (2) oculogyric crises; (3) ophthalmoplegia; (4) obsessive-compulsive behavior; (5) akinetic mutism; (6) central respiratory irregularities; and (7) somnolence and/or sleep inversion.

Parkinsonism may occasionally accompany viral encephalitides [89]. Table 4.3 lists the viruses known to cause encephalitis with or without associated parkinsonism.

Table 4.3   Causes of viral encephalitis

Virus	Parkinsonism	Author
California encephalitis (LaCrosse virus)	Not reported	
Coxsackie virus	Acute	Walters [128]
	Acute, transient	Posner et al. [129]
Cytomegalovirus	Not reported	Giraldi et al. [130]
Eastern equine encephalitis (EEE)	Not reported	
Herpes virus	Not reported	Ickenstein [131]
Human immunodeficiency virus	Secondary to opportunistic infection	Nath et al. [91]; Carrazana et al. [92]; Navia et al. [93]; Noel et al. [4]; Maggi et al. [96]; De la Fuente et al. [107] Singer et al. [108]; Werring and Chaudhuri [109]
	Part/feature of HIV encephalopathy	De Mattos et al. [97]; Mirsattari et al. [98]
Epstein–Barr virus	Acute, transient	Hsieh et al. [132]
Influenza virus	Acute, transient	Isgreen et al. [133]
Japanese B encephalitis	Followed acute phase without interval	Shiraki et al. [134]
	Chronic phase with interval	Ishii et al. [135]
	Acute, persistent	Shoji et al. [136]
	Acute, transient	Pradhan et al. [137]
Lymphocytic choriomeningitis	Acute, transient	Scheid et al. [138]
	Chronic, persistent	Adair et al. [139]
Mumps	Not reported	
Murray valley encephalitis	Reported	Bennett et al. [140]
Papovavirus	Not reported	
Poliovirus	Acute, transient	Bickerstaff and Clarke [141]; Thieffrey [142]
	Acute	Barrett et al. [143]; Duvoisin and Yahr [64]
	Parkinsonism in late life with history of polio as a child/young adult	Vincent and Myers [144];
Rubella	Not reported	
Rubeola, measles	Post-measles, transient	Mellon et al. [145]; Meyer [146]
Russian spring-summer encephalitis, European tick-borne encephalitis	Acute, transient	Henner and Hantal [147, 148]
	Tremor only	Radsel-Medvescek et al. [149]
St. Louis encephalitis	Tremors	Cerna et al. [150]; Wasay et al. [151]
	Dystonia with tremor as sequelae	Finley [152]; Finley and Rigs [153]
Varicella-zoster virus	Not reported	
Venezuelan equine encephalitis	Not reported	
Western equine encephalitis	Reported	Fulton and Burton [154]
	Chronic, persistent	Mulder et al. [155]

In most instances, parkinsonism associated with viral infection occurs during the acute encephalitic phase or shortly thereafter. If the patient survives, the parkinsonism is usually transient, although it can take several months to resolve. Unlike EP or PEP, oculogyric crises, ophthalmoplegia, cranial neuropathies, or psychiatric/ behavioral disturbances are rare.

In HIV-infected patients, parkinsonism may develop from exposure to dopamine blockers (such as prolonged use of metoclopramide); secondary to opportunistic infections (toxoplasmosis, progressive multifocal leukoencephalopathy, tuberculosis) affecting the basal ganglia [91–96]; or as part of HIV encephalopathy in the absence of opportunistic infections [97, 98]. The parkinsonian syndrome is often unresponsive to levodopa [99]. Rarely parkinsonism is associated with nonviral infectious agents: spirochetes (neurosyphilis and Lyme disease), mycoplasma pneumoniae, and opportunistic infections accompanying HIV. Most reported cases of parkinsonism from spirochetal [100, 101] and mycoplasma [102–106] infections present with acute onset and improve markedly with appropriate treatment, despite the severity of the initial clinical presentation. Of the five reported cases with mycoplasma, the presenting extrapyramidal features were parkinsonism and/or dystonia, accompanied by seizures in three cases. All patients were children or young adults, and in all cases, MRI revealed selective involvement of the corpus striatum except for one case with concomitant involvement of the substantia nigra and pallidum [103]. One patient [102] experienced severe dyskinesias and dystonia with levodopa therapy, but symptoms gradually resolved.

In patients with acquired immunodeficiency syndrome (AIDS), parkinsonism, hemichorea-athetosis, and ballismus have been described with opportunistic infection. Parkinsonism, in particular, has been reported with cerebral toxoplasmosis [93, 95], progressive multifocal leukoencephalopathy [107, 108], and cerebral tuberculosis [109]. All but one case presented with bilateral lesions in the basal ganglia. One patient with mycobacterium tuberculosis involving the left lentiform nucleus only developed parkinsonism when the right lentiform nucleus was superinfected with toxoplasma [96]. There is only one reported case of parkinsonism following herpes ophthalmicus [110]. A 5-year-old boy developed isolated fever 15 days after a measles vaccine shot and then developed persistent parkinsonism. MRI showed hyperintense signal affecting the substantia nigra bilaterally. He responded to levodopa but dyskinesias appeared even at low doses [111]. The only other reported case was that of a 38-year-old man who experienced fever, sweats, palpitations, diplopia, and leg tremor within hours of receiving the last of three tetanus vaccinations. Within 1 week, he developed severe parkinsonism with resting tremor, generalized rigidity, and bradykinesia, which responded well to levodopa and a dopamine agonist. Unlike the previous case, parkinsonism was transient [112].

Neuropathology and Imaging

The pathological features of ED differ from those of other viral encephalitides (usually characterized by diffuse brain congestion and edema). In ED, pathology typically consists of non-hemorrhagic involvement of the gray matter, preferentially in the midbrain. Although the brainstem and basal ganglia bear the brunt of the burden, the cerebral cortex and spinal cord can be affected as well. The pathological hallmark of the disease is cytoplasmic inclusions of neurofibrillary tangles (NFTs) within the substantia nigra (SN), associated with severe neuronal loss [69, 113, 114]. Lewy bodies are not present. In the chronic state (PEP), inflammation is often replaced with degeneration of neurons and gliosis throughout the central nervous system, particularly the midbrain [115]. NFTs occur in the absence of senile plaques [65, 116]. Unlike Alzheimer's disease, they do not stain for alpha synuclein or amyloid [117], but similar to progressive supranuclear palsy, they are ubiquitinated and tau-positive on immunohistochemistry [118, 119].

MRI findings from cases of parkinsonism associated with viral encephalitis as well as ED/PEP like cases usually reveal bilateral, symmetrical basal ganglia involvement, predominantly with signal hyperintensities in the SN but may also involve the striatum and lenticular nucleus [120]. When symptoms resolve, these MRI lesions can be transient as well. On fluorodopa positron emission tomography, PEP differs from idiopathic PD. Uptake in the putamen of PEP patients is homogeneously reduced, without the anterior–posterior gradient typically seen in PD [90, 121]. This may be due to the more diffuse involvement of the SN pars compacta in PEP compared to the ventrolateral predominance in PD.

Evaluation

A young patient with acute or subacute onset of parkinsonism associated with a febrile illness should have a complete blood count, and blood chemistries including liver, renal, thyroid function tests, antinuclear antibodies, erythrocyte sedimentation rate, chest radiography, electrocardiogram, and blood and urine cultures. CSF should be sent for cell count, glucose, protein, and extra tubes for CSF gram and acid-fast bacilli stain, VDRL, Lyme titers, serologies (for herpes simplex virus, herpes zoster, mumps, measles, adenovirus, enterovirus, cytomegalovirus, Epstein–Barr virus, toxoplasmosis, etc.), and state-run encephalitis PCR panels. Serum ceruloplasmin, 24-h urine copper and heavy metals, toxicology, HIV test, tuberculin-purified protein derivatives test, and serum VDRL may be necessary. An EEG may define seizure activity and helps grade the level of encephalopathy. Brain imaging with contrast can define ring-enhancing or granulomatous lesions. Rarely, duodenal biopsy (to rule out Whipple's disease), blood smear (for malaria), and CSF 14-3-3 protein (for prion disease) may be of value.

Treatment

Comments on Patient 1
This patient had been taking trifluoperazine and lithium, both of which may cause parkinsonism, but she had been taking both for many years, had not had an increase

in dose recently, and her lithium level was not elevated. Since her symptoms occurred 2 days after surgery, a direct result of the surgery was unlikely. Meperidine may trigger severe reactions with MAO inhibitors, but this has not been reported with the drugs she was taking. The absence of any fever argued strongly against serotonin syndrome or NMS. The fact that she was awake, blinked to threat, moved in response to pain, had a non-focal exam, and a normal brain CT pointed to a probable psychiatric cause. Given the history of bipolar disease requiring an antipsychotic, catatonia was considered, and in fact she met criteria for this syndrome. After a baseline EEG was obtained, which was normal, an infusion of lorazepam was given. Two minutes later she awoke and was manic. This confirmed the diagnosis of catatonia and pointed to the need for more aggressive psychiatric treatment. When the effects of the lorazepam wore off within a few hours, she became catatonic again.

Establishing the etiology of acute parkinsonism is of paramount importance. NMS is treatable, usually with levodopa or dopamine agonists. In cases of profound rigidity and fever, the patient may be paralyzed or treated with dantrolene sodium. Unlike malignant hyperthermia, the muscles in NMS are normal, hence responsive to depolarizing drugs. Catatonia often responds to intravenous lorazepam [53]; however, patients may require prolonged treatment to prevent recurrence. Patients who do not respond to lorazepam should be considered for electroconvulsive therapy which has been reported as successful in treating this disorder as well as NMS.

🔑 IV lorazepam may be therapeutic and diagnostic for catatonia.

Toxic, metabolic, infectious, post-infectious, and structural akinetic rigid syndromes are usually not responsive to symptomatic therapies. Levodopa requires conversion to dopamine by intact nigral cells, suggesting that dopamine agonists may be more effective when the nigra is fully depleted. Unfortunately, the general experience with dopaminergic agents in akinetic rigid syndromes is that levodopa works faster and has fewer side effects; we therefore advocate trials of levodopa for all parkinsonian syndromes except NMS, where a dopamine agonist is our drug of choice. When levodopa is not helpful, we advocate a trial of amantadine 200–400 mg/day in patients with normal renal function. Although amantadine has anti-influenza properties, there is no reason to believe it is useful for other viral syndromes. Dopamine agonists should be initiated at low doses and slowly titrated. Since patients with acute parkinsonism may improve on their own, it may be difficult to gauge the response to a slowly increasing dose of dopamine agonists. Once a patient has improved, our general approach is to slowly taper the medicines, as many patients improve spontaneously.

Comments on Patient 2

This 15-year-old girl developed acute parkinsonism immediately following a presumed viral encephalitis. Measles antibody titers suggested a resolving measles infection. Her parkinsonism gradually resolved over 3 months and was not associated with oculogyric crisis, ophthalmoplegia, myoclonus, or other movement disorders. The presentation is therefore not consistent with ED or PEP. In addition to supportive measures during the acute encephalopathic phase, delivery of the appropriate antibiotic/antiviral agent may suffice to resolve parkinsonism associated with known viral or bacterial encephalitis. When symptoms persist, levodopa alone or in combination with other adjunctive anti-PD agents may be used. Anticholinergic drugs [122], amantadine [123], bromocriptine, and deprenyl [124] have all been reported to augment levodopa response.

ED and PEP patients are extremely sensitive to anti-PD drugs, with dyskinesias and motor and psychic fluctuations occurring even at very low doses. Calne et al. [125] reported a 6-week double-blind, placebo-controlled trial of levodopa in 40 PEP patients, with frequent adverse events among those who received levodopa. Patients experienced chorea, tics, respiratory crises, excess sweating, and psychiatric disturbances. Only a minority gained useful and enduring benefit of levodopa throughout the study. Sacks [126] reported an enormous range of levodopa-induced behavioral and motor abnormalities where patients alternated between a severe "off" state and an emotionally labile "on" state. Unlike PD where patients often chose to be "on" with dyskinesias, PEP patients preferred to be "off" to avoid emotional lability. Similarly, Duvoisin [127] reported 63% of patients with increased involuntary movements and 33% with psychic manifestations among 26 PEP patients treated with levodopa. Slower titration enabled some patients to enjoy a sustained response. There is one report of PEP in which oculogyric crises resolved and tremor and rigidity improved with unilateral thalamotomy [67]. Since parkinsonism in PEP is probably progressive, or, at the very least, persistent, and since patients experience extreme motor fluctuations on low-dose levodopa, stimulation of the subthalamic nucleus might also be an option.

Conclusion

Acute parkinsonism is a frightening and serious movement disorder emergency that may occur due to a variety of causes. Identification of the cause and institution of appropriate treatment can not only improve patients' outcome but may also even be life-saving.

References

1. Friedman JH. Drug induced parkinsonism. In: Lang AE, Weiner WJ, editors. Drug-induced movement disorders. Mt Kisco: Futura Press; 1992. p. 41–84.
2. Fahn S, Przedborski S. Parkinsonism. In: Rowland LP, editor. Merritt's textbook of neurology. 11th ed. Philadelphia: Lippincott Williams and Wilkins; 2005. p. 828–46.
3. Caligiuri MP, Ellwanger J. Motor and cognitive aspects of motor retardation in depression. J Affect Disord. 2000;47:83–93.
4. Hymas N, Lees A, Bolton D, et al. The neurology of obsessional slowness. Brain. 1991;114:2203–33.
5. Curran T, Lang AE. Parkinsonian syndromes associated with hydrocephalus: case reports, a review of the literature and pathophysiological hypotheses. Mov Disord. 1994;9:508–20.

6. Sakurai T, Kimura A, Yamada M, et al. Rapidly progressive parkinsonism that developed one year after ventriculoperitoneal shunting for idiopathic aqueductal stenosis: a case report. Brain Nerve. 2010;62:527–31.
7. Lees AJ. Secondary Parkinson's syndrome. In: Jankovic JJ, Tolosa E, editors. Parkinson's disease and movement disorders. 5th ed. Philadelphia: Lippincott Williams and Williams; 2007. p. 213–24.
8. Boccker H, Weindl A, Leenders K, et al. Secondary parkinsonism due to focal substantia nigra lesions: a PET study with (^{18}F)FDG and (^{18}F)fluorodopa. Acta Neurol Scand. 1996;93:387–92.
9. Stern G. The effects of lesions in the substantia nigra. Brain. 1966;89:449–78.
10. Hunter R, Smith J, Thomson T, Dayan AD. Hemiparkinsonism with infarction of the ilpsilateral substantia nigra. Neuropathol Appl Neurobiol. 1978;4:297–301.
11. Kim JS. Involuntary movements after anterior cerebral artery territory infarction. Stroke. 2001;32:258–61.
12. Nagaratnam N, Davies D, Chen E. Clinical effects of anterior cerebral artery infarction. J Stroke Cerebrovasc Dis. 1998;7:391–7.
13. Dick JP, Benecke R, Rothwell JC, et al. Simple and complex movements in a patient with infarction of the right supplementary motor area. Mov Disord. 1986;1:255–66.
14. Russmann H, Vingerhoets F, Ghika J, et al. Acute infarction limited to the lenticular nucleus: clinical, etiologic and topographic features. Arch Neurol. 2003;60:351–8.
15. Turjanski N, Pentland B, Lees AJ, Brooks DJ. Parkinsonism associated with acute intracranial hematomas: an (^{18}F)Dopa positron-emission tomography study. Mov Disord. 1997;12:1035–8.
16. Orta Daniel SJ, Ulises RO. Stroke of the substantia nigra and parkinsonism as the first manifestation of systemic lupus erythematosis. Parkinsonism Relat Disord. 2008;14:367–9.
17. Wang JD, Huang CC, Hwang YH, et al. Manganese induced parkinsonism: an outbreak due to an unrepaired ventilation control system in a ferromanganese smelter. Br J Ind Med. 1989;46:856–9.
18. Feldman RG. Manganese. In: Occupational and environmental medicine. Philadelphia: Lippincott Raven Press; 1999. p. 168–88.
19. Sohn YH, Jeong Y, Kim HS, Im JH, Kim JS. The brain lesion responsible for parkinsonism after carbon monoxide poisoning. Arch Neurol. 2000;57:1214–8.
20. Perry GF. Occupational medicine forum. What are the potential delayed health effects of high level carbon monoxide exposure? J Occup Med. 1994;36:595–7.
21. Shprecher D, Mehta L. The syndrome of delayed post-hypoxic leukoencephalopathy. NeuroRehabilitation. 2010;26:65–72.
22. Okuda B, Iwamoto Y, Tachibana H, Sugita M. Parkinsonism after acute cadmium poisoning. Clin Neurol Neurosurg. 1997;99:263–5.
23. Barbosa ER, Comerlatti LR, Haddad MS, Scaff M. Parkinsonism secondary to ethylene oxide exposure: case report. Arq Neurosiquiatr. 1992;50:531–3.
24. Laplane D, Attal N, Sauron B, et al. Lesions of the basal ganglia due to disulfiram neurotoxicity. J Neurol Neurosurg Psychiatry. 1992;44:925–9.
25. Messing B. Extrapyramidal disturbance after cyanide poisoning. J Neural Transm Suppl. 1991;33:141–7.
26. Pentore R, Venneri A, Nichelli P. Accidental choke-cherry poisoning: early symptoms and neurological sequelae of an unusual case of cyanide intoxication. Ital J Neurol Sci. 1996;17:233–5.
27. Langston JW, Ballard P, Tetrud JW, Irwin I. Chronic parkinsonism in humans due to a product of meperidine analogue synthesis. Science. 1983;219:979–80.
28. Leopold NA, Bara-Jimenez W, Hallett M. Parkinsonism after a wasp sting. Mov Disord. 1999;14:122–7.
29. Agarwal V, Singh R, Chauhau S, J'Cruz S, Thakur R. Parkinsonism following a honey bee sting. Indian J Med Sci. 2006;60:24–5.

30. Bogolepov NK, Luzhetskaya TA, Fedin AI, et al. Allergic encephalomyelopolyradiculoneu-ritis from a wasp sting (clinico-patholo report). Zh Nevropatol Psikhiatr Im SS Korsakova. 1978;78:187–91.
31. Shandling M, Carlen PL, Lang AE. Parkinsonism in alcohol withdrawal: a follow-up study. Mov Disord. 1990;4:36–9.
32. Carlen PL, Lee MA, Jacob M, Livishitz O. Parkinsonism provoked by alcoholism. Ann Neurol. 1981;9:84–6.
33. Lang AE, Marsden CD, Obeso JA, Parkes JD. Alcohol and Parkinson disease. Ann Neurol. 1982;12:254–6.
34. San Luciano M, Saunders-Pullman R. Substance abuse and movement disorders. Curr Drug Abuse Rev. 2009;2:273–8.
35. Tinker R, Anderson MG, Anand P, et al. Pontine myelinolysis presenting with acute parkin-sonism as a sequel of corrected hyponatremia. J Neurol Neurosurg Psychiatry. 1990;53:87–9.
36. Dickoff DJ, Rapps M, Yahr MD. Striatal syndrome following hyponatremia and its rapid cor-rection. Arch Neurol. 1988;45:112–4.
37. Bernardini GL, Mancall EL. Central pontine myelinolysis. In: Rowland LP, editor. Merritt's neurology. 11th ed. Philadelphia: Lippincott Williams and Wilins; 2005. p. 965–7.
38. Hawker K, Lang AE. Hypoxic-ischemic damage of the basal ganglia: case reports and a review of the literature. Mov Disord. 1990;5:219–24.
39. Straussberg R, Shahar E, Gat R, Brand N. Delayed parkinsonism associated with hypotension in a child undergoing open-heart surgery. Dev Med Child Neurol. 1993;35:1007–14.
40. Li JY, Lai PH, Chen CY, et al. Postanoxic parkinsonism: clinical radiologic and pathologic correlation. Neurology. 2000;55:591–3.
41. Gillman PK. Neuroleptic malignant syndrome: mechanisms, interactions and causality. Mov Disord. 2010;25:1780–90.
42. Carbone JR. The neuroleptic malignant syndrome and serotonin syndromes. Emerg Clin North Am. 2000;18:317–25.
43. Susman VL. Clinical management of neuroleptic malignant syndrome. Psychiatry Q. 2001;72:325–6.
44. Perrin E, Anand E, Dyachkova Y, et al. A prospective observational study of the safety and effectiveness of intramuscular psychotropic treatment in acutely agitated patients with schizophrenia and bipolar mania. Eur Psychiatry. 2012;27(4):234–9.
45. Lockman LA, Sung JH, Krivit W. Acute parkinsonian syndrome with demyelinating leuko-encephalopathy in bone marrrow transplant recipients. Pediatr Neurol. 1991;7:457–63.
46. Devinsky O, Lemann W, Evans AC, et al. Akinetic mutism in a bone marrow transplant recipient following total-body irradiation and amphotericin B chemoprophylaxis: a positron emission tomographic and neuropathologic study. Arch Neurol. 1987;44:414–7.
47. Chuang C, Constantino A, Balmaceda C, et al. Chemotherapy-induced parkinsonism respon-sive to levodopa: an under-recognized entity? Mov Disord. 2003;18:328–31.
48. Lima MA, Maradei S, Maranhao FP. Cyclosporin-induced parkinsonism. J Neurol. 2009;245:674–5.
49. Bhatt MH, Elias MA, Mankodi AK. Acute and reversible parkinsonism due to organophos-phate pesticide intoxication: five cases. Neurology. 1999;52(7):1467.
50. Shahar E, Goshen E, Tauber Z, Lahat E. Parkinsonian syndrome complicating systemic lupus erythematosus. Pediatr Neurol. 1998;18:456–8.
51. Francis A. Catatonia: diagnosis, classification and treatments. Curr Psychiatry Rep. 2010;12:180–5.
52. Friedman JH. Stereotypy and catatonia. In: Jankovic JJ, Tolosa E, editors. Parkinson's disease and movement disorders. 5th ed. Baltimore: Williams and Wilkins; 2007. p. 468–80.
53. Bush G, Fink M, Petrides G, et al. Catatonia: 2. Treatment with lorazepam and electroconvul-sive therapy. Acta Psychiatr Scand. 1996;93:137–43.
54. Factor SA, Podskalny GD, Molho ES. Psychogenic movement disorders: frequency, clinical profile and characteristics. J Neurol Neurosurg Psychiatry. 1994;59:406–12.

55. Trimble MR. Clinical presentations in neuropsychiatry. Semin Clin Neuropsychiatry. 2002;7:11–7.
56. Lang AE, Koller WC, Fahn S. Psychogenic parkinsonism. Arch Neurol. 1995;52:802–10.
57. Koller WC, Findley LI. Psychogenic tremors. Adv Neurol. 1990;53:271–5.
58. Von Economo C. Encephalitis lethargica. Wien Klin Wochenschr. 1917;30:581–5.
59. Urechia CL. Dix cas d'encephalite epidemique avec autopsie. Arch Inter Neurol. 1921;2:65–78.
60. Cruchet R, Moutier F, Calmette A. Quarante cas d'encephalo-myelite subaigue. Bull Mem Soc Med d'Hop. 1917;41:614–6.
61. Etienne G. Myelities aigues epidemiques. Deux épidémies militares. Rev Neurol. 1917;24:375–6.
62. Watson AJ. Origin of encephalitis lethargica. Chin Med J. 1928;42:427–32.
63. Von Economo C. Encephalitis lethargica: its sequelae and treatment (translated by K.O. Newman). London: Oxford University Press; 1931. p. I–XIV. 1–200.
64. Duvoisin RC, Yahr MD. Encephalitis and parkinsonism. Arch Neurol. 1965;12:227–39.
65. Geddes JF, Hughes AJ, Lees AJ, Daniel SE. Pathological overlap in cases of parkinsonism associated with neurofibrillary tangles. Brain. 1993;116:281–2.
66. Wilson SAK. Epidemic encephalitis. In: Neurology, vol. 1. Baltimore: Williams and Wilkins; 1940. p. 118–65.
67. Morrison PJ, Patterson VH. Cranial dystonia (Meige syndrome) in postencephalitic parkinsonism. Mov Disord. 1992;7:90–1.
68. Wenning GK, Jellinger K, Litvan I. Supranuclear gaze palsy and eyelid apraxia in postencephalitic parkinsonism. J Neural Transm. 1997;104:845–65.
69. Litvan I, Jankovic J, Goetz CG. Accuracy of the clinical diagnosis of postencephalitic parkinsonism: a clinicopathologic study. Eur J Neurol. 1998;5:451–7.
70. Vilensky JA, Gilman S, McCall S. A historical analysis of the relationship between encephalitis lethargica and post-encephalitic parkinsonism: a complex rather than a direct relationship. Mov Disord. 2010;25:116–23.
71. Duncan AG. The sequelae of encephalitis lethargica. Brain. 1924;47:76–108.
72. Calne DB, Lees AJ. Late progression of post-encephalitic Parkinson syndrome. Can J Neurol Sci. 1988;15:135–8.
73. Vieregge P, Reinhardt V, Hoft B. Is progression in postencephalitic Parkinson's disease late and age-related? J Neurol. 1991;238:299–303.
74. Ravenholt RT, Foege WH. 1918 Influenza, encephalitis lethargica, parkinsonism. Lancet. 1982;2:860–2.
75. Laidlaw PP. Epidemic influenza: a virus disease. Lancet. 1935;1:1118–24.
76. Casals J, Elizan TS, Yahr MD. Postencephalitic parkinsonism—a review. J Neural Transm. 1998;105:645–76.
77. Gamboa ET, Wolf A, Yahr MD, et al. Influenza virus antigen in postencephalitic parkinsonism brain. Arch Neurol. 1974;31:228–32.
78. Martilla RJ, Halomen P, Rinne UK. Influenza virus antibodies in parkinsonism. Comparison of postencephalitic and idiopathic Parkinson patients and matched controls. Arch Neurol. 1977;34:99–100.
79. Elizan T, Schwartz J, Yahr MD, Casals J. Antibodies against arboviruses in postencephalitic and idiopathic Parkinson's disease. Arch Neurol. 1978;35:257–60.
80. Takahashi M, Yamada T, Nakajima S, et al. The substantia nigra is a major target for neurovirulent influenza A virus. J Exp Med. 1995;181:2161–9.
81. Elizan TS, Casals J, Yahr MD. Antineurofilament antibodies in postencephalitic and idiopathic Parkinson's disease. J Neurol Sci. 1983;59:341–7.
82. Elizan TS, Yahr MD. Histocompatibility antigens and postencephalitic parkinsonism. J Neurol Neurosurg Psychiatry. 1983;46:688–93.
83. Lees AJ, Stern GM, Compston DAS. Histocompatibility antigens and post-encephalitic parkinsonism. J Neurol Neurosurg Psychiatry. 1982;45:1060–1.

84. Williams A, Houff S, Lees A, Calne DB. Oligoclonal banding in the cerebrospinal fluid of patients with postencephalitic parkinsonism. J Neurol Neurosurg Psychiatry. 1979;42:790–2.
85. Rail D, Scholtz C, Swash M. Postencephalitic parkinsonism: current experience. J Neurol Neurosurg Psychiatry. 1981;44:670–6.
86. Clough CG, Plaitakis A, Yahr MD. Oculogyric crises and parkinsonism: a case of recent onset. Arch Neurol. 1983;40:36–7.
87. Johnson J, Lucey PA. Encephalitis lethargica, a contemporary cause of catatonic stupor: a report of two cases. Br J Psychiatry. 1987;151:550–2.
88. Howard RS, Lees AJ. Encephalitis lethargica. A report of four recent cases. Brain. 1987;110:19–33.
89. Misra UK, Kalita J. Spectrum of movement disorders in encephalitis. J Neurol. 2010;257:2052–8.
90. Ghaemi M, Rudolf S, Schmulling S, Bamborschke S, Heiss WD. FDG- and Dopa-PET in postencephalitic parkinsonism. J Neural Transm. 2000;107.1289–93.
91. Cree BC, Bernardini GL, Hays AP, Lowe G. A fatal case of coxackievirus B4 meningoencephalitis. Arch Neurol. 2003;60:107–8.
92. Nath A, Jankovic J, Pettigrew LC. Movement disorders and AIDS. Neurology. 1987;37:37–41.
93. Carranzana EJ, Rossitch E, Samuels MA. Parkinsonian symptoms in a patient with AIDS and cerebral toxoplasmosis. J Neurol Neurosurg Psychiatry. 1989;12:1445–7.
94. Navia BA, Petito CK, Gold JWM, et al. Cerebral toxoplasmosis complicating the acquired immunodeficiency syndrome: clinical and neuropathological findings in 27 patients. Ann Neurol. 1986;19:224–38.
95. Noel S, Gaillaume MP, Telerman-Toppet N, et al. Movement disorders due to cerebral Toxoplasma gondii infection in patients with the acquired immunodeficiency syndrome (AIDS). Acta Neurol Belg. 1992;92:148–56.
96. Maggi P, de Mari M, Moramarco A, Fiorentino P, Lamberti P, Angarano G. Parkinsonism in a patient with AIDS and cerebral opportunistic granulomatous lesions. Neurol Sci. 2002;21:173–6.
97. De Mattos JP, Rosso AL, Correa RD, et al. Involuntary movements and AIDS: report of seven cases and review of the literature. Arq Neuropsiquiatr. 1993;51:491–7.
98. Misattari SM, Power C, Nath A. Parkinsonism with HIV infection. Mov Disord. 1998;13:684–9.
99. Cardoso F. HIV-related movement disorders: epidemiology, pathogenesis and management. CNS Drugs. 2002;16:663–8.
100. Sandyk R. Parkinsonism secondary to neurosyphilis: a case report. S Afr Med J. 1983;23:665–6.
101. Garcia-Moreno JM, Izquierdo G, Chacon J, Angulo S, Borobio MV. Neuroborreliosis in a patient with progressive supranuclear paralysis: an association or a cause? Rev Neurol. 1997;25:1919–21.
102. Zambrino CA, Zorzi G, Lanzi G, Uggetti C, Egitto MC. Bilateral striatal necrosis associated with mycoplasma pnuemoniae infection in an adolescent: clinical and neurodiagnostic follow-up. Mov Disord. 2000;15:1023–6.
103. Al-Mateen M, Gibbs M, Dietrch R, Mitchell WG, Menkes JH. Encephalitis lethargica-like illness in a girl with mycoplasma infection. Neurology. 1988;38:1155–8.
104. Saitoh S, Wada T, Narita M, et al. Mycoplasma pneumoniae infection may cause striatal lesions leading to acute neurological dysfunction. Neurology. 1993;43:2150–1.
105. Kim JS, Choi IS, Lee MC. Reversible parkinsonism and dystonia following probable mycoplasma pneumoniae infection. Mov Disord. 1995;10:510–2.
106. Brandel J, Noseda G, Agid Y. Mycoplasma pneumoniae postinfectious encephalomyelitis with bilateral striatal necrosis. Mov Disord. 1996;11:333–5.
107. Singer C, Berger JR, Bowen BC, Bruce JH, Weiner WJ. Akinetic-rigid syndrome in a 13-year old girl with HIV-related progressive multifocal leukoencephalopathy. Mov Disord. 1993;8:113–6.
108. Werring DJ, Chaudhuri KR. HIV-related progressive multifocal leukoencephalopathy presenting with an akinetic-rigid syndrome. Mov Disord. 1996;11:758–61.

109. De la Fuente J, Bordon J, Moreno JA, et al. Parkinsonism in an HIV-infected patient with hypodense cerebral lesion. Tuber Lung Dis. 1996;77:191–2.
110. Strong G. Parkinson's syndrome following herpes ophthalmicus. Br Med J. 1952;1:533.
111. Fenichel GM. Postvaccinal parkinsonism. Mov Disord. 1993;8:253.
112. Reijneveld JC, Taphoorn MJB, Hoogenraad TU, Van Gijn J. Severe but transient parkinsonism after tetanus vaccination. J Neurol Neurosurg Psychiatry. 1997;63:258–9.
113. McCall S, Henry JM, Reid AH, Taubenberger JK. Influenza RNA not detected in archival brain tissues from acute encephalitis lethargica cases or in postencephalitic parkinson cases. J Neuropathol Exp Neurol. 2001;60:696–704.
114. Krusz JC, Koller WC, Ziegler DK. Historical review: abnormal movements associated with epidemic encephalitis lethargica. Mov Disord. 1987;2:137–41.
115. Elizan TS, Casals J. Astrogliosis in von Economo's and postencephalitic Parkinson's diseases supports probable viral etiology. J Neurol Sci. 1991;105:131–4.
116. Hof PR, Charpiot A, Delacourte A, et al. Distribution of neurofibrillary tangles and senile plaques in the cerebral cortex in postencephalitic parkinsonism. Neurosci Lett. 1992;139:10–4.
117. Josephs KA, Parisi JE, Dickson DW. Alpha-synuclein studies are negative in postencephalitic parkinsonism of von Economo. Neurology. 2002;59:645–6.
118. Ikeda K, Akiyama H, Kondo H, Ikeda K. Anti-tau-positive glial fibrillary tangles in the brain of post-encephalitic parkinsonism of Economo type. Neurosci Lett. 1993;162(1–2):176–8.
119. Wong KT, Allen IV, McQuaid S, McConnell R. An immunohistochemical study of neurofibrillary tangle formation in post-encephalitic parkinsonism. Clin Neuropathol. 1996;15:22–5.
120. Shen WC, Ho YJ, Lee SK, Lee KR. MRI of transient post-encephalitic parkinsonism. J Comput Assist Tomogr. 1994;18:155–9.
121. Caparros-Lefebvre D, Cabaret M, Godefroy O, et al. PET study and neuropsychological assessment of a long-lasting post-encephalitic parkinsonism. J Neural Transm. 1998;105:489–95.
122. Solbrig MV, Nashef L. Acute parkinsonism in suspected herpes simplex encephalitis. Mov Disord. 1993;8:233–4.
123. Savant CS, Singhal BS, Jankovic J, Khan MAK, Virani A. Substantia nigra lesions in viral encephalitis. Mov Disord. 2003;18:213–27.
124. Alves RSC, Barbosa ER, Scaff M. Postvaccinal parkinsonism. Mov Disord. 1992;7:178–80.
125. Calne DB, Stern GM, Laurence DR. L-dopa in postencephalitic parkinsonism. Lancet. 1969;1:744–6.
126. Sacks O. Awakenings. New York: Harper Perennial; 1990.
127. Duvoisin RC, Lobo-Antunes J, Yahr MD. Response of patients with post-encephalitic parkinsonism to levodopa. J Neurol Neurosurg Psychiatry. 1972;35:487–95.
128. Walters JH. Postencephalitic parkinson syndrome after meningoencephalitis due to coxackie virus group B, type 2. N Engl J Med. 1960;263:744–7.
129. Posner CM, Huntley CJ, Poland JD. Para-encephalitic parkinsonism. Acta Neurol Scand. 1969;45:199–215.
130. Giraldi C, Mazzoni M, Morgantini PG, Lunardi CV. Parkinsonian syndrome during viral encephalitis. Riv Neurol. 1991;61:183–5.
131. Ickenstein GW, Klotz JM, Langorh HD. Virus encephalitis with symptomatic parkinsonian syndrome, diabetes insipidus and panhypopituitarism. Fortschr Neurol Psychiatr. 1999;67:476–81.
132. Hsieh JC, Lue KH, Lee YL. Parkinson-like syndrome as the major presenting symptom of Epstein-Barr virus encephalitis. Arch Dis Child. 2002;87:358–9.
133. Isgreen WP, Chutarian AM, Fahn S. Sequential parkinsonism and chorea following "mild" influenza. Trans Am Neurol Assoc. 1976;101:56–9.
134. Shiraki H, Goto A, Narabayashi H. Etat passe et present de l'encephalite Japonnaise au Japon. Rev Neurol (Paris). 1963;108:633–96.
135. Ishii T, Marsushita M, Hamada S. Characteristic residual neuropathological features of Japanese B encephalitis. Acta Neuropathol (Berl). 1977;38:181–6.
136. Shoji H, Watanabe M, Itoh S, Kuwahara H, Hattori F. Japanese encephalitis and parkinsonism. J Neurol. 1993;240:59–60.

137. Pradham S, Pandey N, Shashank S, et al. Parkinsonism due to predominant involvement of the substantia nigra in Japanese encephalitis. Neurology. 1999;53:1781–6.
138. Scheid W, Ackerman R, Felgenhauer K. Lymphozytare choriomeningitis unter dem bild der Encephalitis lethargica. Dtsch Med Wochenschr. 1968;93:940–3.
139. Adair CV, Gould RL, Smadel JE. Aseptic meningitis, a disease of diverse etiology: clinical and etiological studies of 854 cases. Ann Intern Med. 1953;39:675–704.
140. Bennett NM. Murray Valley encephalitis, 1947: clinical features. Med J Aust. 1976;2:446–50.
141. Bickerstaff ER, Cloake PCP. Mesencephalitis and rhombencephalitis. Br Med J. 1951;2:77–81.
142. Thieffrey S. Enterovirus et maladies du systeme nerveux: revisiou critique et experience personnelle. Rev Neurol (Paris). 1963;108:753–76.
143. Barrett AM, Gairdner D, McFarlan AM. An outbreak of encephalitis possibly due to poliomyitis virus. Br Med J. 1952;1:1317–22.
144. Vincent FM, Myers WG. Poliomyelitis and parkinsonism. N Engl J Med. 1978;298:688–9.
145. Mellon AF, Appleton RE, Gardner Medwin D, Aynsley-Green A. Encephalitis lethargica-like illness in a 5 year old. Dev Med Child Neurol. 1991;33:153–6.
146. Meyer B. Encephalitis after measles with severe parkinsonian rigidity: recovery. Br Med J. 1943;1:508.
147. Henner K, Hanzal F. Encephalite tchecoslavaque a tiques. Rev Neurol (Paris). 1957;96:384–408.
148. Henner K, Hanzal F. Les encephalities europeenes a tiques. Rev Neurol (Paris). 1963;108:697–752.
149. Radsel-Melvescek A, Marolt-Gomicek M, Pouse-Trojar M, Gajsek-Zima M. Late sequelae after tick-borne meningoencephalitis in patients treated at the hospital for infectious diseases at University Medical Centre of Ljubljana during the period 1974–1975. Zentralbl Bakteriol. 1980;9(suppl):281–4.
150. Cerna F, Mehrad B. JP Luby, et al. St. Louis encephalitis and the substantia nigra: MR imaging evaluation. Am J Neuroradiol. 1999;20:1281–3.
151. Wasay M, Diaz-Arastia R, Suss R, et al. St. Louis encephalitis: a review of 11 cases in a 1995 Dallas, Texas epidemic. Arch Neurol. 2000;57:114–8.
152. Finley KH. Postencephalitic manifestations of viral encephalitides. In: Fields WS, Blattner RJ, editors. Viral encephalitis. Springfield: Charles C Thomas; 1958. p. 69–94.
153. Finley KH, Riggs N. Convalescence and sequelae. In: Monath TP, editor. St. Louis encephalitis. Washington, DC: American Public Health Association; 1980. p. 535–50.
154. Fulton JC, Burton AN. After effects of WEE infection in man. Canad MAJ. 1953;69:268–72.
155. Mulder DW, Parrot M, Thaler M. Sequelae of western equine encephalitis. Neurology. 1951;1:318–27.

Parkinsonism-Hyperpyrexia Syndrome in Parkinson's Disease

Daniel E. Huddleston and Stewart A. Factor

Patient Vignette

A 44-year-old right-handed man with a 14-year history of Parkinson's disease (PD) presented to the emergency department (ED) with acute onset of fever, confusion, rapidly progressive difficulty with ambulation and dysphagia. He originally developed PD at age 30 with left arm tremor and slowness. Work-up for secondary parkinsonism was unrevealing, and treatment was initiated first with anticholinergic agents and then levodopa. Within 4 years, he had developed bilateral symptoms and signs. Motor fluctuations and complications emerged within 5 years of onset, with related anxiety and behavioral problems as well. He required high doses of dopaminergic agents for the last 8 years. After 13 years he underwent deep brain stimulation (DBS) surgery, with bilateral leads placed in the subthalamic nuclei. They were operational as of the last office visit. DBS surgery led to improved off times and improved dyskinesia but allowed only minimal changes in levodopa dose.

The emergency occurred approximately 1-year post surgery. He had been fully able to communicate, perform activities of daily living and ambulate 48 h prior to ED presentation. He had recently been incarcerated, and during his confinement his medication doses were abruptly and substantially diminished for unclear reasons. His usual dosing schedule included carbidopa/levodopa (C/L) 25/100 one tablet

Supplementary Information The online version of this chapter (https://doi.org/10.1007/978-3-030-75898-1_5) contains supplementary material, which is available to authorized users.

D. E. Huddleston
Department of Neurology, Emory University School of Medicine, Atlanta, GA, USA

S. A. Factor (✉)
Movement Disorders Program, Vance Lanier Chair for Neurology, Emory University School of Medicine, Atlanta, GA, USA
e-mail: sfactor@emory.edu

every 2 h starting at 6:00 a.m. to 8 pm, with two tablets at 10:00 p.m., midnight and 2:00 a.m. In addition, he was also prescribed the dopamine agonist pergolide 1 mg three times/day, and quetiapine 25 mg five tablets per day. In the ED, the patient appeared acutely ill. He was febrile, with a temperature of 101 °F, heart rate of 100 bpm, blood pressure of 140/90, and respiratory rate of 24. He was awake but confused and unable to follow commands or intelligibly communicate. His mucus membranes were dry. He appeared diffusely stiff with severe rigidity of the neck and limbs. A coarse tremor was present in both arms, but no other involuntary movements were seen. No signs of trauma were found. Pupils were symmetrical and reactive to light, and fundoscopic exam was normal. Reflexes were present and symmetric with no pathologic reflexes. Laboratory studies revealed a white blood cell count (WBC) of 16,000 cells/mm^3, blood urea nitrogen of 39 mg/dl, and normal red blood cell indices. No iron indices were measured. Creatine kinase (CK) was >4000. A cranial CT revealed bilateral DBS leads without acute pathology. A lumbar puncture with CSF analysis was normal.

The diagnosis of parkinsonism-hyperpyrexia syndrome was made. A nasogastric tube was placed, and levodopa and pergolide were re-instituted with intravenous fluids. Despite treatment his condition worsened, with medically refractory hypertension, respiratory distress, seizures, and ultimately renal failure. He expired 3 days after presentation. Postmortem examination revealed bilateral pulmonary emboli with infarction. Examination of the brain revealed marked depigmentation of the substantia nigra and the locus coeruleus, with Lewy bodies confirming the diagnosis of PD.

Introduction

Neuroleptic malignant syndrome (NMS) is a potentially fatal drug-induced movement disorder that was first described by Delay and associates in 1960 [1, 2]. These authors reported it as the "most serious but also rarest and least known of complications of neuroleptic chemotherapy" [2]. Since the 1980s, it has been a considerable concern in relation to the treatment of psychiatric patients because of its potentially high mortality rate of 5–20% [3, 4]. The characteristic clinical features include hyperthermia, muscle rigidity, dysautonomia, and mental status change. Hyperthermia is present in nearly all cases of NMS, and muscle rigidity is reported in more than 90% of patients [3–7]. Alterations in mental status can range from fluctuating alertness, to agitation and delirium, to frank stupor or coma [6, 8]. Muteness is also seen although less commonly than catatonia. Unstable blood pressure, cardiac arrhythmia, dyspnea, pulmonary edema, and bladder incontinence are common signs of dysautonomia; diastolic hypertension may be a specific feature [3]. Several laboratory abnormalities support the diagnosis including elevated creatine kinase (CK), elevated white blood cell count (WBC), and diminished serum iron [3]. The core features of NMS have been recognized in patients exposed to other agents such as dopamine depletors (tetrabenazine) [9], and in a related syndrome (serotonin syndrome) associated with exposure to serotonin-specific reuptake inhibitors [10, 11].

In 1981, a similar disorder was described in a patient with PD triggered by sudden withdrawal of dopaminergic medications, specifically levodopa, amantadine, and biperiden. The syndrome seen in PD was reported under a variety of different names, including NMS, neuroleptic malignant-like syndrome (NMLS) [12, 13], levodopa-withdrawal hyperthermia, parkinsonism-hyperpyrexia syndrome (PHS) [14], lethal hyperthermia [15], dopaminergic malignant syndrome [16], acute dopamine depletion syndrome [17], and akinetic crisis (although this syndrome includes worsening of parkinsonism due to medical issues such as infection or trauma which may be pathophysiologically different from changes due to medication withdrawal) [18]. PHS is the most specific and clinically descriptive term and the one currently most accepted for this disorder. As we will show, levodopa withdrawal is not the only cause of this entity, and the word dopaminergic pertains to any NMS-like syndrome. It is important to draw a distinction between true NMS and PHS. From this point forward, when discussing this syndrome in parkinsonian patients we will use the term PHS. This chapter will review the clinical entity of PHS and discuss its management. Interest in this syndrome has been on the rise in recent years, evidenced by the publication of several review articles on the subject [7, 18–22]. We will also discuss two other less common PD emergencies, deep brain stimulation-withdrawal syndrome and dyskinesia-hyperpyrexia syndrome.

Clinical Features

Although PHS is rare, primarily reported as case reports and series, several situations have been found to be common triggers [23]. The scenario initially reported was during a "levodopa holiday" [13, 24–26]. These cases were all reported in the 1980s when drug holidays were still utilized for therapeutic purposes. They were recommended in patients with intractable "off" periods and psychosis, although their utility was controversial [27, 28]. Drug holidays often involved rapid reduction and complete cessation of dopaminergic medication. Patients would remain off for up to 14 days, despite well-known risks associated with immobility such as aspiration pneumonia and pulmonary embolism. Drug holidays fell out of favor long ago and are no longer utilized therapeutically; however, there are situations where dopaminergic medications are discontinued which pose an equal risk. In several reports, the medications were abruptly stopped by the patients themselves because of dysphagia or side effects, misunderstanding medication instructions or a desire to try alternative treatments [12, 16, 17, 23]. In one case the medications were stopped because physicians thought the patient had psychogenic parkinsonism [17]. PHS has also been seen in PD patients with partial withdrawal of dopaminergic therapy, or when medication regimens were substantially changed. Iwuagwa et al. [29] described a case with onset linked to discontinuing the COMT inhibitor tolcapone. When the patient became confused, the treating physician thought this was exacerbated by levodopa; after it was stopped, PHS symptoms escalated. Cunningham et al. [30] described a patient who developed hyperthermia, rigidity, and dysautonomia when immediate release levodopa was switched to controlled release and bromocriptine was tapered off from 40 mg/day to zero in just a few days. Peak serum levodopa levels are notably lower with controlled release formulations than immediate release. Keyster et al. [17] reported a similar case where PHS occurred when a patient was switched from levodopa to bromocriptine.

Never abruptly reduce or discontinue levodopa or dopamine agonists in PD patients.

Another situation where PHS has been reported is in PD patients treated for a coexisting psychiatric disorder with neuroleptics. One such patient with schizophrenia and PD treated with neuroleptics for their primary psychotic disorder became gravely ill after cessation of anti-parkinsonian medications [31]. In another case, a patient admitted to the hospital for drug-induced psychosis had their levodopa stopped and haloperidol started at the same time. It is not unreasonable to refer to these cases as NMS also since it is unclear if symptoms started because of dopaminergic drug withdrawal or neuroleptic initiation, or both. Severe "off" periods associated with motor fluctuations can also trigger such events. Pfeiffer and Sucha [15] reported a single patient developing repeated PHS features with "off" episodes. Events occurred for years, lasting 1 or 2 h and clearing when he turned "on". He ultimately died during a severe episode associated with a fever of 107 °F.

Three other scenarios have been reported in single cases that occurred without change in medication regimen. One involved peri-menstrual "off" times with symptoms of PHS [32]. In this case, it is believed that elevated estrogen and progesterone levels may have decreased CNS dopaminergic stimulation in a manner similar to cutting medication doses. Another case involved metabolic alteration, particularly hypernatremia [33]; the mechanism by which this caused PHS is unclear. In a third case a patient in the intensive care unit developed the symptoms of PHS after his enteric feeding was changed from a formulation with lower protein content to one with higher protein content [34]. The PHS cleared after the enteric feeding formulation was switched back to the formulation with lower protein content. His home regimen of PD medications was continued unchanged throughout his course. In this case the development of PHS was attributed to decreased absorption of his levodopa caused by increased protein content in his enteric nutrition. Despite these cases and others like them, it should be noted that PHS, for the most part, refers to a disorder that occurs with withdrawal of CNS dopaminergic stimulation. Metabolic changes and infection may increase the risk of PHS. However, while they can on their own cause worsening of parkinsonian symptoms, it is unclear if they do so via the same mechanism. Therefore, we propose that the term PHS should indicate the presence of NMS-like constellation of symptoms in the setting of dopaminergic drug withdrawal.

PHS and Deep Brain Stimulation

Our patient vignette suggests an additional risk for PHS in PD patients. DBS of the subthalamic nucleus (STN) is commonly used in advanced fluctuating PD. When performed properly it leads to a substantial decrease in "off" time and severity. This improvement can in turn lead to a decrease in levodopa requirement by about 37% [35]. Some authors advocate discontinuing levodopa altogether [36], but others have voiced concern regarding this objective and the risk of PHS [37]. Our patient had STN DBS implanted and had medications abruptly stopped, although not as part of the programming plan. He developed PHS and secondary pulmonary embolism, which was ultimately fatal. The DBS did not prevent PHS, and therefore it docs not appear to be protective with respect to PHS.

⚊⚊ The decision to completely eliminate levodopa after STN DBS requires careful thought.

Other scenarios leading to PHS surrounding STN DBS have been described. Some relate to medication changes and some to abrupt disruption of the stimulation itself. For those where the symptoms occur due to withdrawal of the DBS itself, it is referred to as "deep brain stimulation-withdrawal syndrome (DBS-WDS)" [38]. In one case report the authors describe onset of PHS following medication withdrawal preoperatively in preparation for DBS surgery the night before [39]. Another patient developed PHS immediately after implantation of bilateral STN DBS. Adjunctive medications, ropinirole, entacapone, and amantadine had been gradually tapered and stopped 1 day preoperatively. Levodopa was held overnight, one dose was given during surgery between implantation of the sides, and it was restarted in the evening. Nevertheless, he developed high fever, rigidity, tachycardia, drowsiness, and elevated CK. Symptoms progressed over 16 days, including the development of renal failure, and the patient ultimately expired [40]. In yet another scenario, a patient had her dopaminergic medications lowered substantially after STN DBS resulted in severe dyskinesias. As the dyskinesias subsided, around day 24 she developed PHS which ultimately led to fatal myocardial infarction [41]. Rajan et al. [42] reported PHS in two patients when their IPG reached "end-of-life" status. In both cases replacement was delayed, but once completed improvement was seen within days. Similar cases have been reported with one case of PHS occurring as the patient was prepared for IPG replacement [43, 44]. The symptoms improved within hours of IPG reimplantation and programming. Reuter et al. [38] reported PHS or DBS-WDS in five patients explanted due to lead infection. One case report (see Case 4 in Section IV below) describes a patient who developed PHS repeatedly after his STN DBS was turned off for recurrent stimulation-associated manic episodes [45]. Longer duration of PD and longer duration DBS stimulation may be risk factors for DBS-WDS [38]. The mechanism by which DBS withdrawal causes DBS-WDS is unknown. One might assume that stopping DBS would have an equivalent effect of dopaminergic drug withdrawal. However, it appears that increasing the levodopa dose does not improve DBS-WDS [43]. This would suggest a different mechanism from PHS due to drug withdrawal. This disorder has been primarily reported with STN DBS and not pallidal DBS. It has been suggested this may relate to the absence of medication withdrawal with the later [42].

PHS Epidemiology

The frequency of PHS in PD has not been studied formally, but the disorder appears to be rare and is likely underreported [22]. We identified more than 80 cases reported in the literature. The details of the cases were varied. One paper was a therapeutic trial that included 40 cases [46]; two papers reported 11 cases each [16, 47]; two reports described three cases each [13, 17], and the rest were single case reports. With one of the larger cohorts, Serrano-Duenas [16] reported that 11 cases accounted for 3.6% of his PD patient population and 0.04% of total patient consultations for PD. In the study by Sato et al. [46], 40 cases were seen over a 3-year period. One study of akinetic crisis observed that it occurred in 30 of 756 cohort patients followed a mean of 14.3 ± 2.7 years of follow-up (overall incidence 2.8/1000 person years [PYs]) but 2.7/1000 PYs for non-familial PD and six in the 142 patients with familial PD (3.0/1000 PYs) [48]. This study also demonstrated that genetic mutation carriers (POLG1, PINK1, LRRK2, GBA) had a substantially higher incidence at 21.2/1000 PYs (seen in 6 of 20 patients) [48]. Although these categories (akinetic crisis and PHS) are not identical, we would expect that they overlap substantially. These findings suggest that PHS may be more prevalent than previously recognized.

In a hospital-based study (single hospital) of consecutive PD admissions between April 2009 and March 2015, there were 164 admissions involving 136 patients, with 40 of these admissions (involving 38 patients) being considered emergencies. Six of these 40 had PHS (15% of emergencies and 4% of total admissions over 6 years) [49]. This represents about one admission with PHS per year. PHS was the most common reason for admission among those with disease duration <5 years in elderly individuals with later onset PD. The PHS reported in this study occurred in the background of dehydration as a result of depression and anxiety. Patients developing PHS were male (47 of 83 [56%] reported) or female, with duration of PD ranging from 2 to 16 years and baseline levodopa dose at time of onset ranged from 200 to 2100 mg/day. Not all patients have motor complications, but this appears to enhance risk. In the report by Ueda et al. [47], only 4 of 11 cases were experiencing this problem at the onset of PHS. The mortality rate was 4% in one study [50] and as high as 23% in another [48]. The later study included worsening of parkinsonism due to medical issues such as infection.

PHS Clinical Syndrome

The clinical features of PHS are nearly identical to NMS, and the clinical presentation seems fairly stereotyped [11]. The time of onset of symptoms after change in dopaminergic therapy ranged from 18 h to 7 days [51]. The initial feature in most patients is severe rigidity along with tremor, with rapid progression to an immobile state [16, 17, 47]. Within 72–96 h, most patients are hyperpyrexic with altered mental status ranging from agitation and confusion to stupor and coma. Autonomic signs include tachycardia, tachypnea, labile blood pressure, urinary incontinence, pallor, and diaphoresis. In some cases, hyperthermia, mental status changes, and autonomic dysfunction may occur from the outset along with worsening of parkinsonism [47]. Temperature as high as 107 °F has been reported [13, 15]. Laboratory findings usually reveal leukocytosis (as high as 26,000) and elevated CK (ranging from 260 to 50,000 in reported cases). There have been no reports of iron levels that were altered in NMS [3]. Respiratory distress is not uncommon, and mechanical ventilation may be necessary [24, 31]. Mutism, as part of the mental status derangement, was reported by several authors [12, 30, 33]. Other neurological features include seizures [25] and myoclonus [14].

Although this description seems very similar to NMS, there appear to be some differences. Serrano-Duenas [16] performed a comparison looking at 11 PHS patients and 21 NMS patients. They found that the latency to onset of symptoms after the inciting event was twice as long (93 h versus 49 h) for PHS than NMS. In addition, in PHS the elevation of CK and WBC was significantly less robust. The duration of hospitalization was also shorter (8.4 versus 12.2 days). As expected, PHS patients were older than the NMS group. These findings suggest that NMS is a more aggressive disorder than PHS, and carries a poorer prognosis. As with NMS, PHS may be associated with serious long-term sequelae. Some patients only partially recover from the event and are left with significantly worsened PD [16, 17]. In one case a patient at Hoehn and Yahr stage 2 prior to the incident became wheelchair-bound (stage 5) afterward [16]. Medical complications are also a concern. Deep venous thrombosis is a serious complication and may ultimately result in pulmonary emboli (as occurred in our illustrative case). Several patients have developed aspiration pneumonia during a bout of PHS and two cases developed renal failure [13, 17], complications well described in NMS. Finally, several of the reported cases were fatal [13, 15, 24, 52]. Two died in hyperthermic coma with no other explanation, one died with aspiration pneumonia and renal failure and one from pulmonary embolism [52]. The longer the duration of the event, the greater the mortality [48].

O━━━🔑 PHS is clinically similar to NMS, although PHS may be less malignant.

Illustrative Cases from the Literature

The following four cases from the literature illustrate PHS, three from drug with-drawal and one related to DBS. In addition, Table 5.1 summarizes the time frame involved in development of PHS after dopaminergic drug withdrawal, and recovery after therapy in six representative cases [16, 17].

Case 1 [17]

A 75-year-old man with a diagnosis of PD was treated with immediate release car-bidopa/levodopa (C/L) 25/100, one tablet three times per day for 1 year. When

Table 5.1 Summary of selected clinical cases from two publications [16, 17] illustrating the time frames involved in onset and recovery of PHS

Patient demographics	Medication discontinued	Clinical features within 24 h	Clinical features within 96 h	Improvement within 24 h	Improvement within 96 h
75-year-old man with PD for 1 year	C/L 300 mg/d	None reported	Weak, rigid, tremulous, diaphoretic	None reported	Full resolution within 5 days
67-year-old woman with PD and schizophrenia	C/L 250 mg/ qid	Febrile (41.2 °C) mute, tremulous, rigid	Same	Afebrile, improved sensorium	Full resolution within 48 h
64-year-old man with PD for 7 years	C/L 250 mg/q.i.d. Benz. 2 mg/d Trihex. 4 mg/d	Tremulous, rigid	Febrile (39.4 °C) Mute, confused, severe tremor and rigidity	Less rigid and tremulousness, improved sensorium	Progressive improvement without return to baseline after 10 days
74-year-old woman with PD (H&Y III)	C/L 750 mg/d Seleg. 10 mg/d	Rigid, unable to ambulate or feed self	Febrile (37.9 °C) Stupor, severe rigidity	Afebrile, alert, much less rigid	Progressive improvement without return to baseline after 10 days
69-year-old man with PD (H&Y II)	C/L 750 mg/d Bromo. 7.5 mg/d	Severe rigidity, unable to ambulate	Febrile (38.7 °C) Somnolent, severe rigidity	Afebrile, alert, much less rigid	Progressive improvement without return to baseline after 10 days
69-year-old woman with PD (H&Y IV)	C/L 1125 mg/d Seleg. 10 mg/d	Febrile, severe rigidity, unable to ambulate	Febrile (39.2 °C) Stupor, severe rigidity	Afebrile, alert, much less rigidity	Progressive improvement without return to baseline after 10 days

C/L carbidopa/levodopa, *Ama.* amantadine, *Seleg.* selegiline, *Bromo.* bromocriptine, *H&Y* Hoehn and Yahr amantadine 100 mg was added for symptomatic benefit, the patient mistakenly discontinued his C/L. Within 5 days he became tremulous, weak, pale, diaphoretic, and dyspneic. Amantadine was increased without clinical benefit. It was discovered that C/L had been discontinued and it was restarted but only at twice daily dosing. Over the ensuing week, the patient became progressively confused, resulting in the cessation of C/L. Within 48 h, he worsened considerably and because of continued confusion 9 mg of haloperidol was given. Soon after, the patient became mute, agitated, and severely rigid with a diffuse coarse tremor. Laboratory review revealed leukocytosis, hypernatremia, and an elevated CK (452 U/L). Within 5 h of this evaluation, the patient's temperature rose to 38.5 °C. Bromocriptine (2.5 mg every 6 h) was started, and within 72 h the patient's condition markedly improved. C/L was subsequently restarted, and the patient fully recovered.

Case 2 [16]

A 74-year-old woman abruptly stopped taking her anti-parkinsonian medication. She had advanced disease (Hoehn and Yahr stage 3), and had been taking C/L 750 mg/d, selegiline 10 mg/d and propranolol 80 mg/d. She decided to begin an alternative natural treatment for PD and did not discuss this first with her treating physician. Within a short time, she became markedly rigid and was unable to walk or feed herself. Within 96 h she was diaphoretic, somnolent, febrile (37.9 °C), rigid and stuporous and had a serum CK of 759 U/L on presentation to a local hospital. A diagnosis of PHS due to abrupt medication withdrawal was made, a nasogastric tube was placed and dopaminergic medication was restarted. Within 9 h she became alert, and rigidity lessened within 15 h. On discharge 9 days later, rigidity was worse than prior to the incident.

Case 3 [24]

A 51-year-old man with a 9-year history of PD was admitted to the hospital because of severe levodopa-induced dyskinesias. His medications on admission included C/L 25/250 three times per day and diphenhydramine 50 mg four times per day. C/L was reduced by one half for 3 days, and then stopped altogether (drug holiday) and diphenhydramine was cut to BID. Two days later the dyskinesias stopped and were replaced by rigidity, bradykinesia, and tremor. On the third day, his temperature rose to 38.2 °C, heart rate of 120/min, respiratory rate 28/min, and he was diaphoretic. The temperature increased further to 40.4 °C by day 10 and he remained confused and disoriented. Anti-PD medications were restarted, and intravenous fluids and low-dose heparin were begun. By day 10 CK was 260 U/l and on day 14 WBC was 13,200/mm^3. Work-up for infection was negative, and antibiotics were initiated empirically. Despite therapy, he remained febrile and stuporous. He was intubated and placed on a ventilator but died in hyperthermic coma on day 15 after discontinuing medications.

Case 4 [45]

A 60-year-old man with a 17-year history of PD developed severe motor fluctuations and dyskinesias 9 years after disease onset. He was levodopa-responsive and underwent bilateral subthalamic nucleus (STN) DBS placement. With stimulation his motor symptoms improved, but he also developed mania. His mania increased 2 years after the DBS placement and he was admitted to the hospital where the stimulators were turned off in light of the mania, which was attributed to the stimulation. On the third hospital day, the patient's manic symptoms disappeared but he developed somnolence, immobility, and rigidity. He became febrile with a temperature of 38.7 °C. Heart rate was 120, white blood cell 12,600/μL, and serum CK was elevated to 1878 U/L. PHS was considered, treatment with medical therapy was initiated and by day 6 in the hospital the patient was afebrile with normal mental status. DBS was then turned back on and the patient had improvement in rigidity and akinesia. However, over the next several years he experienced several more episodes of mania, which did not respond adequately to antipsychotic drugs or DBS stimulation site adjustment. During each episode his DBS had to be turned off, and each time this was done he experienced recurrence of PHS which responded each time to IV fluids followed by the reintroduction of DBS. His most recent manic episode was reversed by lowering the voltage of the stimulation, not completely turning it off, without the emergence of PHS.

Risk Factors and Pathogenesis

In practice, many PD patients have their doses of dopaminergic medications decreased or stopped and yet only a very small fraction experience PHS. On the other hand, some patients are susceptible enough to develop this with minor medication changes or wearing off. There have been attempts to evaluate potential risk factors for the development of PHS in PD patients [47, 53, 54]. The most ambitious of these was a study by Ueda [47], examining clinical and neurochemical features over a 3-year period in 98 consecutive hospitalized PD patients. Demographics, disease severity, and cerebrospinal fluid monoamine metabolites including HVA, MHPG, and 5-HIAA were evaluated. Eleven of the 98 had a history of PHS (either remote or leading to the study admission). The PHS group had significantly worse parkinsonism and a greater daily levodopa dose. No difference was seen between groups with respect to gender, age, duration of disease, or maximum levodopa dose. HVA spinal fluid levels were significantly lower in the PHS group, the only feature independently related to the occurrence of PHS. A second study by the same group [53] examined CSF HVA levels in nine patients during and after an episode of PHS, and compared them to 12 PD patients with simple worsening of PD with discontinuing medications. HVA levels were significantly lower in the PHS group. The authors suggested that the lower baseline level left a "narrow safety margin," leading to an increased susceptibility to the occurrence of PHS. Other studies [54] suggest that the presence of motor fluctuations, psychosis, and dehydration prior to the event represents other possible risks. Overall, it appears that those with more severe disease and more profound dopaminergic depletion are at greater risk. Support for this comes from the ELLDOPA trial where 361 early PD subjects treated with up to 600 mg of levodopa for 9 months were withdrawn over a few days. No cases of PHS occurred [55].

It is generally accepted that alterations in dopaminergic transmission in the brain are the primary pathogenic mechanism of NMS [3, 56]. Abnormalities in muscle membrane function, changes in peripheral and central sympathetic outflow, and alterations in central serotonin metabolism have also been implicated [3]. The occurrence of PHS (which exhibits the same clinical phenomena seen in NMS) with dopaminergic drug withdrawal in PD indicates that a hypodopaminergic state alone is sufficient to trigger this syndrome. The clinical features of PHS can be explained by central dopamine depletion. The motor features of PHS are exaggerated PD symptoms related to decreased dopaminergic activity in the nigrostriatal system. It has been shown on FP/CIT SPECT scans that during an episode of akinetic crisis (five patients) and NMS (one patient), there is almost complete suppression of binding in the putamen and severely reduced or no uptake in the caudate of the patients demonstrating aspects of "burst striatum" pattern [57]. These findings suggest that there is profound presynaptic dopaminergic dysfunction during AC or NMS; dopamine presynaptic transporter activity is suppressed and inefficient and that this dysfunction may recover during follow-up in surviving patients. The role of dopamine in thermal regulation is also well known. These dopamine pathways within the hypothalamus include the preoptic area, the anterior hypothalamus concerned with thermal detection, and the posterior hypothalamus involved with generation of effector signals. The thermosensitive neurons respond to local changes in blood temperature as well as to afferent information from peripheral thermosensors. Dopamine and dopamine agonists modulate hypothalamic temperature regulation, while dopamine receptor antagonists block this ability [3]. Dopaminergic depletion can also explain mental status changes through modulation of mesolimbic and mesocortical pathways [3].

Treatment

PHS is a neurological emergency. The key to treatment is early recognition of the syndrome and rapid reintroduction of withdrawn anti-parkinsonian medication (Table 5.2). If there is no history of medication schedule alteration, then other causes must be sought including the use of neuroleptics or inadvertent shutting off of their DBS device (drained battery for example). When discontinuation of medication is the cause, the drug most commonly responsible is levodopa, and it should be re-instituted first, via nasogastric tube if necessary. Since PHS has occurred in two patients because of poor absorption of levodopa relating to diet this is an important consideration. If the syndrome developed after DBS shutdown or adjustment (DBS-WDS), reversing these changes is recommended. If it relates to IPG failure, then replacement should be completed as soon as possible, even in the situation of the

Table 5.2 Steps in the management of PMS in PD

Recognition of the disorder
Verification of patients' medication regimen/compliance
Reintroduction of anti-parkinsonian medications
Supportive measures anti-pyretics/cooling blankets
   Re hydration
   ICU monitoring/management (see text)
Clinical evaluation for possible co-morbid conditions
Bromocriptine 2.5 mg po t.i.d., titrated by 2.5 mg t.i.d./daily as necessary
Dantrolene sodium 10 mg/kg/d IV in divided doses (t.i.d./q.i.d.) as necessary
Apomorphine 2 mg SC every 3 h as necessary (if no nasogastric tube access, or use as adjunct)

patient being acutely ill, since standard treatments related to PHS including adding more levodopa do not seem to be effective [43, 44]. Beyond that, the treatment is similar to NMS with supportive therapy, including re-hydration with intravenous fluids, treatment of hyperthermia with anti-pyretics and cooling blankets, as well as supportive measures such as mechanical ventilation, cardiovascular monitoring, intravenous access, nasogastric suctioning/feeding, and prevention of thrombophlebitis [43]. Metabolic evaluation and work-up to exclude infection are necessary. Since these patients are at risk for infection, such as aspiration pneumonia, it is reasonable to initiate antibiotic therapy while the work-up is under way. Additional medical therapy with bromocriptine or other dopamine agonists and dantrolene should be considered, although there have been no controlled trials. Bromocriptine is orally administered, with an initial dose of 2.5 mg t.i.d., titrated for effect in increments of 2.5 mg t.i.d. every 24 h. Dantrolene, a muscle relaxant initially used to treat malignant hyperthermia, is a parental compound typically dosed as 10 mg/kg/day in three to four divided doses. Apomorphine administered subcutaneously is also useful in the treatment of PHS when medication administration orally or via nasogastric tube is not feasible [58–60]. Apomorphine may also be useful as an adjunctive therapy for PHS along with levodopa [59]. With proper therapy symptoms will reverse in 10 h to 7 days. Most of the patients described ultimately required a fairly lengthy hospital stay (5–22 days). Studies informing the treatment of PHS have generally been case reports and small case series, and larger randomized trials are needed to better establish optimal therapy for PHS.

One study examined the use of methylprednisolone pulse therapy as an added regimen for PHS in PD [46]. In a randomized trial, all patients received levodopa, bromocriptine, and dantrolene sodium and patients were randomized to receive placebo or 1000 mg of methylprednisolone daily for 3 days. Results suggested that steroid pulse therapy might shorten the course of the illness, perhaps by as much as 10 days, although notable overlap between groups was seen. This is the only double blind, placebo-controlled trial in PHS or NMS, and further investigation is warranted.

Dyskinesia-Hyperpyrexia Syndrome

We chose to also include "dyskinesia-hyperpyrexia syndrome" (DHS) in this chapter as it is another PD emergency relevant to the topic. DHS is rarer than PHS, and only a few cases have been reported. In contrast to PHS, it occurs due to increased dopaminergic activity leading to acute onset, severe and continuous dyskinesia with rhabdomyolysis, hyperpyrexia, and altered mental status. The mechanism is unclear but likely relates to excessive, non-physiological central dopaminergic replacement in the striatum. It has been reported in association with medication changes and has also occurred spontaneously. DHS has developed on a background of oral (pulsatile) levodopa treatment and enteral continuous infusion. Some patients have recurrent episodes [61, 62]. In one case, a patient with a 16-year history of PD treated with enteral levodopa/carbidopa, safinamide and amantadine had ropinirole XL added to the regimen to treat restless leg syndrome. The patient developed severe dyskinesias, hyperpyrexia, and substantially elevated CK and WBC. The patient required cessation of all medications and endotracheal intubation and sedation before the symptoms subsided approximately 24 h later. Medications were ultimately reintroduced with return of prior function [63]. Another case occurred on the background of 19 years of STN-DBS. Motor fluctuations and dyskinesias were previously well controlled. He spontaneously developed severe dyskinesias on a hot July day. He had hyperpyrexia and tachycardia and an elevated CK. Oral dopaminergic medications were adjusted, and the stimulation amplitude was decreased. Dyskinesias improved in hours to days [64]. Longer duration disease and motor fluctuations appear to be important risk factors [63, 64]. It can be triggered by therapeutic changes, infections, dehydration, or trauma. Ambient heat, in combination with hyperactivity, has been invoked as possible triggers. The role of ambient heat is well illustrated by a case where a patient with 16 years of PD complicated by motor fluctuations and dyskinesias would develop DHS, eight episodes over three summers [62]. The episodes included severe dyskinesia, hyperthermia, and elevated CK and WBC and eventually ceased during treatment with enteral L-dopa infusion. Treatment includes intensive supportive care and reducing dopaminergic therapy.

Conclusion

PHS is a neurological emergency caused by the abrupt withdrawal of dopaminergic therapy or alterations in DBS parameters (referred to as DBS-WDS) that has the potential to end in fatality. In all likelihood, it is under-recognized and more common than the literature might suggest. There are several ways to prevent PHS. First, drug holidays are no longer considered an appropriate treatment approach in PD. If reduction in dopaminergic therapy is needed, gradual reduction is mandated, and patients should be made aware of the possible occurrence of PHS. This applies to patients with multiple system atrophy, progressive supranuclear palsy, and cortico-basal degeneration [65]. When lowering doses patients need to remain adequately hydrated. In addition, patients should be advised not to stop medications on their own and the dangers should be spelled out. It is important to avoid the use of standard neuroleptics in these patients since they are already at risk for NMS or PHS. Even atypical antipsychotics have the potential to lead to NMS in PD. The agents best tolerated by PD patients are quetiapine and clozapine [66], but they should also be prescribed with caution. Although patients with more severe disease and those taking larger daily levodopa doses are at greater risk [47, 53, 54], even patients with early PD taking low doses of levodopa can develop PHS. Once the syndrome occurs, recognition is paramount and rapid re-introduction of dopaminergic medications imperative. One other syndrome to be vigilant of is DHS. Although this disorder is related to a hyperdopaminergic state, it also leads to severe dyskinesias with fever, muscle breakdown, and renal failure. This disorder is exceedingly rare.

References

1. Delay J, Pichot P, Lemperiere T, Elissalde B, Peigne F. A non-phenothiazine and non-reserpine major neuroleptic, haloperidol, in the treatment of psychoses. Ann Med Psychol (Paris). 1960;118(1):145–52.
2. Delay J, Denicker P. Drug induced extrapyramidal syndromes. In: Vinken P, Bruyun G, editors. Handbook of clinical neurology. Amsterdam: North Holland; 1968. p. 258–9.
3. Factor SA. Neuroleptic malignant syndrome. In: Factor SA, et al., editors. Drug induced movement disorders. 2nd ed. Massachusetts: Blackwell Futura; 2005. p. 174–212.
4. Caroff SN, Campbell EC. Drug-induced extrapyramidal syndromes: implications for contemporary practice. Psychiatr Clin N Am. 2016;39:391–411.
5. Shalev A, Munitz H. The neuroleptic malignant syndrome: agent and host interaction. Acta Psychiatr Scand. 1986;73:337–47.
6. Rosebush P, Stewart T. A prospective analysis of 24 episodes of neuroleptic malignant syndrome. Am J Psychiatry. 1989;146:717–25.
7. Robottom BJ, Weiner WJ, Factor SA. Movement disorders emergencies. Part 1: Hypokinetic disorders. Arch Neurol. 2011;68:567–72.
8. Kurlan R, Hamill R, Shoulson I. Neuroleptic malignant syndrome. Clin Neuropharmacol. 1984;7:109–20.
9. Burke RE, Fahn S, Mayeux R, Weinberg H, Louis K, Willner JH. Neuroleptic malignant syndrome caused by dopamine-depleting drugs in a patient with Huntington disease. Neurology. 1981;31:1022–5.
10. Sternbach H. The serotonin syndrome. Am J Psychiatry. 1991;148:705–13.
11. Factor SA, Burkhard PR, Caroff S, et al. Recent developments in drug-induced movement disorders: a mixed picture. Lancet Neurol. 2019;18:880–90.
12. Toru M, Matsuda O, Makiguchi K, Sugano K. Neuroleptic malignant syndrome-like state following a withdrawal of antiparkinsonian drugs. J Nerv Ment Dis. 1981;169:324–7.
13. Friedman JH, Feinberg SS, Feldman RG. A neuroleptic malignantlike syndrome due to levodopa therapy withdrawal. JAMA. 1985;254:2792–5.

14. Gordon PH, Frucht SJ. Neuroleptic malignant syndrome in advanced Parkinson's disease. Mov Disord. 2001;16:960–2.
15. Pfeiffer RF, Sucha EL. "On-off"-induced lethal hyperthermia. Mov Disord. 1989;4:338–41.
16. Serrano-Duenas M. Neuroleptic malignant syndrome-like, or--dopaminergic malignant syndrome--due to levodopa therapy withdrawal. Clinical features in 11 patients. Parkinsonism Relat Disord. 2003;9:175–8.
17. Keyser DL, Rodnitzky RL. Neuroleptic malignant syndrome in Parkinson's disease after withdrawal or alteration of dopaminergic therapy. Arch Intern Med. 1991;151:794–6.
18. Onofrj M, Bonanni L, Cossu G, Manca D, Stocchi F, Thomas A. Emergencies in parkinsonism: akinetic crisis, life-threatening dyskinesias, and polyneuropathy during L-Dopa gel treatment. Parkinsonism Relat Disord. 2009;15(Suppl 3):S233–6.
19. Newman EJ, Grosset DG, Kennedy PG. The parkinsonism-hyperpyrexia syndrome. Neurocrit Care. 2009;10:136–40.
20. Kipps CM, Fung VS, Grattan-Smith P, de Moore GM, Morris JG. Movement disorder emergencies. Mov Disord. 2005;20:322–34.
21. Munhoz RP, Scorr LM, Factor SA. Movement disorders emergencies. Curr Opin Neurol. 2015;28:406–12.
22. Grover S, Sathpathy A, Reddy SC, Mehta S, Sharma N. Parkinsonism-hyperpyrexia syndrome: a case report and review of literature. Ind J Psychiatry. 2018;60:499–503.
23. Alty J, Robson J, Duggan-Carter P, Jamieson S. What to do when people with Parkinson's disease cannot take their usual oral medications. Pract Neurol. 2016;16:122–8.
24. Sechi GP, Tanda F, Mutani R. Fatal hyperpyrexia after withdrawal of levodopa. Neurology. 1984;34:249–51.
25. Figa-Talamanca L, Gualandi C, Di Meo L, Di Battista G, Neri G, Lo RF. Hyperthermia after discontinuance of levodopa and bromocriptine therapy: impaired dopamine receptors a possible cause. Neurology. 1985;35:258–61.
26. Hirschorn KA, Greenberg HS. Successful treatment of levodopa-induced myoclonus and levodopa withdrawal-induced neuroleptic malignant syndrome. A case report. Clin Neuropharmacol. 1988;11:278–81.
27. Mayeux R, Stern Y, Mulvey K, Cote L. Reappraisal of temporary levodopa withdrawal ("drug holiday") in Parkinson's disease. N Engl J Med. 1985;313:724–8.
28. Factor SA, Molho ES, Podskalny GD, Brown D. Parkinson's disease: drug-induced psychiatric states. Adv Neurol. 1995;65:115–38.
29. Iwuagwu CU, Riley D, Bonoma RA. Neuroleptic malignant-like syndrome in an elderly patient caused by abrupt withdrawal of tolcapone, a-catechol-o-methyl transferase inhibitor. Am J Med. 2000;108:517–8.
30. Cunningham MA, Darby DG, Donnan GA. Controlled-release delivery of L-dopa associated with nonfatal hyperthermia, rigidity, and autonomic dysfunction. Neurology. 1991;41:942–3.
31. Henderson VW, Wooten GF. Neuroleptic malignant syndrome: a pathogenetic role for dopamine receptor blockade? Neurology. 1981;31:132–7.
32. Mizuta E, Yamasaki S, Nakatake M, Kuno S. Neuroleptic malignant syndrome in a parkinsonian woman during the premenstrual period. Neurology. 1993;43:1048–9.
33. Cao L, Katz RH. Acute hypernatremia and neuroleptic malignant syndrome in Parkinson disease. Am J Med Sci. 1999;318:67–8.
34. Bonnici A, Ruiner CE, St-Laurent L, Hornstein D. An interaction between levodopa and enteral nutrition resulting in neuroleptic malignant-like syndrome and prolonged ICU stay. Ann Pharmacother. 2010;44:1504–7.
35. Deep-Brain Stimulation for Parkinson's Disease Study G, Obeso JA, Olanow CW, et al. Deep-brain stimulation of the subthalamic nucleus or the pars interna of the globus pallidus in Parkinson's disease. N Engl J Med. 2001;345:956–63.
36. Vingerhoets FJ, Villemure JG, Temperli P, Pollo C, Pralong E, Ghika J. Subthalamic DBS replaces levodopa in Parkinson's disease: two-year follow-up. Neurology. 2002;58:396–401.

37. Kleiner-Fisman G, Saint-Cyr JA, Miyasaki J, Lozano A, Lang AE. Subthalamic DBS replaces levodopa in Parkinson's disease. Neurology. 2002;59:1293–4. author reply 1294
38. Reuter S, Deuschl G, Berg D, Helmers A, Falk D, Witt K. Life-threatening DBS withdrawal syndrome in Parkinson's disease can be treated with early reimplantation. Parkinsonism Relat Disord. 2018;56:88–92.
39. Kim JH, Kwon TH, Koh SB, Park JY. Parkinsonism-hyperpyrexia syndrome after deep brain stimulation surgery: case report. Neurosurgery. 2010;66:E1029.
40. Govindappa ST, Abbas MM, Hosurkar G, Varma RG, Muthane UB. Parkinsonism hyperpyrexia syndrome following deep brain stimulation. Parkinsonism Relat Disord. 2015;21:1284–5.
41. Urasaki E, Fukudome T, Hirose M, Nakane S, Matsuo H, Yamakawa Y. Neuroleptic malignant syndrome (parkinsonism-hyperpyrexia syndrome) after deep brain stimulation of the subthalamic nucleus. J Clin Neurosci. 2013;20:740–1.
42. Rajan R, Krishnan S, Kesavapisharady KK, Kishore A. Malignant subthalamic nucleus-deep brain stimulation withdrawal syndrome in Parkinson's disease. Move Disord Clin Pract. 2016;3:288–91.
43. Azar J, Elinav H, Safadi R, Soliman M. Malignant deep brain stimulator withdrawal syndrome. BMJ Case Rep. 2019;12:e229122.
44. Liu CJ, Crnkovic A, Dalfino J, Singh LY. Whether to proceed with deep brain stimulator battery change in a patient with signs of potential Sepsis and Parkinson hyperpyrexia syndrome: a case report. A&A Practice. 2017;8:187–91.
45. Kadowaki T, Hashimoto K, Suzuki K, Watanabe Y, Hirata K. Case report: recurrent parkinsonism-hyperpyrexia syndrome following discontinuation of subthalamic deep brain stimulation. Mov Disord. 2011;26:1561–2.
46. Sato Y, Asoh T, Metoki N, Satoh K. Efficacy of methylprednisolone pulse therapy on neuroleptic malignant syndrome in Parkinson's disease. J Neurol Neurosurg Psychiatry. 2003;74:574–6.
47. Ueda M, Hamamoto M, Nagayama H, Otsubo K, Nito C, Miyazaki T, et al. Susceptibility to neuroleptic malignant syndrome in Parkinson's disease. Neurology. 1999;52:777–81.
48. Bonanni L, Onofrj M, Valente EM, Manzoli L, De Angelis MV, Capasso M, et al. Recurrent and fatal akinetic crisis in genetic-mitochondrial parkinsonisms. Eur J Neurol. 2014;21:1242–6.
49. Fujioka S, Fukae J, Ogura H, Mishima T, Yanamoto S, Higuchi MA, et al. Hospital-based study on emergency admission of patients with Parkinson's disease. Eneurologicalsci. 2016;4:19–21.
50. Mizuno Y, Takubo H, Mizuta E, Kuno S. Malignant syndrome in Parkinson's disease: concept and review of the literature. Parkinsonism Relat Disord. 2003;9(Suppl 1):S3–9.
51. Granner MA, Wooten GF. Neuroleptic malignant syndrome or parkinsonism hyperpyrexia syndrome. Semin Neurol. 1991;11:228–35.
52. Factor SA. Fatal Parkinsonism-hyperpyrexia syndrome in a Parkinson's disease patient while actively treated with deep brain stimulation. Mov Disord. 2007;22:148–9.
53. Ueda M, Hamamoto M, Nagayama H, Okubo S, Amemiya S, Katayama Y. Biochemical alterations during medication withdrawal in Parkinson's disease with and without neuroleptic malignant-like syndrome. J Neurol Neurosurg Psychiatry. 2001;71:111–3.
54. Yamawaki Y, Ogawa N. Successful treatment of levodopa-induced neuroleptic malignant syndrome (NMS) and disseminated intravascular coagulation (DIC) in a patient with Parkinson's disease. Intern Med. 1992;31:1298–302.
55. Fahn S, Oakes D, Shoulson I, Kieburtz K, Rudolph A, Lang A, et al. Levodopa and the progression of Parkinson's disease. N Engl J Med. 2004;351:2498–508.
56. Genis D. Neuroleptic malignant syndrome: impaired dopaminergic systems? Neurology. 1985;35:1806.
57. Martino G, Capasso M, Nasuti M, Bonanni L, Onofrj M, Thomas A. Dopamine transporter single-photon emission computerized tomography supports diagnosis of akinetic crisis of parkinsonism and of neuroleptic malignant syndrome. Medicine (Baltimore). 2015;94:e649.
58. Douglas A, Morris J. It was not just a heatwave! Neuroleptic malignant-like syndrome in a patient with Parkinson's disease. Age Ageing. 2006;35:640–1.

59. Bonuccelli U, Piccini P, Corsini GU, Muratorio A. Apomorphine in malignant syndrome due to levodopa withdrawal. Ital J Neurol Sci. 1992;13:169–70.
60. Colosimo C, Merello M, Albanese A. Clinical usefulness of apomorphine in movement disorders. Clin Neuropharmacol. 1994;17:243–59.
61. Baek MS, Lee HW, Lyoo CH. A patient with recurrent dyskinesia and hyperpyrexia syndrome. J Mov Disord. 2017;10:154–7.
62. Herreros-Rodriguez J, Sanchez-Ferro A. Summertime dyskinesia-hyperpyrexia syndrome: the "dual heat" hypothesis. Clin Neuropharmacol. 2016;39:210–1.
63. Acebron Sanchez-Herrera F, Garcia-Barragan N, Estevez-Fraga C, Martinez-Castrillo JC, Lopez-Sendon Moreno JL. Dyskinesia-hyperpyrexia syndrome under continuous dopaminergic stimulation. Parkinsonism Relat Disord. 2017;36:103–4.
64. Novelli A, Di Vico IA, Terenzi F, Sorbi S, Ramat S. Dyskinesia-hyperpyrexia syndrome in Parkinson's disease with deep brain stimulation and high-dose levodopa/carbidopa and entacapone. Parkinsonism Relat Disord. 2019;64:352–3.
65. Konagaya M, Goto Y, Matsuoka Y, Konishi T, Konagaya Y. Neuroleptic malignant syndrome-like condition in multiple system atrophy. J Neurol Neurosurg Psychiatry. 1997;63:120–1.
66. Friedman JH, Factor SA. Atypical antipsychotics in the treatment of drug-induced psychosis in Parkinson's disease. Mov Disord. 2000;15:201–11.

Neuroleptic Malignant Syndrome

6

Stanley N. Caroff, Stephan C. Mann, Kenneth A. Sullivan, and E. Cabrina Campbell

Patient Vignettes

Patient 1

A 16-year-old woman had been well with no psychiatric history until 1 week prior to admission. She developed difficulty sleeping and bizarre behavior including assaultiveness, sobbing, undressing in public, and thoughts of suicide, prompting admission. On examination, she was labile, agitated, and delusional and experienced tactile, visual, and auditory hallucinations. Neurological exam revealed impaired recall, dyscalculia, and right-sided sensory deficits. Haloperidol (2 mg) orally b.i.d. was started, and she also received 5 mg intramuscularly for worsening agitation. Within a few hours, she developed a temperature of 39.8 °C, tachycardia, diaphoresis, board-like rigidity with cogwheeling, tremors, and mutism. A generalized seizure was observed. Despite administration of diphenylhydantoin, steroids, diazepam, benztropine, and three electroconvulsive treatments, she remained rigid and unresponsive with temperatures rising to 40.5 °C. Laboratory examination revealed elevated serum creatine kinase (CK) (44,000 IU) and peripheral leukocytosis. Serial EEGs showed diffuse generalized slowing, and CT scan of the head was normal. Lumber puncture on three occasions revealed 30–70 WBC/mm^3 (98% lymphocytes) with normal pressure, glucose, and protein suggesting encephalitis due to a viral or atypical pathogen, but cultures, stains, serology, and polymerase chain reaction for viral antigens were negative. Haloperidol was discontinued, and

S. N. Caroff (✉) · K. A. Sullivan · E. C. Campbell
Department of Psychiatry, Corporal Michael J. Crescenz VA Medical Center and the University of Pennsylvania Perelman School of Medicine, Philadelphia, PA, USA
e-mail: caroffs@pennmedicine.upenn.edu

S. C. Mann
Private Practice, Harleysville, PA, USA

© Springer Nature Switzerland AG 2022
S. J. Frucht (ed.), *Movement Disorder Emergencies*, Current Clinical Neurology,
https://doi.org/10.1007/978-3-030-75898-1_6

dantrolene and amantadine were administered. Over 2 weeks, she became alert, verbal, and ambulatory, while memory deficits and dysarthria resolved after 6 months.

Patient 2

A 65-year-old man with a history of alcohol dependence was admitted with abdominal pain and nausea. Observation of a mass on an MRI scan of the abdomen led to surgery for a perforated diverticulum. Postoperatively, he appeared restless, agitated, and delirious. He received haloperidol (2 mg) and lorazepam (2 mg) intravenously every 2 h. Within 24 h, he became unresponsive, tachycardic, hypotensive, tremulous, rigid, and febrile with temperature reaching 41.5 °C. Laboratory examination revealed hypoxia, metabolic acidosis, elevated serum CK (21,500 IU), and leukocytosis. An EEG showed diffuse generalized slowing, and a CT scan of the head demonstrated mild cortical atrophy. Haloperidol was discontinued, but he developed sudden respiratory arrest requiring intubation. Lorazepam was continued, and dantrolene and bromocriptine were administered. Subsequently, he was treated for acute renal failure and disseminated intravascular coagulation. He gradually improved over 4 weeks but continued to exhibit persistent dysarthria and mild ataxia several months later.

Introduction

Neuroleptic malignant syndrome (NMS) was first identified by Delay and colleagues during early trials of haloperidol [1]. Although subsequently studied in France and Japan [2, 3], NMS remained obscure for an additional two decades until a cascade of hundreds of published clinical reports increased recognition and confirmed acceptance of NMS as a severe drug reaction associated with dopamine-receptor blocking agents used primarily as antipsychotics [4–9]. The resistance and prolonged delay in acceptance of NMS as an iatrogenic condition occurred in part because it was often misdiagnosed as a form of malignant catatonia attributed to psychosis or schizophrenia, leading to tragic and fatal consequences of continued or even more aggressive antipsychotic treatment [6, 10].

In subsequent years, the accumulation of published clinical observations enabled a more precise definition of NMS, clarified risk factors and treatment strategies, renewed interest in related hyperthermic disorders, and shed light on the pathophysiology of the syndrome. Increased awareness facilitating early diagnosis, more conservative use of antipsychotic medications, and the introduction of newer antipsychotics with fewer neurological side effects have reduced the incidence and mortality of NMS. Nevertheless, the evaluation, differential diagnosis, and treatment of NMS in medical as well as psychiatric settings remain unfamiliar to most practicing physicians. This is alarming given that antipsychotics are increasingly promoted and prescribed to an expanding number of patients, and that NMS remains potentially lethal if unrecognized, underscoring the need for increased awareness of this serious drug reaction.

Epidemiology

Incidence

Although NMS occurs relatively infrequently, the widespread use of dopamine-receptor blocking agents in medicine and psychiatry suggests that the absolute number of cases may be significant. For example, data from the US Agency for Healthcare Research and Quality indicate that about 2000–2500 cases of NMS are diagnosed annually in hospitals in the United States. Annual healthcare costs of $70 million and a mortality rate of 10% underscore the continuing public health impact of this drug reaction (http://hcup.ahrq.gov/HCUPnet.asp).

The incidence of NMS varies depending on the sample size and risk of the population studied, prescribing practices and methods of case ascertainment [11]. There is marked heterogeneity in methodology among incidence studies of NMS. Combining data from published studies of NMS occurring among groups of psychiatric patients treated with antipsychotics, we previously estimated the incidence of NMS to be about 0.2%, while other early estimates reported in the literature ranged even higher [7]. In a meta-analysis of 26 published studies of the incidence of NMS, a pooled mean incidence of 140/141,291 (0.099%) was calculated [11]. However, more recent rates in two large-scale prescription database studies were reported as 0.02%, equivalent to one case developing in 5000 patients receiving antipsychotics [12, 13]. There is a significant correlation between the estimated incidence of NMS in various studies and the size of the sample population at risk [11], suggesting that the lower frequency of NMS in the large database studies may be closest to the true incidence of the disorder. The apparent reduction in incidence of NMS reported over time, which may not be statistically significant [11], could be the result of more conservative dosing of antipsychotics, minimizing risk factors, early recognition of incipient cases, and the widespread use of newer and less potent antipsychotic drugs. As an example of the effect of drugs with less affinity for the dopamine receptor, Stubner et al. found a tenfold lower incidence of NMS with clozapine compared with haloperidol [12].

Risk Factors

Several studies have been conducted to identify risk factors for the syndrome [14–16]. NMS has been reported in both sexes and all age and ethnic groups implying that anyone exposed to dopamine-receptor blocking agents is at risk. Although recent studies have revealed that NMS is most often reported in young adults with a peak between 20 and 25 years of age, in males by a ratio of 3:2, and in patients of non-white ethnicities [16, 17]; differences and prejudices in the rates of underlying psychotic diagnoses and prescribing practices may have biased these findings. NMS is rarely reported among children, but recent reviews indicate that youngsters, especially male adolescents, may be affected [18–21]. Although elevated environmental heat and humidity have been proposed as contributing factors in a few cases, NMS occurs independent of ambient conditions. NMS is not limited to specific neuropsychiatric diagnoses. It has developed in patients treated with antipsychotics for diverse psychiatric illnesses, as well as in patients without any evidence of brain or behavioral disorders who received dopamine-receptor antagonists (e.g., promethazine, droperidol, prochlorperazine, metoclopramide) for agitation, sedation, or gastrointestinal disorders [22]. Previous authors have proposed an increased risk of NMS in patients with schizophrenia, mood disorders, developmental disorders, organic brain syndromes, pre-existing catatonia, and disorders affecting the basal ganglia [8, 23, 24]. Adults with intellectual disabilities may be highly susceptible and were three times as likely as controls to develop NMS when treated with antipsychotics in one retrospective study [25]. There have been several reports of NMS in patients with anti-N-methyl-D-aspartate receptor (NMDAR) encephalitis who received antipsychotics [24, 26–28]. It is unclear whether autoimmune impairment of NMDA receptors per se imparts special risk of NMS, or whether patients with encephalitis and other inflammatory brain diseases are at high risk regardless of etiology. Several systemic and metabolic factors have been correlated with the risk of NMS including exhaustion, agitation, dehydration, low serum iron, and use of physical restraints [2, 7, 8, 29].

Although the occurrence of NMS among family members has been reported [16, 30], studies of genetic risk have been limited to association studies of targeted genes in relatively small patient samples. Suspected pathogenic polymorphisms have been investigated in dopamine and other neurotransmitter receptor genes [31–35], in genes coding for cytochrome enzymes associated with antipsychotic metabolism [36], and in ryanodine-receptor genes associated with risk of malignant hyperthermia [37–39], all with conflicting results. Further large case–control studies including genome-wide association studies will be needed to confirm population frequencies possibly implicating multiple genetic variants with respect to NMS that could ideally enable screening for risk prior to antipsychotic treatment.

Pharmacologically, about 15–20% of patients who develop NMS experienced a similar episode during prior exposure to neuroleptics, suggesting a possible trait susceptibility with limited penetrance of the disorder [40]. Virtually all classes of drugs that induce dopamine-receptor blockade have been associated with NMS . This includes all dopamine-receptor blocking antipsychotics, with higher potency antipsychotics associated with greater risk; haloperidol has accounted for about half of all reported cases [12]. Although newer, less potent antipsychotics have clearly been associated with NMS in clinical reports, the incidence of NMS has been less than with haloperidol and older antipsychotics in reviews and database studies [12, 17, 21, 41, 42]. However, a possible signal of relative risk has been reported for aripiprazole in two of three retrospective studies [17, 21, 43]. In addition, clinical manifestations of NMS associated with newer antipsychotics, especially clozapine, have often been described as atypical, with less severe and prominent neurological features of rigidity and tremor [43, 44]. Research on emerging agents that may have antipsychotic effects apart from dopamine-blocking mechanisms, e.g., pimavanserin [45] and trace amine-associated receptor-1 agonists [46], could lead to further decline in risk of NMS and other drug-induced movement disorders.

NMS cases, including some that were fatal, have also been reported in association with other dopamine-receptor blocking drugs prescribed by medical and surgical practitioners [22]. These include prochlorperazine, metoclopramide, droperidol, and promethazine [47, 48]. Haloperidol is also frequently used in medical and critical care settings for management of agitation and delirium. We believe that cases of NMS in these settings remain seriously under-reported and under-recognized [22, 49, 50]. Tetrabenazine used to treat hyperkinetic movement disorders, e.g., Huntington's disease, tardive dyskinesia, in addition to two other recently approved vesicular monoamine transporter-2 (VMAT-2) inhibitors (valbenazine and deutetrabenazine), may increase the risk of NMS by presynaptic dopamine depletion [51]. Rare cases of NMS have been reported primarily with tetrabenazine, which also has weak dopamine-receptor blocking properties, but it is possible that combinations of dopamine depleting and dopamine-receptor blocking drugs could act synergistically in triggering NMS.

NMS is not a result of overdosage with antipsychotics, usually occurring within the therapeutic range. However, several studies have suggested that patients who develop NMS are more likely to have received relatively higher doses, more rapid titration, more parenteral injections, and polypharmacy with multiple antipsychotics compared to controls [14, 15]. The relative risk of NMS with long-acting depot antipsychotics has been controversial, with some concerns regarding greater incidence or a more prolonged course. However, a recent report found no association between depot administration and NMS in general, except for the use of older first-generation depot antipsychotics, primarily flupenthixol [17]. A recent report from a company clinical trial database of only one case of NMS among 5008 patients treated with long-acting depot paliperidone was indeed complicated by concurrent treatment with flupenthixol [52]. It is currently unknown whether or not adjunctive or concomitant medications (e.g., antiparkinsonian drugs, benzodiazepines, or lithium) increase or decrease the risk of NMS. Recently, the FDA required manufacturers of antidepressants to add a warning to their package labeling about NMS-like reactions associated with these drugs when used either alone or in combination with antipsychotics. Concurrent administration of antipsychotics and other drugs, including lithium, SSRIs, or SNRIs may increase the risk of NMS, but alternatively these events could be instances of serotonin syndrome [53]. It is important to realize that the association of these risk factors with rare cases of NMS does not outweigh the benefits of antipsychotic therapy for the vast majority of patients for whom they are properly indicated [9].

Pathophysiology

Although the lack of an accepted animal model of NMS has limited efforts to clarify mechanisms, several lines of clinical evidence support a reduction in dopamine activity in the brain as the trigger underlying NMS [8, 54]. All drugs implicated in NMS share the property of dopamine-receptor blockade. Clinical studies indicate that the risk of NMS correlates with dose, potency, rate, and route of administration of dopamine antagonists [14]. Dopaminergic drugs have been administered empirically and found to be effective therapy for NMS in some studies [55–57]. Most convincingly by analogy, patients with Parkinson's disease have developed a syndrome that is indistinguishable from NMS following abrupt withdrawal of dopamine agonists or levodopa known as the parkinsonism-hyperpyrexia syndrome. Patients with lesions interrupting dopamine pathways have developed a syndrome of akinetic mutism and hyperthermia resembling NMS. Studies of neurotransmitter metabolites in cerebrospinal fluid obtained from patients with acute NMS reveal central dopamine hypoactivity as a possible trait marker for NMS, based on comparatively low concentrations of the dopamine metabolite homovanillic acid [58, 59]. A few preliminary studies have also suggested abnormalities in dopamine-receptor genes of patients who recovered from NMS episodes, although results have not been consistently replicated [8]. Studies of clinical correlates of frontal-subcortical circuits provide a framework within which individual NMS symptoms may be mapped to perturbations in specific dopamine pathways [54]. Finally, changes in dopamine pathways in response to stress may be implicated as an additional state-related cofactor involved in the triggering of NMS [54].

Although the evidence for a central role of dopaminergic mechanisms in the pathophysiology of NMS is persuasive, other primary or secondary mechanisms have been proposed. These include a relative excess of glutaminergic transmission secondary to dopamine blockade, effects of low serum iron on dopamine receptor function, effects of reduced activity of gamma aminobutyric acid, and dysregulation of the sympathetic nervous system [29, 54, 59–61]. Finally, even though NMS and malignant hyperthermia induced by anesthetics (MH) differ in initial pharmacologic triggering mechanisms—MH attributed to a primary pharmacogenetic defect in skeletal muscle rather than a centrally driven process in NMS—their similar clinical presentations as hypermetabolic syndromes suggest potential parallels. Clinical reports of NMS episodes following administration of antipsychotics in patients with MH susceptibility, pre-existing myopathies, or unexplained CK elevations lend support to overlapping or convergent mechanisms between NMS and MH [8, 22, 62, 63]. Although nonspecific, the effect of dantrolene in reducing skeletal muscle metabolism and heat production has been beneficial in NMS as well as MH crises [55, 56, 64–66]. This clinical evidence combined with reported pharmacologic effects of antipsychotics on CK levels, membrane permeability, calcium regulation and contractility in skeletal muscle are intriguing and merit further investigation [67].

Clinical Characteristics

Prodromal Signs

In addition to the development of reliable risk factors, it would be useful to identify early signs of NMS in order to abort the progression of the syndrome by discontinuing triggering drugs. Although occasional cases of NMS may have a fulminant onset within hours after drug administration, the initial progression of symptoms is usually insidious, occurring over days. Neurologic signs of muscle rigidity and altered mental status occur early, followed by autonomic changes and hyperthermia; in over 80% of cases in which a single presenting sign was reported, rigidity or mental status changes constituted the initial manifestation [68]. Other prodromal signs may include obtundation, catatonia, tachycardia, tachypnea, labile blood pressure, dysarthria, dysphagia, diaphoresis, sialorrhea, incontinence, rigidity, myoclonus, tremors, low-grade fevers, or serum CK elevations. Clinicians should be prepared to diagnose NMS early and to document the rationale for cessation versus continuation of antipsychotic therapy. However, these early signs are not specific for NMS, do not necessarily progress to NMS, and do not invariably precede the syndrome [7].

Signs and Symptoms

Clinical features of NMS are listed in Table 6.1. NMS may be conceptualized as a form of drug-induced hyperthermia or hypermetabolism, usually associated with profuse sweating. Extreme temperature elevations represent a medical emergency

Table 6.1   Clinical features of NMS

Administration of dopamine-receptor blocking agents
Signs and symptoms
Hyperthermia (>38 °C)
Muscle rigidity ± cogwheeling
Tremor and myoclonus
Mental status changes (stupor, mutism, and delirium)
Autonomic instability (tachycardia and labile blood pressure)
Tachypnea and dyspnea
Diaphoresis, sialorrhea, and incontinence
Dysarthria and dysphagia
Associated laboratory findings
Muscle enzyme elevations (CK, LDH, transaminases, and aldolase), myoglobinuria, leukocytosis, metabolic acidosis, hypoxia, low serum iron, elevated serum catecholamines, and slowing on EEG
Complications
Cardiorespiratory arrest, acute renal failure, rhabdomyolysis, pulmonary emboli, aspiration pneumonia, disseminated intravascular coagulation, limb contractures, and ischemic brain damage
Exclusion of other central, systemic, and toxic causes of hyperthermia

and predispose to complications, including irreversible brain damage if not reduced immediately. There are few disorders that result in extreme elevations in temperature, signifying an underlying disruption of thermoregulatory systems, as occurs in NMS due to drug effects on hypothalamic centers; thus, the diagnosis of NMS is more likely in a patient with very high temperatures, whereas the differential diagnosis in a patient with low-grade temperature elevations is quite broad. Generalized rigidity, often described as "lead-pipe," is a core feature of NMS and is usually associated with rhabdomyolysis. Cogwheeling, spontaneous and action myoclonus of multifocal distribution, and tremors are often described, along with other movement disorders. Mental status changes include clouding of consciousness ranging from stupor to coma, delirium, or new-onset catatonia. The classic NMS patient appears awake but dazed, stuporous, and mute. Autonomic activation and instability are common, manifested by tachycardia, oscillations in blood pressure, and tachypnea. The extent and severity of symptoms may vary significantly between individuals.

O━━━🔑 The classic appearance of a patient with NMS is a dazed, stuporous, mute patient, with high fever, generalized rigidity, and autonomic instability.

Laboratory Evaluation

Although several laboratory abnormalities have been reported in NMS, none are specific or pathognomonic for the diagnosis [8]. Instead, a comprehensive laboratory evaluation is essential in excluding other causes of hyperthermia and detecting medical illnesses. Serum CK is usually moderately elevated in up to 90% of cases but occasionally reaches extraordinary levels reflecting massive rhabdomyolysis [66, 69]. Rhabdomyolysis is multifactorial in origin, stemming from rigidity, immobility, hyperthermia, ischemia, and possibly direct drug effects on skeletal muscle. Although elevations in CK are not specific to NMS, monitoring of the enzyme level remains important as a measure of the severity of rhabdomyolysis and the attendant risk of renal failure. Rhabdomyolysis is also manifested by increases in serum myoglobin, aldolase, transaminases, and lactic acid dehydrogenase concentrations. Other frequently described laboratory abnormalities include metabolic acidosis, hypoxia, decreased serum iron concentrations, elevated serum catecholamines, electrolyte abnormalities, leukocytosis with or without a left shift, and coagulopathies including those associated with disseminated intravascular coagulation.

Nonfocal generalized slowing on EEG, consistent with encephalopathy, has been reported in over half of NMS cases [40]. Brain imaging studies, cerebrospinal fluid examination, and sepsis evaluation are typically negative, allowing for the exclusion of other causes of fever and neurologic deterioration [40]. A few patients with NMS have recently been reported to exhibit reversible MRI lesions with transiently restricted diffusion in the splenium of the corpus callosum [70]. These radiological findings resolved after recovery and appear to represent a nonspecific "splenial lesion syndrome" associated with diverse causes of encephalopathy. In a recent study, a patient with NMS showed significant reduction in caudate and putamen binding of the presynaptic dopamine transporter on single-photon emission computerized tomography, suggesting the possibility of diagnostic imaging if further replicated [71].

Diagnostic Criteria

Although a number of rating scales and diagnostic criteria have been proposed [8, 72, 73], the degree of agreement between them is only modest [74]. To address this issue, an international, multispecialty panel of NMS experts was convened recently to reach a consensus using a standardized Delphi process to identify the clinical features that are most valuable in making a diagnosis of NMS and to develop a priority point scoring system to quantify the relative importance of each criterion (Table 6.2) [75]. The key features of NMS that were agreed upon included: exposure to a dopamine antagonist or dopamine agonist withdrawal, within the past 72 h; hyperthermia (>100.4 °F or >38.0 °C on at least two occasions, measured orally); muscle rigidity; mental status alteration (reduced or fluctuating level of consciousness); CK elevation (at least four times upper limit of normal); evidence of sympathetic nervous system lability and hypermetabolism; and a negative work-up for infectious, toxic, metabolic, or other neurologic causes. In a subsequent validation study comparing the International Expert Consensus (IEC) criteria with DSM-IV-TR and consultant opinions on 221 clinician-initiated calls to a national

Table 6.2 International Expert Consensus NMS Diagnostic Criteria [75]

Diagnostic criterion	Priority score
Exposure to dopamine antagonist, or dopamine agonist withdrawal, within past 72 h	20
Hyperthermia (>100.4 °F or >38.0 °C on at least two occasions, measured orally)	18
Rigidity	17
Mental status alteration (reduced or fluctuating level of consciousness)	13
CK elevation (at least four times upper limit of normal)	10
Sympathetic nervous system lability, defined as at least two of the following:	10
Blood pressure elevation (systolic or diastolic ≥25% above baseline)	
Blood pressure fluctuation (≥20 mmHg diastolic change or ≥25 mmHg systolic change within 24 h)	
Diaphoresis	
Urinary incontinence	
Hypermetabolism, defined as heart rate increase (≥25% above baseline) and respiratory rate increase (≥50% above baseline)	5
Negative work-up for infectious, toxic, metabolic, and neurologic causes	7
Total	100

Reprinted with permission from Gurrera et al. [76]. https://journals.lww.com/psychopharmacology/toc/2017/02000
CK creatine kinase

telephone consultation service (www.nmsis.org), a threshold score of 74 achieved the highest agreement (sensitivity, 69.6%; specificity, 90.7%) [76].

Clinical Course and Outcome

NMS results from neurochemical changes induced by antipsychotics or other dopamine-receptor blockers during the initial stages of treatment or after dosages are increased. In a review by Caroff and Mann [40], 16% of patients developed NMS within 24 h of initiating neuroleptic treatment, 66% by 1 week, and 96% within the first 30 days. It would be unusual for NMS to develop later than 1 month after treatment initiation, unless the dose was increased or another antipsychotic was added. Only 4% of reported cases developed NMS beyond 30 days. Conversely, once antipsychotics were discontinued, NMS is self-limited barring complications. Following discontinuation of oral antipsychotics, the mean recovery time has been estimated at 7–10 days [7]. About 63% of patients recover within 1 week and nearly all within 30 days [40].

In some cases, the course of NMS may be prolonged. For example, patients receiving long-acting depot antipsychotics may remain ill nearly twice as long [7]. Occasional patients may develop a residual catatonic-parkinsonian state that can persist for weeks to months if left untreated after the acute hyperthermic and hyper-metabolic symptoms of NMS subside [77]. Although dopamine agonists and benzo-diazepines have been advocated for treatment of this residual state, electroconvulsive therapy (ECT) appears to be more rapidly effective with reduced mortality in reported series [77]. Early diagnosis and intervention have contributed to a decline in the mortality rate, but not all patients recover from NMS. Fatalities may occur as a result of sudden cardiorespiratory arrest, aspiration pneumonia, pulmonary emboli, acute renal failure, or disseminated intravascular coagulation. Findings at autopsy are usually nonspecific and variable, depending on complications. Persistent clinical sequelae of NMS are rare in patients who recover. However, cases of amnestic syndromes, extrapyramidal and cerebellar disorders, peripheral neuropathy, myopathy, and contractures have been reported.

Evaluation and Differential Diagnosis

The differential diagnosis of NMS encompasses a broad range of disorders presenting with encephalopathy, neurological signs, and fever, necessitating a thorough medical and neurologic evaluation. Despite careful investigation, the cause of the syndrome in some patients may remain unclear or reflect multiple determinants. Other disorders that can resemble NMS include primary disorders of the brain and systemic disorders that secondarily affect brain function. Among the former are infectious encephalitis, structural lesions, and rare cases of nonconvulsive status epilepticus [7, 8].

We have been consulted on several cases resembling the patient described in our first clinical vignette in which a patient with underlying encephalitis is initially misdiagnosed with a psychiatric condition and then develops NMS following administration of antipsychotics [24, 28]. Behavioral symptoms typical of orbito-frontal lobe (lability, disinhibition, and akinetic mutism) and temporal lobe (rage, terror, fear, and foreboding) syndromes that are uncharacteristic of psychiatric disorders were observed in the first patient and with subtle focal neurological signs may serve as "red flags" for underlying encephalitis in such cases [27]. Most often, a causative pathogen is not identified, or these cases are found to represent autoimmune or paraneoplastic encephalitides [78]. Recent reports of anti-N-methyl-D-aspartate receptor (NMDAR) encephalitis have renewed interest in the possibility that patients with this or other forms of encephalitis have antipsychotic sensitivity [26, 27]. These observations led us to underscore the importance of considering encephalitis in the differential diagnosis of patients who present with the new onset of psychosis and develop NMS after treatment with antipsychotics. Such cases imply that encephalitic patients in general may be at increased risk for NMS and other drug-induced movement disorders.

⊶━━▀ Patients with NMDA receptor-mediated encephalitis are likely at greater risk for developing NMS.

Advanced stages of psychotic disorders associated with excited or stuporous catatonia (delirious mania or malignant catatonia) can progress to exhaustion, hyperthermia, and death [79, 80]. Although the incidence of malignant catatonia has decreased, it still occurs and can be indistinguishable from NMS. Indeed, NMS has been conceptualized as a drug-induced iatrogenic form of malignant catatonia. In either NMS or malignant catatonia, antipsychotics should be discontinued because most NMS episodes are self-limited and should subside within 2 weeks after drug discontinuation, and in idiopathic malignant catatonia, antipsychotics appear to be ineffective and even detrimental. In contrast, ECT appears to be the treatment of choice in malignant catatonia and may be effective in NMS as well [57, 81].

In relation to systemic disorders, patients with common and benign forms of anti-psychotic-induced parkinsonism or catatonia may develop fever from coincident infections or dehydration and be mistakenly diagnosed as having NMS. Antipsychotics have also been associated with rhabdomyolysis alone without other features of NMS, and the relationship between these two drug-induced phenomena is unclear. Hyperthermia may be observed in patients with thyrotoxicosis and pheochromocytoma, which can be distinguished from NMS by the absence of rigidity. Systemic lupus erythematosus or other autoimmune diseases affecting the brain may present with fever and neurologic signs. Cases of NMS-like episodes responsive to dantrolene in diabetic patients with hyperglycemic hyperosmolar syndrome have been reported, especially in children [82, 83]. Exertional or classic heatstroke may develop in patients during hot weather and may be confused with NMS [84]. Furthermore, antipsychotic treatment may predispose to heatstroke by blocking thermoregulatory heat loss pathways. Unlike NMS, muscle rigidity is unusual in heatstroke.

Diverse toxins and drugs have been associated with hyperthermia and must be considered in the differential diagnosis of NMS. Volatile anesthetics and succinylcholine are associated with MH during surgery, which can be confused with NMS if antipsychotics are administered perioperatively [22]. Although NMS has been reported before and after surgery, it appears unlikely to develop intraoperatively in contrast to MH. Furthermore, centrally derived muscle rigidity associated with NMS can be reversed by neuromuscular blockade, whereas rigidity associated with MH reflects a defect within skeletal muscle that does not respond to paralyzing agents.

Abrupt withdrawal of levodopa or dopamine agonists in patients with Parkinson's disease has resulted in the parkinsonism-hyperpyrexia syndrome indistinguishable from NMS, reflecting the same mechanism of acute dopamine deficiency [85]. A similar syndrome has been observed after device failure or explantation of deep brain stimulation devices in Parkinson's disease patients [86]. Abrupt discontinuation of oral or intrathecal administration of the GABAergic agent, baclofen, can produce a similar syndrome, which has also been observed after intrathecal instillation of contrast materials. Illegal stimulants (amphetamines, 3,4-methylenedioxym ethamphetamine, and cocaine) and hallucinogens have been associated with hyperthermia, seizures, rigidity, rhabdomyolysis, and death. Anticholinergic drugs used to treat extrapyramidal disorders can result in atropinic toxicity manifested by fever without rigidity. Withdrawal states, such as delirium tremens, can also be difficult to distinguish from NMS, especially if antipsychotics have been administered to control agitation or psychotic symptoms. Increasingly, chemicals and supplements obtained "over-the-internet" (2,4-dinitrophenol, cathinones) have induced NMS-like toxic syndromes. Finally, serotonin syndrome is often considered in the differential of NMS and has been increasingly reported in association with serotonergic agents introduced for the treatment of depression or migraine headaches, and subsequently expanded to use in many disorders [87]. Although serotonin syndrome can present as an NMS-like hypermetabolic state in its most severe form associated with monoamine oxidase inhibitors (including antidepressants, linezolid, methylene blue, and St. John's wort), it usually presents with milder and more transient symptoms indicative of an agitated delirium.

Our second vignette illustrates the need to exclude several of these conditions before settling on the diagnosis of NMS. This is a particularly challenging task in critical care units where fever commonly occurs as a result of infections or other conditions. It is unusual for MH to occur postoperatively and, therefore, MH was an unlikely diagnosis in this case. In contrast, NMS has been reported in the context of antipsychotic treatment of postoperative agitation. Furthermore, this patient was alcohol dependent raising the possibility of a withdrawal reaction. Although CK elevations can be observed in alcoholics as well as in patients with NMS, the characteristic rigidity of NMS is not a typical feature of alcohol withdrawal. However, we have previously suggested that patients with severe withdrawal from alcohol or sedatives may be at increased risk of developing NMS after antipsychotics are administered [8]. Both clinical vignettes illustrate the fact that NMS is a diagnosis of exclusion, stemming from antipsychotic-induced effects on the brain.

> NMS is a diagnosis of exclusion, requiring a high index of suspicion.

Treatment

The mainstay of treatment of NMS includes risk reduction, early diagnosis, cessation of dopamine-receptor blocking medications (and/or dopamine depleting medications), and provision of intensive medical and nursing care [9, 57]. There is less evidence and consensus concerning the comparative efficacy of specific pharmacologic agents and ECT in the treatment of NMS. This derives from the fact that with early recognition and prompt cessation of antipsychotics, NMS is a self-limited disorder in most cases, regardless of the specific therapy that is employed. Furthermore, there are no controlled treatment trials. It is difficult to compare any specific treatments because NMS is rare, self-limited, heterogeneous and unpredictable in onset, progression, and outcome. Nevertheless, there are rational theories and empirical clinical data that lead to consideration of specific pharmacologic agents and ECT in the treatment of NMS.

Based on available evidence, we recommend that specific treatment of NMS should be individualized and based empirically on the character, duration, and severity of clinical signs and symptoms (Table 6.3) [9, 57, 88]. In many cases, supportive care alone after drug cessation with close monitoring for progression of symptoms or complications may be sufficient until recovery occurs. While anticholinergic drugs are effective in relieving drug-induced parkinsonism, they impair heat loss by sweating and are therefore contraindicated in NMS. Benzodiazepines are effective in reversing catatonia, easy to administer, and can be tried initially in most cases. Trials of bromocriptine, amantadine, or other dopamine agonists may be a reasonable next step in patients with moderate symptoms of NMS that include prominent parkinsonian signs, or when withdrawal of dopamine agonists (e.g., amantadine) are implicated as an etiology [89]. Although amantadine enhances dopamine transmission, it is also a noncompetitive NMDA receptor antagonist that may be its predominant effect at therapeutic doses [90]. When severe symptoms render treatment by the oral route impractical, nasogastric tube access, intravenous, or subcutaneous administration of dopamine agonists, e.g., lisuride or apomorphine, may be an option [91]. In addition, newer dopamine agonists developed for transdermal delivery may facilitate administration of dopaminergic drugs under extreme circumstances (e.g., rotigotine).

Anticholinergics are contraindicated in NMS.

Dantrolene appears to be beneficial primarily when significant rigidity and severe hyperthermia develop as manifestations of a full-blown hypermetabolic state [55, 56, 64–66]. As an inhibitor of skeletal muscle rigidity and hypermetabolism by enhancing sequestration of calcium in sarcoplasmic reticulum via the ryanodine receptor, dantrolene has been associated with rapid reduction of extreme temperature elevations in many clinical reports. None of the above medications have been reliably effective in all reported NMS cases in which they have been administered, and they are often administered in more severe or refractory cases after supportive management has failed to reduce symptoms [92]. Furthermore, positive drug effects

Table 6.3 Proposed treatment algorithm for NMS [9]

Woodbury stage [88]	Clinical presentation	Supportive care	First-line interventions	Second-line interventions
Stage I: drug-induced parkinsonism	Rigidity; tremor	Discontinue, reduce or switch antipsychotics	Anticholinergic agents	
Stage II: drug-induced catatonia	Rigidity; mutism; stupor	Discontinue, reduce, or switch antipsychotics	Lorazepam (1–2 mg i.m. or i.v. every 4–6 h)	
Stage III: mild or early NMS	Mild rigidity; catatonia or confusion; temperature >38 °C (100.4 °F); heart rate >100 bpm	Discontinue antipsychotics; carefully monitor for progression; correct risk factors	Lorazepam (1–2 mg i.m. or i.v. every 4–6 h)	
Stage IV: moderate NMS	Moderate rigidity; catatonia or confusion; temperature 38–40 °C (100.4–104 °F); heart rate 100–120 bpm	Discontinue antipsychotics, manage fluids, initiate cooling measures, correct risk factors, provide intensive care	Lorazepam (1–2 mg i.m. or i.v. every 4–6 h), bromocriptine (2.5–5 mg p.o. or by nasogastric [NG] tube every 8 h), or amantadine (100 mg p.o. or by NG tube every 8 h)	Consider electroconvulsive therapy (6–10 bilateral treatments)
Stage V: severe NMS	Severe rigidity; catatonia or coma; temperature >40 °C (104 °F); heart rate >120 bpm	Discontinue antipsychotics, manage fluids, initiate cooling measures, correct risk factors, provide intensive care	Dantrolene (1–2.5 mg/kg i.v. every 6 h. for 48 h), bromocriptine (2.5–5 mg p.o. or by NG tube every 8 h), or amantadine (100 mg p.o. or by NG tube every 8 h)	Consider electroconvulsive therapy (6–10 bilateral treatments)

are usually reported during the first few days of treatment of NMS, whereas delayed administration is unlikely to produce a response.

If symptoms of NMS persist despite supportive care and pharmacotherapy, ECT may be effective even late in the course. ECT may be preferred if idiopathic malignant catatonia cannot be excluded, if NMS symptoms are refractory to other measures, in patients with prominent catatonic features, and in patients who develop a residual catatonic-parkinsonian state or remain psychotic after NMS has resolved [57, 77, 79, 81].

Among patients who recover from NMS, there may be a 30% risk of recurrent episodes following subsequent antipsychotic rechallenge [7]. However, the majority of patients who require antipsychotic therapy can be safely treated, provided precautions are taken. Reports of previous NMS episodes should be checked for accuracy, indications for antipsychotics clearly documented, alternative medications considered, informed consent discussed with, obtained and documented from patients and families, risk factors reduced, at least 2 weeks allowed to elapse following recovery before rechallenge, low doses of low potency conventional antipsychotics or newer antipsychotics titrated gradually after a test dose, and patients carefully monitored for incipient signs of NMS.

Patients who have experienced an episode of NMS are at increased risk for a second episode after antipsychotic rechallenge.

Additional resources on NMS can be obtained from the Neuroleptic Malignant Syndrome Information Service (NMSIS; www.nmsis.org).

Conclusion

Antipsychotics and other dopamine-receptor blocking agents are highly effective and safe medications that have achieved widespread use in medicine and psychiatry. However, they have been associated with NMS in about 0.02% of patients who receive them. Significant progress has been achieved in recognizing, managing, and understanding this drug reaction since it was first described over 60 years ago. Introduction of newer antipsychotics with reduced liability for neurological side effects, conservative prescribing guidelines, reduction of proposed risk factors, and education of staff has reduced the incidence of this disorder. Early diagnosis, cessation of dopamine-receptor blockers or dopamine depletors, prompt medical intervention, and consideration of specific remedies can reduce morbidity and mortality when NMS occurs. It is essential for all physicians and other providers to become familiar with the diagnosis and treatment of this uncommon but potentially lethal drug reaction.

References

1. Delay J, Pichot P, Lemperiere T, Elissade B, Peigne F. Un neuroleptique majeur non-phenothiazine et non-reserpinique, l'haloperidol, dans le traitement des psychoses. Ann Med Psychol (Paris). 1960;118:145–52.
2. Itoh H, Ohtsuka N, Ogita K, Yagi G, Miura S, Koga Y. Malignant neuroleptic syndrome-its present status in Japan and clinical problems. Folia Psychiatr Neurol Jpn. 1977;31:565–76.
3. Bourgeois M, Tignol J, Henry P. Syndrome malin et morts subite au cours des traitements par neuroleptiques simple and retard. Ann Med Psychol. 1971;2:729–46.
4. Caroff SN. The neuroleptic malignant syndrome. J Clin Psychiatry. 1980;41(3):79–83.
5. Meltzer HY. Rigidity, hyperpyrexia and coma following fluphenazine enanthate. Psychopharmacologia. 1973;29(4):337–46.
6. Weinberger DR, Kelly MJ. Catatonia and malignant syndrome: a possible complication of neuroleptic administration. J Nerv Ment Dis. 1977;165:263–8.
7. Caroff SN, Mann SC. Neuroleptic malignant syndrome. Med Clin North Am. 1993;77(1):185–202.

8. Caroff SN. Neuroleptic malignant syndrome. In: Mann SC, Caroff SN, Keck PE, Lazarus A, editors. Neuroleptic malignant syndrome and related conditions. 2nd ed. Washington, DC: American Psychiatric Press, Inc.; 2003. p. 1–44.
9. Strawn JR, Keck PE Jr, Caroff SN. Neuroleptic malignant syndrome. Am J Psychiatry. 2007;164(6):870–6.
10. Kinross-Wright VJ. Trifluoperazine and schizophrenia. In: Brill H, editor. Trifluoperazine:clinical and pharmacologic aspects. Philadelphia: Lea & Febiger; 1958. p. 62–70.
11. Gurrera RJ, Simpson JC, Tsuang MT. Meta-analytic evidence of systematic bias in estimates of neuroleptic malignant syndrome incidence. Compr Psychiatry. 2007;48(2):205–11.
12. Stubner S, Rustenbeck E, Grohmann R, Wagner G, Engel R, Neundorfer G, et al. Severe and uncommon involuntary movement disorders due to psychotropic drugs. Pharmacopsychiatry. 2004;37(Suppl 1):S54–64.
13. Spivak B, Maline DI, Kozyrev VN, Mester R, Neduva SA, Ravilov RS, et al. Frequency of neuroleptic malignant syndrome in a large psychiatric hospital in Moscow. Eur Psychiatry. 2000;15(5):330–3.
14. Keck PE Jr, Pope HG Jr, Cohen BM, McElroy SL, Nierenberg AA. Risk factors for neuroleptic malignant syndrome. A case-control study. Arch Gen Psychiatry. 1989;46(10):914–8.
15. Berardi D, Amore M, Keck PE Jr, Troia M, Dell'Atti M. Clinical and pharmacologic risk factors for neuroleptic malignant syndrome: a case-control study. Biol Psychiatry. 1998;44(8):748–54.
16. Gurrera RJ. A systematic review of sex and age factors in neuroleptic malignant syndrome diagnosis frequency. Acta Psychiatr Scand. 2017;135:398–408.
17. Su YP, Chang CK, Hayes RD, Harrison S, Lee W, Broadbent M, et al. Retrospective chart review on exposure to psychotropic medications associated with neuroleptic malignant syndrome. Acta Psychiatr Scand. 2014;130(1):52–60.
18. Silva RR, Munoz DM, Alpert M, Perlmutter IR, Diaz J. Neuroleptic malignant syndrome in children and adolescents. J Am Acad Child Adolesc Psychiatry. 1999;38(2):187–94.
19. Neuhut R, Lindenmayer JP, Silva R. Neuroleptic malignant syndrome in children and adolescents on atypical antipsychotic medication: a review. J Child Adolesc Psychopharmacol. 2009;19(4):415–22.
20. Croarkin PE, Emslie GJ, Mayes TL. Neuroleptic malignant syndrome associated with atypical antipsychotics in pediatric patients: a review of published cases. J Clin Psychiatry. 2008;69(7):1157–65.
21. Kimura G, Kadoyama K, Brown JB, Nakamura T, Miki I, Nisiguchi K, et al. Antipsychotics-associated serious adverse events in children: an analysis of the FAERS database. Int J Med Sci. 2015;12(2):135–40.
22. Caroff SN, Rosenberg H, Mann SC, Campbell EC, Gliatto MF. Neuroleptic malignant syndrome in the perioperative setting. Am J Anesthesiol. 2001;28:387–93.
23. White DA, Robins AH. Catatonia: harbinger of the neuroleptic malignant syndrome. Br J Psychiatry. 1991;158:419–21.
24. Caroff SN, Mann SC, McCarthy M, Naser J, Rynn M, Morrison M. Acute infectious encephalitis complicated by neuroleptic malignant syndrome. J Clin Psychopharmacol. 1998;18(4):349–51.
25. Sheehan R, Horsfall L, Strydom A, Osborn D, Walters K, Hassiotis A. Movement side effects of antipsychotic drugs in adults with and without intellectual disability: UK population-based cohort study. BMJ Open. 2017;7(8):e017406.
26. Sarkis RA, Coffey MJ, Cooper JJ, Hassan I, Lennox B. Anti-N-methyl-D-aspartate receptor encephalitis: a review of psychiatric phenotypes and management considerations: a report of the American Neuropsychiatric Association Committee on Research. J Neuropsychiatry Clin Neurosci. 2019;31(2):137–42.
27. Caroff SN. Phenomenology and Management of Encephalitis. J Neuropsychiatry Clin Neurosci. 2019;31(4):399.
28. Caroff SN, Mann SC, Gliatto MF, Sullivan KA, Campbell EC. Psychiatric manifestations of acute viral encephalitis. Psychiatr Ann. 2001;31:193–204.

29. Rosebush PI, Mazurek MF. Serum iron and neuroleptic malignant syndrome. Lancet. 1991;338(8760):149–51.
30. Otani K, Horiuchi M, Kondo T, Kaneko S, Fukushima Y. Is the predisposition to neuroleptic malignant syndrome genetically transmitted? Br J Psychiatry. 1991;158:850–3.
31. Kishida I, Kawanishi C, Furuno T, Kato D, Ishigami T, Kosaka K. Association in Japanese patients between neuroleptic malignant syndrome and functional polymorphisms of the dopamine D(2) receptor gene. Mol Psychiatry. 2004;9(3):293–8.
32. Mihara K, Kondo T, Suzuki A, Yasui-Furukori N, Ono S, Sano A, et al. Relationship between functional dopamine D2 and D3 receptors gene polymorphisms and neuroleptic malignant syndrome. Am J Med Genet B Neuropsychiatr Genet. 2003;117B(1):57–60.
33. Suzuki A, Kondo T, Otani K, Mihara K, Yasui-Furukori N, Sano A, et al. Association of the TaqI A polymorphism of the dopamine D(2) receptor gene with predisposition to neuroleptic malignant syndrome. Am J Psychiatry. 2001;158(10):1714–6.
34. Ram A, Cao Q, Keck PE Jr, Pope HG Jr, Otani K, Addonizio G, et al. Structural change in dopamine D2 receptor gene in a patient with neuroleptic malignant syndrome. Am J Med Genet. 1995;60(3):228–30.
35. Kawanishi C, Hanihara T, Shimoda Y, Suzuki K, Sugiyama N, Onishi H, et al. Lack of association between neuroleptic malignant syndrome and polymorphisms in the 5-HT1A and 5-HT2A receptor genes. Am J Psychiatry. 1998;155(9):1275–7.
36. Kato D, Kawanishi C, Kishida I, Furuno T, Suzuki K, Onishi H, et al. Effects of CYP2D6 polymorphisms on neuroleptic malignant syndrome. Eur J Clin Pharmacol. 2007;63(11):991–6.
37. Sato T, Nishio H, Iwata M, Kentotsuboi TA, Miyazaki T, et al. Postmortem molecular screening for mutations in ryanodine receptor type 1 (RYR1) gene in psychiatric patients suspected of having died of neuroleptic malignant syndrome. Forensic Sci Int. 2010;194(1–3):77–9.
38. Russell T, Riazi S, Kraeva N, Steel AC, Hawryluck LA. Ecstacy-induced delayed rhabdomyolysis and neuroleptic malignant syndrome in a patient with a novel variant in the ryanodine receptor type 1 gene. Anaesthesia. 2012;67(9):1021–4.
39. Miyatake R, Iwahashi K, Matsushita M, Nakamura K, Suwaki H. No association between the neuroleptic malignant syndrome and mutations in the RYR1 gene associated malignant hyperthermia. J Neurol Sci. 1996;143(1–2):161–5.
40. Caroff SN, Mann SC. Neuroleptic malignant syndrome. Psychopharmacol Bull. 1988;24(1):25–9.
41. Ananth J, Parameswaran S, Gunatilake S, Burgoyne K, Sidhom T. Neuroleptic malignant syndrome and atypical antipsychotic drugs. J Clin Psychiatry. 2004;65(4):464–70.
42. Anzai T, Takahashi K, Watanabe M. Adverse reaction reports of neuroleptic malignant syndrome induced by atypical antipsychotic agents in the Japanese Adverse Drug Event Report (JADER) database. Psychiatry Clin Neurosci. 2019 Jan;73(1):27–33.
43. Belvederi Murri M, Guaglianone A, Bugliani M, Calcagno P, Respino M, Serafini G, et al. Second-generation antipsychotics and neuroleptic malignant syndrome: systematic review and case report analysis. Drugs R D. 2015;15(1):45–62.
44. Sarkar S, Gupta N. Drug information update. Atypical antipsychotics and neuroleptic malignant syndrome: nuances and pragmatics of the association. BJPsych Bull. 2017;41(4):211–6.
45. Nasrallah HA, Fedora R, Morton R. Successful treatment of clozapine-nonresponsive refractory hallucinations and delusions with pimavanserin, a serotonin 5HT-2A receptor inverse agonist. Schizophr Res. 2019;208:217–20.
46. Koblan KS, Kent J, Hopkins SC, Krystal JH, Cheng H, Goldman R, et al. A non-D2-receptor-binding drug for the treatment of schizophrenia. N Engl J Med. 2020;382(16):1497–506.
47. Lau Moon Lin M, Robinson PD, Flank J, Sung L, Dupuis LL. The safety of prochlorperazine in children: a systematic review and meta-analysis. Drug Saf. 2016;39(6):509–16.
48. Lau Moon Lin M, Robinson PD, Flank J, Sung L, Dupuis LL. The safety of metoclopramide in children: a systematic review and meta-analysis. Drug Saf. 2016;39(7):675–87.
49. Escobar-Vidarte MF, Loaiza-Osorio S, Messa AA, Macias GE. Neuroleptic malignant syndrome in pregnancy: case report and literature review. J Matern Fetal Neonatal Med. 2019;32(14):2438–41.

50. Sato I, Onishi H, Kawanishi C, Yamada S, Ishida M, Kawakami K. Neuroleptic malignant syndrome in patients with cancer: a systematic review. BMJ Support Palliat Care. 2020 Sep;10(3):265–70.
51. Caroff SN. Risk of neuroleptic malignant syndrome with vesicular monoamine transporter inhibitors. Clin Psychopharmacol Neurosci. 2020;18(2):322–6.
52. Kane JM, Correll CU, Delva N, Gopal S, Savitz A, Mathews M. Low incidence of neuroleptic malignant syndrome associated with paliperidone palmitate long-acting injectable: a database report and case study. J Clin Psychopharmacol. 2019;39(2):180–2.
53. Stevens DL. Association between selective serotonin-reuptake inhibitors, second-generation antipsychotics, and neuroleptic malignant syndrome. Ann Pharmacother. 2008;42(9):1290–7.
54. Mann SC, Caroff SN, Fricchione G, Campbell EC. Central dopamine hypoactivity and the pathogenesis of neuroleptic malignant syndrome. Psychiatr Ann. 2000;30:363–74.
55. Rosenberg MR, Green M. Neuroleptic malignant syndrome. Review of response to therapy. Arch Intern Med. 1989;149(9):1927–31.
56. Sakkas P, Davis JM, Janicak PG, Wang ZY. Drug treatment of the neuroleptic malignant syndrome. Psychopharmacol Bull. 1991;27(3):381–4.
57. Davis JM, Caroff SN, Mann SC. Treatment of neuroleptic malignant syndrome. Psychiatr Ann. 2000;30:325–31.
58. Ueda M, Hamamoto M, Nagayama H, Okubo S, Amemiya S, Katayama Y. Biochemical alterations during medication withdrawal in Parkinson's disease with and without neuroleptic malignant-like syndrome. J Neurol Neurosurg Psychiatry. 2001;71(1):111–3.
59. Nisijima K, Ishiguro T. Cerebrospinal fluid levels of monoamine metabolites and gamma-aminobutyric acid in neuroleptic malignant syndrome. J Psychiatr Res. 1995;29(3):233–44.
60. Gurrera RJ. Sympathoadrenal hyperactivity and the etiology of neuroleptic malignant syndrome. Am J Psychiatry. 1999;156(2):169–80.
61. Kornhuber J, Weller M, Riederer P. Glutamate receptor antagonists for neuroleptic malignant syndrome and akinetic hyperthermic parkinsonian crisis. J Neural Transm. 1993;6:63–72.
62. Portel L, Hilbert G, Gruson D, Favier JC, Gbikpi-Benissan G, Cardinaud JP. Malignant hyperthermia and neuroleptic malignant syndrome in a patient during treatment for acute asthma. Acta Anaesthesiol Scand. 1999;43(1):107–10.
63. Sato T, Hara T, Takeichi M. A case of neuroleptic malignant syndrome with a history of general anesthesia. Hum Psychopharmacol. 1992;7:351–3.
64. Yamawaki S, Yano E, Uchitomi Y. Analysis of 497 cases of neuroleptic malignant syndrome in Japan. Hiroshima J Anesth. 1990;26:35–44.
65. Tsutsumi Y, Yamamoto K, Matsuura S, Hata S, Sakai M, Shirakura K. The treatment of neuroleptic malignant syndrome using dantrolene sodium. Psychiatry Clin Neurosci. 1998;52(4):433–8.
66. Nisijima K, Shioda K. Temporal changes in serum creatine kinase concentration and degreee of muscle rigidity in 24 patients with neuroleptic malignant syndrome. Neuropsychiatr Dis Treat. 2013;9:853–9.
67. Caroff SN, Mann SC, Sullivan KA, Macfadden W. Drug-induced hypermetabolic syndromes. In: Ohnishi ST, Ohnishi T, editors. Malignant hyperthermia. Boca Raton: CRC Press; 1994. p. 118–32.
68. Velamoor VR, Norman RM, Caroff SN, Mann SC, Sullivan KA, Antelo RE. Progression of symptoms in neuroleptic malignant syndrome. J Nerv Ment Dis. 1994;182(3):168–73.
69. Masi G, Milone A, Viglione V, Mancini A, Pisano S. Massive asymptomatic creatine kinase elevation in youth during antipsychotic drug treatment: case reports and critical review of the literature. J Child Adolesc Psychopharmacol. 2014;24(10):536–42.
70. Gasparini A, Poloni N, Caselli I, Ielmini M, Callegari C. Reversible splenial lesion in neuroleptic malignant syndrome. Panminerva Med. 2018;60(3):134–5.
71. Martino G, Capasso M, Nasuti M, Bonanni L, Onofrj M, Thomas A. Dopamine transporter single-photon emission computerized tomography supports diagnosis of akinetic crisis of parkinsonism and of neuroleptic malignant syndrome. Medicine. 2015;94(13):e649.

72. Sachdev PS. A rating scale for neuroleptic malignant syndrome. Psychiatry Res. 2005;135(3):249–56.
73. American Psychiatric Association. Neuroleptic malignant syndrome. Diagnostic and statistical manual of mental disorders. Washington, DC: American Psychiatric Press, Inc.; 1994. p. 739–42.
74. Gurrera RJ, Chang SS, Romero JA. A comparison of diagnostic criteria for neuroleptic malignant syndrome. J Clin Psychiatry. 1992;53(2):56–62.
75. Gurrera RJ, Caroff SN, Cohen A, Carroll BT, DeRoos F, Francis A, et al. An international consensus study of neuroleptic malignant syndrome diagnostic criteria using the Delphi method. J Clin Psychiatry. 2011 Sep;72(9):1222–8.
76. Gurrera RJ, Mortillaro G, Velamoor V, Caroff SN. A validation study of the international consensus diagnostic criteria for neuroleptic malignant syndrome. J Clin Psychopharmacol. 2017;37(1):67–71.
77. Caroff SN, Mann SC, Keck PE Jr, Francis A. Residual catatonic state following neuroleptic malignant syndrome. J Clin Psychopharmacol. 2000;20(2):257–9.
78. Kayser MS, Kohler CG, Dalmau J. Psychiatric manifestations of paraneoplastic disorders. Am J Psychiatry. 2010;167(9):1039–50.
79. Mann SC, Caroff SN, Bleier HR, Welz WK, Kling MA, Hayashida M. Lethal catatonia. Am J Psychiatry. 1986;143(11):1374–81.
80. Fricchione G, Mann SC, Caroff SN. Catatonia, lethal catatonia and neuroleptic malignant syndrome. Psychiatr Ann. 2000;30:347–55.
81. Mann SC, Caroff SN, Bleier HR, Antelo RE, Un H. Electroconvulsive therapy of the lethal catatonia syndrome. Convuls Ther. 1990;6(3):239–47.
82. Ahuja N, Palanichamy N, Mackin P, Lloyd A. Olanzapine-induced hyperglycaemic coma and neuroleptic malignant syndrome: case report and review of literature. J Psychopharmacol. 2010;24(1):125–30.
83. Zeitler P, Haqq A, Rosenbloom A, Glaser N, Drugs and Therapeutics Committee of the Lawson Wilkins Pediatric Endocrine Society. Hyperglycemic hyperosmolar syndrome in children: pathophysiological considerations and suggested guidelines for treatment. J Pediatr. 2011;158(1):9–14. e1-2
84. Mann SC, Boger WP. Psychotropic drugs, summer heat and humidity, and hyperpyrexia: a danger restated. Am J Psychiatry. 1978;135(9):1097–100.
85. Huddleston DE, Factor SA. Parkinsonism-hyperpyrexia syndrome in Parkinson's disease. In: Frucht SJ, editor. Movement disorder emergencies; diagnosis and treatment. Current clinical neurology. 2nd ed. New York: Human Press; 2013. p. 29–42.
86. Caroff SN. Parkinsonism-hyperthermia syndrome and deep brain stimulation. Can J Anaesth. 2017;64(6):675–6.
87. Keck PE Jr, Arnold LM. The serotonin syndrome. Psychiatr Ann. 2000;30:333–43.
88. Woodbury MM, Woodbury MA. Neuroleptic-induced catatonia as a stage in the progression toward neuroleptic malignant syndrome. J Am Acad Child Adolesc Psychiatry. 1992;31(6):1161–4.
89. Fryml LD, Williams KR, Pelic CG, Fox J, Sahlem G, Robert S, et al. The role of amantadine withdrawal in 3 cases of treatment-refractory altered mental status. J Psychiatr Pract. 2017;23(3):191–9.
90. Caroff SN, Jain R, Morley JF. Revisiting amantadine as a treatment for drug-induced movement disorders. Ann Clin Psychiatry. 2020;32(3):198–208.
91. Rodriguez ME, Luquin MR, Lera G, Delgado G, Salazar JM, Obeso JA. Neuroleptic malignant syndrome treated with subcutaneous lisuride infusion. Mov Disord. 1990;5(2):170–2.
92. Rosebush P, Stewart T. A prospective analysis of 24 episodes of neuroleptic malignant syndrome. Am J Psychiatry. 1989;146(6):717–25.

Malignant Catatonia

7

Stephan C. Mann, Stanley N. Caroff,
and E. Cabrina Campbell

Patient Vignette

A 27-year-old female with bipolar disorder had been off psychiatric medications for 6 months. One week prior to admission, she developed elevated mood, pressured speech, and flight of ideas. She grew markedly agitated, talked constantly, paced relentlessly, and refused food or drink. On admission, she was confused and intensely hyperactive with periods of hostile verbal outbursts and responded to auditory hallucinations. She exhibited muscular rigidity, posturing, echolalia, and echopraxia. Temperature was 39 °C with tachycardia, tachypnea, profuse diaphoresis, and blood pressure of 170/120 mm Hg. Laboratory abnormalities showed leukocytosis and elevation in creatinine phosphokinase (CK). Lumbar puncture, EEG, and CT scan of the head were normal. Over the next 24 h, she lapsed into stupor with increased rigidity and a fever of 40.2 °C. The diagnosis of malignant catatonia associated with a manic episode was made and electroconvulsive therapy (ECT) initiated. Body temperature and other vital signs returned to normal after the first bilateral ECT treatment. She received one bilateral ECT treatment daily for the next 5 days with three more over the next week with marked improvement in all symptoms.

S. C. Mann (✉)
Private Practice, Harleysville, PA, USA

S. N. Caroff · E. C. Campbell
Department of Psychiatry, Corporal Michael J. Crescenz VA Medical Center and the
University of Pennsylvania Perelman School of Medicine, Philadelphia, PA, USA

© Springer Nature Switzerland AG 2022
S. J. Frucht (ed.), *Movement Disorder Emergencies*, Current Clinical Neurology,
https://doi.org/10.1007/978-3-030-75898-1_7

Introduction

Catatonia is a syndrome of striking motor and behavioral abnormalities that may occur in association with diverse neuromedical, drug-induced, and psychiatric illnesses. Furthermore, catatonia may be conceptualized as a continuum, with milder forms at one end (termed *simple* or *benign*) and more severe forms, involving hyperthermia and autonomic dysfunction (termed *malignant*), at the other [1]. In 1934, Stauder [2] described *lethal catatonia* characterized by extreme motor excitement followed by stuporous exhaustion, coma, cardiovascular collapse, and death. The entire course involved progressive hyperthermia, autonomic dysfunction, clouding of consciousness, and prominent catatonic features. In cases ending in death, the paucity of findings was puzzling and in sharp contrast to the catastrophic clinical manifestations. In fact, this disorder had been discussed previously by Calmeil (1832) [3] and Bell (1849) [4] and was the subject of numerous North American and foreign publications during the pre-antipsychotic drug era. Other names used to describe this same disorder included *Bell's mania, acute delirious mania, delirium acutum, delire aigu, psychotic exhaustion syndrome*, and *Scheid's cyanotic syndrome*, among others [5–8]. More recently, stressing that not all cases are fatal, Philbrick and Rummans [1] have promulgated the term *malignant catatonia* (MC).

In this chapter, we review the historical and modern world literature on MC. On the basis of this review, we conclude that MC represents a currently under-recognized but potentially fatal neuropsychiatric disorder. Our data indicate that MC, like benign catatonia, represents a syndrome rather than a specific disease that may occur in association with diverse neuromedical illnesses as well as with psychiatric disorders. Current data suggest that a substantial proportion of MC cases previously attributed to schizophrenia were more likely linked to autoimmune encephalitis, particularly anti-N-methyl-D-aspartate receptor (NMDAR) encephalitis [9]. Neuroleptic malignant syndrome (NMS), a life-threatening complication of antipsychotic drug treatment [6, 10], may be viewed as an antipsychotic drug-induced toxic or iatrogenic subtype of MC. The hypothesis that simple catatonia, MC, and NMS share a common pathophysiology involving reduced dopaminergic neurotransmission within the basal ganglia-thalamocortical circuits underscores their identity as variants of a larger unitary catatonic syndrome. Recognition of the clinical features of MC and an appreciation of its diverse etiologies are essential for the effective management of patients who develop this catastrophic reaction.

Clinical Presentation: Pre-antipsychotic Drug Era

Despite the diversity of nomenclature, there is considerable consistency to early accounts of MC [5–8]. A prodromal phase was observed in most but not all cases, lasting an average of 2 weeks, and involved insomnia, anorexia, and labile mood. In roughly 90% of cases, the disease proper began with a phase of intense motor excitement that then continued almost without interruption (as exemplified by the Patient Vignette). Features of this excited phase included refusal of foods and fluids, clouding of consciousness, tachycardia, tachypnea, cyanosis, labile or elevated blood pressure, and profuse perspiration. Acrocyanosis and spontaneous hematomas of the skin were frequently noted. At times, excitement might be interrupted by periods of catatonic stupor and rigidity. Other catatonic signs, such as mutism, catalepsy, posturing, echolalia, and echopraxia were often present. Thought processes became increasingly disorganized and speech grew progressively incoherent. Auditory and visual hallucinations accompanied by bizarre delusions were frequently prominent.

In this "classic" excited phase of MC, excitement was always associated with hyperthermia that could attain levels approaching 43.3 °C prior to the final stuporous phase of MC. This presentation differs phenomenologically from NMS in that although NMS is often preceded by a period of hyperactivity, hyperthermia first emerges concomitantly with, or shortly after, the onset of stupor and rigidity. The excited phase of MC was noted to vary in duration but lasted an average of 8 days [11].

In the final phase of MC, excitement gave way to stuporous exhaustion and extreme hyperthermia, often followed by coma, cardiovascular collapse, and death [5]. In all of Stauder's 27 cases [2], rigidity of the skeletal muscles was described during this terminal stupor, similar to that seen in NMS. Although other accounts of MC echoed the findings of Stauder, some reports described flaccid muscles in contrast to NMS [6]. About 10% of cases reported during the pre-antipsychotic drug era involved hyperthermia and a primarily stuporous course unassociated with a preceding hyperactive phase. During the pre-antipsychotic drug era, MC was reported fatal in 75–100% of cases [5]. It was observed to occur predominantly in young adults between the ages of 18 and 35 and involved women roughly seven times more often than men. During this period, MC was estimated to account for 0.25–3.5% of admissions to psychiatric hospitals and occurred with equal frequency throughout the seasons [5]. Stauder [2] and others reported findings consistent with a familial pattern of occurrence.

Kraepelin [12], who called this disorder delirium acutum, considered it a nonspecific syndrome that could occur as an outgrowth of neuromedical illness as well as the major psychoses. In contrast, most early French authors viewed MC as an unusual but deadly form of encephalitis preferentially involving the hypothalamus [13]. Subsequent to Stauder's [2] publication, however, MC was increasingly seen as confined to the major psychoses, although Stauder himself never fully dismissed the possibility that some or all of his patients may have had encephalitis. Most German and American authors emphasized lack of autopsy findings that could account for death, with the CNS abnormalities reported by the French either unconfirmed or deemed trivial. Bronchopneumonia and other infections were considered "opportunistic," occurring in an already exhausted and compromised host.

Contemporary Presentation

In 1986, we conducted a computerized search of the PubMed database and identified 292 MC cases reported between 1960 and 1985 [5]. In 2013 [8], we added 107 cases found in the literature between 1986 and 2010 and reported on the total 399 cases identified over a 50-year period. Since then, we have reviewed 105 cases published between 2011 and 2020 [14–113], thus extending our series to 504 MC cases. Most patients had received antipsychotic drugs at some point during their treatment. All cases involved hyperthermia, since its presence is required for a diagnosis of MC.

Gender was specified in 450 of the full series of 504 MC cases; in 280 (62%) of the cases, the patient was a female. This indicates that women continue to be disproportionately affected, although the trend now appears somewhat moderated compared to the pre-antipsychotic drug era. Mean age of occurrence was 32, compared with 25 during the pre-antipsychotic drug era. Mortality, which had exceeded 75% during the pre-antipsychotic drug era and was still at 60% between 1960 and 1985, has fallen to 10% in cases reported between 1986 and 2020. This decline in mortality is striking and presumably reflects enhanced awareness of MC, early diagnosis, and rapid institution of appropriate treatment. Nevertheless, MC continues to represent a potentially lethal disorder. MC has been estimated to occur in 0.07% of psychiatric admissions or annually in 0.0004% of community adults [5].

Table 7.1 summarizes the clinical features of MC. Along with catatonic stupor and hyperactivity, they have hyperthermia, altered consciousness, and autonomic instability manifested by diaphoresis, tachycardia, labile or elevated blood pressure, and varying degrees of cyanosis. Catatonic signs aside from stupor and excitement continue to be noted. One large series [114] identified 62 patients with psychogenic MC and reported that each exhibited at least three catatonic features. In our most

Table 7.1 Clinical features of malignant catatonia

Signs and symptoms
  Hyperthermia
  Catatonic excitement and/or stupor
  Other catatonic features (e.g., mutism, negativism, catalepsy, posturing, echolalia, echopraxia, and staring)
  Muscular rigidity (variable)
  Altered consciousness
  Autonomic instability
    Profuse diaphoresis
    Tachycardia
    Labile or elevated blood pressure
    Tachypnea and cyanosis (variable)
Positive laboratory findings
  Most consistent-CPK elevation, leukocytosis
  Less consistent low serum iron levels, elevated serum creatinine, hyponatremia, hypernatremia, dehydration, lymphocytic pleocytosis, EEG-generalized slowing, epileptic activity, delta brush, MRI hyperintensities in cortical and subcortical brain regions
Outgrowth of diverse neuromedical, drug-induced, and psychiatric conditions

Copyright 2005, Humana Press Inc. (adapted from [7] with permission)

recent 105 MC cases, muscle rigidity was present in 64 of the 79 (81%) cases in which muscle tone was characterized. Among these recent cases, CK was elevated in 41 of the 48 patients (85%) and leukocytosis was present in 19 of 35 (54%). A reduction in serum iron, which has been associated with both MC and NMS [115], was reported in the single case in which serum iron level was measured.

In 60 (15%) of the 399 MC cases reported during the 50-year period between 1960 and 2010 [8], a neuromedical illness was believed to have initiated the full syndromic picture of MC. Infectious causes predominated, in particular, acute and postinfectious viral encephalitis and bacterial septicemia with cerebrovascular disorders, normal pressure hydrocephalus, and various metabolic and toxic disorders accounting for additional cases. Two cases were associated with anti-NMDAR encephalitis and two with paraneoplastic limbic encephalitis. This 15% figure for organic MC was similar to that found in our previous reports [5–8], as well as in surveys of simple or benign organic catatonia in general hospital settings [116]. During the 50-year period between 1960 and 2010, 339 (85%) of the 399 MC cases reported were considered the outgrowth of a psychiatric disorder, diagnosed as schizophrenia in 127 cases, mania in 22 cases, major depression in 31 cases, psychotic disorder not otherwise specified in 22 cases, and "periodic catatonia" in 10 cases.

However, our most recent 105 MC cases reported during the nine years between 2011 and 2020 differ markedly in this regard. Eighty of 105 (76%) are now attributed to neuromedical illness whereas only 25 (24%) are associated with a psychiatric disorder. Table 7.2 lists the causes associated with these 105 MC cases. Symptom profiles and neurodiagnostic findings in these most recent cases contrast distinctly with those of our earlier reports. For example, seizures, observed in only 14 of the 399 cases (3%) prior to 2010, were reported in 38 of the most recent 105 MC cases (36%). Findings rarely seen in earlier cases included cerebrospinal fluid lymphocytic pleocytosis (27%), abnormalities on electroencephalography (slowing, epileptic activity, and delta brush) (73%), and abnormalities on magnetic resonance imaging (hyperintensities in cortical or subcortical brain regions) (18%).

Two principle factors appear to account for this recent inversion in the ratio of neuromedical to psychiatric MC cases: a decline in cases attributed to schizophrenia and a dramatic increase in cases due to autoimmune encephalitis, particularly NMDAR encephalitis. A critical observation regarding MC cases seen as an outgrowth of schizophrenia is that 117 of the 127 cases reported between 1960 and 2010 appeared in the literature prior to 1985 [6]. Previously, we had cautioned that the frequent association of MC with schizophrenia may be spurious, resulting from a continued misconception that catatonic signs imply catatonic schizophrenia, a view more prominent at that time [5]. Furthermore, although methodologic limitations preclude a definitive answer, studies using consistent diagnostic criteria over time support a true decrease in the incidence of benign or simple catatonic schizophrenia [117, 118].

Anti-NMDAR encephalitis, first described in 2007, is a common and severe form of autoimmune encephalitis [9, 119]. It primarily involves young patients with a median age of 21 but can be seen at any age [120]. Like MC, it more commonly

Table 7.2 Etiologies of 105 malignant catatonia cases: 2011–2020

Psychiatric and neurodevelopmental disorders	Reference(s)
Schizophrenia—9 cases	[14–22]
Mania—6 cases	[23–28]
Major depressive disorder—5 cases	[29–32]
Brief psychotic disorder—2 cases	[33, 34]
Schizoaffective disorder—1 case	[25]
Autistic spectrum disorder—2 cases	[25, 35]
Autoimmune disorders	
NMDA receptor encephalitis —40 cases	[36–75]
GABA-A receptor encephalitis—2 cases	[76, 77]
LGI1 receptor encephalitis—2 cases	[37, 78]
Progressive encephalomyelitis with rigidity and myoclonus—1 case	[79]
Systemic lupus erythematosus—4 cases	[80–83]
Hashimoto's encephalopathy—2	[84, 85]
Sjogren's syndrome—2 cases	[86, 87]
Infectious disorders	
Viral encephalitis	
Dengue virus —1 case	[88]
Herpes simplex virus type 1—1 case	[89]
Unspecified—3 cases	[90–92]
Encephalitis lethargica —2 cases	[93, 94]
Mycoplasma pneumonia encephalitis —1 case	[95]
Neurobrucellosis encephalitis —1 case	[96]
Sepsis-associated encephalopathy—1 case	[97]
Toxic and drug-related disorders	
Clozapine withdrawal—3 cases	[98–100]
Amantadine withdrawal—1 case	[101]
Lorazepam withdrawal—1 case	[102]
Dexamethasone induced—1 case	[103]
Lithium toxicity—1 case	[104]
Cocaine-induced leukoencephalopathy—1 cases	[105]
Bath salts abuse—1 case	[106]
Methadone overdose—1 case	[25]
Disulfiram overdose—1 case	[107]
3-methoxyphencyclidine intoxication—1 case	[108]
Synthetic cannabinoid intoxication—1 case	[109]
Cyclosporine A-related neurotoxicity—1 case	[110]
Parkinsonism-hyperpyrexia syndrome—1 case	[111]
Post-surgical-paroxysmal sympathetic hyperactivity—1 case	[112]
Surgical removal of lesion near hypothalamus—1 case	[113]

affects women (80%), a percentage of whom will have an ovarian teratoma [121]. Early in its course, anti-NMDAR encephalitis possesses a remarkable capacity to mimic psychiatric disorders [122]. Dalmau et al. [123] reported that 77% of anti-NMDAR encephalitis cases were seen initially by a psychiatrist. Prompt recognition is critical as the condition is treatable and can be diagnosed serologically.

Gurrera [122] retrospectively identified 230 adult cases of anti-NMDAR encephalitis associated with prominent psychiatric symptoms and scored them for the presence of clinical features. Regarding the manifestations of MC, catatonic features were present in 45.7%, autonomic dysfunction in 45.7%, fever in 28.3%, and reduced arousal in 30%. This symptom profile clearly predicts that a certain percentage of anti-NMDAR cases with prominent psychiatric symptoms should meet criteria for MC. Frequently observed neurologic features included seizures (60.4%), orofacial dyskinesias (39.1%), dyskinesias involving other body parts (36.1%), memory disturbance (34.8%), and impaired language/aphasia (25.7%).

Other recent studies have explored the frequency of catatonia in anti-NMDAR encephalitis. Serra-Mestres and associates [121] retrospectively applied the Bush-Frances Catatonia Screening Instrument (BFCSI) to 189 anti-NMDAR encephalitis patients identified in a systematic literature search; catatonia was present in 60%. Additionally, autonomic dysfunction was found in 58% of patients who were catatonic compared to 38% who were not. Furthermore, the first prospective study has now been conducted [124]. It assessed the presence of catatonia in 58 anti-NMDAR encephalitis patients entering an inpatient research unit using both the BFCSI and the Braunig Catatonia Rating Scales and identified catatonia in 70.6% of cases.

🔑 Anti-NMDA receptor-mediated encephalitis is a frequent cause of malignant catatonia.

In a paper exploring evidence for immune dysregulation in catatonia, Rogers and associates [125] conducted a systematic literature search for autoimmune disorders causing catatonia. Similar to our observations regarding MC, they found that 72% (249/346) of all cases of autoimmune catatonia reported were due to anti-NMDAR encephalitis. They observed that catatonia described in anti-NMDAR encephalitis cases is often of the MC variety and tends to co-occur in association with psychosis or mania. This led them to propose that MC represents an entity that could be largely accounted for by autoimmune disorders such as anti-NMDAR encephalitis. We would contend that the causes of MC are multiple and diverse. Nevertheless, our findings appear consistent with the impression that autoimmune encephalitis, particularly anti-NMDAR encephalitis, may account for many MC cases previously attributed to psychosis or schizophrenia, MC cases viewed as an outgrowth of viral encephalitis where no causative pathogen is identified, and, as Rogers and associates suggest, cases previously ascribed to encephalitis lethargica.

The Malignant Catatonia Syndrome

Our review of the modern world literature supports Kraepelin's [12] conceptualization of MC as a nonspecific syndrome that may occur in association with diverse neuromedical, drug-induced, and psychiatric disorders. Table 7.3 summarizes known causes of the MC syndrome. Consistent with this view of MC as a nonspecific syndrome, it is appropriate to consider the relationship between MC and NMS. Among the total 504 contemporary MC cases, the "classic" excited form

Table 7.3 Disorders associated with malignant catatonia syndrome

Psychiatric and neurodevelopmental disorders
   Schizophrenia
   Bipolar disorder
   Schizoaffective disorder
   Brief psychotic disorder
   Periodic catatonia
   Autistic spectrum disorder
   Prader–Willi syndrome
Autoimmune disorders
   NMDA receptor encephalitis
   GABA A receptor encephalitis
   LGI1-receptor encephalitis
   Progressive encephalomyelitis with rigidity
   Systemic lupus erythematosus
   Hashimoto's encephalopathy
   Sjogren's syndrome
   Addison's disease
   Multiple sclerosis
Infectious disorders
   Viral encephalitis—acute and postinfectious
   Human immunodeficiency virus encephalopathy
   Viral hepatitis
   Encephalitis lethargica
   Bacterial meningoencephalitis
   Bacterial septicemia
   Borrelia encephalitis
   General paresis
   Mycoplasma pneumonia encephalitis
   Neurobrucellosis encephalitis
   Typhoid fever
   Chagas' encephalitis
   Cerebral malaria
Cerebrovascular disorders
   Basilar artery thrombosis
   Bilateral hemorrhagic infarction of the anterior cingulated gyri
   Bilateral hemorrhagic lesions of temporal lobes
Other central nervous system disorders
   Normal-pressure hydrocephalus
   Seizure disorders
   Autonomic (diencephalic) epilepsy
   Petit mal status
   Cerebral anoxia
Tumors
   Periventricular diffuse pinealoma
   Glioma of the third ventricle
   Glioma involving the splenium of the corpus callosum
   Angioma of the midbrain
Head trauma
   Closed head trauma
   Surgical removal of lesions near the hypothalamus
   Post-surgical-paroxysmal sympathetic hyperactivity

Table 7.3 (continued)

Metabolic disorders
   Cushing's disease
   Uremia
   Wernicke's encephalopathy
Toxic and drug-related disorders
   Amantadine withdrawal
   Clozapine withdrawal
   Barbiturate withdrawal
   Clonazepam withdrawal
   Lorazepam withdrawal
   Lithium toxicity
   Dexamethasone-induced
   Methadone overdose
   Disulfiram overdose
   Cyclosporine A-related neurotoxicity
   Cocaine-induced leukoencephalopathy
   Bath salts abuse
   3-Methoxyphencyclidine intoxication
   Synthetic cannabinoid intoxication
   Tetraethyl lead poisoning
   Intrathecal administration of ziconotide
   Toxic epidermal necrolysis
   Temporomandibular joint surgery
   Renal transplantation
   Parkinsonism-hyperpyrexia syndrome
   Neuroleptic malignant syndrome

Copyright 1986, American Journal of Psychiatry, American Psychiatric Association (adapted from [5] with permission), and Copyright 2019, Lancet Psychiatry (adapted from [125] with permission from Elsevier Ltd)

(clinical vignette) involving extreme hyperactivity and progressive hyperthermia prior to the onset of stupor has continued to predominate with 61% of cases presenting in this fashion. However, 39% of patients exhibited a primarily stuporous course. This represents a change from the pre-antipsychotic drug era when only about 10% of MC cases were presented in this fashion. Furthermore, a selective analysis of the 105 cases reported since 2011 indicates a reversal in this trend with only 43% presenting as excited and 57% exhibiting a primarily stuporous course.

In many of these cases involving a stuporous course, stupor and hyperthermia developed only following the initiation of antipsychotic drug treatment, giving rise to questions concerning the differentiation of MC from NMS. Furthermore, the clinical features of the classic excited form of MC, once stupor emerges, appear equally difficult to distinguish from those of NMS. Viewing MC as a syndrome, we have suggested that NMS represents an antipsychotic drug-induced toxic or iatrogenic subtype of MC. Accordingly, the emergence of NMS as a subtype of MC could help explain the increased percentage of primarily stuporous MC cases reported in the contemporary literature. Furthermore, anti-NMDAR encephalitis, by far the single most frequent cause of MC in cases reported since 2011, appears to entail an extraordinarily high risk for NMS that could prove critical in explaining the current dominance of the primarily stuporous presentation in our most recent cases. In one study [126], NMS was diagnosed or suspected in 22% of anti-NMDAR encephalitis patients exposed to antipsychotic drugs. Another report suggested that as many as 18 of 33 (55%) patients with anti-NMDAR encephalitis developed suspected NMS upon exposure to antipsychotic drugs [127]. These rates dramatically exceed recent estimates of NMS as occurring in about 0.02 percent of psychiatric patients treated with antipsychotics.

A number of authors have concurred with our conceptualization of NMS as a drug-induced subtype of MC [1, 128]. Fricchione [129] suggested a close relationship between catatonic states triggered by antipsychotics and those that are not, and proposed that antipsychotic drug-induced catatonia is to simple catatonia what NMS is to MC. Koch and associates [130] provided further evidence for overlap among catatonia, MC, and NMS. Among 16 patients with NMS, 15 met clinical and research criteria for catatonia. Furthermore, in each of their cases, there was a strong positive correlation between the severity of NMS and the number of catatonic signs reported, strengthening the argument for a relationship between the disorders and consistent with a view of NMS as a severe variant of catatonia.

In contrast, other authors have argued that simple catatonia, MC, and NMS are distinct clinical entities. Both Castillo and associates [131] and Fleischhacker and associates [132] proposed that excited or agitated behavior points to a diagnosis of MC. However, agitation is commonly a feature of the psychosis preceding NMS for which antipsychotic drugs were originally used. Castillo and associates [132] maintained that prominent muscle rigidity might be a distinguishing feature. However, patients with agitated catatonia usually receive medications early in treatment. Accordingly, if rigidity is present, it may be difficult to know whether this represents NMS or drug-related extrapyramidal symptoms superimposed on MC. Based on our review, we concur with Fricchione and colleagues' [129, 133] conclusion that aside from a few differences in presentation, catatonia, MC, and NMS appear to be variants of a larger unitary catatonic syndrome.

Pathogenesis

There is evidence for involvement of several neurotransmitter systems in the pathogenesis of catatonia including dopamine, glutamate, gamma-aminobutyric acid, and serotonin. On biochemical grounds, motor symptoms in catatonia appear modulated by dopamine [134]. A consideration of the role of dopamine further supports a view of catatonia, MC, and NMS as subtypes of the same disorder. A number of authors have posited a key role for dopaminergic hypoactivity in triggering both simple catatonia and MC [6, 129, 133]. Furthermore, there is compelling clinical evidence implicating antipsychotic drug-induced dopamine receptor blockade in the pathogenesis of NMS [135]. Our group [6, 135], along with Fricchione and colleagues [129, 133], have proposed that the onset of simple catatonia, MC, and NMS coincides with a reduction in dopaminergic activity within the basal ganglia-thalamocortical circuits. As elucidated by Alexander and associates [136, 137], these circuits represent one of the brain's principal organizational networks underlying brain–behavior relationships. Five circuits connecting the basal ganglia with their associated areas in the cortex and thalamus have been identified and are named according to their cortical site of origin (Fig. 7.1). They include the "motor circuit," the "oculomotor circuit," the "dorsolateral prefrontal circuit," the "lateral orbitofrontal circuit," and the "anterior cingulate-medial orbitofrontal circuit." Each circuit involves the same member structures, including an origin in a specific area of the frontal cortex; projections to the striatum (putamen, caudate, and ventral striatum); connections to the globus pallidus interna and the substantia nigra pars reticulata, which, in turn, project to specific thalamic nuclei; and a final link back to the frontal area from which they originated, thus creating a feedback loop.

Dopamine is in a key position to influence activity in each of the circuits. Mesocortical dopamine pathways project directly to circuit areas of origin in the supplementary motor area, frontal eye fields, and the three prefrontal cortical areas. Additionally, dopamine modulates each circuit through its projections to the striatum [138]. The motor, the anterior cingulate-medial orbitofrontal circuit, and the lateral orbitofrontal circuits represent the most likely candidates for involvement in the pathogenesis of simple catatonia, MC, and NMS.

Specifically, the onset of hypodopaminergia in the motor circuit may underly muscular rigidity [6–8, 135]. In addition, hypodopaminergia developing in the anterior cingulate-medial orbitofrontal circuit could participate in causing diminished responsiveness, akinesia and mutism, and contribute to hyperthermia and autonomic dysfunction. Bilateral lesions of this circuit have been associated with akinetic mutism, which involves severe hypomotility, diminished arousal and mutism, and has been mistaken for simple catatonia [138]. Furthermore, certain cases of akinetic mutism have presented with hyperthermia and autonomic dysfunction, making them difficult to distinguish from MC and NMS [6, 8, 135]. In this regard, it is of considerable interest that the anterior cingulate-medial orbitofrontal circuit contains a spur from the ventral pallidum to the lateral hypothalamus [139]. This suggests that reduced dopamine activity could cause hyperthermia and autonomic dysfunction in MC and NMS by disrupting anterior cingulate-medial orbitofrontal circuit transmission to the lateral hypothalamus.

Finally, hypodopaminergia involving the lateral orbitofrontal subcortical circuit may mediate selected catatonic features observed in simple catatonia, MC, and NMS. Dysfunction in the lateral orbitofrontal region has been associated with utilization and imitation behaviors [140]. These behaviors involve automatic imitation of the gestures and actions of others or inappropriate use of objects such as tools or utensils. Utilization and imitation behaviors reflect enslavement to environmental cues [140] and share striking clinical similarities with catatonic features such as echopraxia, echolalia, and geigenhalten, all of which are viewed as stimulus bound or motor preservative phenomena consistent with frontal lobe dysfunction [140]. Utilization and imitation behaviors may also occur in association with dorsolateral prefrontal circuit dysfunction.

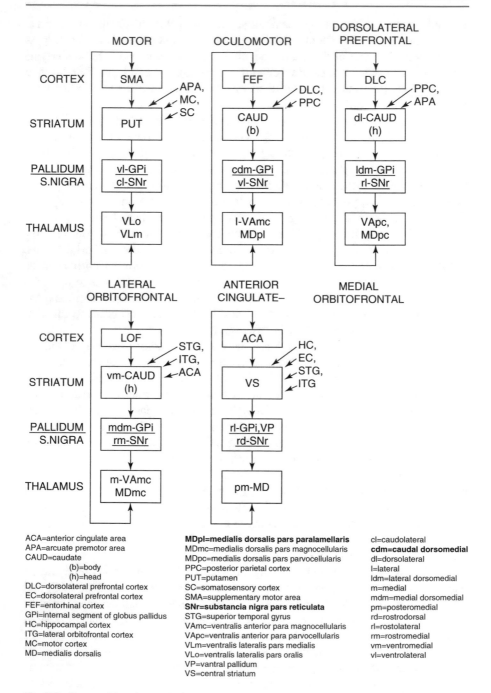

Fig. 7.1 Proposed basal ganglia-thalamocortical circuits. Parallel organization of the five basal ganglia-thalamocortical circuits. Each circuit engages specific regions of the cerebral cortex, striatum, pallidum, substantia nigra, and thalamus. (Adapted with permission from Alexander et al. [136])

We have proposed that in addition to dopamine-2 receptor blockade, NMS is the product of pre-existing central dopamine hypoactivity that represents a trait vulnerability marker for this disorder, coupled with state-related downward adjustments in the dopamine system occurring in response to acute or repeated exposure to stress [6, 8, 135]. Here, we suggest that such state- and trait-related factors are also critical in causing hypodopaminergia in the frontal subcortical circuits in simple catatonia, MC, and NMS. A number of lines of evidence indicate that certain individuals may exhibit baseline hypodopaminergia, including reduced homovanillic acid (HVA) levels in post-NMS patients; reduced striatal HVA levels or lack of elevated HVA to dopamine ratios in patients who died from MC or NMS; lower cerebrospinal fluid HVA levels and more severe baseline parkinsonian symptoms in patients with Parkinson's disease following recovery from NMS; and reports of abnormalities in the dopamine-2 receptor gene in NMS [6, 8, 135].

Furthermore, the enhanced responsiveness of the dopamine system to stress may be implicated as a state-related co-factor predisposing to simple catatonia, MC, and NMS. In particular, the dopaminergic innervation of the medial prefrontal cortex in the rat is unique in that it is activated by very mild stressors such as limited foot shock or conditioned fear [141]. In addition, there are considerable data indicating a functional interdependence of dopamine systems innervating the medial prefrontal cortex and subcortical dopamine systems; changes in the medial prefrontal cortex dopamine system appear to have an inverse relationship with dopamine turnover in the dorsal and ventral striatum [142]. Consistent with this, lesions of the mesocortical dopamine pathway to the medial prefrontal cortex in the rat result in increased indexes of subcortical dopamine functioning [142].

Conversely, increased mesocortical dopaminergic neurotransmission to the medial prefrontal cortex has been associated with decreased indexes of subcortical dopamine functioning [142, 143]. Accordingly, if stress activates the stress-sensitive mesocortical dopaminergic pathway to the medial prefrontal cortex, it could have feedback effects in both the dorsal and ventral striata, rendering these areas hypodopaminergic and predisposing to MC and NMS in individuals with pre-existing central dopaminergic hypoactivity.

Management

Effective management hinges on early recognition of this disorder. Excluding neuromedical or drug-induced causes of MC is critical before assigning a psychiatric etiology. The potential for severe autonomic symptoms and the high rate of medical complications dictate early institution of intensive medical care focusing on fluid replacement, temperature reduction, and support of cardiac, respiratory, and renal functions. Careful monitoring to prevent complications, particularly aspiration pneumonia, thromboembolism, and renal failure is essential. Many clinicians, not recognizing the syndrome they are witnessing, are apt to treat MC patients with antipsychotic drugs. However, the bulk of evidence indicates that the dopamine receptor blocking effects of both first- and second-generation antipsychotics are likely to aggravate MC episodes, as in NMS where continuation of antipsychotic drug treatment clearly increases the likelihood of death. Antipsychotics should be withheld whenever MC is suspected. A treatment algorithm is shown in Fig. 7.2.

Benzodiazepines have been highly effective in the treatment of simple catatonia, including antipsychotic drug-induced catatonia [133]. Philbrick and Rummans [1] observed that the benefits of benzodiazepines in MC appeared less uniform than in simple catatonia but were nonetheless impressive at times. They asserted that even a partial response might be beneficial to retard the progression of MC until more definitive treatment can be instituted. Van Den Eede and associates [144] suggested that lorazepam be started at 2–4 mg per day (PO, IM, IV) and increased to 8–16 mg per day if simple catatonia does not resolve in 2 days. For MC, however, they proposed that lorazepam be initiated at 8–16 mg per day. Fricchione and associates [133] suggested that if simple catatonia proves unresponsive to lorazepam after 5 days of treatment, ECT should become a consideration. In MC, however, these researchers argued against a 5-day wait and urged that ECT be started expeditiously if lorazepam does not briskly reverse the MC process.

Indeed, ECT is a safe and effective treatment for MC occurring as an outgrowth of a psychiatric disorder [1, 145]. Although controlled studies are lacking, case reports and series of consecutive cases indicate excellent results with its use. Among 50 patients reported in four large series [1, 5, 145], 40 of 41 patients treated with

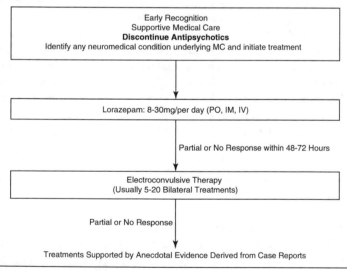

Fig. 7.2 Proposed treatment algorithm for malignant catatonia. (Adapted with permission from Fricchione et al. [133]. Copyright 1997, Sage Publications Inc)

ECT survived. In contrast, only five of nine who received antipsychotics and supportive care survived. However, ECT appears effective only if initiated before severe progression of MC symptoms. Sedvic [146] stressed that the onset of coma or a temperature exceeding 41 °C predicts a poor response even to ECT. Arnold and Stepan [11] found that of 19 patients starting ECT within 5 days of the onset of hyperthermia, 16 survived, whereas in 14 patients starting treatment beyond this point, ECT had no effect in preventing a fatal outcome. Although earlier protocols called for particularly intensive treatment [11], recent trials have indicated that ECT can be efficacious when given once or twice daily or every other day for a total of 5–20 treatments (usually bilateral). Substantial improvement often becomes evident after 1–4 treatments [145].

⊙━━▼ Lorazepam and ECT are safe and effective treatments for MC.

Several investigators have suggested that ECT in combination with dantrolene, a drug that inhibits contraction and heat production in muscle, represents the optimal treatment for MC [5–8]. Other cases have reported successful treatment with dantrolene alone; the dopamine agonist bromocriptine combined with dantrolene and ECT; bromocriptine and benzodiazepines; dantrolene and bromocriptine [5–8]; the NMDA antagonist and dopamine agonist amantadine [26, 147]; and the NMDA antagonist memantine combined with lorazepam [74]. Successful treatment with transcranial magnetic stimulation (rTMS) has been observed in one case [90]. Lastly, intravenous propofol has been reported effective as an interim measure until ECT can be instituted [148], considered a superior anesthetic for MC during ECT [150], and proposed as capable of "lysing" MC on its own [28, 149, 150]. In MC occurring as an outgrowth of a neuromedical illness, specific treatment must be directed at the underlying disorder. Nevertheless, in our full series of 504 MC cases, ECT has been reported as highly effective in treating MC complicating a diversity of neuromedical conditions [1, 5–8, 145]. In such cases, the efficacy of ECT appears largely independent of the underlying condition and improvement is likely to be transient if the neuromedical condition persists. If, however, the underlying disorder either remits or is corrected, permanent recovery may be possible. Along these lines, ECT has been used effectively in stabilizing MC (and NMS) in anti-NMDA receptor encephalitis, permitting definitive measures such as tumor removal (if indicated) and sequential immunotherapies to take effect [49, 151].

Conclusion

MC represents a life-threatening neuropsychiatric disorder described long before the introduction of modern antipsychotic drugs. A review of the world literature on MC indicates that although the incidence of the condition may have declined since the pre-antipsychotic drug era, it continues to occur but is under-recognized. MC represents a syndrome rather than a specific disease and may develop as an outgrowth of diverse neuromedical illnesses as well as with psychiatric disorders. Among 399 MC cases reported during the 50-year period between 1960 and 2010,

339 (85%) were attributed to a psychiatric condition and only 60 (15%) to a neuro-medical condition. In contrast, among our most recent 105 MC cases reported during the nine years between 2011 and 2020, 80 (76%) are now attributed to neuromedical illness and only 25 (24%) are associated with a psychiatric disorder. These findings are striking but appear consistent with the impression that anti-NMDAR encephalitis may now account for many MC cases previously attributed to psychosis or schizophrenia, MC cases viewed as an outgrowth of viral encephalitis where no pathogen was identified, and MC cases previously ascribed to encephalitis lethargica.

Also, from a perspective of MC as a syndrome, NMS may be conceptualized as an antipsychotic drug-induced toxic or iatrogenic subtype of MC. The hypothesis that simple catatonia, MC, and NMS share a common pathophysiology involving reduced dopaminergic neurotransmission within the basal ganglia-thalamocortical circuits underscores their identity as variants of a larger unitary catatonic syndrome. ECT appears to be the preferred treatment for MC. Antipsychotic drugs should be withheld whenever MC is suspected. Recognition of the clinical features of MC and an appreciation of its diverse etiologies are essential for the effective management of patients who develop this catastrophic reaction.

References

1. Philbrick KL, Rummans TA. Malignant catatonia. J Neuropsychiatry Clin Neurosci. 1994;6(1):1–13.
2. Stauder KH. Die todliche Katatonie. Arch Psychiatr Nervenkr. 1934;102:614–34.
3. Calmeil LF. Dictionnaire de Medecine ou Repertoire General des Sciences. Medicales sous le Rapport Theorique et Practique. 2nd ed. Paris: Bechet; 1832.
4. Bell LV. On a form of insanity resembling some advanced stages of mania and fever. Am J Insan. 1849;6:97–127.
5. Mann SC, Caroff SN, Bleier HR, Welz WK, Kling MA, Hayashida M. Lethal catatonia. Am J Psychiatry. 1986;143(11):1374–81.
6. Mann SC. Malignant catatonia. In: Mann SC, Caroff SN, Keck Jr PE, Lazarus A, editors. The neuroleptic malignant syndrome and related conditions. 2nd ed. Washington, DC: American Psychiatric Publishing Inc.; 2003. p. 121–43.
7. Mann SC, Caroff SN, Campbell EC, Bleier HR, Greenstein RA. Malignant catatonia. In: Frucht SJ, Fahn S, editors. Movement disorder emergencies: diagnosis and treatment. Totowa: Humana Press; 2005. p. 53–67.
8. Mann SC, Caroff SN, Bleier HR, Campbell EC. Malignant catatonia. In: Frucht SJ, editor. Movement disorder emergencies: diagnosis and treatment. 2nd ed. New York: Humana Press; 2013. p. 59–74.
9. Dalmau J, Graus F. Antibody-mediated encephalitis. N Engl J Med. 2018;378(9):840–51.
10. Caroff SN. The neuroleptic malignant syndrome. J Clin Psychiatry. 1980;41(3):79–83.
11. Arnold OH, Stepan H. Untersuchungen zur Frage der akuten todlichen Katatonie. Wien Z Nervenheilkd Grenzgeb. 1952;4:235–58.
12. Kraepelin E. In: Johnstone T, editor. Lectures on clinical psychiatry. 2nd ed. New York: William Wood; 1905.
13. Ladame C. Psychose aigue idiopathique ou foudroyante. Schweizer Archiv fur Neurologic und Psychiatre. 1919;5:3–28.

14. Karacetin G, Bayer R, Demir T. Successful treatment of benzodiazepine-resistant malignant catatonia with electroconvulsive therapy. J Neuropsychiatry Clin Neurosci. 2012;24(1):E48.
15. Wong S, Hughes B, Pudek M, Dailin L. Malignant catatonia mimicking pheochromocytoma. Case Rep Endocrinol. 2013;2013:815821. https://doi.org/10.1155/2013/815821.
16. Nisijima K. Increased biogenic catecholamine and metabolite levels in two patients with malignant catatonia. Neuropsychiatr Dis Treat. 2013;9:1171–4.
17. Hobo M, Uezato A, Nishiyama M, Suzuki M, Kurata J, Makita K, et al. A case of malignant catatonia with idiopathic pulmonary arterial hypertension treated by electroconvulsive therapy. BMC Psychiatry. 2016;16:130. https://doi.org/10.1186/s12888-016-0835-4.
18. Duncan MD, Vazirani SS. An unusual rapid response call: malignant catatonia. Am J Med. 2016;129(7):678–80.
19. Park J, Tan J, Krzeminski S, Hazeghazam M, Bandiamuri M, Carlson RW. Malignant catatonia warrants early psychiatric-critical care collaborative management: two cases and literature review. Case Rep Crit Care. 2017;2017:1951965. https://doi.org/10.1155/2017/1951965.
20. Ohi K, Kuwata A, Shimada T, Yasuyama T, Nitta Y, Uehara T, et al. Response to benzodiazepines and the clinical course in malignant catatonia associated with schizophrenia. Medicine (Baltimore). 2017;96(16):e6566. https://doi.org/10.1097/MD.0000000000006566.
21. Ghaziuddin N, Hendricks M, Patel P, Wachtel LE, Dhossche DM. Neuroleptic malignant syndrome/malignant catatonia in child psychiatry: literature review and a case series. J Child Adolesc Psychopharmacol. 2017;27(4):359–65.
22. Kurose S, Koreki A, Funayama M, Takahashi E, Kaji M, Ogyu K, et al. Resting-state hyperperfusion in whole brain: a case of malignant catatonia that improved with electric convulsion therapy. Schizophr Res. 2019;210:287–8.
23. Ozan E, Aydin EF. Challenges in diagnosing and treating malignant catatonia and its fatal consequences. J Neuropsychiatry Clin Neurosci. 2014;26(1):E52.
24. Wachtel L, Commins E, Park M, Rolider N, Stephens R, Reti I. Neuroleptic malignant syndrome and delirious mania as malignant catatonia in autism: prompt relief with electroconvulsive therapy. Acta Psychiatr Scand. 2015;132(4):319–20.
25. Dessens F, van Passen J, van Westerloo DJ, van der Wee N, van Vliet IM, Van Noorden MS. Electroconvulsive therapy in the intensive care unit for the treatment of catatonia: a case series and review of the literature. Gen Hosp Psychiatry. 2016;38:37–41.
26. Maki M, Kato O, Kunimatsu J, Sato T, Fujie S. Significant response to amantadine in a patient with malignant catatonia. Eur Psychiatry. 2016;33(S1):S336.
27. Onofrei C, Singh R, Sears C. 1821: diagnostic challenges and treatment of malignant catatonia with electroconvulsive therapy. Crit Care Med. 2016;44(12):530.
28. Bellani M, Zanette G, Zovetti N, Barillari M, Del Piccolo L, Brambilla P. Adult mild encephalitis with reversible splenial lesion associated with delirious mania: a case report. Front Psych. 2020;11:79. https://doi.org/10.3389/fpsyt.2020.00079.
29. Adams G, Brown A, Burnside R, Tandy D, Lowe K, Malhotra A, et al. A undiagnosed stupor in the acute medical unit: a case of malignant catatonia. Q J Med. 2015;108(4):335–6.
30. Matias DFM, de Mello AS, Riera R, Teixeira de Gois A. Malignant catatonia responsive to low doses of lorazepam: case report. Sao Paulo Med J. 2016;134(2):176–9.
31. Shenai N, White CD, Azzam PN, Gopalan P, Solai LK. Practical and legal challenges to a electroconvulsive therapy in malignant catatonia. Harv Rev Psychiatry. 2016;24(3):238–41.
32. Hirayama I, Inokuchi R, Hiruma T, Doi K, Morimura N. Malignant catatonia mimics tetanus. Clin Pract Cases Emerg Med. 2018;2(4):369–70.
33. Buvanaswari P. Behaviour changes with autonomic disturbances-malignant catatonia? Eur Psychiatry. 2015;30(Supplement 1):1264.
34. Averna R, Battaglia C, Labonia M, Riccioni A, Vicari S. Catatonia in adolescence: first onset psychosis or anti-NMDAR encephalitis? Clin Neuropharmacol. 2019;42(4):136–8.
35. Hefter D, Topor CE, Gass P, Hirjak D. Two sides of the same coin: a case report of first-episode catatonic syndrome in a high-functioning autism patient. Front Psych. 2019;10:224. https://doi.org/10.3389/fpsyt.2019.00224.

36. Consoli A, Ronen K, An-Gourfinkel I, Barbeau M, Marra D, Costedoat-Chalumeau N, et al. Malignant catatonia due to anti-MNDA-receptor encephalitis in a 17-year old girl: case report. Child Adolesc Psychiatry Ment Health. 2011;5(1):15. https://doi.org/10.118 6/1753-2000-5-15.

37. Wingfield T, McHugh C, Vas A, Richardson A, Wilkens E, Boninton A, et al. Autoimmune encephalitis: a case series and comprehensive review of the literature. Q J Med. 2011;104(11):921–31.

38. Achour NB, Youssef-Turki IB, Messelmani M, Kraoua I, Yaacoubi J, Klaa H, et al. Anti-NMDA receptor encephalitis mimicking a primary psychiatric disorder in a 13-year-old girl. Turk J Psychiatry. 2012;24(2):145–7.

39. Finke C, Kopp UA, Pruss H, Dalmau J, Wandinger K-P, Ploner CJ. Cognitive deficits following anti-NMDA receptor encephalitis. J Neurol Neurosurg Psychiatry. 2012;83(2):195–8.

40. Haththotuwa HR, Malhas L, Jagadeeswaran A. Anti-NMDA receptor encephalitis an intensive care perspective. J Intensive Care Soc. 2012;13(2):147–50.

41. McCarthy A, Dineen J, McKenna P, Keogan M, Sheehan J, Lynch T, et al. Anti NMDA receptor encephalitis with associated catatonia during pregnancy. J Neurol. 2012;259(12):2632–5.

42. Obligar P, Ortiz M, Lee L. Rapid response of methylprednisone in a 14 year old male with proven anti-NMDA receptor encephalitis. Philipp J Neurol. 2012;16(1):54–5.

43. Di Capua D, Garcia-Ptacek S, Garcia-Garcia ME, Abarrategui B, Porta-Etessam J, Garcia-Morales I. Extreme delta brush in a patient with anti-NMDAR encephalitis. Epileptic Disord. 2013;15:461–4.

44. Wilson JE, Shuster J, Fuchs C. Anti-NMDA receptor encephalitis in a 14-year-old female presenting as malignant catatonia-medical and psychiatry approach to treatment. Psychosomatics. 2013;54(6):585–9.

45. Young PJ, Baker S, Cavazzoni E, Erickson SJ, Krishnan A, Kruger PS, et al. A case series of critically ill patients with anti-NMDA receptor encephalitis. Crit Care Resusc. 2013;15(1):8–14.

46. Serban-Pereteanu AS, Trasca D, Stefanescu VC, Bustan M, Zurac S, Cojocaru IM. Anti-NMDA receptor encephalitis in a young woman: a diagnostic challenge. Rom J Neurol. 2014;8(4):200–11.

47. Acien P, Ruiz-Macia E, Acien M, Martin-Estefania C. Mature ovarian teratoma-associated limbic encephalitis. J Obstet Gynaecol. 2015;35(3):317–9.

48. Hur J. Fever of unknown origin: an unusual presentation of anti-NMDA receptor encephalitis. Infect Chemother. 2015;47(2):129–32.

49. Jones KC, Schwartz AC, Hermida AP, Kahn DA. A case of anti-NMDA receptor encephalitis treated with ECT. J Psychiatr Pract. 2015;21(5):374–80.

50. Kiani R, Lawden M, Eames P, Critchley P, Bhaumik S, Odedra S, et al. Anti-NMDA-receptor encephalitis presenting with catatonia and neuroleptic syndrome in patients with intellectual disability and autism. BJPsych Bull. 2015;39(1):32–5.

51. Koksal A, Baybas S, Mutluay B, Altunkaynak Y, Keskek A. A case of NMDAR encephalitis missed diagnosed as post partum psychosis and neuroleptic malignant syndrome. Neurol Sci. 2015;36(7):1257–8.

52. Simabukuro MM, de Andrade Freitas CH, Castro LHM. A patient with a long history of relapsing psychosis and mania presenting with anti-NMDA receptor encephalitis 10 years after first episode. Dement Neuropsychol. 2015;9(3):311–4.

53. Afanasiev V, Brechemier M-L, Boisseau W, Ducoudray R, Mayer M-E, Meyronet D, et al. Anti-NMDA receptor antibody encephalitis and neuroendocrine pancreatic tumor: causal link? Neurology. 2016;87(1):112–3.

54. Aulicka S, Horak O, Mrazova L, Mikolasek P, Strba J, Krbkova L, et al. Malignant catatonia due to anti-NMDA-receptor encephalitis in a 15-year-old girl: case report and summary of current knowledge. Neuropsychiatry (London). 2016;6(4):136–41.

55. Halbert RK. Anti-N-Methyl-D-Aspartate receptor encephalitis: a case study. J Neurosci Nurs. 2016;48(5):270–3.

56. Milovac Z, Santini M, Pisk SV, Caratan S, Gorsic V, Filipcic E. Acute psychosis-anti-NMDA receptor encephalitis phase. Psychiatr Danub. 2016;28(3):301–3.
57. Rozier M, Morita D, King M. Anti-N-Methyl-D-Aspartate receptor encephalitis: a potential mimic of neuroleptic malignant syndrome. Pediatr Neurol. 2016;63:71–2.
58. Splendiani A, Felli V, Di Sibio A, Gennarelli A, Patriarca L, Stratta P, et al. Magnetic resonance imagining and magnetic resonance spectroscopy in a young male patient with anti-N-methyl-D-aspartate receptor encephalitis and uncommon cerebellar involvement: a case report with review of the literature. Neuroradiol J. 2016;29(1):30–5.
59. Vargas RJ, Farid H, Goldenson RP, Fairchild AH, Dorton BJ, Bromley BS. Ovarian teratomas and Anti-N-Methyl-D-Aspartate receptor encephalitis: why sonography first? J Ultrasound Med. 2016;35(4):852–4.
60. Ziplow J, Chadha T, Wen A. 1834: psychosis seizures and autonomic instability in a teenage girl with an ovarian mass. Crit Care Med. 2016;44(12):534.
61. Bota RG, Groysman L, Momii A. Catatonia as a syndrome characterized by GABAergic interneuronal dysfunction mediated by NMDA receptors. Br J Med Med Res. 2017;19(11):1–6.
62. Doden T, Sekijima Y, Ikeda J, Ozawa K, Ohashi N, Kodaira M, et al. Postpartum anti-N-Methyl-D-aspartate receptor encephalitis: a case report and literature review. Intern Med (Tokyo). 2017;56(3):357–62.
63. Hermans T, Santens P, Matton C, Oostra K, Heylens G, Herremans S, et al. Anti-NMDA receptor encephalitis: still unknown and underdiagnosed by physicians and especially psychiatrists? Acta Clin Belg. 2017;73(5):364–7.
64. Liang Z, Yang S, Sun X, Li B, Li W, Liu Z, et al. Teratoma-associated anti-NMDAR encephalitis. Two cases report and literature review. Medicine (Baltimore). 2017;96:e9177.
65. Sivarooban V, Yogitagavari Y, Che CK, Lee CW. Organic disorder with neuropsychiatric symptoms-case report of anti-NMDA receptor encephalitis with neuropsychiatric manifestations. Malaysian J Psychiatry Ejournal. 2017;26(1):37–42.
66. Tsutsui K, Takaki M, Omori Y, Imai Y, Nishino S, Tanaka K, et al. N-Methy-D-aspartate receptor antibody could be the cause of catatonic symptoms in psychiatric patients: case reports and methods for detection. Neuropsychiatr Dis Treat. 2017;13:339–45.
67. Voice J, Ponterio JM, Lakhi N. Psychosis secondary to an incidental teratoma: a "heads-up" for psychiatrists and gynecologists. Arch Womens Ment Health. 2017;20(5):703–7.
68. Vasenina EE, Levin OS, Gan'kina OA, Chimagomedova AS, Levikov DI. Auto immune anti-NMDA receptor encephalitis. Neurosci Behav Phys. 2018;48(6):650–6.
69. Amugoda C, Foroush NC, Akhlaghi H. Anti-NMDAR encephalitis: higher suspicious needed for earlier diagnosis (Case report, literature review and diagnostic criteria). Neurol Med. 2019:7476254. https://doi.org/10.1155/2019/7476254.
70. Ford B, McDonald A, Srinivasan S. Anti-NMDA receptor encephalitis: a case study and illness overview. Drugs Context. 2019;8:212589. https://doi.org/10.7573/dic.212589.
71. Moussa T, Afzal K, Cooper J, Rosenberger R, Gerstle K, Wagner-Weiner L. Pediatric anti-NMDA receptor encephalitis with catatonia: treatment with electroconvulsive therapy. Pediatr Rheumatol. 2019;17:8. https://doi.org/10.1186/s12969-019-0310-0.
72. Schermann H, Ponomareva IV, Gennadievich V, Yakushev KB, Sherman MA. Clinical variants of limbic encephalitis. SAGE Open Med Case Rep. 2019;7:1–10. https://doi.org/10.1177/2050313X19846042.
73. AlShimemeri S, Alsaeed M, Lai J, Uy C. Delayed N-methyl-D-aspartate receptor encephalitis relapse. Can J Neurol Sci. 2020;47(2):264–6. https://doi.org/10.1017/cjn.2019.332.
74. Ramirez-Bermudez J, Restrepo-Martinez M, Diaz-Victoria AR, Espinola-Nadurille ME. Memantine as an adjunctive therapy in a patient with anti-NMDA receptor encephalitis. J Clin Psychopharmacol. 2019;40(1):92–3. https://doi.org/10.1097/JCP.0000000000001145.
75. Sokhi DS, Bhogal OS. Autoimmune encephalitis is recognized as an important differential diagnosis in a Kenyan tertiary referral center. BMJ Mil Health. 2020; https://doi.org/10.1136/jramc-2019-001338.

76. Nikolaus M, Knierim E, Meisel C, Kreye J, Pruss H, Schnabel D, et al. Severe GABA A receptor encephalitis without seizures: a paediatric case successfully treated with early immunomodulation. Eur J Paediatr Neurol. 2018;22(3):558–62.
77. Samra K, Rogers J, Mahdi-Rogers M, Stanton B. Catatonia with GABA A receptor antibodies. Pract Neurol. 2020;20:139–43.
78. Carneiro S, Fernades I, Abuowda Y, Oliveria AA, Santos C, Palos A, et al. Anti-vgkc antibody-associated limbic encephalitis presenting with recurrent catatonia. Eur Psychiatry. 2015;30(Supp 1):812.
79. Xu Z, Prasad K, Yeo T. Progressive encephalomyelitis with rigidity and myoclonus in an intellectually disabled patient mimicking neuroleptic malignant syndrome. J Mov Disord. 2017;10(2):99–101.
80. Mon T, L'Ecuyer S, Farber NB, White AJ, Baszis KW, Hearn JK, et al. The use of electroconvulsive in a patient with juvenile systemic lupus erythematosus and catatonia. Lupus. 2012;21(14):1575–81.
81. Ali A, Taj A. Misbah-uz-Zehra. Lupus catatonia in a young girl who presented with fever and altered sensorium. Pak J Med Sci. 2014;30(2):446–8.
82. Strohmayer K. D47 case vignette in critical care: a case of malignant catatonia due to central nervous system involvement of systemic lupus erythematosus (sle) necessitating treatment in the intensive care unit (icu). Am J Respir Crit Care Med. 2014;189:A6128.
83. Jones M, Gausche E, Reed E. A case of neuropsychiatric lupus with severe malignant catatonia that improves with daily electroconvulsive therapy. J Neuropsychiatry Clin Neurosci. 2016;28(1):e19–20. https://doi.org/10.1176/appi.neuropsych.15080211.
84. Bharadwaj B, Sugaparaneetharan A, Rajkumar RP. Graves' disease presenting with catatonia: a probable cause of encephalopathy associated with autoimmune thyroid disease. Acta Neuropsychiatr. 2012;24(6):374–9.
85. Saito T, Saito R, Suwa H, Yakushiji F, Takezawa K, Nakamura M. Differences in the treatment response to antithyroid drugs versus electroconvulsive therapy in a case of recurrent catatonia due to Graves' disease. Case Rep Psychiatry. 2012:868490. https://doi.org/10.1155/2012/868490.
86. Rosado SN, Silveira V, Reis AI, Gordinho A, Noronha C. Catatonia and psychosis as manifestations of primary Sjogren's syndrome. Eur J Case Rep Intern Med. 2018;5(6):000855. https://doi.org/10.12890/2018_000855.
87. Mischel NA, Mooneyham GLC, Lau C, Van Mater H, Weiner RD. Non-N-methyl-D-aspartate autoimmune encephalopathy and catatonia treatment with electroconvulsive therapy: a pediatric case series and treatment guidelines. Psychosomatics. 2020; https://doi.org/10.1016/j.psym.2019.12.005.
88. Aggarwal A, Kumar P, Faridi MMA. Neurological manifestation as presenting feature of dengue infection. J Pediatr Neurosci. 2015;10:76–7.
89. Halder A, Biswas A. Multifactorial organic etiological agents causing catatonia: a learning experience. Int J Educ Psychol Res. 2015;1:301–3.
90. Kate MP, Raju D, Vishwanathan V, Khan FR, et al. Successful treatment of refractory organic catatonic disorder with repetitive transcranial magnetic stimulation (rTMS) therapy. J Neuropsychiatry Clin Neurosci. 2011;22(3):E2–3.
91. Shukla L, Narayanaswamy JC, Gopinath S, Math SB. Electroconvulsive therapy for the treatment of organic catatonia due to viral encephalitis. J ECT. 2012;28(3):E-27–E28. https://doi.org/10.1097/YCT.0b013e31824e9228.
92. Saini SM, Eu CL, Yahya WNN, Rahman AHA. Malignant catatonia secondary to viral menigoencephalitis in a young man with bipolar disorder. Asia Pac Psychiatry. 2013;5(Supp 1):55–8.
93. Vadala SF, Pellegrini D, Silva ED, Minarro D, Finn BC, Bruetman JE, et al. Lethargic encephalitis. Report of one case. Rev Med Chile. 2013;141(4):531–4.
94. Bigman DY, Bobrin BD. Von Economo's disease and post-encephalitic parkinsonism responsive to carbidopa and levodopa. Neuropsychiatr Dis Treat. 2018;14:927–31.

95. Becker MA, Cannon J, Certa KA. A case of mycoplasma pneumonia encephalopathy presenting as mania. Psychosomatics. 2020; https://doi.org/10.1016/j.psym.2020.02.004.
96. Aghamollaii V, Ahmadinejad Z, Mohammadian F, Mirsepassi Z. Catatonic state as a rare presentation of neurobrucellosis: a case report. Iran J Psychiatry Behav Sci. 2019;13(3):e95824. https://doi.org/10.5812/ijpbs.95824.
97. Hocker SE, Wijdicks EFM. Neurological complications of sepsis. Continuum (Minneapolis, MN). 2014;20(3):598–613.
98. Kanagasundram S, Chengappa KNR. Meningoencephalitis or clozapine withdrawal catatonia or both in a patient with schizophrenia. Acta Neuropsychiatr. 2011;23(2):85–7.
99. Koch A, Reich K, Wielopolski J, Clepce M, Fischer M, Cornhuber J, et al. Catatonic dilemma in a 33-year-old woman: a discussion. Case Rep Psychiatry. 2013:542303.
100. Bilbily J, McCollum B, de Leon J. Catatonia secondary to sudden clozapine withdraw: a case with three repeated episodes and a literature review. Case Rep Psychiatry. 2017:2402731. https://doi.org/10.1155/2017/2402731.
101. Fryml LD, Williams KR, Pelic CG, Fox J, Sahlem G, Robert S, et al. The role of amantadine withdrawal in 3 cases of treatment-refractory altered mental status. J Psychiatr Pract. 2017;23(3):191–9.
102. Amos JJ. Lorazepam withdrawal-induced catatonia. Ann Clin Psychiatry. 2012;24(2):170–1.
103. Dada MU, Oluwole L, Obadeji A, Ajayi OA. Dexamethasone induced psychosis presenting with catatonic features. Afr J Psychiatry. 2011;14:316–8.
104. Clough Z, Henry R, Ekelund A. Delirium associated with therapeutic levels of lithium in bipolar disorder. Prog Neurol Psychiatry. 2014;18(2):10–2.
105. van Esch AMJ, Fest A, Hoffland BS, Janzing JGE, Steens SCA, Esselink RAJ, et al. Toxic leukoencephalopathy presenting as lethal catatonia. J Addict Med. 2019;13(3):241–4.
106. Keary CJ, Nejad SH, Rasimas JJ, Stern TA. Intoxications associated with agitation, tachycardia, hypertension, and fever: differential diagnosis, evaluation, and management. Prim Care Companion CNS Disord. 2013;15(3):PCC.12f01459. https://doi.org/10.4088/PCC.12f01459.
107. Kumar KK, Bondade S, Sattar FA, Singh N. Malignant catatonia and neuroleptic malignant syndrome in relation to disulfiram overdose. Indian J Psychol Med. 2016;38(4):344–7.
108. Johansson A, Lindstedt D, Roman M, Thelander G, Nielson EI, Lennborn U, et al. A nonfatal intoxication and seven deaths involving the dissociative drug 3-MeO-PCP. Forensic Sci Int. 2017;275(6):76–82.
109. Bulbena-Cabre A, DiGenova P, Sigel P, Dunn NR, Swift RG. Synthetic cannabinoid intoxication presenting as malignant catatonia: a case report. Int J Ment Health Addict. 2020;18(3):582–6.
110. Heekin RD, Bradshaw K, Calarge CA. First known case of catatonia due to cyclosporine A-related neurotoxicity in a pediatric patient with steroid-resistant nephrotic syndrome. BMC Psychiatry. 2019;19:123. https://doi.org/10.1186/s12888-019-2107-6.
111. Rojas PG, Morton L. An unusual case of fever and altered mental status. JAMDA. 2020;21(3):B4. https://doi.org/10.1016/j.jamda.2020.01.019.
112. Lee S, Jun GW, Jeon SB, Kim CJ, Kim JH. Paroxysmal sympathetic hyperactivity in brain-compressing huge benign tumors: clinical experience and literature review. Springerplus. 2016;5:340. https://doi.org/10.1186/s40064-016-1898-x.
113. Rengers E, Pop-Purceleanu M, Rietveld L, van der Weyer RW, Frenzael T. Recognize malignant catatonia early: it is well treatable! A case report and review of the literature. Neth J Crit Care. 2017;25(2):67–70.
114. Singerman S, Raheja R. Malignant catatonia-a continuing reality. Ann Clin Psychiatry. 1994;6(4):259–66.
115. Lee JW. Serum iron in catatonia and neuroleptic syndrome. Biol Psychiatry. 1998;44(6):499–507.
116. Oldham MA. The probability that catatonia in the hospital has a medical cause the relative proportions of its causes: a systematic review. Psychosomatics. 2018;59(4):333–40.

117. Caroff SN, Mann SC, Campbell EC, Sullivan KA. Epidemiology. In: Caroff SN, Mann SC, Francis A, Fricchione G, editors. Catatonia: from psychopathology to neurobiology. Washington, DC: American Psychiatric Press; 2004. p. 15–31.
118. Stompe T, Ortwein-Swoboda G, Ritter K, Schanda H, Friedman A. Are we witnessing the disappearance of catatonic schizophrenia? Compr Psychiatry. 2002;43:167–74.
119. Dalmau J, Tuzun E, Wu H-Y, Masjuan J, Rossi JE, Voloschin A, et al. Paraneoplastic anti-N-methyl-D-aspartate receptor encephalitis associated with ovarian teratoma. Ann Neurol. 2007;61(1):25–36.
120. Tanguturi YC, Cundiff AW, Fuchs C. Anti-N Methyl d-aspartate receptor encephalitis and electroconvulsive therapy. Literature review and future directions. Child Adolesc Psychiatric Clin N Am. 2019;28:79–89.
121. Serra-Mestres J, Villagrasa-Blasco B, Thacker V, Jaimes-Albornoz W, Sharma P, Isetta M. Catatonia in N-methyl-d-aspartate receptor antibody encephalitis: phenomenological characteristics from a systematic review of case reports. Gen Hosp Psychiatry. 2020;64:9–16.
122. Gurrera RJ. Frequency and temporal sequence of clinical features in adults with anti-NMDA receptor encephalitis presenting with psychiatric symptoms. Psychol Med. 2019;49:2709–16.
123. Dalmau J, Gleichman AJ, Hughes EG, Rossi JE, Peng X, Lai M, et al. Anti-NMDA-receptor encephalitis: case series and analysis of effects of antibodies. Lancet Neurol. 2008;7(12):1091–8.
124. Espinola-Nadurille M, Flores-Rivera J, Rivas-Alonso V, Vargas-Canas S, Fricchione GL, Bayliss L, et al. Catatonia in patients with anti-NMDA receptor encephalitis. Psychiatry Clin Neurosci. 2019;73(9):574–80.
125. Rogers JP, Pollak TA, Blackman G, David AS. Catatonia and the immune system: a review. Lancet Psychiatry. 2019;6:620–30.
126. Sarkis RA, Coffey MJ, Cooper JJ, Hassan I, Lennox B. Anti-N-Methyl-D-Aspartate receptor encephalitis: a review of psychiatric phenotypes and management considerations: a report of the American Neuropsychiatric Committee on Research. J Neuropsychiatry Clin Neurosci. 2019;31(2):137–42.
127. Lejuste F, Thomas L, Picard G, Desestret V, Ducray F, Rogemond V, et al. Neuroleptic intolerance in patients with anti-NMDAR encephalitis. Neurol Neuroimmunol Neuroinflamm. 2016;3:e280.
128. Fink M, Taylor MA. Catatonia: a clinician's guide to diagnosis and treatment. Cambridge: Cambridge University Press; 2003.
129. Fricchione GL. Neuroleptic catatonia and its relationship to psychogenic catatonia. Biol Psychiatry. 1985;20(3):304–13.
130. Koch M, Chandragiri S, Rizvi S, Petrides G, Francis A. Catatonic signs in neuroleptic malignant syndrome. Compr Psychiatry. 2000;41(1):73–5.
131. Castillo E, Rubin RT, Holsboer-Trachsler E. Clinical differentiation of lethal catatonia and neuroleptic malignant syndrome. Am J Psychiatry. 1989;146(3):324–8.
132. Fleischhacker WW, Unterweger B, Kane JM, Hinterhuber H. The neuroleptic malignant syndrome and its differentiation from lethal catatonia. Acta Psychiatr Scand. 1990;81(1):3–5.
133. Fricchione G, Bush G, Fozdar M, Frances A, Fink M. Recognition and treatment of the catatonic syndrome. J Intensive Care Med. 1997;12(3):135–47.
134. Hirjak D, Kubera KM, Wolf RC, Northoff G. Going back to Kahlbaum's psychomotor (and GABAergic) origins. Is catatonia more than just a motor and dopaminergic syndrome? Schizophr Bull. 2020;46(2):272–85.
135. Mann SC, Caroff SN, Fricchione G, Campbell EC. Central dopamine hypoactivity and the pathogenesis of neuroleptic malignant syndrome. Psychiatric Ann. 2000;30(5):363–74.
136. Alexander GE, DeLong MR, Strick PL. Parallel organization of functionally segregated circuits linking basal ganglia and cortex. Ann Rev Neurosci. 1986;9:357–81.
137. Alexander GE, Curtcher MD, DeLong MR. Basal ganglia-thalamocortical circuits: parallel substrates for motor, oculomotor, "prefrontal" and "limbic" functions. Prog Brain Res. 1991;85:119–46.

138. Cummings JL. Frontal-subcortical circuits and human behavior. Arch Neurol. 1993;50(8):873–80.
139. Deutch AY, Bourdelais AJ, Zahm DS. The nucleus accumbens core and shell: accumbal compartments and their functional attributes. In: Kalivas PW, Barnes CD, editors. Limbic motor circuits and neuropsychiatry. Boca Raton: CRC Press; 1993. p. 163–75.
140. Taylor MA. Catatonia: a review of a behavioral neurologic syndrome. Neuropsychiatry Neuropsychol Behav Neurol. 1990;3(1):48–72.
141. Thierry AM, Tassin JP, Blanc G, Glowinski J. Selective activation of the mesocortical dopamine system by stress. Nature. 1976;263:242–4.
142. Weinberger DR. Implications of normal brain development for the pathogenesis of schizophrenia. Arch Gen Psychiatry. 1987;44(7):660–9.
143. Pycock CL, Kerwin RW, Carter CJ. Effects of lesion of cortical dopamine terminals on subcortical dopamine receptors in rats. Nature. 1980;286:74–6.
144. Van Den Eede F, Van Hecke J, Van Dalfsen A, Van den Bossche B, Cosyns P, Sabbe BGC. The use of atypical antipsychotics in the treatment of catatonia. Eur Psychiatry. 2005;20(5–6):422–9.
145. Mann SC, Caroff SN, Bleier HR, Antelo RE, Un H. Electroconvulsive therapy of the lethal catatonia syndrome. Convuls Ther. 1990;6(3):239–47.
146. Sedvic V. Psychoses endangering life. Cesk Psychiatr. 1981;77:38–41. (In Czech)
147. Northoff G, Lins H, Boker H, Danos P, Bogerts B. Therapeutic efficacy of N-methyl-D-aspartate antagonist amantadine in febrile catatonia. J Clin Psychopharmacol. 1999;19(5):484–6.
148. Schonfeldt-Lecuona C, Cronemeyer M, Hiesener L, Connemann BJ, Gahr M, Sartorius A, et al. Comparison of international guidelines with regard to the treatment of malignant catatonia. Pharmacopsychiatry. 2020;53(1):14–20.
149. Alfson ED, Awosika OO, Singhal T, Fricchione GL. Lysis of catatonic withdrawal by propofol in a bone-marrow transplant recipient with adenovirus limbic encephalitis. Psychosomatics. 2013;54(2):192–5.
150. Fox FL, Bostwick JM. Propofol sedation of refractory delirious mania. Psychosomatics. 1997;38(3):288–90.
151. Coffey MJ, Cooper JJ. Electroconvulsive therapy in anti-N-methyl-D-aspartate receptor encephalitis. J ECT. 2016;32(4):225–9.

Serotonin Syndrome

8

Mark Forrest Gordon, Adena N. Leder,
and Laura A. Ketigian

Patient Vignettes

Patient 1

A 19-year-old male college student with a history of depression began treatment with sertraline 8 months ago. He has been compliant and is tolerating the treatment well. He presents to the emergency department with diaphoresis, agitation, confusion, dysarthria, staggering gait, and occasional myoclonic jerks in the lower extremities. He is accompanied by a friend, who admits the patient ingested 3,4-methylenedioxymethamphetamine (MDMA) at a college party a few hours earlier.

Patient 2

A 50-year-old female with fibromyalgia, depression, and anorexia currently takes duloxetine and mirtazapine. Tramadol was recently added for her chronic pain. She

Supplementary Information The online version of this chapter (https://doi.org/10.1007/978-3-030-75898-1_8) contains supplementary material, which is available to authorized users.

M. F. Gordon
Specialty Clinical Development, Teva Pharmaceuticals, West Chester, PA, USA

A. N. Leder
Adele Smithers Parkinson's Disease Treatment Center, New York Institute of Technology—College of Osteopathic Medicine, Old Westbury, NY, USA

L. A. Ketigian (✉)
New York Institute of Technology—College of Osteopathic Medicine, Old Westbury, NY, USA
e-mail: lketigia@nyit.edu

© Springer Nature Switzerland AG 2022
S. J. Frucht (ed.), *Movement Disorder Emergencies*, Current Clinical Neurology,
https://doi.org/10.1007/978-3-030-75898-1_8

arrives at the emergency department presenting with anxiety, diaphoresis, tachycardia, and diarrhea. On physical exam, she is found to have tremor and hyperreflexia.

Introduction

In 1960, Oates and Sjoerdsma [1] first identified the serotonin syndrome (SS) in depressed patients. These patients exhibited diaphoresis, mental status changes, restlessness, ataxia, and lower-extremity hyperreflexia. The authors attributed this syndrome to increased levels of serotonin from concurrent use of L-tryptophan and monoamine oxidase inhibitors (MAOIs). The serotonin syndrome has three manifestations: cognitive, autonomic, and neuromuscular, as outlined in Table 8.1 [2]. Each of these groups may present with varying degrees of symptoms. When diagnosing serotonin syndrome, at least one feature from each group should be present. Rarely, serotonin syndrome causes high fever, seizures, nystagmus, oculogyric crisis, opisthotonos, dysarthria, and paresthesias. It is important to also consider nontraditional initial presentations of serotonin syndrome, such as diffuse body pain as described in a case report by Guo et al. [3].

Criteria for Diagnosis of Serotonin Syndrome

In 1991, based on an analysis of 12 literature reports (10 case reports and 2 case series) of 38 cases of serotonin syndrome, Sternbach [4] proposed provisional criteria for the diagnosis of serotonin syndrome. Diagnosis by Sternbach's criteria

Table 8.1 Clinical manifestations of the serotonin syndrome [2]

Clinical manifestations	Features
Cognitive and behavioral	Confusion/disorientation
	Agitation/irritability
	Coma/unresponsiveness
	Hallucinations (visual and auditory)
Autonomic excitation	Hyperthermia
	Diaphoresis
	Sinus tachycardia
	Hypertension
	Dilated pupils
	Nausea
	Flushing
Neuromuscular features	Myoclonus (especially in the legs)
	Hyperreflexia (in the legs more than the arms)
	Muscle rigidity
	Restlessness/hyperactivity
	Tremor
	Ataxia
	Extensor plantar responses

included three of the following clinical features in the setting of a serotonergic agent, assuming other etiologies have been ruled out and excluding neuroleptic drug use: mental status changes, agitation, myoclonus, hyperreflexia, diaphoresis, shivering, tremor, diarrhea, incoordination, and fever. However, the Hunter Serotonin Toxicity Criteria (HSTC) proposed by Dunkley [5] in 2003 has widely replaced Sternbach's criteria due to its increased sensitivity (84% from 75%) and specificity (97% from 96%) for the diagnosis when compared to the gold standard diagnosis by a medical toxicologist [5, 6]. These criteria were validated in a retrospective study of over 2000 overdoses of one or more serotonergic agents [7–9].

The HSTC decision rules state that in the presence of a serotonergic agent, one of the five following criteria must be met [5]:

1. Spontaneous clonus
2. Inducible clonus *and* agitation *or* diaphoresis
3. Ocular clonus *and* agitation *or* diaphoresis
4. Tremor *and* hyperreflexia
5. Hypertonia *and* hyperthermia (temperature >38 °C) *and* ocular clonus *or* inducible clonus

The HSTC demonstrated that clonus and hyperreflexia are the most important signs required to diagnose serotonin syndrome; however, they may be masked by muscle rigidity [5, 6]. Hyperreflexia is more pronounced in the lower extremities, with clonus lasting for a few seconds in the patellar tendons compared to the upper extremities, where there is only a slight increase in the brachioradialis reflex [10]. Ocular clonus refers to rhythmic involuntary eye movements in all directions. It can include coarse or fine oscillations of the eye that can be constant or prompted by rapid eye movements [11]. Patients may even display moderate neck extension and simultaneous repetitive head rotation [10].

🔑 Clonus and hyperreflexia in the lower extremities help differentiate serotonin syndrome from neuroleptic malignant syndrome at the bedside.

"Serotonin syndrome," more recently termed "serotonin toxicity" (ST) to better reflect that the condition is due to toxic effects of serotonin, is caused by excess serotonin (5-hydroxytryptamine [5-HT]) in the central nervous system [7, 8, 12]. This excess CNS serotonin can be due to several pharmacological mechanisms, including inhibition of the metabolism of serotonin (MAOIs), prevention of the reuptake of serotonin in nerve terminals (serotonin reuptake inhibitors), and increased serotonin precursors (tryptophan) or serotonin release (serotonin-releasing agents) [7]. The resulting excess CNS serotonin acts on serotonin receptors and produces the clinical effects. The exact role of the various serotonin receptors is not completely clear, but there is good evidence that the severe life-threatening clinical effects such as rigidity and hyperthermia are mostly mediated by 5-HT2A receptors.

Serotonin toxicity is characterized by neuromuscular excitation (clonus, hyperreflexia, myoclonus, rigidity, and tremor), autonomic stimulation (hyperthermia, tachycardia, tachypnea, diaphoresis, and flushing), and alteration in mental state (anxiety, agitation, and confusion). Depending on the degree to which intrasynaptic serotonin is elevated in the central nervous system, serotonin toxicity can be mild (serotonergic features that may or may not concern the patient and may be underdiagnosed), moderate (toxicity that causes significant distress and deserves treatment but is not life-threatening), or severe and life-threatening (a medical emergency characterized by rapid onset of severe hyperthermia, muscle rigidity, and multisystem organ failure) (Fig. 8.1) [7, 8, 11].

The most common cause of serotonin syndrome is intentional overdose with antidepressant medications [13]. Certain combinations of serotonergic agents produce more severe forms of serotonin syndrome than others (see Fig. 8.1) [11]. A greater increase in 5-HT levels and a higher incidence of fatalities from serotonin toxicity occur when combining an MAOI with paroxetine, a potent and highly selective serotonin reuptake inhibitor (SSRI), as compared to an MAOI with fluoxetine (a weaker SRI). Severe toxicity resulting in death most commonly occurs with combinations of MAOIs and SSRIs or MAOIs and serotonin releasers, such as amphetamine [7, 8]. However, more recently serotonin toxicity has been reported with monotherapy of serotonergic agents even with therapeutic doses [13, 14]. A case series by Moss et al. reported 35% of their serotonin syndrome cases were due

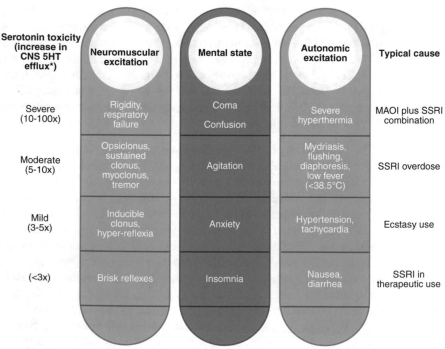

Serotonin toxicity (increase in CNS 5HT efflux*)	Neuromuscular excitation	Mental state	Autonomic excitation	Typical cause
Severe (10-100x)	Rigidity, respiratory failure	Coma / Confusion	Severe hyperthermia	MAOI plus SSRI combination
Moderate (5-10x)	Opsiclonus, sustained clonus, myoclonus, tremor	Agitation	Mydriasis, flushing, diaphoresis, low fever (<38.5°C)	SSRI overdose
Mild (3-5x)	Inducible clonus, hyper-reflexia	Anxiety	Hypertension, tachycardia	Ecstasy use
(<3x)	Brisk reflexes	Insomnia	Nausea, diarrhea	SSRI in therapeutic use

CNS = central nervous system; 5HT = 5-hydroxytryptamine; MAOI =monoamine oxidase inhibitor; SSRI = selective serotonin reuptake inhibitor
*Approximate extent of increase in CNS 5HT efflux seen with animal models

Fig. 8.1 Spectrum of serotonin syndrome presentation [11]

to a single offending agent, with bupropion as the most common [13]. Serotonin syndrome generally presents abruptly and can progress quickly, especially in patients taking a combination of serotonergic medications. The length of an episode of serotonin syndrome partly depends on pharmacokinetic properties of the implicated drug, such as the duration of action and elimination half-life [8].

☐━━☞ Compared to neuroleptic malignant syndrome, serotonin syndrome usually presents acutely over several hours.

Neurochemistry

Serotonin (5-HT), as illustrated in Fig. 8.2, is a monoamine neurotransmitter that is synthesized from the amino acid tryptophan. Tryptophan is transported into the brain from the plasma. Since tryptophan is one of the eight essential amino acids, the body cannot synthesize tryptophan from other amino acids, and it must be ingested with food. Foods that are high in tryptophan include dairy products, beef, poultry, barley, brown rice, fish, soybeans, legumes, and peanuts [5]. Once inside the serotonergic neuron in the central nervous system and the enterochromaffin cells of the gastrointestinal tract, dietary tryptophan undergoes enzymatic conversion to form 5-HT (Fig. 8.3) [15]. The rate-limiting step of the pathway is the production of 5-hydroxytryptophan (5-HTP) by tryptophan hydroxylase. Serotonin is a monoamine present throughout the body. Ninety-nine percent of total body serotonin is located intracellularly [16]. Most of the body's serotonin is located in the periphery stored in platelets and enterochromaffin cells, modulating GI motility as well as vascular and hemodynamic functions [6, 17, 18]. Only 1–2% of its entire body content is in the central nervous system, playing a role in wakefulness, attention, aggression, appetite, emesis, affective and sexual behavior, motor tone, and thermoregulation [6, 18]. Serotonin is unable to cross the blood–brain barrier. The primary metabolic pathway for serotonin is degradation by monoamine oxidase (MAO), especially by the MAO-A form. The major metabolite of MAO metabolism of

Fig. 8.2 The chemical structure of serotonin

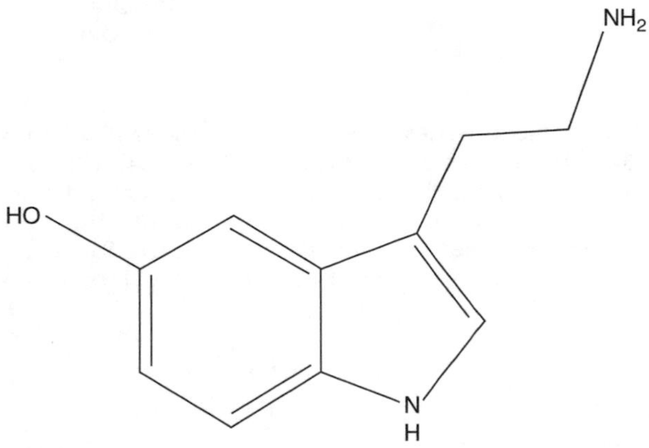

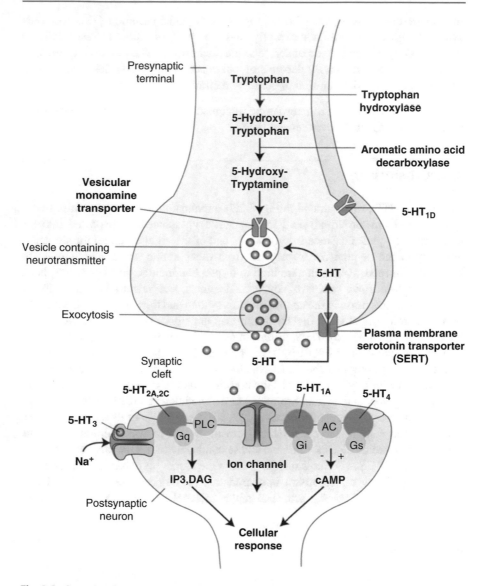

Fig. 8.3 Steps involved in the synthesis and release of serotonin. The distribution of some 5-HT receptors on different components of the serotonergic synapse is also shown; AC, adenylyl cyclase; cAMP, cyclic adenosine monophosphate; DAG, diacylglycerol; G_i, G_s, G_q, different G-proteins; IP3, inositol trisphosphate; 5-HT$_{1A}$, 5-HT$_{1D}$, 5-HT$_{2A}$, 5-HT$_{2C}$, 5-HT$_3$, 5-HT$_4$, different 5-HT receptors [15]. (Reprinted with permission from Siegel A, Sapru HN. Neurotransmitters. In: Essential Neuroscience. 2nd ed. Philadelphia: Wolters Kluwer/Lippincott Williams & Wilkins Health; 2011)

Table 8.2 Serotonin receptor classification [17]

Serotonin receptor family	Subtypes	Receptor type
5-HT$_1$	5-HT$_{1A}$	G$_i$
	5-HT$_{1B}$	
	5-HT$_{1D}$	
	5-HT$_{1E}$	
	5-HT$_{1F}$	
5-HT$_2$	5-HT$_{2A}$	G$_q$
	5-HT$_{2B}$	
	5-HT$_{2C}$	
5-HT$_3$	–	Cys-loop
5-HT$_4$	–	G$_s$
5-HT$_5$	5-HT$_{5A}$	G$_i$
	5-HT$_{5B}$	
5-HT$_6$	–	G$_s$
5-HT$_7$	–	G$_s$

serotonin is 5-hydroxyindoleacetic acid (5HIAA), which is excreted primarily in the urine.

At least 14 different serotonin receptors have been identified [17, 19, 20]. There are seven types of receptors (5-HT$_1$–5-HT$_7$), some of which include subtypes (Table 8.2) [17]. The 5-HT$_1$, 5-HT$_2$, 5-HT$_4$, 5-HT$_5$, 5-HT$_6$, and 5-HT$_7$ receptor families are single-subunit proteins that are members of the G-protein-coupled receptor (GPCR) superfamily. GPCRs are characterized by the presence of seven transmembrane domains, an intracellular carboxy terminus, and an extracellular amino terminus. It is the interaction of the receptor with the G-protein that allows the receptor to modulate the activity of different effector systems, such as ion channels, phospholipase C, and adenylyl cyclase [7].

The 5-HT$_1$ receptor family contains receptors that are negatively coupled to adenylyl cyclase (activation of these receptors down-regulates cyclic AMP) and includes the 5-HT$_{1A}$ receptor (see Fig. 8.3) [15]. The 5-HT$_{1A}$ receptor is coupled via G-proteins to two distinct effector systems: (1) the inhibition of adenylyl cyclase activity and (2) the opening of potassium channels, which results in neuronal hyperpolarization.

The serotonin autoreceptors and the serotonin transporter limit the availability of serotonin in the synapse. The 5-HT$_{1A}$ and 5-HT$_{1D}$ serotonin receptors are presynaptic receptors that act as autoreceptors to prevent further 5-HT release when they sense the presence of 5-HT. Additionally, the highly selective serotonin transporter (SERT), located on the presynaptic membrane, removes serotonin from the synaptic cleft (see Fig. 8.3) [15]. Once transported into the presynaptic neuron, serotonin is recycled back into presynaptic vesicles where it is protected from metabolism. The abundance of serotonin in the synaptic cleft is the major determinant of the strength and duration of signaling on the postsynaptic serotonin receptor. Binding of serotonin to its autoreceptor and the activity of the SERT, both of which are located on the presynaptic membrane, control the availability of serotonin in the synaptic cleft. As noted by Mohammad-Zadeh [16], the negative feedback created by stimulation of the 5-HT autoreceptor decreases further release of serotonin, while the SERT actually removes serotonin from the synaptic cleft.

Several serotonin receptors are postsynaptic, including 5-HT_{1A}, 5-HT_{1D}, 5-HT_{2A}, and 5-HT_{2C}. These receptors are responsible for postsynaptic nerve stimulation or inhibition. Previously, both 5-HT_{1A} and 5-HT_{2A} were implicated in the serotonin syndrome; however, Gillman [12] states that activation of the 5-HT_{2A} receptor (not the 5-HT_{1A} receptor) is needed to cause a serious serotonin syndrome. For example, hyperthermia, the primary risk of serious morbidity and death in serotonin syndrome, is mediated in a dose-related manner by the action of 5-HT or 5-HT agonists on 5-HT_{2A} receptors and is ameliorated or prevented by 5-HT_{2A} antagonists, such as cyproheptadine but not by 5-HT_{1A} antagonists [12].

Serotonin syndrome is directly related to the synaptic concentration of serotonin and the concentration-dependent action of serotonin at postsynaptic serotonin 5-HT_{2A} receptors [8, 12]. Gillman [12] states that serotonin syndrome is not "an idiosyncratic response, but a predictable and inevitable result of toxicity (mediated via the final common pathway of elevated intrasynaptic serotonin)." The evidence implicating serotonin in causing the serotonin syndrome is largely based on animal (rat) models, including radioligand binding studies [19]. Human studies have been anecdotal, and the mechanism of serotonin syndrome in humans remains unproven.

Neuroanatomy

Within the central nervous system, serotonin is synthesized and stored in the presynaptic neurons (i.e., serotonergic neurons, pineal gland, and catecholaminergic neurons). Serotonin is located in nine groups of cell bodies isolated to reticular formation of the pons and midbrain [16, 17]. Serotonergic neurons are restricted to midline structures of the brainstem. Most serotonergic cells overlap with the distribution of the raphe nuclei in the brainstem. A rostral group (B6–8 neurons) project to the thalamus, hypothalamus, amygdala, striatum, and cortex. The largest group of serotonergic cells is B7, which is continuous with a smaller group of serotonergic cells, B6. Groups B6 and B7 together comprise the dorsal raphe nucleus. A more caudal group (B1–4 neurons) of serotonergic cells is found in the mid-pons to caudal medulla and projects to other brainstem neurons, the cerebellum and the spinal cord. In the medulla, serotonergic neurons lie in the nuclei raphe magnus, raphe obscurus, and raphe pallidus, which give rise to descending spinal projections.

The principal ascending fibers arise from serotonin-containing cell bodies located in the dorsal (supratrochlear) and median (superior central) nucleus of the raphe nuclei. The major ascending pathway from the rostral raphe nuclei passes through the ventral tegmental area and joins the medial forebrain bundle in the lateral hypothalamus. The superior central nucleus is particularly associated with serotonergic fibers projecting to the interpeduncular nucleus, the mammillary bodies, and the hippocampal formation. Ascending projections from the caudal raphe nuclei are less numerous and distribute to the superior colliculus, the pretectum, and the nuclei of the posterior commissure. Ascending serotonergic pathways from the superior central nucleus project mainly to mesolimbic structures, such as the hippocampus and the septal nuclei, while the dorsal nucleus of the raphe has major projections to the neostriatum and substantia nigra.

The Role of Serotonin

Serotonin has been implicated in appetite, emotion, nociception, motor, cognitive, and autonomic (sympathetic) function. Studies of the firing rate of serotonergic soma in the raphe nuclei suggest that serotonin (5-HT) modulates the nervous system. Serotonergic activity correlates with behavioral arousal, motor output, circadian rhythm, neuroendocrine function, appetite, and sleeping. Precursors of 5-HT, releasing agents, reuptake inhibitors, and receptor agonists and antagonists have been used to assess serotonergic function [7].

Epidemiology

Serotonin syndrome is an iatrogenic disorder related to drugs that augment serotonin transmission. It occurs in patients treated for depression (the most common group), bipolar affective disorder, obsessive compulsive disorder, eating disorders with depression, Parkinson's disease, migraines, HIV/AIDS, and sepsis, as well as in patients who are drug abusers. Serotonin syndrome may occur in pediatric and adult patients. The patient's age and sex are not known to predispose to the development of serotonin syndrome. Serotonin syndrome contributes to 2% of all bedside consults made by medical toxicologists [13].

Drugs Associated with Serotonin Syndrome

There are many serotonergic drugs reported to produce serotonin syndrome. Table 8.3 [2, 6, 8, 17, 21] lists mechanisms of action and names of serotonergic drugs. There are several drug mechanisms that cause excess serotonin, such as increased serotonin synthesis and release, inhibited serotonin metabolism and reuptake, activation of serotonin receptors, and inhibition of CYP450 enzymes by SSRIs. Severe serotonin toxicity (serotonin syndrome) generally occurs with combinations of serotonergic drugs (often acting at different sites), most commonly including a serotonin reuptake inhibitor and an MAOI [7]. Less severe toxicity occurs with other combinations, overdoses, and even single-drug therapy in susceptible individuals.

Table 8.3 Mechanisms of action and names of serotonergic agents [2, 6, 8, 17, 21]

Mechanism	Class	Drugs implicated in serotonin syndrome
Inhibit serotonin synthesis	Dietary supplement	L-Tryptophan
Inhibit serotonin metabolism	Anxiolytics	Buspirone
	Herbal supplements	St. John's Wort (*Hypericum perforatum*)
	Monoamine oxidase inhibitors	Clorgyline, furazolidone, iproniazid, isocarboxazid, linezolid, methylene blue, moclobemide, pargyline, phenelzine, procarbazine, rasagiline, safinamide, selegiline, Syrian rue, tedizolid, and tranylcypromine
Increase serotonin release	Amphetamines + derivatives	Dexfenfluramine, fenfluramine, and phentermine
	Antidepressants (atypical)	Mirtazapine
	Cold remedies	Dextromethorphan
	Drugs of abuse	Cocaine, methylenedioxymethamphetamine (MDMA; Ecstasy)
	Opiates (not all)	Meperidine, oxycodone, and tramadol
	Parkinson disease Treatment/amino acid	Levodopa
Inhibit serotonin uptake	Amphetamines + derivatives	Dexfenfluramine, fenfluramine, and phentermine
	Antidepressants (atypical)	Bupropion, nefazodone, and trazodone
	Antiemetics	Granisetron and ondansetron
	Antihistamines	Chlorpheniramine
	Anxiolytics	Buspirone
	Cold remedies	Dextromethorphan
	Drugs of abuse	Cocaine, methylenedioxymethamphetamine (MDMA; Ecstasy)
	Herbal supplements	St. John's Wort (*Hypericum perforatum*)
	Opiates (not all)	Fentanyl, levomethorphan, levorphanol, meperidine, methadone, pentazocine, pethidine, propoxyphene, tapentadol, and tramadol
	Selective norepinephrine Reuptake inhibitors (SNRIs)	Desvenlafaxine, duloxetine, milnacipran, sibutramine, and venlafaxine
	Selective serotonin reuptake inhibitors (SSRIs)	Citalopram, escitalopram, fluoxetine, fluvoxamine, paroxetine, and sertraline
	Tricyclic antidepressants (TCAs)	Amitriptyline, amoxapine, clomipramine, desipramine, doxepin, imipramine, maprotiline, nortriptyline, protriptyline, and trimipramine
Serotonin receptor agonists	Antidepressants (atypical)	Mirtazapine and trazodone
	Antiemetic/prokinetic agents	Metoclopramide
	Anxiolytics	Buspirone
	Drugs of abuse	Lysergic acid diethylamide (LSD)
	Ergot derivatives	Dihydroergotamine, ergotamine, and methylergonovine
	Mood stabilizers	Lithium
	Opiates (not all)	Fentanyl and meperidine
	Triptans	Almotriptan, eletriptan, frovatriptan, naratriptan, rizatriptan, sumatriptan, and zolmitriptan

Table 8.3 (continued)

Mechanism	Class	Drugs implicated in serotonin syndrome
Serotonin receptor (5-HT2A) antagonists	Second-generation antipsychotics	Aripiprazole, clozapine, olanzapine, quetiapine, and risperidone
CYP450 microsomal oxidase interactions	CYP2D6	*Inhibitors*: fluoxetine and sertraline *Substrates*: Dextromethorphan, oxycodone, phentermine, risperidone, and tramadol
	CYP3A4	*Inhibitors*: ciprofloxacin and ritonavir *Substrates*: methadone, oxycodone, and venlafaxine
	CYP2C19	*Inhibitors*: fluconazole *Substrates*: citalopram
Modulators	Antidepressants (atypical)	Bupropion
	Parkinson's disease treatments	Amantadine, and levodopa

An overdose with a serotonin reuptake inhibitor rarely, if ever, causes fatal serotonin toxicity. Life-threatening serotonin toxicity generally occurs only when MAOIs are combined with either serotonin reuptake inhibitors (selective or nonselective) or serotonin releasers, such as amphetamine or the recreational drug MDMA. Death can also occur from a large overdose of an older irreversible MAOI (i.e., tranylcypromine) alone. The newer reversible MAOIs (i.e., moclobemide) do not cause serotonin toxicity alone in overdose [8].

Selected Patient Profiles

The following patient populations are at increased risk of developing serotonin toxicity, based on their use of certain medications or other substances with serotonergic properties. The clinician should be especially mindful of the co-administration of serotonergic medications or other substances. When evaluating a patient with clinical features of neuromuscular excitation, autonomic stimulation, and/or altered mental state, the identification that the patient falls into one of these profiles and is using one or more serotonergic medications or other substances should prompt the clinician to consider the diagnosis of serotonin syndrome.

The Patient with Psychiatric Disease

Antidepressants are the most common class of drugs to produce serotonin syndrome. Specifically, MAOI, selective and nonselective serotonin reuptake inhibitors, and tricyclic antidepressants (TCAs) cause the serotonin syndrome, but atypical antidepressants should also be used with caution when considering this toxicity. Buckley et al. [11] reported about 15% of SSRI toxicities leading to cases of moderate serotonin syndrome. Fluoxetine has unique pharmacokinetics, which makes it prone to cause serotonin syndrome. The half-life of fluoxetine is 1–4 days, but its active metabolite, norfluoxetine, has a half-life of 7–14 days. To decrease the risk of serotonin syndrome, when discontinuing fluoxetine a patient should wait 5 weeks before starting another serotonergic agent [22] or an MAO-I [23]. Durson [24] reported a patient who developed serotonin syndrome while taking carbamazepine and fluoxetine.

O━━━▼ Due to the long elimination half-life of fluoxetine, care should be taken before switching to another SSRI.

Lithium may enhance the serotonergic effect of serotonin reuptake inhibitors (SRIs), potentially increasing the risk of serotonin syndrome when lithium and SRIs are used concomitantly, compared to when SRIs are used alone. We identified two reports of patients taking lithium and venlafaxine (an antidepressant with dual selective reuptake inhibition) who developed serotonin syndrome, possibly due to lithium's increasing the serotonergic effect of venlafaxine or diminishing its renal excretion [8, 25, 26]. Furthermore, patients with end-stage renal disease who are on SSRIs and hemodialysis are at risk of serotonin syndrome due to decreased renal excretion of serotonergic agents [6, 17].

The serotonin syndrome is most commonly the result of the interaction between serotonergic agents and MAOIs. MAO-A has greater affinity for serotonin, whereas MAO-B has a higher affinity for dopamine. Classical MAOIs produce irreversible inhibition of MAO enzyme activity. MAO enzyme activity is regenerated in approximately 2 weeks due to the gradual production of uninhibited MAO enzyme. Therefore, when a patient changes from an MAOI to a different class of serotonergic agents, a 2-week period must elapse between the two drugs. Serotonin syndrome may also occur with moclobemide ("RIMA"), a reversible inhibitor of monoamine oxidase-A [27].

Combining MAOIs with serotonin selective or nonselective reuptake inhibitors or serotonin releasers may precipitate a rapid deterioration to life-threatening and sometimes fatal serotonin toxicity [8]. Depending on their serotonin reuptake inhibitor potency, TCAs combined with MAOIs can also precipitate life-threatening serotonin toxicity. Clomipramine, one of the most potent TCAs, has serotonergic effects at both therapeutic levels and in overdose. When combined with MAOIs, clomipramine is known to cause serotonin toxicity and consequential death. Imipramine also has clinically significant serotonergic potency. Amitriptyline, a less potent SRI, is not known to cause symptoms of serotonin toxicity if taken in overdose. Amitriptyline can be combined with an MAOI without the risk of serotonergic side effects or serotonin toxicity [8].

Electroconvulsive therapy (ECT) is a treatment for depression that may, although uncommon, precipitate serotonin syndrome, especially when performed in a patient taking serotonergic agents [28–30]. Case reports have been published involving serotonin syndrome in the presence of ECT with paroxetine [28], ECT with lithium [29] and ECT with trazodone, bupropion, and quetiapine [30]. Potential mechanisms include ECT causing increased blood–brain barrier permeability, increasing the risk of serotonin toxicity in the presence of a serotonergic agent [28], as well as transient hypersensitivity to serotonergic agents [29] or modulation of serotonin transmission and receptors [30]. As it is common for patients receiving ECT for depression to be taking serotonergic antidepressants, physicians should be aware of this potential reaction. Interestingly, a few case reports suggest that serotonin syndrome may also *benefit* from ECT. For example, Nisijima [31] reported a depressed patient with diaphoresis, tremor, and myoclonus who was diagnosed with serotonin syndrome by Sternbach's criteria. The patient was refractory to medical therapies. The serotonin syndrome resolved, and the depression lessened with ECT. More research is needed regarding ECT and serotonin syndrome. Physicians should be aware of ECT's potential precipitation of serotonin syndrome, as well as its potential use as a treatment for serotonin syndrome.

The Patient with Parkinson's Disease

Increased concentrations of dopamine in the CNS can induce the serotonin syndrome by indirect serotonin release. Patients with Parkinson's disease (PD) may theoretically have an increased risk of serotonin syndrome due to the high rate of depression among PD patients. In clinical practice, many PD patients concurrently use an antidepressant and a dopaminergic agent. Levodopa and selegiline (an MAO-B inhibitor) have classically been associated with serotonin syndrome. However, a review by Aboukarr et al. [32] investigated the risk of serotonin syndrome in Parkinson's patients taking an SSRI and MAO-B inhibitor. Serotonin syndrome is most common with SSRIs and nonselective MAO inhibitors, or selective MAO-A inhibitors, due to the rise of serotonin in the CNS. MAO-B inhibitors at low doses selectively inhibit the breakdown of dopamine; only at high doses (>10 mg per day), MAO-B inhibitors lose selectivity and additionally inhibit MAO-A, leading to serotonin syndrome risk. The study concluded that selegiline or rasagiline can safely be used concomitantly with an SSRI, given the MAO-B inhibitor is at a therapeutic dose, and the SSRI is given at the low end of its therapeutic range. Of all the cases and studies reviewed, serotonin syndrome in response to MAO-B inhibitors and SSRIs was rare; therefore, the benefits of this drug combination outweigh the risk of serotonin syndrome for Parkinson's patients with depression [32]. Fernandes [33] reported a diagnosis of possible serotonin syndrome in a 76-year-old woman with a 10-year history of PD treated with carbidopa/levodopa and entacapone. After a 4-day accidental overdose of rasagiline, 4 mg per day, she developed agitation, loss of consciousness, labile blood pressure, tachycardia, fever, and a tremor "not typical of Parkinson's."

Toyama and Iacono [34] suggested that parkinsonian patients might be protected from the serotonin syndrome by decreased serotonergic functioning, shown by loss of serotonergic neurons and decreased serotonin metabolites. A chart reviewed by Waters [35] on 23 patients receiving combined fluoxetine and selegiline, and another chart review by Toyama [34] on 25 patients receiving combined SSRI and selegiline both revealed no serious side effects.

The Patient with a Severe Infection

Linezolid, an antibiotic of the oxazolidone family, is a reversible, nonselective MAOI used in the treatment of vancomycin-resistant *Enterococcus faecium* infections, nosocomial pneumonia caused by *Staphylococcus aureus* (methicillin-susceptible and resistant strains), or *Streptococcus pneumoniae* (including multidrug resistant strains), and skin infections caused by *Staphylococcus aureus* (methicillin-susceptible and resistant strains), *Streptococcus pyogenes*, or *Streptococcus agalactiae* [36]. Linezolid should not be used in patients taking any medication that inhibits MAO-A or MAO-B or within 2 weeks of taking such medication [36]. Serotonin syndrome has been described from the interaction of linezolid and SSRIs such as citalopram, sertraline, paroxetine, and fluoxetine [36, 37]. It has also been described in a case of linezolid with methadone, which, while both are weak serotonergic agents less likely to cause toxicity, is important for physicians to consider when encountering a patient with potential serotonin syndrome [38].

The Patient with Pain

Some narcotic analgesics, such as the phenylpiperidine series opioids (including dextromethorphan, fentanyl, meperidine, methadone, propoxyphene, and tramadol), are weak serotonin reuptake inhibitors (increase CNS serotonin) and can precipitate life-threatening serotonin toxicity reactions when combined with other serotonin modulators, especially MAOIs and SSRIs [8]. Some opioids, such as tramadol, have the potential to cause serotonin syndrome as monotherapy, whether due to overdose, reduced tramadol metabolism, or deficient 5-HT uptake [9]. A comprehensive overview of opioids and serotonin syndrome by Baldo reports 20.3% of 74 investigated cases of toxicity were due to SSRIs and opioids [18]. Most commonly these cases are associated with dextromethorphan, fentanyl, meperidine, methadone, oxycodone, and tramadol; however, cases have also been linked with alfentanil, remifentanil, sufentanil, hydrocodone, hydromorphone, morphine, naltrexone, pentazocine, and tapentadol while in combination with other serotonergic agents [13, 18]. With the March 2016 FDA Drug Safety Communication warning of the association of the entire class of opioids with serotonin syndrome, physician awareness of this interaction is imperative for proper patient care [18]. Zornberg [39] described a patient taking meperidine and selegiline who developed possible serotonin syndrome. Meperidine, dextromethorphan, and tramadol are contraindicated in patients using an MAOI, including selegiline, and should be used with caution in patients using other serotonergic drugs.

Duloxetine and milnacipran are serotonin and noradrenaline reuptake inhibitors. Duloxetine is indicated for the management of fibromyalgia, diabetic peripheral neuropathic pain, and chronic musculoskeletal pain [40]. Milnacipran is indicated for the management of fibromyalgia [41]. The concomitant use of these drugs with MAOIs is contraindicated. If concomitant treatment with a 5-hydroxytryptamine receptor agonist (triptan) is clinically warranted, careful observation of the patient is advised, particularly during treatment initiation and dose increases. The concomitant use of these drugs with serotonin precursors (such as tryptophan) is not recommended. Due to the risk of serotonin syndrome, caution is advised when using these drugs with certain narcotic analgesics that are serotonin reuptake inhibitors, such as tramadol. Yacoub [42] described a patient with depression treated with paroxetine (a selective serotonin reuptake inhibitor) who 8 days after adding on milnacipran for fibromyalgia developed altered mental status, autonomic dysfunction, and skeletal muscle rigidity, diagnosed as serotonin syndrome. The authors hypothesized that the concomitant use of these two serotonergic agents produced serotonin syndrome.

The Recreational Drug Abuser

3,4-Methylenedioxymethamphetamine (MDMA, "molly") or Ecstasy has become one of the most popular recreational drugs over the past 25 years. MDMA, a synthetic amphetamine, increases serotonin availability by stimulating its release from presynaptic terminals and preventing its reuptake. In addition to serotonin, MDMA is thought to affect other neurotransmitters, including dopamine. Initially in the 1980s, MDMA was used as a psychotherapeutic adjunct but it soon became a drug of abuse. Its popularity is likely due to its positive effect on mood and sense of well-being. There are several administration routes: oral, injection, smoking, and nasal. According to Parrot [43], about 85–90% of recreational Ecstasy users reported an increase in body temperature, sweating, dehydration, bruxism, and trismus. Deaths at UK "rave" parties were attributed to serotonin syndrome following ingestion of MDMA [44]. The factors that may contribute to death from MDMA ingestion are unknown; however, they may include dosage, individual sensitivity, tolerance, variability in drug metabolism, and concomitant use of antidepressants or other recreational drugs including cocaine, amphetamines, cannabis, or alcohol.

A main concern is the use of MDMA in depressed patients already taking SSRIs. Increased rates of depression in the pediatric and adolescent populations have led to a rise in SSRI use. Furthermore, patients with psychiatric illness may have increased risk of substance abuse, increasing the likelihood of combining antidepressant, and substance use [45]. Some users purposely ingest concomitant SSRIs and MDMA with the misconceptions that it will lead to a greater euphoric effect and that the SSRI will actually be neuroprotective against MDMA [45]. Dobry [45] explains the mechanism of serotonin syndrome in MDMA users. Apart from its effects on the synapse and variability in drug metabolism, MDMA can lead to liver necrosis, consequently reducing liver function and reducing the ability to clear SSRIs and MDMA, increasing the chance of serotonin syndrome. Second, hyperthermia from MDMA use leads to dehydration, which stimulates the body to release in vitro serotonin for thermodynamic regulation [45]. Therefore, both endogenous and exogenous serotonin release in this scenario puts this population at risk for serotonin syndrome.

Dextromethorphan (DXM) is a cough suppressant found in over-the-counter (OTC) cold medications. DXM may be abused in high doses by adolescents to generate euphoria, visual and auditory hallucinations, and dissociative "out of body" experiences similar to those caused by the hallucinogens phencyclidine (PCP) and ketamine. Illicit use of DXM is referred to on the street as "Robo-tripping" or "skit-tling." These terms are derived from the most commonly abused products: Robitussin and Coricidin [46]. Annually about one million US youth and young adults (age 12–25 years) misuse OTC cough and cold medicines that contain DXM [47]. The Drug Abuse Warning Network (DAWN ED) reports that nearly 8000 emergency department visits in the USA each year were associated with the nonmedical use of DXM during 2006–2008 [48]. DXM potentiates serotonin levels. Recreational usage of products containing DXM can lead to serotonin syndrome. Schwartz [49] described two cases of serotonin syndrome associated with supra-therapeutic doses of DXM and therapeutic levels of an SSRI. An additional concern from abuse of DXM-containing products is the development of potential toxicity from the other ingredients, such as delayed hepatotoxicity from acetaminophen, increased blood pressure from pseudoephedrine, and central nervous system, cardiovascular and anti-cholinergic toxicity from antihistamines. The abuse of DXM in high doses with alcohol or other drugs is particularly dangerous and potentially lethal [46].

Other recreational drugs to be aware of in association with serotonin syndrome include mephedrone (4-MMC), cathinone, methylenedioxypyrovalerone (MDPV, "bath salts"), methylone (MDMC), butylone (βk-MBDB), methamphetamine, cocaine, lysergic acid diethylamide (LSD, "acid"), 251-NBOMe, psilocybin ("magic mushrooms"), and 2,5-dimethoxy-4-bromophenethylamine (2-CB) [13, 50]. The first known case report of intoxication with 2-CB, a phenethylamine, in an 18-year-old male resulted in severe brain edema and serotonin syndrome diagnosed with the HSTC [50]. There have been no reported cases to date of serotonin syndrome in relation to N,N-dimethyltryptamine (DMT), salvia divinorum, or methoxetamine (MXE) [13].

Genetic Polymorphisms and Drug Interactions with CYP-450

Genetic polymorphisms of CYP2D6 of the CYP-450 system produce differences in an individual's ability to metabolize certain drugs, including DXM (dextromethorphan), MDMA, TCAs, tramadol, and SSRIs, including fluoxetine and paroxetine [9, 45]. For instance, CYP2D6 metabolizes dextromethorphan to dextrorphan, its active metabolite. Poor metabolizers via CYP2D6 produce less dextrorphan, experience a higher risk of developing adverse effects (e.g., nausea, vomiting, and dysphoria) from DEX, and are less likely to abuse DXM. Conversely, extensive metabolizers via CYP2D6 produce more dextrorphan, experience more of the euphoric and mind-altering effects, and are more likely to abuse DXM [51]. Genetic variation may also exist in the SERT gene for serotonin transport, or in the 5-HT2A and 5-HT-3B receptors, playing a role in the risk of serotonin syndrome [6].

Further attention should be placed on drug interactions within the CYP-450 system (Table 8.4) [52]. For patients with polypharmacy, recognizing drugs that are substrates, inducers, and inhibitors of CYP enzymes is imperative for preventing adverse drug reactions, such as serotonin syndrome. For example, patients who

Table 8.4 CYP-450 interactions of some serotonergic agents [52]

CYP enzyme	Substrates	Inducers	Inhibitors
1A2	Duloxetine	–	Fluvoxamine
2B6	Bupropion, methadone, selegiline, and sertraline	–	Paroxetine and sertraline
2C9		–	Fluvoxamine
2D6	Clozapine, codeine, desipramine, dextromethorphan, fluoxetine, haloperidol, hydrocodone, oxycodone, paroxetine, risperidone, selegiline, tricyclic antidepressants, and venlafaxine	–	Bupropion, fluoxetine, and paroxetine
3A4	Alfentanil, buspirone, cocaine, and methadone	St. John's Wort	–

co-administer DXM with drugs that may inhibit CYP2D6 (e.g., dextromethorphan itself, venlafaxine, amitriptyline, and fluoxetine) have a higher risk of adverse effects and are less likely to abuse the drug. Forget [53] recommends avoiding DXM in patients taking a tricyclic antidepressant or other inhibitors of CYP2D6. Further reports have been made of patients experiencing serotonin syndrome via CYP-3A4 inhibition by ciprofloxacin, a fluoroquinolone antibiotic, in patients taking serotonergic agents, as well as CYP-2C19 inhibition by fluconazole, an antifungal, in a patient taking citalopram [6].

The Patient with Human Immunodeficiency Virus

Human Immunodeficiency Virus (HIV)-positive patients are also at risk for developing serotonin syndrome due to CYP-450 interactions. Since depression is prevalent among HIV-positive patients, they often take serotonin reuptake inhibitors. Drugs that inhibit the metabolism of serotonin reuptake inhibitors can produce serotonin syndrome. Antiretroviral therapy inhibits serotonin metabolism via the cytochrome P450 enzymes. Although ritonavir specifically inhibits the 2D6 isoenzyme, the exact mechanism of inhibition remains unknown as many of the antiretrovirals inhibit the 3A4 rather than 2D6 isoenzyme. DeSilva [54] described five cases of serotonin syndrome that occurred in HIV-positive patients who were taking fluoxetine with protease inhibitors and non-nucleoside reverse transcriptase inhibitors. Fluoxetine is metabolized by P450 2D6 to an active metabolite, norfluoxetine, which is then further metabolized by 2D6. Fluoxetine has been associated with serotonin syndrome likely due to its very long half-life.

The Patient with Cough

Dextromethorphan is an antitussive agent in many over-the-counter cough medications. Doctors need to be aware that since dextromethorphan is an opioid with serotonin reuptake inhibitor activity, it has the potential to cause serotonin toxicity in patients taking MAOIs.

The Patient with Migraine Headaches

Serotonin syndrome in patients with migraines is questionable. The pathophysiology of migraine is thought to involve the neurotransmitter serotonin. It has been hypothesized that patients with recurrent migraines have chronically low systemic 5-HT. Agents that increase serotonin in the CNS are effective in treating migraine. Sumatriptan selectively activates the 5-HT_{1D} receptors. Dihydroergotamine (DHE), another 5-HT agonist, is more potent at the 5-HT_{1A} than the 5-HT_{1D} receptor. Triptans are high-affinity agonists at $5\text{-HT}_{1B}/5\text{-HT}_{1D}/5\text{-HT}_{1F}$ subtype receptors with lower affinity for 5-HT_{1A} receptors. Available evidence supports a model of serotonin syndrome due to activation of 5-HT_{2A} receptors, with some questionable involvement of 5-HT_{1A} receptors. Additionally, the SSRIs, which are used for migraine prophylaxis, inhibit serotonin reuptake. In 2006, the United States Food and Drug Administration (FDA) [55] warned about the potential life-threatening risk of serotonin syndrome when triptans are used with SSRIs or SNRIs. This alert was based on a total of 29 cases (reported to the FDA or derived from the published literature) of presumptive SS occurring in association with the combination of triptans and SSRIs.

In an American Headache Society Position Paper [56], Evans (2010) reviewed the potential risk of serotonin syndrome (based on the Sternbach's criteria or the Hunter Serotonin Toxicity Criteria) when combining triptans with other serotonergic agents. Of the 29 cases used as the basis for the FDA alert, 10 cases actually met Sternbach's criteria for diagnosing serotonin syndrome. No cases fulfilled the Hunter criteria for serotonin toxicity. The study concluded that the currently available evidence does not support limiting the use of triptans with SSRIs or SNRIs or the use of triptan monotherapy, due to concerns for serotonin syndrome.

A retrospective cross-sectional study from 2014 to 2018 by Roblee et al. [57] reviewed clinical outcomes of intentional overdoses with triptans and ergotamines, concluding that the toxidrome of these agents did not include serotonin syndrome. Similarly, a review by Orlova et al. [58] of patients taking concomitant triptans and SSRI/SNRIs from 2001 to 2014 determined a low risk of serotonin syndrome with coprescription of these agents. Of the 19,017 patients reviewed, 17 suspected cases of serotonin syndrome were identified, with only one actually meeting Hunter criteria for serotonin syndrome [58]. Due to the suspected mechanisms of triptans and ergotamines, serotonin syndrome may still be considered in patients with migraine headaches; however, in light of the stated research, this reaction may be less common than previously indicated.

Methylene Blue and the Surgical Patient

Methylene blue (MB; methylthioninium chloride), a potent inhibitor of MAO-A, is a phenothiazine derivative used in medicine for staining in parathyroid procedures and urological procedures and in the treatment of methemoglobinemia, ifosfamide toxicity, and perioperative vasoplegic shock in cardiac surgery [59]. In patients taking serotonergic agents, such as antidepressants, the administration of MB poses a risk of serotonin syndrome. Most commonly, serotonin syndrome from MB administration occurs via parenteral routes, but one case of serotonin syndrome by oral administration of MB has been described and should be considered [59].

MB is most commonly used for parathyroid surgery where it accumulates in the target tissue to assist surgical identification. Ng and Cameron [60] presented a literature review that identified nine case reports and two retrospective reviews; 26 patients developed an acute confusional state after MB infusion; 24 of these patients were taking an SRI, and one was taking clomipramine. Serotonin syndrome was a possible diagnosis in all 25 of these patients. They concluded that serotonin reuptake inhibitors could interact with MB to cause a serious adverse reaction consistent with serotonin syndrome.

Less commonly, yet still worth consideration, is the potential for serotonin syndrome in cardiac patients undergoing surgery. Cardiac patients are often depressed and prescribed SSRIs. MB is utilized preoperatively in these patients to control vasoplegic shock and can precipitate serotonin syndrome in this population [59, 61]. Reports of serotonin syndrome from MB use in urological procedures have also been reported [59].

The Pediatric Patient

Serotonin syndrome must be considered in the pediatric population, now that behavioral disorders are more frequently treated with serotonergic formulations. Additionally, unintentional exposures of children to serotonergic drugs may occur due to the rising number of serotonergic antidepressants being prescribed to adults. Children and adolescents may present differently than adults, more commonly presenting with symptoms of headache, anxiety, nervousness, insomnia, agitation, and sedation [45]. Several case reports describe children who developed the serotonin syndrome after overdosing on serotonergic antidepressants and even while on therapeutic doses of these drugs, sometimes in combination with other serotonergic drugs [62, 63].

Dextromethorphan, an opioid with serotonin reuptake inhibitor activity, is widely used in cough syrups. It should be given cautiously to children who take behavior-modifying medications since it may trigger a serotonin syndrome.

The Patient Who Uses Herbal Remedies

In addition to traditional prescription antidepressants, herbal antidepressants may also cause serotonin syndrome. In general, due to lack of standardization, herbal remedies vary in potency and side effects [64]. The mechanism of St. John's Wort (*Hypericum perforatum*) is not entirely clear. It is hypothesized that certain constituents of St. John's Wort, most notably hypericin and hyperforin, may reduce the expression of serotonin receptors, increase the numbers of 5-HT_{1A} and 5-HT_{2A} receptors, inhibit synaptosome serotonin uptake, and induce certain CYP-450 enzymes [64, 65]. The biggest risk of serotonin syndrome with St. John's Wort is when it is ingested concomitantly with SSRIs; therefore, this should be avoided [65]. However, Parker [66] reported a patient who developed cognitive and autonomic symptoms following 10 days of monotherapy with St. John's Wort. Other herbal remedies that may also increase the activity of serotonin include black seed oil [67], ginseng, Brewer's yeast, and yohimbine.

Differential Diagnosis

Serotonin syndrome is often misdiagnosed as it can easily be mistaken for other pathological processes. Since there are no laboratory tests to diagnose serotonin syndrome, physicians should be aware of the appropriate symptomatology so as to exclude other causes and obtain an accurate diagnosis. A comprehensive differential diagnosis for serotonin syndrome is as follows [6, 9, 11]:

- Neuroleptic malignant syndrome (NMS)
- Malignant hyperthermia
- Anticholinergic poisoning
- Heatstroke
- Serotonergic discontinuation syndrome
- Central hyperthermia
- Cerebral vasculitis
- Thyroid storm
- Delirium
- Delirium tremens
- Sympathomimetic overdose
- Meningitis
- Encephalitis
- Tetanus
- Alcohol or drug withdrawal
- Nonconvulsive seizures
- Stiff person syndrome

Table 8.5 compares signs and symptoms of the top differentials when considering a patient with serotonin syndrome [10].

Table 8.5 Manifestations of severe serotonin syndrome and related clinical conditions

Condition	Medication history	Time needed for condition to develop	Vital signs	Pupils	Mucosa	Skin	Bowel sounds	Neuromuscular tone	Reflexes	Mental status
Serotonin syndrome	Proserotonergic drug	<12 h	Hypertension, tachycardia, tachypnea, and hyperthermia (>41.1 °C)	Mydriasis	Sialorrhea	Diaphoresis	Hyperactive	Increased, predominantly in lower extremities	Hyperreflexia and clonus (unless masked by increased muscle tone)	Agitation and coma
Anticholinergic "toxidrome"	Anticholinergic agent	<12 h	Hypertension (mild), tachycardia, tachypnea, and hyperthermia (typically, 38.8 °C or less)	Mydriasis	Dry	Erythema, hot, and dry to touch	Decreased or absent	Normal	Normal	Agitated and delirium
Neuroleptic malignant syndrome	Dopamine antagonist	1–3 days	Hypertension, tachycardia, tachypnea, and hyperthermia (>41.1 °C)	Normal	Sialorrhea	Pallor, diaphoresis	Normal or decreased	"Lead-pipe" rigidity, present in all muscle groups	Bradyreflexia	Stupor, alert, mutism, and coma
Malignant hyperthermia	Inhalational anesthesia	30 min to 24 h after administration of inhalational anesthesia or succinylcholine	Hypertension, tachycardia, tachypnea, and hyperthermia (can be as high as 46.0 °C)	Normal	Normal	Mottled appearance and diaphoresis	Decreased	Rigor mortis-like rigidity	Hyporeflexia	Agitation

From Boyer EW, Shannon M. The Serotonin Syndrome. N Engl J Med. 2005;352(11):1112–20. Copyright © 2005 Massachusetts Medical Society. Reprinted with permission from Massachusetts Medical Society

A Common Mistake: Misdiagnosis of Serotonin Syndrome as Neuroleptic Malignant Syndrome

Neuroleptic malignant syndrome (NMS) is another lethal disorder that is most often seen in psychiatric patients. A similar disorder is also seen in parkinsonian patients when withdrawing dopaminergic agents. The mechanism is thought to be blockade of central dopamine receptors in the basal ganglia and hypothalamus and blockade of peripheral postganglionic sympathetic neurons in smooth muscle. The clinical picture may mimic that of serotonin syndrome. The American Psychiatric Association's Diagnostic and Statistical Manual of Mental Disorders (DSM-IV-TR) [68] defines NMS as the development of severe muscle rigidity and elevated temperature in association with two or more of the following: diaphoresis, dysphagia, tremor, incontinence, changes in level of consciousness, mutism, tachycardia, elevated or labile blood pressure, leukocytosis, and laboratory evidence of muscle injury (elevated creatinine phosphokinase).

The clinician must be able to distinguish between serotonin syndrome and neuroleptic malignant syndrome because the management is different. Serotonin syndrome treatment is reviewed below, while NMS is treated with dopaminergic agents. Sun-Edelstein [8] noted that attempts to use bromocriptine to treat patients with misdiagnosed neuroleptic malignant syndrome who actually had serotonin syndrome triggered a worsening of serotonergic signs and symptoms. Since ergots, such as bromocriptine, also have 5-HT_2 antagonist activity, the relationship of bromocriptine to the development of serotonin syndrome is uncertain.

Laboratory Studies

There are no specific laboratory studies that will help to positively identify serotonin syndrome. The gold standard is diagnosis by a medical toxicologist [6, 9]. Since serotonin syndrome is largely a diagnosis of exclusion, the following laboratory data can be useful to eliminate other causes of disease and to identify any complications of serotonin syndrome:

- Complete blood count (CBC)
- Serum electrolytes
- Blood urea nitrogen (BUN) and creatinine
- Creatine phosphokinase
- Liver function tests
- Blood culture
- Urinalysis and urine culture
- Coagulation studies
- Toxicology screen
- Cerebrospinal fluid (CSF) analysis and culture
- Head computed tomography (CT)
- Brain magnetic resonance imaging (MRI)
- Electroencephalogram (EEG)

Additionally, it is not necessary to demonstrate increased drug levels of the serotonergic agents. In fact, the majority of patients do not have elevated drug levels. The serotonin metabolite, 5-HIAA, can be measured but does not aid in diagnosing serotonin syndrome. In neuroleptic malignant syndrome, serum creatinine kinase and polymorphonuclear leukocytes are generally increased, whereas in serotonin syndrome these levels are either normal or mildly increased. Carcinoid syndrome, which can mimic the serotonin syndrome, can be ruled out by checking 5-HIAA, the marker for carcinoid. An EEG may be necessary to rule out seizures.

Complications of serotonin syndrome include: rhabdomyolysis (from muscle rigidity), hypoxia (from respiratory muscle rigidity or coma), disseminated intravascular coagulation (from multiple organ failure), metabolic acidosis (from seizures or ventricular tachycardia), aspiration pneumonia (from decreased level of consciousness), arrhythmias, respiratory failure, respiratory arrest, coma, and death [6, 9]. Hyperthermia increases the morbidity and mortality from serotonin syndrome [31]. The hyperthermia has been attributed to activation of the 5-HT_{2A} receptor [31].

Management of the Patient

Serotonin syndrome must be promptly recognized. Misdiagnosis, inability to recognize the rapid progression of the syndrome, and adverse pharmacological therapy effects may be potential management problems faced by physicians [10]. A thorough review of the patient's past medical history, prescriptions, over-the-counter medications, and dietary supplement use should be conducted. Treatment considerations are often complex, as the therapy chosen will depend upon the severity of the serotonin syndrome.

Table 8.6 reviews the management of serotonin syndrome.

An Overview

Supportive care is initiated to stabilize vital signs and control agitation, hyperthermia, and autonomic dysfunction, which are commonly manifested as fluctuations in

Table 8.6 Management of serotonin syndrome

Prompt recognition
Supportive care to control agitation, hyperthermia, and autonomic dysfunction
Discontinuation of all serotonergic agents
Intensive care unit monitoring, if needed
External cooling
Muscular paralysis with neuromuscular blocking agents
Mechanical ventilation
Sedation and muscle relaxation with intravenous benzodiazepine
Nonspecific serotonin receptor blockers, such as cyproheptadine, chlorpromazine, and methysergide
Electroconvulsive therapy may be considered

blood pressure and heart rate [10]. Supportive management includes maintaining oxygen saturation ≥93%, IV hydration, cardiac monitoring, external cooling, sedation with benzodiazepines as needed, and observation for ≥6 h [9, 11]. All serotonergic agents must be discontinued. The severity and rapidity of symptoms help determine the management. The clinician may consider pharmacotherapy with a benzodiazepine and/or nonspecific serotonin receptor blockers, such as cyproheptadine, chlorpromazine, and methysergide. Supportive therapy, discontinuation of serotonergic drugs, and administration of benzodiazepines often alleviate mild cases of serotonin syndrome [10]. In more severe cases, intensive care unit monitoring and treatment may be necessary. Interventions such as external cooling, muscular paralysis with neuromuscular blocking agents, endotracheal intubation and mechanical ventilation, control of autonomic instability, hemodynamic instability, and sedation with an intravenous benzodiazepine may be indicated.

The Role of Benzodiazepines

Benzodiazepines, such as lorazepam or diazepam, are integral to the treatment of mild-to-moderate serotonin syndrome [10]. In a case series by Moss [13], benzodiazepines were the most common treatment for serotonin syndrome, used in 67% of cases. Benzodiazepines may have a protective role due to nonspecific inhibitory effects on serotonergic transmission. Benzodiazepines also treat muscle hypertonia. Aside from benzodiazepines, other agents that may modify serotonergic excess include nonspecific serotonin receptor blockers, such as cyproheptadine, chlorpromazine, and methysergide. Drugs that have anticholinergic properties, such as haloperidol, should be avoided.

The Role of Serotonin Receptor Blockers

Oral Cyproheptadine

Due to the currently accepted mechanism for the development of serotonin syndrome, treatment with a $5\text{-}HT_{2A}$ antagonist is advised. Cyproheptadine is a first-generation histamine-1 receptor-blocking agent with nonspecific antagonist properties at $5\text{-}HT_{1A}$, $5\text{-}HT_{2B}$, $5\text{-}HT_{2C}$, $5\text{-}HT_3$, $5\text{-}HT_6$, and $5\text{-}HT_7$ receptors, and weak anticholinergic properties [17]. The dose of cyproheptadine that binds 85% to 95% of serotonin receptors is 12 mg orally (or crushed and administered through a nasogastric tube) initially, with 2 mg every 2 h until symptoms resolve, followed by a maintenance dose of 4–8 mg every 6 h with a maximum of 32 mg in 24 h [6, 8, 17]. Patients with serotonin syndrome often respond within hours of receiving 4–8 mg of cyproheptadine by mouth [69]. Cyproheptadine is available only in tablet and liquid forms; there is no parenteral formulation. Cyproheptadine may cause sedation, which can be useful for the agitation in SS [10]. Physicians should be aware of other side effects of cyproheptadine such as urinary retention, tachycardia, sedation, hyperthermia, and delirium [70].

While cyproheptadine is advised for serotonin syndrome, it is not always used and its effect in preventing mortality is questioned. Moss [13] notes its use in about 15% of cases, most of which were severe. In a case series by Nguyen et al. [70], out of 288 cases, cyproheptadine was not recommended in 28% cases and was recommended but not administered in 48% of cases. Those who did receive cyproheptadine were older, more frequently intubated and sedated, and often critical care patients as compared with those who did not. The efficacy of cyproheptadine in these cases is unclear, and its effectiveness may have been influenced by polypharmacy, duration of serotonergic drug use, duration and severity of symptoms, complications, and ability to correctly diagnose serotonin syndrome in a timely manner [70]. This study did not find a significant association between cyproheptadine use and the severity of patient outcome; therefore, supportive care remains the most important treatment of serotonin syndrome, and adverse effects versus the benefit of cyproheptadine should be weighed before deciding upon its use.

Intravenous Chlorpromazine

If charcoal has already been given, intravenous chlorpromazine must be administered rather than cyproheptadine. Currently, chlorpromazine that shows nanomolar affinity for cloned human 5-HT_{2A} receptors is the only intravenous 5-HT_{2A} antagonist that is effective in the treatment of serotonin toxicity [8, 10]. The initial dose of chlorpromazine is 12.5–25 mg intravenously, followed by 25 mg orally or intravenously every 6 h, although higher doses have been used with apparent safety and effectiveness. Chlorpromazine treatment should be preceded by fluid loading as it can precipitate hypotension through α (alpha)-2 adrenoceptor antagonism. Patients who require acute parenteral therapy for the serotonin syndrome are often hypertensive and are not ambulatory, so the risk of orthostatic hypotension is minimized.

Chlorpromazine should be avoided if the drugs that precipitate serotonin toxicity have pronounced cardiotoxic or epileptogenic properties (i.e., venlafaxine), as it may aggravate those symptoms. Chlorpromazine, as a neuroleptic, may cause hyperthermia as an idiosyncratic response and thus potentially aggravate the hyperthermia of serotonin syndrome. Chlorpromazine should not be given to a patient with neuroleptic malignant syndrome as it may worsen the condition [8, 10].

Induction of Paralysis

As Boyer and Shannon [10] noted, paralysis should be performed with nondepolarizing agents such as vecuronium. Etomidate and succinylcholine may be used to induce paralysis; however, succinylcholine should be avoided in patients with possible arrhythmia due to hyperkalemia from rhabdomyolysis. The use of dantrolene in animal models of serotonin syndrome has not shown efficacy [6].

Treatment of Hyperthermia

In serotonin syndrome, the appropriate therapy for hyperthermia is neuromuscular paralysis, as the hyperthermia results from excess muscle activity rather than an alteration in the hypothalamic temperature set point. Consequently, antipyretic drugs are not typically needed to treat the fever during serotonin toxicity. Physical restraints should be avoided since they may increase the isometric muscle contractions associated with lactic acidosis and hyperthermia.

Treatment of Autonomic Instability

Symptomatic treatment is needed in patients with serotonin syndrome with fluctuating blood pressure, cardiac effects, and hemodynamic instability. Low doses of direct acting sympathomimetics (phenylephrine, norepinephrine, and epinephrine) should be used to treat hypotension from MAO inhibitor effects. If hypertension and tachycardia persist, short-acting cardiovascular drugs (esmolol and nitroprusside) can be administered. Propranolol, a long-acting beta blocker, should be avoided due to the risk of hypotension and shock in the setting of autonomic instability. Propranolol may also mask tachycardia, which is important for monitoring treatment response [6].

Treatment of the Pediatric Patient

The treatment of serotonin syndrome in children is similar to that in adults. Recognition of the syndrome and discontinuation of the offending agent(s) are critical. Supportive care, maintenance of high urine output, and prevention of rhabdomyolysis are crucial. Cyproheptadine is recommended in severe cases of serotonin syndrome in children. Dosages of cyproheptadine need to be adjusted according to the child's age and/or size.

The Prognosis

The prognosis for serotonin syndrome may vary depending on the severity of disease. This condition is both preventable and treatable. The prognosis of serotonin syndrome is generally good if there is prompt recognition, with improvement often within 24 h of symptom onset [10]. Mild cases warrant observation for 6–12 h to manage symptoms of clonus, hypertension, and anxiety. Moderate cases may require hospitalization for cardiac monitoring. Severe cases often call for admission to the intensive care unit (ICU).

Opioids and antiemetics are commonly added to patient regiments in the ICU. Patients admitted to the ICU, for reasons both related and unrelated to serotonin syndrome, who continue outpatient serotonergic prescriptions and are started on new serotonergic agents may precipitate or worsen serotonin syndrome [71].

Without treatment and discontinuation of serotonergic agents, the prognosis may not be as favorable. The syndrome may be present for longer periods in cases involving serotonergic drugs with long duration of action, active metabolites, or long half-lives [8, 10].

Prevention

To decrease the risk of serotonin syndrome, it is important to avoid prescribing more than one serotonergic agent. If it becomes necessary to do so, the lowest effective dose should be prescribed, and the patient should be monitored closely for serotonin syndrome [72]. MAOIs should not be used with other serotonergic agents. When switching agents, a 5-week washout period is necessary after discontinuing fluoxetine, and a 2-week washout period is necessary after discontinuing an MAO-I. Regular monitoring of the patient after dosage increases and with continued use of the serotonergic agents is imperative [72].

When prescribing a serotonergic agent, it is important to obtain a clear history of other drugs or herbs that the patient is currently taking or has recently discontinued (and record the date of cessation). Increased knowledge of the serotonin syndrome, including potential offending serotonergic agents and selected genetic polymorphisms of the hepatic P450 system (e.g., CYP2D6 enzyme), and the recognition of regimens of multiple serotonergic agents can reduce the risk of serotonin syndrome [10]. If serotonin syndrome occurs, clinicians should discontinue the offending agent(s) and allow a substantial washout period (usually, about 3 weeks) before restarting any necessary serotonergic agents [71].

Conclusion

Serotonin syndrome is an uncommon but potentially life-threatening condition related to excess serotonergic activity. The clinical features seen in serotonin syndrome represent a concentration-dependent range of toxicity due to an increase in the intrasynaptic concentration of serotonin in the central nervous system [5]. The critical serotonin receptor required for activation of serotonin toxicity is the 5-HT_{2A} receptor. Increased awareness of serotonin syndrome and possible offending agents may reduce the risk of this syndrome or promote earlier recognition and treatment. Fortunately, knowledge of drug mechanisms, pharmacology, and interactions can help prevent this syndrome. Since the implicated medications are employed in various clinical situations, health-care providers must be familiar with the agents associated with serotonin syndrome. Prompt identification and management of suspected cases are necessary.

Authors' Statements

Any opinion(s) expressed by Dr. Gordon are his personal opinion(s) and do not necessarily reflect the position of Teva Pharmaceuticals.

Any opinion(s) expressed by Dr. Leder are her personal opinion(s) and do not necessarily reflect the position of the New York Institute of Technology College of Osteopathic Medicine.

Any opinion(s) expressed by Laura Ketigian are her personal opinion(s) and do not necessarily reflect the position of the New York Institute of Technology College of Osteopathic Medicine.

References

1. Oates JA, Sjoerdsma A. Neurologic effects of tryptophan in patients receiving a monoamine oxidase inhibitor. Neurology. 1960;10:1076–8.
2. Mills KC. Serotonin syndrome. Am Fam Physician. 1995;52:1475–82.
3. Guo MH, Monir RL, Wright A, Holland NP. Case of serotonin syndrome initially presenting as diffuse body pain. Am J Case Rep. 2018;19:1227–31.
4. Sternbach H. The serotonin syndrome. Am J Psychiatry. 1991;148:705–13.
5. Dunkley EJC, Isbister GK, Sibbritt D, Dawson AH, Whyte IM. Hunter serotonin toxicity criteria: a simple and accurate diagnostic decision rule for serotonin toxicity. Q J Med. 2003;96:635–42.
6. Volpie-Abadie J, Kaye AM, Kaye AD. Serotonin syndrome. Ochsner J. 2013;13(4):533–40.
7. Isbister GK, Buckley NA, Whyte IM. Serotonin toxicity: a practical approach to diagnosis and treatment. Med J Aust. 2007;187:361–5.
8. Sun-Edelstein C, Tepper SJ, Shapiro RE. Drug-induced serotonin syndrome: a review. Expert Opin Drug Saf. 2008;7:587–96.
9. Beakley BD, Kaye AM, Kaye AD. Tramadol, pharmacology, side effects, and serotonin syndrome: a review. Pain Physician. 2015;18(4):395–400.
10. Boyer EW, Shannon M. The serotonin syndrome. N Engl J Med. 2005;352(11):1112–20.
11. Buckley NA, Dawson AH, Isbister GK. Serotonin syndrome. BMJ. 2014;348(6):g2159.
12. Gillman PK. Triptans, serotonin agonists, and serotonin syndrome (serotonin toxicity): a review. Headache. 2010;50:264–72.
13. Moss MJ, Hendrickson RG. Serotonin toxicity. J Clin Psychopharmacol. 2019;39(6):628–33.
14. Duignan KM, Quinn AM, Matson AM. Serotonin syndrome from sertraline monotherapy: a caese report. Am J Emerg Med. 2019;38(8):1695, e5.
15. Siegel A, Sapru HN. Neurotransmitters. In: Essential neuroscience. 2nd ed. Philadelphia: Wolters Kluwer/Lippincott Williams & Wilkins Health; 2011. p. 121.
16. Mohammad-Zadeh LF, Moses L, Gwaltney-Brant SM. Serotonin: a review. J Vet Pharmacol Ther. 2008;31:187–99.
17. Scotton WJ, Hill LJ, Williams AC, Barnes NM. Serotonin syndrome: pathophysiology, clinical features, management, and potential future directions. Int J Tryptophan Res. 2019;12 https://doi.org/10.1177/1178646919873925.

18. Baldo BA. Opioid analgesic drugs and serotonin toxicity (syndrome): mechanisms, animal models, and links to clinical effects. Arch Toxicol. 2018;92(8):2457–73.
19. Van Oekelen D, Megnes A, Meert T, et al. Functional study of rat 5-HT$_{2A}$ receptors using antisense oligonucleotides. J Neurochem. 2003;85:1087–100.
20. Barnes NM, Andrade R, Bockaert J, et al. 5-Hydroxytryptamine receptors, introductory chapter. International Union of Basic and Clinical Pharmacology (IUPHAR) database (IUPHAR-DB). http://www.iuphar-db.org/DATABASE/FamilyIntroductionForward?familyId=1. Last modified on 2011-04-18. Accessed 04 May 2011.
21. Gillman PK. A review of serotonin toxicity data: implications for the mechanisms of antidepressant drug action. Biol Psychiatry. 2006;59:1046–51.
22. Kennedy SH, McKenna KF, Baker GB. Monoamine oxidase inhibitors. In: Sadock BJ, Sadock VA, editors. Kaplan & Sadock's comprehensive textbook of psychiatry. 7th ed. Philadelphia: Lippincott Williams & Wilkins; 2000. p. 2398–407.
23. Prozac (fluoxetine hydrochloride) Prescribing Information, Eli Lilly and Company, Indianapolis; 2009. http://www.prozac.com/Pages/index.aspx. Accessed 05 Mar 2011.
24. Durson SM, Mathew VM, Reveley MA. Toxic serotonin syndrome after fluoxetine plus carbamazepine. Lancet. 1993;342:442–3.
25. Mekler G, Woggon B. A case of serotonin syndrome caused by venlafaxine and lithium. Pharmacopsychiatry. 1997;30:272–3.
26. Adan-Manes J, Novalbos J, López-Rodríguez R, Ayuso-Mateos JL, Abad-Santos F. Lithium and venlafaxine interaction: a case of serotonin syndrome. J Clin Pharm Ther. 2006 Aug;31(4):397–400.
27. Gillman PK. Serotonin syndrome: clomipramine too soon after moclobemide. Int Clin Psychopharmacol. 1997;12:339–42.
28. Okamoto N, Sakamoto K, Yamada M. Transient serotonin syndrome by concurrent use of electroconvulsive therapy and selective serotonin reuptake inhibitor: a case report and review of the literature. Case Rep Psychiatry. 2012;2012:1–3.
29. Deuschle M, Böhringer A, Meyer-Lindenberg A, Sartorius A. Electroconvulsive therapy induces transient sensitivity for a serotonin syndrome: a case report. Pharmacopsychiatry. 2016;50(01):41–2.
30. Cheng Y-C, Liang C-M, Liu H-C. Serotonin syndrome after electroconvulsive therapy in a patient on trazodone, bupropion, and quetiapine. Clin Neuropharmacol. 2015;38(3):112–3.
31. Nisijima K, Nibuya M, Kato S. Toxic serotonin syndrome successfully treated with electroconvulsive therapy. J Clin Psychopharmacol. 2002;22:338–9.
32. Aboukarr A, Giudice M. Interaction between monoamine oxidase B inhibitors and selective serotonin reuptake inhibitors. Can J Hosp Pharm. 2018;71(3)
33. Fernandes C, Reddy P, Kessel B. Rasagiline-induced serotonin syndrome (letter to the editor). Mov Disord. https://doi.org/10.1002/mds.23649.
34. Toyama SC, Iacono RP. Is it safe to combine a selective serotonin reuptake inhibitor with selegiline? Ann Pharmacother. 1994;28:405.
35. Waters CH. Fluoxetine and selegiline–lack of significant interaction. Can J Neurol Sci. 1994;21:259–61.
36. Zyvox (linezolid) Prescribing Information, Pfizer, distributed by Pharmacia & Upjohn Company, NY, NY, 2010. http://www.pfizer.com/products/rx/rx_product_zyvox.jsp. Accessed 05 Mar 2011.
37. Morales N, Vermette H. Serotonin syndrome associated with linezolid treatment after discontinuation of fluoxetine. Psychosomatics. 2005;46:274–5.
38. Mastroianni A. Gianfranco Ravaglia. Serotonin syndrome due to co-administration of linezolid and methadone. Infez Med. 2017;25(3):263–6.
39. Zornberg GL, Bodkin JA, Cohen BM. Severe adverse interaction between pethidine and selegiline. Lancet. 1991;337:246.
40. Cymbalta (duloxetine hydrochloride) Prescribing Information, Eli Lilly and Company, Indianapolis, IN, April 22, 2011. http://www.cymbalta.com/index.jsp?WT.seg_1=Branded&DCSext.ag=BrandGeneral&WT.mc_id=CymDPNA14120001&WT.srch=1. Accessed 06 May 2011.

41. Savella (milnacipran hydrochloride) Prescribing Information, Forest Pharmaceuticals, Inc; 2009. http://www.savella.com/index.aspx. Accessed 06 May 2011.
42. Yacoub HA, Johnson WG, Souayah N. Serotonin syndrome after administration of milnacipran for fibromyalgia. Neurology. 2010;74:699.
43. Parrott AC. Recreational Ecstasy/MDMA, the serotonin syndrome, and serotonergic neurotoxicity. Pharmacol Biochem Behav. 2002;71:837–44.
44. Randall T. Ecstasy-fueled "rave" parties become dances of death for English youths. JAMA. 1992;268:1505–6.
45. Dobry Y, Rice T, Sher L. Ecstasy use and serotonin syndrome: a neglected danger to adolescents and young adults prescribed selective serotonin reuptake inhibitors. Int J Adolesc Med Health. 2013;25(3):193–9.
46. Drugs and Chemicals of Concern: dextromethorphan. U.S. Department of Justice, Drug Enforcement Administration, Office of Diversion Control; 2010. http://www.deadiversion.usdoj.gov/drugs_concern/dextro_m/dextro_m.htm. Accessed 09 Apr 2011.
47. Substance Abuse and Mental Health Services Administration. Office of Applied Studies. The NSDUH report: misuse of over-the-counter cough and cold medications among persons aged 12 to 25. 2008. Available at http://www.oas.samhsa.gov/2k8/cough/cough.cfm. Accessed 09 Apr 2011.
48. Ball, JK, Albright, V. Substance Abuse and Mental Health Services Administration, Office of Applied Studies. Emergency department visits involving dextromethorphan. The New DAWN report 2006; 32:1. Available at http://www.oas.samhsa.gov/DAWN/dextromethorphan.cfm. Accessed 10 Apr 2011.
49. Schwartz AR, Pizon AF, Brooks DE. Case series: dextromethorphan-induced serotonin syndrome. Clin Toxicol. 2008;46:771–3.
50. Spoelder AS, Louwerens JKG, Krens SD, Jager N, Lecouffe NE, Ruijter W, et al. Unexpected serotonin syndrome, epileptic seizures, and cerebral edema following 2,5-dimethoxy-4-bromophenethylamine ingestion. J Forensic Sci. 2019;64(6):1950–2.
51. Andersen IB. Dextromethorphan abuse in adolescence: a rising trend. California Poison Control System, 2007, slides accessed from www.csam-asam.org/pdf/misc/DXM_CSAM_9_07.ppt. Accessed 10 Apr 2011.
52. Katzung BG, Trevor AJ. Drug biotransformation. In: Basic & clinical pharmacology. 13th ed. New York: McGraw-Hill Education; 2015. p. 62.
53. Forget P, le Polain de Waroux B, Wallemacq P, Gala JL. Life-threatening dextromethorphan intoxication associated with interaction with amitriptyline in a poor CYP2D6 metabolizer: a single case re-exposure study. J Pain Symptom Manag. 2008 Jul;36(1):92–6.
54. DeSilva KE, Le Flore DB, Marston BJ, Rimland D. Serotonin syndrome in HIV-infected individuals receiving antiretroviral therapy and fluoxetine. AIDS. 2001;15:1281–5.
55. Anon. US Food and Drug Administration. Information for healthcare professionals. Selective serotonin reuptake inhibitors (SSRIs), selective serotonin norepinephrine reuptake inhibitors (SNRIs), 5-hydroxytryptamine receptor agonists (triptans). 2006. Available at: http://www.fda.gov/cder/drug/InfoSheets/HCP/triptansHCP.htm
56. Evans RW, Tepper SJ, Shapiro RE, Sun-Edelstein C, Tietjen GE. The FDA alert on serotonin syndrome with use of triptans combined with selective serotonin reuptake inhibitors or selective serotonin-norepinephrine reuptake inhibitors: American headache society position paper. Headache. 2010;50:1089–99.
57. Robblee JV, Butterfield RJ, Kang AM, Smith JH. Triptan and ergotamine overdoses in the United States. Neurology. 2019;94(14):e1460–9.
58. Orlova Y, Rizzoli P, Loder E. Association of coprescription of triptan antimigraine drugs and selective serotonin reuptake inhibitor or selective norepinephrine reuptake inhibitor antidepressants with serotonin syndrome. JAMA Neurol. 2018;75(5):566–72.
59. Zuschlag ZD, Warren MW, Schultz SK. Serotonin toxicity and urinary analgesics: a case report and systematic literature review of methylene blue-induced serotonin syndrome. Psychosomatics. 2018;59(6):539–46.

60. Ng BKW, Cameron AJD. The role of methylene blue in serotonin syndrome: a systematic review. Psychosomatics. 2010;51:194–200.
61. Katzianer D, Chism K, Qureshi AM, Watson R, Massey HT, Boyle AJ, et al. Serotonin syndrome following left ventricular assist device implantation: a report and institution-specific strategy for prevention. J Cardiol Case. 2019;20(6):218–20.
62. Gill M, Lo Vecchio F, Seldan B. Serotonin syndrome in a child after a single dose of fluvoxamine. Ann Emerg Med. 1999;33:457–9.
63. Spirko BA, James FW. Serotonin syndrome: a new pediatric intoxication. Pediatr Emerg Care. 1999;15:440–3.
64. Wilson V, Maulik SK. Herb-drug interactions in neurological disorders: a critical appraisal. Curr Drug Metab. 2018;19(5):443–53.
65. Henderson L, Yue QY, Bergquist C, Gerden B, Arlett P. St John's wort (Hypericum perforatum): drug interactions and clinical outcomes. Br J Clin Pharmacol. 2002;54(4):349–56.
66. Parker V, Wong AIIC, Doon II3, Seeman MV. Adverse reactions to St John's wort. Can J Psychiatr. 2001;46:77–9.
67. Warner ME, Warner PA, Sprung J, Warner MA. Black seed oil and perioperative serotonin syndrome. A A Pract. 2019;13(11):420–2.
68. Task Force on DSM-IV. Diagnostic and statistical manual of mental disorders (DSM-IV-TR). Washington, DC: American Psychiatric Association; 2000.
69. Graudins A, Stearman CB. Treatment of the serotonin syndrome with cyproheptadine. J Emerg Med. 1998;16:615–9.
70. Nguyen H, Pan A, Smollin C, Cantrell LF, Kearney T. An 11-year retrospective review of cyproheptadine use in serotonin syndrome cases reported to the California Poison Control System. J Clin Pharm Ther. 2019;44(2):327–34.
71. Pedavally S, Fugate JE, Rabinstein AA. Serotonin syndrome in the intensive care unit: clinical presentations and precipitating medications. Neurocrit Care. 2013;21(1):108–13.
72. Foong A-L, Grindrod KA, Patel T, Kellar J. Demystifying serotonin syndrome (or serotonin toxicity). Can Fam Physician. 2018;64(10):720–7.

Acute Spinal Rigidity

9

Philip D. Thompson

Patient Vignettes

Patient 1

A 69-year-old woman presented with a 1-year history of low back and leg pain accompanied by progressive difficulty walking. Lumbar surgery was undertaken for spondylolisthesis and canal stenosis. Postoperatively the pain improved but walking continued to deteriorate, and spasms of the back and right leg developed with flexion of the trunk, hip, and knee. Examination revealed a rigid right leg with palpable contractions in all muscle groups, brisk tendon reflexes, and an extensor plantar response. There was no truncal rigidity or sensory loss. Sensory stimulation elicited a brisk flexion withdrawal of the whole leg. Similar flexion spasms of the right leg and hip interfered with her gait. Spinal cord imaging was normal. A glucose tolerance test was abnormal. Antiglutamic acid decarboxylase (AntiGAD) antibodies were not detected. Baclofen improved the rigidity and mobility. One year later her mobility declined again. On this occasion, examination revealed abdominal wall, lumbar paraspinal, and bilateral leg rigidity. The clinical picture was now consistent with stiff person syndrome. AntiGAD antibodies remained negative until 10 years after the initial presentation, at which time she developed stimulus-sensitive brainstem myoclonus in response to auditory stimuli and nose and mantle taps. This case illustrates the focal onset of rigidity in one leg and subsequent evolution of the stiff person syndrome, despite absent antiGAD antibodies.

P. D. Thompson (✉)
The University of Adelaide, Adelaide, SA, Australia
e-mail: philip.thompson@adelaide.edu.au

© Springer Nature Switzerland AG 2022
S. J. Frucht (ed.), *Movement Disorder Emergencies*, Current Clinical Neurology,
https://doi.org/10.1007/978-3-030-75898-1_9

Patient 2

A 68-year-old woman presented with inability to stand or move her legs following a fall. This occurred on the background of a 2-month history of progressive difficulty walking, associated with leg muscle spasm, falls, pain, and altered sensation in the legs. Upper limb and sphincter function were normal. Examination revealed the rigid extension of both legs and plantar flexion of the feet. Voluntary leg movement was impossible and the legs could not be bent by passive manipulation because of rigidity. Tendon taps and cutaneous stimulation elicited prolonged jerking of the legs with prominent crossed reflex responses. Plantar responses were extensor, and magnetic resonance imaging of the spinal cord was normal. Magnetic brain stimulation produced normal responses in leg muscles (indicating intact corticospinal pathways). Peripheral nerve stimulation elicited bursts of muscle activity followed by prolonged tonic activity consistent with exaggerated cutaneomuscular (exteroceptive) reflexes. Multiple investigations were normal or negative, including anti-GAD antibodies. The cerebrospinal fluid contained six monocytes and borderline IgG elevation but no oligoclonal bands. She then developed a right facial sensory disturbance, a left sixth nerve palsy, and then a left conjugate gaze palsy. Intravenous methylprednisolone and oral prednisolone improved the rigidity and gaze palsy. Three weeks later rigidity had subsided, she was able to walk unaided, and tendon reflexes were normal. There has been no recurrence of symptoms over 10 years of follow-up.

This case illustrates leg rigidity as the presenting feature of progressive encephalomyelitis with rigidity (PERM). Severe leg rigidity mimicked paraplegia but electrophysiological testing confirmed that corticospinal tracts were intact. Testing for antiglycine receptor antibodies was not available at the time, but the clinical presentation and subsequent dramatic response to corticosteroids were consistent with an inflammatory, presumed immune-mediated etiology.

The Differential Diagnosis of Rigidity

Rigidity and Basal Ganglia Disease

Rigidity in Parkinson's disease, the striatonigral form of multiple system atrophy, or neuroleptic-induced parkinsonism, is characterized by a uniform increase in muscle tone that is detected as a continuous "lead pipe" resistance to passive movement of a limb. The classic form of parkinsonian rigidity is described as "cog-wheeling." Rigidity in basal ganglia disease is often most prominent in axial muscles. The mechanisms of this increase in tone are poorly understood. Increased muscle tone in dystonia is typically variable and may be related to movement (action dystonia). During movement, co-contraction of antagonist muscle pairs and overflow of muscle activity lead to an increase in muscle tone and twisted or dystonic limb postures. The dystonic postures and excessive muscle contractions subside during rest, although in advanced primary and secondary dystonia there may be a sustained increase in muscle tone that persists in repose.

Increased Tone in Spasticity and the Upper Motor Neuron Syndrome

Hypertonia in spasticity is associated with enhanced monosynaptic muscle stretch reflexes. Increased tone is detected as a "catch" or an abrupt increase in tone felt after rapidly stretching a muscle. This effect is typically velocity dependent, and stretching the muscle at different speeds may be necessary to detect an increase in tone. The increase in tone is followed by a reduction in tone, the "clasp-knife" phenomenon that is best appreciated in the extensor (quadriceps, triceps surae) muscles of the lower limbs. Brisk tendon reflexes and altered cutaneous reflexes, including loss of superficial abdominal reflexes and extensor plantar responses, are also signs of spasticity and the upper motor neuron syndrome.

Frontal Lobe Rigidity

The distinguishing characteristic of frontal rigidity (paratonia) is a progressive increase in muscle tone during limb manipulation. As the amount of resistance encountered increases, greater force is required to move the limb, giving the impression that the patient is not fully relaxed or is voluntarily resisting or opposing the movement imposed by the examiner. This is also referred to as "gegenhalten." Frontal lobe signs including grasp reflexes are useful adjuncts to recognizing frontal rigidity. Rigidity with similar characteristics to paratonia or gegenhalten, accompanied by waxy flexibility and posturing of the limbs, may be the presenting feature of catatonia and the neuroleptic malignant syndrome. Mutism, stupor, and frontal lobe signs are also evident. These conditions are described elsewhere in this book.

Muscle Stiffness and Peripheral Nerve Hyperexcitability

Hypertonia caused by continuous muscle activity due to peripheral neuromuscular hyperexcitability in Isaacs' syndrome is referred to as neuromyotonia. This is accompanied by widespread muscle rippling due to fasciculations and myokymia, and delayed muscle relaxation after voluntary contraction. Tendon reflexes may be absent and, in some cases, other signs of neuropathy are an important clue to the peripheral origin of the syndrome. Characteristic high-frequency electromyographic discharges, also referred to as neuromyotonia and myokymia, are useful in diagnosis.

Primary Muscle Disease and Muscle Stiffness

Myotonia and delayed muscle relaxation in primary muscle disease may present with complaints of muscle stiffness during voluntary movement, although the examination of muscle tone and resistance to passive movement at rest are normal. Some congenital myopathies, muscular dystrophies, and inflammatory myopathies are associated with muscle contractures, (limiting the range of limb movement), which may be misinterpreted as rigidity. Electromyography indicating electrical silence in shortened muscles indicates contracture, and imaging of paraspinal muscles can demonstrate fatty replacement in fibrotic contracture of affected muscles in axial myopathy.

Clinical Features of Spinal Rigidity

Spinal rigidity is attributed to unrestrained discharge of spinal alpha motor neurons, isolated or released from normal inhibitory interneuronal control, causing continuous muscle activity, and co-contraction of antagonist muscle groups. Accordingly, spinal rigidity is also referred to as "alpha" rigidity [1–3]. The continuous motor activity is barely influenced by voluntary effort or stimulation of reflex pathways, further indicating the isolation of spinal interneurones from segmental reflex and descending supraspinal influences. The physiology of spinal rigidity has been studied in experimental canine models of spinal cord ischemia causing selective damage to interneurones in the posterior central spinal gray matter, sparing anterior horn cells [1]. Loss of inhibitory and excitatory interneuronal activity increased motoneuronal excitability resulting in a spontaneous, continuous discharge of spinal motoneurones and continuous muscle contraction and rigidity. The posture of the rigid hindlimbs resembled decerebrate rigidity but was constant without phasic exacerbations and was not influenced by positional change, cutaneous, or noxious stimuli. Dorsal root section did not abolish or prevent the development of spinal rigidity, indicating that the rigidity was not driven by afferent feedback [1]. The continual muscle contraction was followed by muscle contracture after a few days.

The characteristic clinical sign of spinal rigidity is an increase in muscle tone that is more or less uniform throughout the range of passive or attempted voluntary movement. Rigidity can be so intense that passive manipulation of the affected limb is difficult. Severe rigidity is frequently accompanied by abnormal limb posturing with superimposed prolonged spasms, segmental myoclonus, or a jerky tremor. Persistent muscle contraction also leads to contractures and fixed limb deformities. Spinal rigidity is an uncommon clinical phenomenon. Recognizing spinal rigidity can be a challenging clinical task and differentiating spinal rigidity from the many causes of hypertonia (Table 9.1) is usually influenced by the presence of other clinical signs. In most examples of spinal rigidity, other signs of a myelopathy are present. These include segmental muscle wasting and weakness, absent tendon reflexes at the level of the spinal lesion, brisk tendon reflexes below the lesion, extensor plantar responses, and segmental radicular or long tract sensory signs.

Table 9.1 Differential diagnosis of muscle stiffness, rigidity, and spasms caused by conditions affecting the central nervous system. These are to be distinguished from muscle cramps that have peripheral neuromuscular causes. It is always important to exclude muscle contracture (electrically silent) as the cause of a fixed rigid limb posture

Stiffness, rigidity, spasm
Stiff person syndrome (SPS)
Progressive encephalomyelitis with rigidity and myoclonus (PERM)
Spinal rigidity associated with spinal lesions
Akinetic rigid basal ganglia syndromes
Axial torsion dystonia
Frontal rigidity (paratonia, gegenhalten)
Tetanus, strychnine poisoning
Muscle cramps
Benign physiological cramps
Peripheral nerve hyperexcitability syndromes (neuromyotonia)
Schwartz Jampel syndrome
Metabolic myopathies (electrically silent cramps)
Brody disease (electrically silent cramps)
Endocrine myopathies
Muscle contracture
Myopathies with contracture
Inflammatory myopathies (polymyositis)
Ischemic contracture of muscle (Volkmann)
Inherited genetic myopathies
    Rigid spine syndrome (cervical and thoracic spine)
    Bethlem myopathy (elbow, fingers, ankle)
    Emery Dreifuss myopathy (spine, elbows, fingers)

Causes of Spinal Rigidity in Man

Spinal rigidity and spasms have been described in a variety of spinal pathologies (Table 9.2), which share the common feature of predominant and selective involvement of spinal interneurones within the central gray matter of the spinal cord.

Structural Lesions of the Spinal Cord

Rushworth [3] reported a patient in whom an intramedullary astrocytoma infiltrated the central gray matter of the C2-C6 cervical cord. The patient presented with neck pain, a wasted left arm, and a Brown-Sequard syndrome. Over the following months, both arms became weak, areflexic, rigid, adducted, and extended. Spontaneous electromyographic (EMG) activity was recorded in the deltoid, pectoralis major, biceps, and triceps. Muscle stretch evoked an increase in EMG activity in these and the antagonist's muscles. Reciprocal innervation during voluntary shoulder abduction was impaired. The authors concluded that this "alpha rigidity" was due to spontaneous discharge of motoneurones isolated from interneuronal inhibitory control, and therefore insensitive to reflex or voluntary inputs.

Table 9.2 Spinal lesions and myelopathy associated with spinal rigidity

Traumatic spinal injury
Intrinsic spinal tumors
Demyelinating myelopathies and multiple sclerosis
Arteriovenous malformations
Spinal cord ischemia
Necrotizing myelopathy
Syringomyelia

Tarlov [4] described a 38-year-old woman with an intrinsic spinal cyst at the level of T12 who developed the gradual onset of painful flexor spasms over the 8 years following surgical drainage of the cyst. The hips and knees were flexed due to a combination of rigidity and contracture. She was able to flex the hips voluntarily but there was little distal voluntary leg movement. All modalities of sensation were impaired in the legs. Dorsal root section from L2 to L5 produced only a transient reduction in rigidity and spasm. In a further patient with posttraumatic hydromyelia, dorsal rhizotomy (T11-L1) and subsequently T12-L1 spinal cord section failed to relieve painful flexor spasms and rigidity of the legs [5]. Removal of the isolated segment of the spinal cord and associated ventral roots reduced the muscle activity. Pathological examination of the excised spinal cord revealed a reduced number of interneurons in the intermediate zone of the cord at L5. Lourie [6] described a 55-year-old man who presented with stiffness of the hips, pain and numbness in the lower back, scoliosis, board-like rigidity of the abdomen, persistent contraction of lumbar paraspinal muscles, and "plastic" rigidity of the legs with slow leg movements. A spinothalamic sensory loss with sacral sparing suggested an intramedullary spinal cord lesion. There were spontaneous rhythmic contractions of the hip adductor, external oblique, and paraspinal muscles that persisted during sleep, consistent with spinal myoclonus.

Necrotizing Myelopathy

Penry [2] described a patient with "subacute necrotizing myelopathy" and extensive gliosis with the destruction of the posterolateral central gray and white matter in the posterolateral spinal cord between C3 and T8. The initial clinical presentation was of a cervical myelopathy evolving over weeks, with flaccid weakness of the left arm and an asymmetric quadriplegia. Five months later, rigidity and spasms developed in the left arm, which was held in a posture of shoulder abduction and internal rotation, elbow flexion, wrist dorsiflexion, and finger flexion. A curious and distinctive finding was the inability to activate voluntarily the muscles in spasm. Intense EMG discharges in muscles of the left arm were not influenced by muscle stretch or tendon taps.

Tetanus and Strychnine

The rigidity accompanying tetanus may be localized to the site of infection but there is often spread with facial (risus sardonicus) and jaw spasm (trismus or lockjaw). Spasms occur spontaneously or in response to auditory or cutaneous stimulation, spreading throughout the body producing abdominal rigidity and opisthotonic spasms. Spasms and rigidity may be dramatic, building in a crescendo fashion over several seconds, lasting for minutes, and spreading from one site to another. Profound autonomic features including hypertension, tachycardia, and sweating frequently accompany the spasms. Myoclonus and tremor may also occur [7]. Similar spasms occur in strychnine poisoning [8]. Tendon reflexes are brisk. An encephalopathy with decreased consciousness may accompany the spasms of strychnine poisoning. Both tetanus and strychnine disrupt inhibitory glycinergic and GABA release, blocking interneuronal inhibition of motoneurons in the spinal cord, brainstem, and possibly cortex. Prolonged rigidity and spasm can lead to fever, rhabdomyolysis, and acute renal failure.

Spinal Segmental Rigidity and Myoclonus

The capacity of the isolated spinal cord to produce a range of rhythmic activities was documented in traumatic spinal injuries during the First World War [9]. These included jerks and spasms with phasic and tonic elements that resulted in multisegmental movements of the abdomen, pelvis, and legs, and coordinated locomotor-like activities of the legs [9, 10]. Similar rhythmic activities arising from an isolated segment of the spinal cord have been described in traumatic paraplegia [11], spina bifida [12], and experimental encephalomyelitis [13]. Varying combinations of spontaneous motor activities including rigidity and myoclonic or tremulous movements have been described in "spinal myoclonus."

Segmental rigidity and myoclonus affecting one leg were the presenting features of a paraneoplastic syndrome in a 68-year-old woman reported by Roobol [14]. The rigidity was accompanied by a posture of flexion at the knee, plantar flexion of the foot, and extension of the great toe. Thoracic radicular sensory symptoms and signs also were present. Microscopic examination of the spinal cord revealed a reduction in the number of anterior horn cells, and interneurons could not be identified in the lumbar region. Involvement of the central spinal gray matter in ischemic myelopathy may lead to a similar clinical picture. Davis [15] reported the case of a 75-year-old man who presented with bilateral spontaneous and stimulus-sensitive myoclonus of the legs. The myoclonus produced movement of the whole leg involving hip, knee, and plantar flexion. In between the myoclonus, muscle tone in the legs was increased with spasticity and plastic rigidity. Fasciculations were recorded on EMG between spasms but there was no mention of continuous motor activity to explain the rigidity. Pathological examination of the lumbar and sacral spinal segments revealed a selective reduction in the number of small and medium-sized interneurons with relative sparing of the large anterior horn cells. The anterior spinal artery was virtually occluded at the mid-thoracic level.

Spinal Interneuronitis and the Stiff Leg Syndrome

Isolated rigidity and spasms affecting one leg (the "stiff leg syndrome") have been attributed to segmental motoneuronal disinhibition caused by a localized form of spinal interneuronitis [16]. A similar mechanism involving spinal interneurones has been proposed to explain spasms, rigidity, and continuous motor unit activity in an inflammatory myelopathy [17, 18].

Rigidity in the Stiff Person Syndrome

Rigidity, due to continuous motor unit activity, is usually the initial symptom of the stiff person syndrome (SPS) and is often focal (leg) or segmental (leg, trunk). Delay in diagnosis is common and by the time of diagnosis other signs have commonly appeared with rigidity progressing to generalized distribution over a variable period [19]. The initial focal or segmental distribution of rigidity in SPS, confined to the lower trunk and legs, or one leg, is suggestive of segmental spinal rigidity. Rigidity may vary with cutaneous or emotional stimuli. Sudden increases in tone in response to such stimuli can interfere with voluntary movement and lead to falls. Continuous motor unit activity in thoracolumbar paraspinal and abdominal muscles is a characteristic finding and becomes more prominent with time leading to axial stiffness, an exaggerated lumbar lordosis, and "board-like" rigidity of the anterior abdominal wall. Stimulus-sensitive spasms caused by enhanced cutaneomuscular reflexes are superimposed on the rigidity [19]. These occur in response to sensory stimulation of the lower limb and begin with a myoclonic burst followed by a prolonged phase of tonic contraction representing the "spasm." This activity may be misinterpreted as brisk tendon reflexes due to spasticity. Similar responses occur after an unexpected auditory stimulus. Electrophysiological studies demonstrating continuous muscle contraction and enhanced cutaneomuscular reflexes along with serological testing for anti-GAD antibodies are helpful in diagnosis [19]. Repetitive spasms in SPS can be accompanied by dysautonomia with hypertension, tachycardia, and sweating.

The precise nature and anatomical location of the disturbance causing the SPS and associated rigidity are not known [19]. Alterations in the descending brainstem control of muscle tone are evident in the exaggerated startle response, the enhanced cutaneomuscular responses, and similar responses to unexpected supraspinal visual, auditory or emotional stimuli. The continuous muscle activity may reflect disinhibition of spinal motoneurones at a segmental level as discussed for spinal rigidity.

Progressive Encephalomyelitis with Rigidity and Myoclonus

Similarities in the distribution and pattern of rigidity in PERM and SPS were recognized in the early descriptions of PERM, but the subacute onset, a fluctuating progressive course and clinical signs of brainstem involvement such as ophthalmoplegia, dysphagia, gait and limb ataxia, and sensory symptoms were clearly different [20–22]. Both SPS and PERM show pathological evidence of perivascular inflammation in the brainstem and spinal cord consistent with an inflammatory encephalomyelitis [19]. In 2008, Hutchison et al. [23] described a 54-year-old man who presented with "violent" generalized brainstem myoclonus triggered by sensory and auditory stimuli, severe rigidity, and brainstem signs consistent with PERM. There was a cerebrospinal fluid lymphocytosis, anti-GAD antibodies were negative and he improved with immunosuppression. Subsequently, high titers of antiglycine receptor antibodies were identified (investigated on the basis that the prominent brainstem myoclonus was reminiscent of hereditary hyperekplexia due to glycine receptor mutations) [23]. In fact, other similar cases of PERM with prominent brainstem myoclonus had been reported in the literature and referred to as the "jerking stiff man" [24] and symptomatic hyperekplexia [25, 26]. A strong association has since been established between glycine receptor antibodies and the clinical presentation of PERM with a subacute onset over weeks and improvement with immunotherapy through relapses may occur [27]. To date, antibodies are not identified in one third of PERM cases [27, 28]. Between 10% and 20% of patients with antiglycine receptor antibodies have an underlying malignancy [27].

There is a strong association between glycine receptor antibodies and progressive encephalomyelitis with rigidity and myoclonus. The diagnosis of PERM requires a search for an underlying malignancy.

Other Immune Associations of Rigidity

Antiamphiphysin antibodies associated with breast cancer have been associated with SPS typically beginning with upper limb rigidity [29]. The neurological signs may precede the discovery of cancer. Accordingly, the onset of upper limb rigidity in a female should prompt a search for breast malignancy and include follow-up examinations [29]. Other immunological associations with the clinical picture of PERM include antibodies to DPPX [30], gephyrin [31], and anti-Ri antibodies [32] (Table 9.3). Some of these may also represent paraneoplastic syndromes [31, 32]. In addition to rigidity and myoclonus, anti-Ri PERM may exhibit other neurological signs including opsoclonus, ataxia [32], and bulbar (facial, masticatory) rigidity (unpublished personal observations).

A presentation of a unilateral rigid arm in a female patient should prompt an intense search for an underlying breast malignancy.

Table 9.3 Antibodies associated with immune-mediated rigidity presenting with the clinical picture of the stiff person syndrome (SPS) or progressive encephalomyelitis with rigidity and myoclonus (PERM). In a retrospective study of neuroimmunological investigations in 121 patients designated "stiff-person spectrum disorder" the commonest antibodies identified were anti-GAD65 associated with SPS and antiglycine receptor antibodies were associated with "SPS plus" (analogous to PERM) [28]. The other antibodies listed in the table below were detected infrequently and antibodies were not detected in one-third of the patients [28]

Antiglutamic acid decarboxylase (GAD) (SPS) [19, 28]
Antiglycine receptor (PERM) [23, 27, 28]
Antiamphiphysin (paraneoplastic) (SPS) [30]
Antidipeptidyl-peptidase like protein 6 (DPPX) (PERM) [31]
Antigephyrin (PERM) [32]
Anti-Ri (paraneoplastic) (PERM) [33]

Management

The management of acute rigidity and associated movement disorders is based on the identification of the anatomical site of origin of the neurological signs and then the underlying cause. This requires appropriate imaging of the spinal cord. Where structural or inflammatory disease of the spinal cord is identified, treatment revolves around the management of the spinal pathology and cause. Serological studies for anti-GAD and antiglycine receptor antibodies along with electrophysiological testing for enhanced cutaneomuscular reflexes are helpful when SPS or PERM is suspected. Disease-modifying immunological therapies such as intravenous immunoglobulin are effective in SPS [33], but in general immune strategies are more effective in PERM, though relapses can occur [27, 28]. A detailed discussion of the immunotherapy strategies used is beyond the scope of this chapter. In each case, such therapies need to be individually tailored.

Drugs such as baclofen, tizanidine, and diazepam are useful in the symptomatic treatment of spinal rigidity and spasms (Table 9.4). Large doses are often needed and intrathecal baclofen may provide a more effective method of delivery. Abrupt cessation of these drugs must be avoided as this may precipitate a severe exacerbation of rigidity accompanied by acute autonomic failure [34].

Acute withdrawal or interruption of intrathecal baclofen can precipitate a hyperkinetic crisis that can be fatal. Complaints of fever, an abrupt increase in rigidity, or alteration of mental status in a patient with an intrathecal baclofen pump should always prompt immediate evaluation in the emergency room.

Table 9.4 Drugs that may be useful in the treatment of spinal rigidity and spasms

Benzodiazepines: diazepam, clonazepam
GABA analog: baclofen
Centrally acting antiadrenergic: tizanidine, clonidine
Anticonvulsants: gabapentin, valproate
Botulinum toxin injections for focal rigidity, spasm
Immunotherapy: PERM, SPS

Conclusion

Focal or segmental spinal rigidity is an unusual neurologic presentation, one that carries significant implications for diagnosis and treatment. Recognizing this clinical syndrome and initiating the appropriate work-up and treatment can have a profound effect on patients' outcomes.

References

1. Gelfand S, Tarlov IM. Interneurones and rigidity of spinal origin. J Physiol (London). 1959;146:594–617.
2. Penry JK, Hoefnagel D, van den Noort S, Denny-Brown D. Muscle spasm and abnormal postures resulting from damage to interneurones in spinal cord. Arch Neurol. 1960;3:500–12.
3. Rushworth G, Lishman WA, Hughes TJ, Oppenheimer DR. Intense rigidity of the arms due to isolation of motor neurones by a spinal tumour. J Neurol Neurosurg Psychiatry. 1961;24:132–42.
4. Tarlov IM. Rigidity in man due to spinal interneuron loss. Arch Neurol. 1967;16:536–43.
5. Tarlov IM. Deafferentation to relieve spasticity or rigidity: reasons for failure in some cases of paraplegia. J Neurosurg. 1966;25:270–4.
6. Lourie H. Spontaneous activity of alpha motor neurons in intramedullary spinal cord tumor. J Neurosurg. 1968;29:573–80.
7. Warren JD, Kimber TE, Thompson PD. Brainstem myoclonus in generalized tetanus. Mov Disord. 2003;18:1204–6.
8. Case records of the Massachusetts general hospital. N Engl J Med. 2001;344:1232–9.
9. Riddoch G. The reflex functions of the completely divided spinal cord in man, compared with those associated with less severe lesions. Brain. 1917;40:264–401.
10. Pollock LJ, Boshes B, Finkelman I, Chor H, Brown M. Spasticity, pseudospasms and other reflex activities later after injury to the spinal cord. Arch Neurol Psychiatr. 1951;66:537–60.
11. Bussell B, Roby-Brami A, Azouvi P, Biraben A, Yakovleff A, Pierrot-Deselligny E. Myoclonus in a patient with spinal cord transection. Brain. 1988;111:1235–45.
12. Warren JE, Vidailhet M, Kneebone CS, Quinn NP, Thompson PD. Myoclonus in spinal dysraphism. Mov Disord. 2003;18:961–4.
13. Lutterell CN, Bang FB, Luxenberg K. Newcastle disease encephalomyelitis in cats. II: physiological studies on rhythmic myoclonus. Arch Neurol Psych. 1959;81:285–91.
14. Roobol TH, Kazzazz BA, Vecht CHJ. Segmental rigidity and spinal myoclonus as a paraneoplastic syndrome. J Neurol Neurosurg Psychiatry. 1987;50:628–31.

15. Davis SM, Murray NMF, Diengdoh JV, Galea-Debono A, Kocen RS. Stimulus-sensitive spinal myoclonus. J Neurol Neurosurg Psychiatry. 1981;44:884–8.
16. McCombe PA, Chalk JB, Searle JW, Tannenberg AEG, Smith JJ, Pender MP. Progressive encephalomyelitis with rigidity: a case report with magnetic resonance imaging findings. J Neurol Neurosurg Psychiatry. 1989;52:1429–31.
17. Brown P, Quinn NP, Barnes D, Wren DR, Marsden CD. Spinal rigidity following acute myelitis. Mov Disord. 1997;12:1056–9.
18. Brown P, Rothwell JC, Marsden CD. The stiff leg syndrome. J Neurol Neurosurg Psychiatry. 1997;62:31–7.
19. Meinck H-M, Thompson PD. The stiff man syndrome and related conditions. Mov Disord. 2002;17:853–66.
20. Kasperek S, Zebrowski S. Stiff man syndrome and encephalomyelitis. Arch Neurol. 1971;24:22–31.
21. Howell DA, Lees AJ, Toghill PJ. Spinal internuncial neurones in progressive encephalomyelitis with rigidity. J Neurol Neurosurg Psychiatry. 1979;42:773–85.
22. Whiteley AM, Swash M, Urich H. Progressive encephalomyelitis with rigidity. Brain. 1976;99:27–42.
23. Hutchison M, Waters P, McHugh J, Gorman G, O'Riordan S, Connolly S, et al. Progressive encephalomyelitis, rigidity and myoclonus: a novel glycine receptor antibody. Neurology. 2008;71:1291–2.
24. Leigh PN, Rothwell JC, Traub M, Marsden CD. A patient with reflex myoclonus and muscle rigidity: "the jerking stiff man syndrome". J Neurol Neurosurg Psychiatry. 1980;43:1125–31.
25. Brown P, Rothwell JC, Thompson PD, Britton TC, Day BL, Marsden CD. The hyperekplexias and their relationship to the normal startle response. Brain. 1991;114:1903–28.
26. Burn DJ, Ball J, Lees AJ, Behan PO, Morgan-Hughes JA. A case of progressive encephalomyelitis with rigidity and positive anti-glutamic acid dehydrogenase antibodies. J Neurol Neurosurg Psychiatry. 1991;54:449–51.
27. Carvajal Gonzalea A, Leite MI, Waters P, Woodhall M, Coutinho E, Balint B, et al. Glycine receptor antibodies in PERM and related syndromes: characteristics, clinical features and outcomes. Brain. 2014;137:2178–92.
28. Martinez-Hernandez M, Arino H, McKeon A, Iizuka T, Titulaer MJ, Simabukuro MM, et al. Clinical and immunological investigations in patients with Stiff Person Spectrum disorder. JAMA Neurol. 2016;73:714–20.
29. Rosin L, De Camilli P, Butler M, Solimena M, Schmitt HP, Morgenthaler N, et al. Stiff man syndrome in a woman with breast cancer: an uncommon central nervous system paraneoplastic syndrome. Neurology. 1998;50:94–8.
30. Balint B, Jarius S, Nagel U, Haberkorn U, Probst C, Blöcker IM, et al. Progressive encephalomyelitis with rigidity and myoclonus. A new variant with DPPX antibodies. Neurology. 2014;82:1521–8.
31. Butler HM, Hatashi A, Ohkoshi N, Villmann C, Becker CM, Feng G, et al. Autoimmunity to gephyrin in stiff man syndrome. Neuron. 2000;26:307–12.
32. Casado JL, Gil-Peralta A, Graus F, Arenas C, Lopez JM, Alberca R. Anti-Ri antibodies associated with opsoclonus and progressive encephalomyelitis with rigidity. Neurology. 1994;44:1521–2.
33. Dalakas MC, Fujii M, Li M, Lutfi B, Kyhos J, McElroy B. High-dose intravenous immune globulin for stiff-person syndrome. N Engl J Med. 2001;345:1870–6.
34. Stayer C, Tronnier V, Dressnandt J, Mauch E, Marquardt G, Rieke K, et al. Intrathecal baclofen therapy for stiff-man syndrome and progressive encephalomyelopathy with rigidity and myoclonus. Neurology. 1997;49:1519–97.

Status Dystonicus

10

Inge A. Meijer and Alfonso Fasano

Patient Vignettes

Patient 1

An 11-year-old boy with dystonic cerebral palsy (CP) presented to the emergency department with progressive worsening of dystonic posturing affecting the trunk, neck, and left arm, as well as difficulty feeding and swallowing. Upon arrival, he was diaphoretic, febrile, and tachypneic, and his creatine kinase level was 500 U/L. His medications at home included baclofen 10 mg TID and trihexyphenidyl 2 mg TID as well as clonazepam 0.5 mg BID. No clear triggers, such as recent infections or medication changes, were identified aside from psychological stressors. He was hospitalized in the pediatric intensive care unit for 5 days while baseline medication was adjusted and was temporarily sedated with propofol and ketamine for complaints of severe pain. Within a 2-week period, he started improving and was discharged with adjusted doses of clonazepam, quetiapine, trihexyphenidyl, and baclofen as well as close psychiatric follow-up.

Supplementary Information The online version of this chapter (https://doi.org/10.1007/978-3-030-75898-1_10) contains supplementary material, which is available to authorized users.

I. A. Meijer
Department of Neurosciences, CHU Sainte Justine, Montreal, QC, Canada

A. Fasano (✉)
Toronto Western Hospital, Movement Disorders Centre, Toronto, ON, Canada
e-mail: alfonso.fasano@uhn.ca

© Springer Nature Switzerland AG 2022
S. J. Frucht (ed.), *Movement Disorder Emergencies*, Current Clinical Neurology,
https://doi.org/10.1007/978-3-030-75898-1_10

Patient 2

An 11-year-old boy initially presented with focal leg dystonia at age 8, which generalized over the following years. He developed subacute worsening of his generalized dystonia involving mainly the trunk and limbs, leading to severe pain and injuries. Rapid genetic evaluation confirmed the diagnosis of DYT1-TOR1A within a week of his admission for SD and enabled urgent deep brain stimulation (DBS) implantation of the globus pallidus pars interna (GPi). Within 2 weeks he was discharged with significant improvement and continued to improve over the following months/years.

Introduction

Status dystonicus (SD) was initially defined as "increasingly frequent and severe episodes of generalized dystonia," which necessitate urgent hospital admission (Fig. 10.1) [1]. In 1982, Jankovic and Penn first reported SD in a child with generalized dystonia (later found to be caused by *TOR1A* mutation) who deteriorated and required muscle paralysis and ventilation [2]. Marsden et al. later described two children with generalized dystonia who presented with life-threatening dystonia which they referred to as "desperate dystonics" [3]. Narayan et al. described an 18-year-old man with predominantly axial dystonia caused by cerebral palsy (CP) who deteriorated markedly after spinal surgery with opisthotonos and dystonic spasms of the legs, abdominal, and respiratory muscles [4]. The term "dystonic storm" was first coined by Vaamonde et al. in 1994 to describe two children with isolated dystonia probably caused by pantothenate kinase-associated neurodegeneration (PKAN) who deteriorated following a febrile illness with generalized tonic spasms and respiratory distress [5]. In 1998, the current definition of SD was described in a case series (1) of 12 cases that included two isolated inherited dystonias, three dyskinetic CPs, three post-traumatic dystonias, one postencephalitic dystonias, one infantile striatal necrosis, one neuroacanthocytosis (presently classified

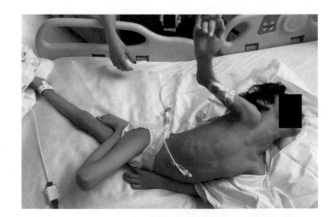

Fig. 10.1 A typical pediatric case of status dystonicus (tonic type) in an 11-year-old girl with idiopathic generalized dystonia of unknown etiology. (Courtesy of Sara Breitbart, Carolina Gorodetsky, and George Ibrahim from The Hospital for Sick Children, Toronto, ON, Canada)

as CHOR-VPS13A), and one unknown acquired dystonia [1]. During the subsequent years, a few other series have been reported including another series of five patients, that defined SD as "episodes of generalized, intense and potentially fatal exacerbation of muscle contractures, usually refractory to traditional pharmacological therapy" [6], and two original cases [7]. Nerrant et al. (2018) described 40 SD cases with mainly genetic dystonia who underwent 58 SD episodes [8]. The largest SD series reported, including 68 patients who presented with 89 SD episodes, further elucidated the clinical spectrum, treatment strategies, and outcome of SD [9]. The second large SD series included predominantly genetic SD cases most likely because of a selection bias for deep brain stimulation (DBS)-implanted cases [8].

Terminology and Definition

Many different terms other than SD have been employed to describe this condition including "dystonic storm" [5], "life-threatening dystonia: [2], "desperate dystonics" [3], and "dystonic state" [10]. It has been suggested that SD is the preferable term as "status" is part of the common neurological culture (e.g., status epilepticus, SE) [11]. The aforementioned definition by Manji et al. describes SD as a life-threatening event associated with the development of one or more of the following: (1) bulbar weakness, (2) respiratory failure, (3) metabolic derangements, and (4) exhaustion and pain [1]. However, this definition is limited by the assumption that SD generally occurs in patients with underlying dystonia and exclusively with generalized involvement. However, even nongeneralized dystonia can be a medical emergency (Table 10.1) and SD has been described also in patients without dystonia at baseline (Fig. 10.2). Therefore, a new definition has more recently been proposed: *"SD is a movement disorder emergency characterized by severe episodes of generalized or focal hyperkinetic movements that have necessitated urgent hospital admission because of the direct life-threatening complication(s) of these*

Table 10.1 Focal/segmental dystonia as emergency

Pathophysiology	Causes	Phenomenology
Primary disorders of CNS	Paroxysmal dystonia	Usually involving a lower limb
Lesions	Basal ganglia stroke (especially putamen)	Usually involving trunk
Drug induced	D2 receptors antagonists (neuroleptic and antiemetics)	Usually involving trunk (e.g., Pisa syndrome) or lower face (e.g., oromandibular dystonia)
Degenerative	Multiple system atrophy	Adductor laryngeal dystonia
Psychiatric	Functional dystonia	Usually involving trunk (e.g., camptocormia) or upper limb
Mimickers	Atlantoaxial subluxation, posterior fossa and cervical cord lesions, retropharyngeal abscess, immune reactions.	Usually involving neck, laryngeal muscles (i.e., stridor), or upper limb (e.g., pseudo-dystonia due to somatosensory deficits).

Abbreviations: *CNS* central nervous system, *SD* status dystonicus

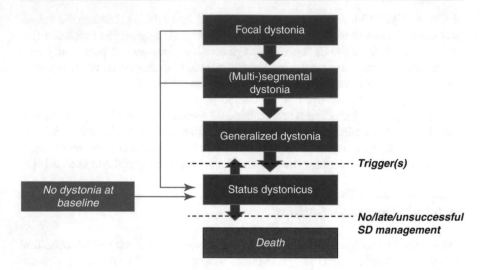

Fig. 10.2 A nosological framework of status dystonicus. In red, the new concepts introduced by the new definition: even nongeneralized dystonia can become a medical emergency and patients without dystonia at baseline (or healthy) can present with a status dystonicus

movements, regardless of the patient's neurological condition at baseline" [11, 12], whereby a movement disorder emergency is defined as *"an event where patients develop a movement disorder over hours or several days, and in which morbidity and even mortality can result from failure to appropriately diagnose and manage the patient"* [13]. In spite of these classification efforts, there are no established diagnostic criteria of SD, in contrast to SE which is defined by its duration of more than 5 min of tonic-clonic seizures [14]; clearly defined criteria that have greatly advanced research in SE.

Prevalence and Phenomenology

SD is characterized by severe, generalized, and continuous hyperkinetic movements, which often occur as the end of a continuum of a relatively rapidly worsening dystonia following a trigger [9]. Sixty to eighty percent of SD occurs in children and adolescents [15] and the majority are male, with dystonia duration of an average of 6 years [9, 16]. A recent review describes 34 pediatric cases from a cohort of 336 dystonic patients who experienced 63 acute dystonic exacerbations, thus suggesting that SD may affect up to 10% of children with dystonia [15]. In addition, 60% of these SD cases initially developed dystonia between age 0–2 years.

Rarely, SD may occur as the first manifestation of an acute onset of a movement disorder, e.g., in Wilson's disease (DYT-*ATP7B*), especially when treatment with penicillamine is initiated [6]. In other cases, SD is "monophasic," i.e., it develops in an otherwise healthy individual, who recovers to a complete healthy baseline after the episode of SD subsides [11]. Although the clinical spectrum of dystonic patients prior to SD is quite heterogenous, the most common underlying conditions include CP, followed by inherited isolated dystonias (mutations in genes such as *TOR1A* or *THAP1*) and degenerative forms of dystonia such as pantothenate kinase-associated neurodegeneration (PKAN) or Wilson's disease (Table 10.2) [17, 18]. With regard to baseline dystonia severity prior to SD, it was shown that 34/63 episodes of dystonia exacerbation were graded with a score of 3 according to the dystonia severity action plan (DSAP) score (unable to tolerate lying down and sleep disturbance without metabolic or airway complications) at the time of presentation before evolving to SD (grade 4 and 5) [19], thus indicating that SD is the climax of a rapidly progressive condition.

Table 10.2 Known genetic causes associated with SD [8, 11, 17]

Gene	Classification	Distinguishing features
DYT-TOR1A	Isolated, AD	Onset in limbs and often generalizes
DYT-THAP1	Isolated, AD	Cervical and laryngeal dystonia
DYT/PARK-TH	Combined, AR	Dopa responsive dystonia, oculogyric crisis
DYT/PARK-TAF1	Combined, X linked	More common in Panay, Philippines (Lubag disease)
PxMD-PNKD	Combined, AD	Paroxysms triggered by voluntary movement, stress, sleep deprivation
MOPED*	Complex, AD	Photosensitive epilepsy
GNAO1	Combined, AD	Refractory epilepsy
DYT-ATP7B-Wilson's disease	Combined, AR	KF rings, Giant Panda MRI sign
GCDH-glutaric aciduria type 1	Combined, AR	Worsening with protein loading, metabolic stressors
DYT/CHOR-MUT-methylmalonic aciduria	Combined, AR	Worsening with protein loading, chronic vomiting
DYT/CHOR-PCCA/PCCB-propionic aciduria	Combined, AR	Worsening with protein loading, chronic vomiting
CPS1-3-methylglutaconic aciduria	Complex, AR	Hyperammonemia
DYT-SUCLA2-succinate-CoA ligase	Complex, AR	Deafness
ETHE1-ethylmalonic encephalopathy	Complex, AR	Petechiae, orthostatic acrocyanosis
ARX	Complex, X linked	History of infantile spasms
HPRT1—Lesch-Nyhan disease	Combined, X linked	Auto mutilation, elevated uric acid
NPC1—Niemann-Pick type C	Combined, AR	Supranuclear gaze palsy, cataplexy
NBIA/DYT-PANK2	Combined, AR	Eye of the tiger sign, peripheral visual loss
DYT/PARK-PLA2G6	Combined, AR	Parkinsonism, neuroaxonal dystrophy
KCNT1	Complex, AD	Epileptic encephalopathy
AT—ataxia telangiectasia	Combined, AR	Telangiectasias, immune deficiency
TIMM8—Mohr-Tranebjaerg	Combined, X linked	Deafness
Leigh disease	Complex, Mitochondrial or nuclear	Multisystemic involvement

(continued)

Table 10.2 (continued)

Gene	Classification	Distinguishing features
SLC19A3-Biotin-thiamine responsive basal ganglia disease	Complex, AR	Epilepsy
NUP62-related disorder	Complex, AR	Infantile bilateral striatal necrosis
MOCS1 or MOCS2—molybdenum cofactor deficiency	Complex, AR	Refractory epilepsy
SUOX—sulfite oxidase deficiency	Complex, AR	Microcephaly

Genetic nomenclature according to [33, 34]
Abbreviations: * gene unknown, *AD* autosomal dominant, *AR* autosomal recessive, *DYT* dystonia, *DYT/Park* dystonia/parkinsonism, *TOR1A* torsin family 1 member A, *THAP* thanatos-associated-domain containing, apoptosis-associated protein 1, *TH* tyrosine hydroxylase, *TAF1* TATA-box binding protein associated factor 1, *PxMD-PNKD* paroxysmal movement disorders-paroxysmal nonkinesigenic dyskinesia, *MOPED* myoclonic occipital photosensitive epilepsy with dystonia, *GNAO1* G protein subunit alpha o1, *ATP7B* ATPase activity, 7 distinct domain, *GCDH* glutaryl-CoA dehydrogenase, *CHOR-MUT* dystonia/chorea-methylmalonyl-CoAmutase, *DYT/CHOR-PCCA/PCCB* dystonia/chorea-propionyl-CoA carboxylase alpha subunit/propionyl-CoA carboxylase beta subunit, carbamoyl-phosphate synthase 1, *SUCLA2* succinate-CoA ligase ADP-forming beta subunit, *ETHE1* ethylmalonic encephalopathy 1, *ARX* aristaless related homeobox, *HPRT1* hypoxanthine phosphoribosyltransferase 1, *NPC1* Niemann-Pick type C1, *PANK2* pantothenate kinase 2, *PLA2G6* phospholipase A2 group VI, *KCNT1* potassium sodium-activated channel subfamily T member 1, *AT* ataxia-telangiectasia, *TIMM8* translocase off inner mitochondrial membrane 8A, *SLC19A3* solute carrier family 19 member 3, *NUP62* nucleoporin 62, *MOCS* molybdenum cofactor synthesis, *SUOX* sulfite oxidase

SD has been classified by Fasano et al. according to four domains: (1) phenomenology (phasic vs tonic), (2) temporal profile (Fig. 10.3), (3) recovery, and (4) outcome of the underlying disease (Table 10.3) [9]. This classification might help outcome prediction, as the tonic subtype (rather than specific etiology of the underlying dystonic disorder) was associated with a worse outcome, i.e., worsening or death at the end of an SD episode [9]. The tonic subtype was most common, but the phasic subtype was more frequent in acquired and monophasic cases of SD, such as in the case of an infective or autoimmune encephalitis. Dystonia in SD may also co-occur with additional hyperkinesias, further complicating timely diagnosis [1, 9, 11]. The associated movement disorders identified in 87.5% of patients most commonly included tremor as well as chorea, myoclonus, bradykinesia, and tics [8].

Differential Diagnosis

Several conditions should be considered in the differential diagnosis of SD, including other movement disorder emergencies described in other chapters (Table 10.4) [20]. Distinguishing these conditions is often challenging especially in an urgent care setting [20]. The main difference is the presence of dystonia and/or chorea with or without additional dyskinesias, which highlights the importance of a thorough clinical examination. It is also important to highlight that the level of consciousness

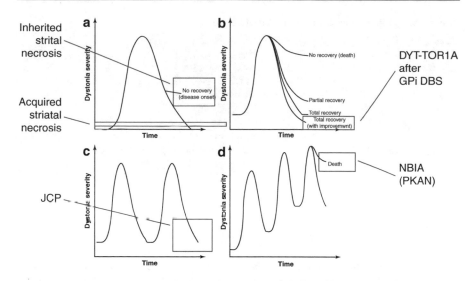

Fig. 10.3 The temporal profile of status dystonicus (SD, with examples in the figure, modified from [11]) can be classified as monophasic (**a** and **b**) or relapsing (**c** and **d**). Type of recovery of each episode and outcome of the underlying disease is described in Table 10.3. SD usually occurs at the end of a continuum of worsening dystonia (**b**, **c**, and **d**) but it can present also as the first manifestation of dystonia (**a**). Two different scenarios are described in picture (**a**): complete recovery (it is usually the case in acquired striatal necrosis) or no recovery after treatment (as it usually happens in inherited striatal necrosis, SD is just the onset of the disease). Picture (**b**) shows those cases where SD occurs once and as worsening of an underlying dystonia. These patients can not recover and die from the episode; partially recover; completely recover or even get better than they were at baseline (i.e., DYT-TOR1A after GPi DBS). Pictures (**c**) and (**d**) show relapsing cases of SD. We could call relapsing-remitting (**c**) those cases where after each episode of SD recover and return to their previous state (i.e., JCP); and relapsing-progressive (**d**) where there is a deterioration in the underlying dystonia after each episode of SD (i.e., PKAN) and eventually may lead to a lack of recovery and potential death. Abbreviations: DYT-TOR1A dystonia-torsin family 1 member A, GPi DBS globus pallidus pars interna deep brain stimulation, NBIA neurodegeneration with brain iron accumulation, PKAN pantothenate kinase-associated neurodegeneration, JCP juvenile cerebral palsy

is normal at the onset of SD and that features such as hyperthermia, CK increase, and autonomic instability are nonspecific and common to most of these emergencies. The underlying condition and medication use are other key factors to consider while establishing a differential diagnosis. Dopamine receptor blockers (DRBs) can cause acute parkinsonism (AP) and acute dystonic reactions (ADRs). Several other medications such as selective serotonin reuptake inhibitors or gabapentin are also known to cause these two conditions [21]. Serotonin syndrome (SS) and neuroleptic malignant syndrome (NMS) are also adverse drug reactions to psychotropic medications [22]. Malignant hyperthermia (MH) is a rare inherited condition often caused by mutations in *RYR1*, which presents similarly to NMS and SS. The triggers for MH are general anesthetics and/or the depolarizing neuromuscular

Table 10.3 Proposed classification of status dystonicus

Phenomenology	Tonic (dystonic)
	Phasic (choreic)
Recovery	Total recovery
	Partial recovery (including disease onset)
	No recovery (death)
Temporal profile (see Fig. 10.3)	Monophasic (including "isolated SD")
	Relapsing-remitting
	Relapsing-progressive
Outcome of the underlying disease	First manifestation of a neurological disorder
	Return to pre-SD severity
	Improvement
	Worsening
	Death

Modified from [9]
Abbreviations: *SD* status dystonicus

blocking agent succinylcholine as well as infections, stress, and exercise [23]. In intrathecal baclofen withdrawal syndrome, the association with sudden discontinuation of baclofen (generally due to pump or catheter issues) is straightforward.

Dyskinesia-hyperpyrexia syndrome (DHS) and parkinsonism-hyperpyrexia syndrome (PHS) are two conditions that should be considered in the differential diagnosis of SD in patients with Parkinson's disease. The main difference between these two entities is that PHS presents as an acute akinetic-rigid syndrome, as opposed to DHS which is hyperkinetic [24]. Lastly, paroxysmal sympathetic hyperactivity (PSH) is characterized by dysautonomia associated with dystonia in patients with severe acquired brain injury [25]. The shared features between these conditions complicate diagnosis and choice of appropriate treatment. It has been argued that many of the aforementioned conditions represent a clinical spectrum of the same entity and that there are too many entities with only subtle clinical differences, generating confusion in the literature and among physicians [11].

⚡ The differential diagnosis of SD is broad, and a wide net should be cast in the initial evaluation of patients.

Triggers

SD is triggered by a precipitating factor in most patients. The most common trigger is infection (51.7%) followed by medication change (30.0%) [9, 26, 27]. A typical example of medication-induced SD is penicillamine-induced SD in Wilson's disease, which has been reported to be lethal [28]. Other triggers include surgical procedure/anesthesia, metabolic disturbances, puberty, protein loading in glutaric aciduria, the failure of an implantable pulse generator for DBS, as well as DBS implantation [9, 17, 29, 30]. Noteworthy, the expanding use of DBS for dystonia patients has contributed to an increasing number of related SD episodes [31, 32].

Table 10.4 Differential diagnosis of status dystonicus

	Myoclonus	Rigidity	Tremor	Dystonia	Decreased LOC *at onset*	Hyperthermia	CK increase	Autonomic dysfunction	Distinguishing features
Status dystonicus	+/−	−	+	+ (dysk)	−	+/−	+	+/−	Different triggers
Status epilepticus	+/−	−	−	+/−	+	−/+	−/+	−/+	Electrophysiological correlation on EEG, hyperthermia if febrile status
Neuroleptic malignant syndrome	−	+	+	−	−/+	+	+	+	DRB use, altered mental status, rigidity
Serotonin syndrome	+	+	+	−/+	−/+	+	+	+	Serotoninergic drugs, hyperreflexia, altered mental status, rigidity
Malignant hyperthermia	−	+	−	−	−/+	+	+	+	Genetic predisposition, specific triggers anesthesia
Acute parkinsonism	−	+	+	−/+	−	−/+	−/+	−/+	Acquired (drugs, toxins, etc.)
Dyskinesia-hyperpyrexia syndrome	−	−	+/−	−/+ (dysk)	−	+	+	+/−	PD patients
Parkinsonism-hyperpyrexia syndrome	+	+		−/+	−	+	+/−	+	PD patients
Paroxysmal autonomic instability with dystonia	−	−	−	+	−/+	+	+	+	Acquired CNS lesions
Intrathecal baclofen withdrawal	−	−	−	−/+	−/+	+/−	+	+	Spasticity
Acute dystonic reactions	−	−	+	+	−	−/+	−/+	−	DRB use Focal dystonia (neck and face)

Modified from [11]

Abbreviations: + present, − absent, +/− may or not be present, *LOC* level of consciousness, *Dysk* dyskinesia, *CK* creatine kinase, *EEG* electroencephalogram, *DRB* dopamine receptors blockers, *PD* Parkinson's disease, *CNS* central nervous system

Table 10.5 The triggers of status dystonicus reported to date

Anesthesia
Autoimmune processes
Diet (protein loading in glutaric aciduria)
Hardware failure (DBS or ITB pump)
Infections
Medication changes
Introduction of, e.g., penicillamine (WD), zinc (WD), dopamine-receptor blockers, clonazepam
Withdrawal of, e.g., penicillamine (WD), dopamine depleting agents, baclofen, lithium
Metabolic disturbances
Puberty
Surgery (including DBS surgery)
Trauma (physical and psychological)

Abbreviations: *DBS* deep brain stimulation, *ITB* intrathecal baclofen, *WD* Wilson's disease

This is usually related to battery depletion and clinically presents with rapid-onset dystonia which can be fatal [17, 31].

No precipitating factor was identified in 32.6–50% of SD diagnoses [8, 9]. The clinical vignette mentioned above can be included in the 30% of SD cases without an identifiable trigger, however psychological stressors and pain should not be overlooked even though they are rarely reported [6]. Table 10.5 summarizes the known triggers reported so far.

 DBS battery failure may precipitate SD, with catastrophic results.

Etiology

Determining the underlying etiology in SD is key to identifying triggers and securing optimal care. There are over 200 causes of dystonia that can be classified according to clinical and etiological features [33]. In addition, the genetic nomenclature of movement disorders has been reviewed recently [34].

SD in Inherited Neurological Syndromes

The inherited subgroup of dystonia can be divided into isolated, combined, and complex dystonia [35]. The most common forms of isolated dystonia are DYT-*TOR1A* (DYT1) and DYT-*THAP1* (DYT6), which are inherited in an autosomal dominant (AD) fashion (see Table 10.1) [36, 37]. DYT-*TOR1A* usually presents with limb dystonia which generalizes over time, whereas DYT-*THAP1* (DYT6) tends to involve mainly cranial and cervical regions. Both forms of dystonia can generalize and have been reported to cause SD. Other causes include dopa-responsive dystonia [34], Lubag disease [36], and paroxysmal nonkinesigenic dyskinesia due to *MR1* gene mutation [38].

The co-occurrence of epilepsy and dystonia further complicates the proper diagnosis of SD as it may be mistaken for SE. At least three epileptic syndromes have been described with SD: myoclonic occipital photosensitive epilepsy with dystonia (MOPED) [39], *ARX* related refractory epilepsy (Ohtahara syndrome), and *GNAO1* encephalopathy [8, 17]. *GNAO1* is important to recognize as these patients respond better to DBS treatment than medical treatment. In addition, chorea as the predominant movement disorder at baseline in *GNAO1* confers a higher risk of developing SD [40]. In addition to the classic isolated and combined causes of genetic dystonia, several degenerative genetic causes can also lead to SD such as Wilson's disease, glutaric aciduria type 1, *ARX,* and Lesch-Nyhan disease (see Table 10.1).

SD in Acquired Neurological Syndromes

The second category of dystonia is classified as acquired dystonias, which are due to a specific cause (perinatal brain injury, infection, drugs, toxic, vascular, neoplastic, or paraneoplastic, brain injury, and psychogenic—now known as functional) [33]. The most common acquired cause underlying SD is CP, which is reported in almost 60% of the acquired dystonia cohort reported by Fasano et al. [9]. Other less common causes include inflammatory or autoimmune conditions, hypoxic-ischemic injury, trauma, and infections [9]. It is important to recognize autoimmune encephalitis such as anti-NMDA-receptor (NMDAR) encephalitis as the underlying cause for SD because treatment should focus on immunomodulatory interventions in addition to supportive treatment [11]. Altered mental status, psychiatric disturbance, seizures, and dyskinesias affecting the orobuccal region are important clues to the diagnosis of this condition [41]. The associated movement disorder is hyperkinetic and usually complex, with dystonia and chorea involving mainly the craniofacial region [42]. Although several etiologies have been highlighted in this chapter, one can assume that any patient with moderate to severe dystonia, including all acquired causes of striatal necrosis, can hypothetically progress to SD [11, 43].

Mechanisms

The understanding of dystonia pathophysiology is steadily growing. Dystonia is presently thought to be caused by an imbalance between excitation and inhibition in the cerebello-thalamo-basal ganglia pathway thereby leading to (1) decreased pallidal inhibition by the indirect pathway, (2) abnormal thalamo-motor-cortical hyperexcitability, (3) loss of sensorimotor integration, and (4) maladaptive plasticity [44]. The cerebellum and the spinal cord have more recently been implicated [45]. It is also thought that the underlying mechanisms may differ between acquired and nonacquired dystonias [46]. Although more is known about dystonia pathophysiology, the mechanisms underlying SD have not yet been identified. Termsarasab and Frucht have proposed increased pallidal output as a potential pathophysiological mechanism for SD [47]. Factors thought to predispose younger individuals to SD include brain immaturity in children, hormonal changes during puberty, and sudden metabolic requests [1, 9]. Simply speaking, although no actual recording of the basal ganglia of SD awake patients is available [27], one can argue that SD pathophysiology is similar to SE because of its shared paroxysmal presentation, genetic overlap, and triggers [11, 48]. Further research is needed to better understand the pathophysiological mechanisms in SD.

Management and Outcome

While an increasing number of papers on SD have been reported, it remains an underrecognized entity with suboptimal treatment [27]. The first proposal for a pharmacological treatment algorithm was published in 1984 by Marsden et al. (the "Marsden cocktail") and is still the mainstay of medical management [3]. The Marsden cocktail consists of benzhexol/trihexyphenidyl, tetrabenazine, and pimozide. However, more recent data indicate that only 10% of SD episodes are successfully treated with this pharmacological approach [9]. In addition, pimozide and other DRBs are rarely used today due to the risk of tardive dystonia, and in fact tetrabenazine and anticholinergics are the most effective in the majority of recovered cases [9].

A recent study reported the benefits of clonidine administered via enteral, intravenous, or transdermal routes in five pediatric cases with SD. The main benefit was decreased use of benzodiazepines, morphine, and propofol, thereby avoiding the need for respiratory support in most cases [49]. Other medications also considered as add-on treatment are baclofen, gabapentin, and levodopa–carbidopa [15]. Nonresponders require additional escalating treatment including sedatives (benzodiazepines, propofol, and barbiturates) and neurosurgical interventions, particularly DBS, although pallidotomy or intrathecal baclofen (ITB) may have a role [9]. Neurosurgery is the most effective treatment strategy, with improvement in 33.7% of SD episodes [9]. It should be considered early in SD if the underlying cause is a confirmed genetic diagnosis known to respond well to DBS, e.g., DYT1-TOR1A [47]. The first ablative surgery used in refractory SD was thalamotomy [1]. Since then, the GPi has become the preferred target for ablative surgery (pallidotomy) and subsequently DBS [10]. Levi and colleagues compared GPi DBS to pallidotomy in a small case series and showed that there was no significant difference in outcome (87.5% and 83.3% response to treatment, respectively) [50]. Their data also suggest that pallidotomy may resolve SD faster than DBS, probably because the latter requires programming.

ITB is another neurosurgical option in SD treatment [4, 51, 52]. Even though beneficial for improving dystonia, ITB often leads to long-term technical complications, which in turn can cause SD [53]. Recently, three cases of SD were reported to respond well to early treatment with short-term intraventricular baclofen (IVB) [54]. The study suggests that the effect may be long lasting as two out of the three patients were able to discontinue the IVB treatment, which reduces the risk of hardware complications. Intrathecal morphine has also been reported as a less commonly used therapeutic avenue if ITB and DBS are not readily available [55].

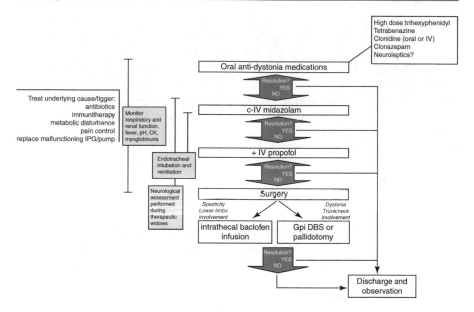

Fig. 10.4 Proposed treatment algorithm in status dystonicus according to disease severity and underlying. Abbreviations: c-IV continuous intravenous, DBS deep brain stimulation, GPi globus pallidus pars interna, IV intravenouscause. (Modified from [3, 7, 11, 19])

Overall, neurosurgical approaches are increasingly being used in the treatment of SD (40.2–65.9%) [56], but their use is limited by the availability of local expertise.

In 2007, Mariotti et al. were the first to propose a treatment algorithm based on the scanty evidence present in the literature [7]. Ten years after, Temrsarasab and Frucht proposed a treatment algorithm according to time of onset: the first 24 h should include supportive therapy and identifying surgical candidates, and that pharmacological treatments for symptomatic control should be adjusted over the following 2- to 4-week period [47]. On the other hand, the ABCD approach by Lumsden et al. describes a stepwise approach to pediatric SD management: (a) address precipitant, (b) begin supportive care, (c) calibrate sedation, and (d) dystonia specific treatment [19]. A combined stepwise algorithm taking into consideration underlying causes, triggers, and disease severity is proposed in Fig. 10.4.

Course and Outcome

The course and outcome of SD are highly variable, but early recognition facilitates aggressive intervention which is thought to potentially prevent progression and favor a better outcome. In a large pediatric cohort, approximately 30% of cases required intensive care unit admission [15]. Subsequent relapses were common with a recurrence risk of 25% in the first year, and up to 38.6% at 27 months. It is important to note that no SD patient was treated with DBS, which can affect long-term outcome [15, 18]. Similar outcomes were reported by Fasano et al. and Lumsden et al.: 36.8–43.2% improved compared to baseline dystonia, 27.3–36.8% returned to baseline, 16.2–18.2% improved but did not return to baseline [9, 19]. In a DBS-treated SD cohort, 62.5% received DBS therapy during an SD episode (25 patients) with resolution in 92% [8]. The mortality rate in SD ranges from 10.3% to 11.4% [9, 56]. Lastly, it is important to highlight the role of SD prevention. Iodice and Pisani suggest regular clinical visits, especially during the first 3 years of life and puberty, prompt management of potential triggers, and early introduction of treatments such as trihexyphenidyl to limit SD episodes [17].

Conclusion

SD is one of the most common emergencies in pediatric movement disorders and requires aggressive multimodal management to prevent worsening and mortality. However, management algorithms are based on expert opinion as no evidenced-based studies are available. SD remains a relatively rare condition that lacks clinical criteria, limiting the number of large studies available. Future standardized studies of dystonia and SD are needed to better define the clinical features in order to develop improved treatment strategies. Nerrant et al. have shown that DBS has revolutionized the treatment of SD, particularly in known genetic responders [8]. However, DBS therapy is limited to experienced centers, and with increased use of DBS, hardware complications as a cause of SD will become more frequent.

Acknowledgments We would like to thank Sara Breitbart, Carolina Gorodetsky, and George Ibrahim from The Hospital for Sick Children (SickKids), Toronto, ON, Canada, for having provided Fig. 10.1 and Ariane Belzile for editing references.

Funding Sources and Conflict of Interest This work was partly funded by the Chair in Neuromodulation and Multidisciplinary care at the University of Toronto and University Health Network (A.F.)

Financial Disclosures IAM has nothing to disclose.

AF received speaker and/or consulting honoraria and/or research support from Abbott, Boston Scientific, Brainlab, Ceregate, Ipsen, and Medtronic.

References

1. Manji H, Howard RS, Miller DH, Hirsch NP, Carr L, Bhatia K, et al. Status dystonicus: the syndrome and its management. Brain. 1998;121(Pt 2):243–52.
2. Jankovic J, Penn AS. Severe dystonia and myoglobinuria. Neurology. 1982;32(10):1195–7.
3. Marsden CD, Marion MH, Quinn N. The treatment of severe dystonia in children and adults. J Neurol Neurosurg Psychiatry. 1984;47(11):1166–73.
4. Narayan RK, Loubser PG, Jankovic J, Donovan WH, Bontke CF. Intrathecal baclofen for intractable axial dystonia. Neurology. 1991;41(7):1141–2.

5. Vaamonde J, Narbona J, Weiser R, Garcia MA, Brannan T, Obeso JA. Dystonic storms: a practical management problem. Clin Neuropharmacol. 1994;17(4):344–7.
6. Teive HA, Munhoz RP, Souza MM, Antoniuk SA, Santos ML, Teixeira MJ, et al. Status dystonicus: study of five cases. Arq Neuropsiquiatr. 2005;63(1):26–9.
7. Mariotti P, Fasano A, Contarino MF, Della Marca G, Piastra M, Genovese O, et al. Management of status dystonicus: our experience and review of the literature. Mov Disord. 2007;22(7):963–8.
8. Nerrant E, Gonzalez V, Milesi C, Vasques X, Ruge D, Roujeau T, et al. Deep brain stimulation treated dystonia-trajectory via status dystonicus. Mov Disord. 2018;33(7):1168–73.
9. Fasano A, Ricciardi L, Bentivoglio AR, Canavese C, Zorzi G, Petrovic I, et al. Status dystonicus: predictors of outcome and progression patterns of underlying disease. Mov Disord. 2012;27(6):783–8.
10. Sobstyl MR, Slawek JW, Zabek M. The neurosurgical treatment of patients in dystonic state – overview of the literature. Neurol Neurochir Pol. 2014;48(1):63–70.
11. Ruiz-Lopez M, Fasano A. Rethinking status dystonicus. Mov Disord. 2017;32(12):1667–76.
12. Lumsden DE, Allen NM. Rethinking status dystonicus: a welcome start to a challenging problem. Mov Disord. 2018;33(2):344.
13. Poston KL, Frucht SJ. Movement disorder emergencies. J Neurol. 2008;255(Suppl 4):2–13.
14. Baxter P. Status dystonicus: under-recognized and under-treated. Dev Med Child Neurol. 2013;55(2):99.
15. Garone G, Graziola F, Nicita F, Frascarelli F, Randi F, Zazza M, et al. Prestatus and status dystonicus in children and adolescents. Dev Med Child Neurol. 2020;62(6):742–9.
16. Allen NM, Lin JP, Lynch T, King MD. Status dystonicus: a practice guide. Dev Med Child Neurol. 2014;56(2):105–12.
17. Iodice A, Pisani F. Status dystonicus: management and prevention in children at high risk. Acta Biomed. 2019;90(3):207–12.
18. Lumsden DE. The spectrum of dystonia severity before status dystonicus. Dev Med Child Neurol. 2020;62(6):668.
19. Lumsden DE, King MD, Allen NM. Status dystonicus in childhood. Curr Opin Pediatr. 2017;29(6):674–82.
20. Kipps CM, Fung VS, Grattan-Smith P, de Moore GM, Morris JG. Movement disorder emergencies. Mov Disord. 2005;20(3):322–34.
21. Iselin-Chaves IA, Grotzsch H, Besson M, Burkhard PR, Savoldelli GL. Naloxone-responsive acute dystonia and parkinsonism following general anaesthesia. Anaesthesia. 2009;64(12):1359–62.
22. Dosi R, Ambaliya A, Joshi H, Patell R. Serotonin syndrome versus neuroleptic malignant syndrome: a challenging clinical quandary. BMJ Case Rep. 2014;2014:bcr2014204154. https://doi.org/10.1136/bcr-2014-204154.
23. Lee MA, McGlinch EB, McGlinch MC, Capacchione JF. Malignant hyperthermia susceptibility and fitness for duty. Mil Med. 2017;182(3):e1854–e7.
24. Gil-Navarro S, Grandas F. Dyskinesia-hyperpyrexia syndrome: another Parkinson's disease emergency. Mov Disord. 2010;25(15):2691–2.
25. Baguley IJ, Perkes IE, Fernandez-Ortega JF, Rabinstein AA, Dolce G, Hendricks HT, et al. Paroxysmal sympathetic hyperactivity after acquired brain injury: consensus on conceptual definition, nomenclature, and diagnostic criteria. J Neurotrauma. 2014;31(17):1515–20.
26. Franzini A, Cordella R, Rizzi M, Marras CE, Messina G, Zorzi G, et al. Deep brain stimulation in critical care conditions. J Neural Transm (Vienna). 2014;121(4):391–8.
27. Marras CE, Rizzi M, Cantonetti L, Rebessi E, De Benedictis A, Portaluri F, et al. Pallidotomy for medically refractory status dystonicus in childhood. Dev Med Child Neurol. 2014;56(7):649–56.
28. Svetel M, Sternic N, Pejovic S, Kostic VS. Penicillamine-induced lethal status dystonicus in a patient with Wilson's disease. Mov Disord. 2001;16(3):568–9.
29. Ruiz-Lopez M, Munhoz RP, Kalia SK, Zorzi G, Nardocci N, Fasano A. Status dystonicus induced by deep brain stimulation surgery. Neurol Sci. 2020;41(3):729–30.

30. Oterdoom DLM, van Egmond ME, Ascencao LC, van Dijk JMC, Saryyeva A, Beudel M, et al. Reversal of status dystonicus after relocation of pallidal electrodes in DYT6 generalized dystonia. Tremor Other Hyperkinet Mov (N Y). 2018;8:530.
31. Rohani M, Munhoz RP, Shahidi G, Parvaresh M, Miri S. Fatal status dystonicus in tardive dystonia due to depletion of deep brain stimulation's pulse generator. Brain Stimul. 2017;10(1):160–1.
32. Sobstyl M, Zabek M, Kmiec T, Slawek J, Budohoski KP. Status dystonicus due to internal pulse generator depletion in a patient with primary generalized dystonia. Mov Disord. 2014;29(2):188–9.
33. Albanese A, Bhatia K, Bressman SB, Delong MR, Fahn S, Fung VS, et al. Phenomenology and classification of dystonia: a consensus update. Mov Disord. 2013;28(7):863–73.
34. Marras C, Lang A, van de Warrenburg BP, Sue CM, Tabrizi SJ, Bertram L, et al. Nomenclature of genetic movement disorders: recommendations of the international Parkinson and movement disorder society task force. Mov Disord. 2016;31(4):436–57.
35. Meijer IA, Pearson TS. The twists of pediatric dystonia: phenomenology, classification, and genetics. Semin Pediatr Neurol. 2018;25:65–74.
36. Balint B, Bhatia KP. Isolated and combined dystonia syndromes – an update on new genes and their phenotypes. Eur J Neurol. 2015;22(4):610–7.
37. Lohmann K, Klein C. Update on the genetics of dystonia. Curr Neurol Neurosci Rep. 2017;17(3):26.
38. Zittel S, Ganos C, Munchau A. Fatal paroxysmal non-kinesigenic dyskinesia. Eur J Neurol. 2015;22(2):e30–1.
39. Sadleir LG, Paterson S, Smith KR, Redshaw N, Ranta A, Kalnins R, et al. Myoclonic occipital photosensitive epilepsy with dystonia (MOPED): a familial epilepsy syndrome. Epilepsy Res. 2015;114:98–105.
40. Schirinzi T, Garone G, Travaglini L, Vasco G, Galosi S, Rios L, et al. Phenomenology and clinical course of movement disorder in GNAO1 variants: results from an analytical review. Parkinsonism Relat Disord. 2019;61:19–25.
41. Titulaer MJ, McCracken L, Gabilondo I, Armangue T, Glaser C, Iizuka T, et al. Treatment and prognostic factors for long-term outcome in patients with anti-NMDA receptor encephalitis: an observational cohort study. Lancet Neurol. 2013;12(2):157–65.
42. Mohammad SS, Fung VS, Grattan-Smith P, Gill D, Pillai S, Ramanathan S, et al. Movement disorders in children with anti-NMDAR encephalitis and other autoimmune encephalopathies. Mov Disord. 2014;29(12):1539–42.
43. Tonduti D, Chiapparini L, Moroni I, Ardissone A, Zorzi G, Zibordi F, et al. Neurological disorders associated with striatal lesions: classification and diagnostic approach. Curr Neurol Neurosci Rep. 2016;16(6):54.
44. Quartarone A, Hallett M. Emerging concepts in the physiological basis of dystonia. Mov Disord. 2013;28(7):958–67.
45. Shakkottai VG, Batla A, Bhatia K, Dauer WT, Dresel C, Niethammer M, et al. Current opinions and areas of consensus on the role of the cerebellum in dystonia. Cerebellum. 2017;16(2):577–94.
46. Kojovic M, Parees I, Kassavetis P, Palomar FJ, Mir P, Teo JT, et al. Secondary and primary dystonia: pathophysiological differences. Brain. 2013;136(Pt 7):2038–49.
47. Termsarasab P, Frucht SJ. Dystonic storm: a practical clinical and video review. J Clin Mov Disord. 2017;4:10.
48. Erro R, Bhatia KP, Espay AJ, Striano P. The epileptic and nonepileptic spectrum of paroxysmal dyskinesias: Channelopathies, synaptopathies, and transportopathies. Mov Disord. 2017;32(3):310–8.
49. Nakou V, Williamson K, Arichi T, Lumsden DE, Tomlin S, Kaminska M, et al. Safety and efficacy of high-dose enteral, intravenous, and transdermal clonidine for the acute management of severe intractable childhood dystonia and status dystonicus: an illustrative case-series. Eur J Paediatr Neurol. 2017;21(6):823–32.

50. Levi V, Zorzi G, Messina G, Romito L, Tramacere I, Dones I, et al. Deep brain stimulation versus pallidotomy for status dystonicus: a single-center case series. J Neurosurg. 2019:1–11. https://doi.org/10.3171/2019.10.JNS191691.
51. Dalvi A, Fahn S, Ford B. Intrathecal baclofen in the treatment of dystonic storm. Mov Disord. 1998;13(3):611–2.
52. Kyriagis M, Grattan-Smith P, Scheinberg A, Teo C, Nakaji N, Waugh M. Status dystonicus and Hallervorden-Spatz disease: treatment with intrathecal baclofen and pallidotomy. J Paediatr Child Health. 2004;40(5–6):322–5.
53. Albright AL, Barry MJ, Shafton DH, Ferson SS. Intrathecal baclofen for generalized dystonia. Dev Med Child Neurol. 2001;43(10):652–7.
54. Ruggiero C, Meccariello G, Spennato P, Mirone G, Graziano S, Gilone M, et al. Early intraventricular baclofen therapy (IVB) for children with dystonic and dysautonomic storm. Childs Nerv Syst. 2019;35(1):15–8.
55. Lopez WO, Kluge Schroeder H, Santana Neville I, Jacobsen Teixeira M, Costa Barbosa D, et al. Intrathecal morphine therapy in the management of status dystonicus in neurodegeneration brain iron accumulation type 1. Pediatr Neurosurg. 2015;50(2):94–8.
56. Lumsden DE, Kaminska M, Ashkan K, Selway R, Lin JP. Deep brain stimulation for childhood dystonia: is 'where' as important as in 'whom'? Eur J Paediatr Neurol. 2017;21(1):176–84.

Posthypoxic Myoclonus and Its Management

11

Giulietta Maria Riboldi

Clinical Vignette

A 24-year-old man with a history of asthma experienced a sudden respiratory arrest while at home. While paramedics were on their way, he arrested and cardiopulmonary resuscitation was started. Circulation was re-established after 5 min. He was transferred to the hospital and admitted to the intensive care unit. On day two of hospitalization, he developed myoclonic jerks affecting mostly the limbs, particularly triggered by sensory stimuli such as noises or touch. As he started regaining consciousness the myoclonus persisted. EEG showed occasional spikes at the vertex, time-locked with the myoclonic jerks. A diagnosis of chronic posthypoxic myoclonus (Lance-Adams syndrome, or LAS) was formulated. Action and intention myoclonus were precipitated by fine tasks and triggered by sensory stimuli. Upon standing, postural laps were present with a tendency to fall if not supported. Cognition was normal. Clonazepam was started with only mild benefit. Eventually, symptoms were successfully controlled with a combination of clonazepam, valproic acid, and levetiracetam. Symptoms mildly improved over time but he required treatment with this multidrug regimen.

Posthypoxic myoclonus (PHM) is a complication occurring in 18–37% of patients who enter coma after cardiopulmonary resuscitation (CPR) from different causes, such as cardiac arrest, surgical complications, respiratory arrest due to asthma attacks, anesthesia, or drug intoxication [1–5]. PHM usually arises in

Supplementary Information The online version of this chapter (https://doi.org/10.1007/978-3-030-75898-1_11) contains supplementary material, which is available to authorized users.

G. M. Riboldi (✉)
Department of Neurology, NYU Langone Health, The Marlene and Paolo Fresco Institute for Parkinson's and Movement Disorders, New York, NY, USA
e-mail: giulietta.riboldi@nyulangone.org

© Springer Nature Switzerland AG 2022
S. J. Frucht (ed.), *Movement Disorder Emergencies*, Current Clinical Neurology,
https://doi.org/10.1007/978-3-030-75898-1_11

patients where cardiopulmonary arrest lasts between 2 and 7 min, or even longer in rare cases [6]. Myoclonic jerks, defined as brief, usually irregular, muscle contractions, may present with different patterns of distribution and rhythmicity depending on the underlying generating pathways. PHM can develop while patients are still in the intensive care units or in delayed fashion days or weeks from the initial event.

An acute form and a chronic form of PHM have been described. Acute PHM has received more attention in the literature due to its dramatic presentation [7]. Chronic PHM (LAS) represents instead a persistent condition that can severely affect the life of surviving patients when residual myoclonus is prominent, requiring appropriate diagnosis and management.

Clinical Features and Diagnostic Assessments

PHM is commonly observed in adults with only a few reports in children before the second decade and in the elderly. This may reflect the higher resistance of younger brains to hypoxia/anoxia, and the susceptibility of the aged population to hypoxia [3, 8, 9]. Few pediatric cases have been described, mostly associated with perinatal anoxia [10–13]. No clear differences in gender distribution have been reported [3]. The diagnosis of PHM is clinical, while neurophysiological and imaging assessments help define the nature and origin of this movement disorder, helping to guide treatment (Table 11.1). Although the distinction between an acute and a chronic form of PHM is universally accepted, there is overlap between the two forms and features such as time of onset and duration are not homogeneously reported in the literature [14].

In the acute form, myoclonus develops 24–48 h after cardiopulmonary arrest, although some cases with onset at 48–72 h from the acute event or even beyond 72 h have been reported [3]. The chronic form of PHM (LAS) is named for the two authors who first described four patients affected by this condition [15]. In LAS myoclonus classically presents once patients regain consciousness [15]. However, cases of LAS where myoclonic manifestations started during coma have been reported, making the distinction between the acute and chronic forms more challenging [6]. Deep sedation, mechanical ventilation, muscle relaxants, and hypothermic treatments can also mask myoclonus in its initial phases, further confounding the distinction between these two entities. Since the prognosis and the treatments for the acute and chronic forms can be very different, distinguishing the two is important. Additional elements that can help differentiate between PHM-subtypes are the distribution, synchronicity, variability, and neurophysiological assessments of myoclonic jerks (i.e., electroencephalogram (EEG), back-averaged EEG, somatosensory evoked potentials (SEPs), and long-latency reflex).

PHM is characterized by cortical and subcortical myoclonus in various combinations. In general, cortical myoclonus, also called cortical reflex myoclonus, presents with distal, focal, or multifocal, asynchronous, variable myoclonic jerks, usually associated with EEG correlates [14, 16]. Myoclonus involves areas with a larger cortical representation, such as face and hands, with a craniocaudal distribution of

Table 11.1 Characteristic diagnostic features in acute and chronic posthypoxic myoclonus

	Acute PHM	Chronic PHM
Time of onset	24–48 h	Upon regaining consciousness
Demographic	Adults	Adults
Type of myoclonus	Subcortical	Cortical and/or subcortical Negative myoclonus (mostly lower limbs)
Clinical features of myoclonus	Generalized, symmetric, proximal, stereotyped, stimulus sensitive Possible myoclonic status (myoclonus lasting continuously >30 min) Cranial nerves: caudocranial involvement Occasionally focal	Focal or multifocal, more distal, action and intentional myoclonus, stimulus sensitive Cranial nerves: craniocaudal involvement Occasionally focal
Additional neurological features	Severe general deterioration Cognitive impairment Frequent seizures	Ataxia Dysarthria Dysphagia Gait impairment Seizure is rare
EEG	Status epilepticus, burst suppression, diffuse slow waves and background, spike-wave activity, alpha coma	Spikes at the vertex or in the contralateral cortical motor area
Additional neurophysiology	EEG abnormalities not time-locked Normal SEPs Normal long latency reflex	± time-locked EEG abnormalities Giant SEPs Prolonged long latency reflex
IMAGING	Nonspecific	Nonspecific (brain MRI) PET scan: increased signal in VL nucleus (thalamus), pontine tegmentum, mesencephalon
PROGNOSIS	Poor (survival up to 10% cases)	Good (rare additional neurological sequela, possible improvement of myoclonus)

The table reports the classical features of the two phenotypes of posthypoxic myoclonus (PHM). Nuances and overlaps are possible as described in the text (such as a later or an earlier onset for acute and chronic PHM, respectively, occasional good outcomes in acute PHM or severe residual myoclonus in chronic PHM)

EEG electroencephalogram, *SEP* somatosensory evoked potentials, *VL* ventrolateral, *PET* positron emission tomography

involvement of cranial nerves [14]. Cortical reflex myoclonus can be triggered by sensory stimuli and voluntary activation [14]. Neurophysiological assessments show time-locked epileptiform discharges at simultaneous EEG-EMG recordings, with electrical activities localized in the central motor cortical areas, giant SEPs, and long-latency response at EMG after peripheral nerve stimulation [3]. Seizures often coexist with this condition [14].

In contrast, subcortical myoclonus (also called "reticular reflex myoclonus") is mostly generalized, symmetrical, stereotyped, and synchronous. Proximal and flexor muscles are mainly involved [14]. Cranial nerves activate in a caudocranial fashion [14]. EEG can present with spikes and waves, but these are not time-locked to jerks, and SEPs are normal [3, 14]. Reticular reflex myoclonus has been reported to originate from the nucleus reticularis gigantocellularis [14]. Analysis of cases of PHM reveals that the acute phenotype mostly stems from subcortical generators, while LAS can be associated with both cortical and subcortical myoclonus [3, 14].

Acute PHM presents with jerks that are usually generalized, spontaneous, or stimulus-induced. Tactile, painful, or auditory stimuli, not uncommon in intensive care units, as well as passive eye opening and closing can all trigger myoclonus. Movements are characterized by symmetric proximal flexion jerks involving the trunk, limbs, and head, triggered by touching or tapping [17, 18]. Acute PHM can also manifest with the so-called status myoclonicus (also referred to as "myoclonic status epilepticus," "status myoclonus," or "myoclonic status") where myoclonus is generalized and continuously persistent for more than 30 min [19]. Status myoclonus can be very disruptive, and whether these episodes should be considered a separate entity or a manifestation of seizures is a subject of debate. In rare cases, isolated stimulus-sensitive myoclonus has been described associated with specific EEG correlates and ominous prognosis [20–25]. In the literature, signs suggestive of cortical myoclonus such as giant SEPs may be hidden by ongoing antiepileptic and sedative treatments [3, 5, 14].

LAS refers to chronic and persistent myoclonus that beings shortly after the acute event, usually when the patient starts to regain consciousness. LAS is rare, with less than 200 cases reported in the literature. Initially described by Lance and Adams in 1963 [15], myoclonus is triggered by muscle activation and intention as well as by sensory stimuli. Negative myoclonus is more frequently present in the lower limbs [14]. Intention myoclonus is significantly worsened by precise movements (such as reaching for a target or pouring water in a cup), although interestingly the same movements can often be pantomimed by these patients without difficulty [15, 26]. Myoclonic jerks occur in volleys or more rarely in isolation, and they usually abate as the patient tries to relax [9, 15]. Chronic PHM can be associated with cerebellar features (ataxia and dysarthria), dysphagia, gait abnormalities, and in some cases cognitive disfunction, usually mild [8, 9, 27, 28]. Gait is significantly impaired by negative myoclonic jerks in the lower limbs on standing, causing postural lapses and falls [15]. Seizures can be present during coma, but only rarely persist [8, 9].

Myoclonus in LAS stems from both cortical and subcortical generators, and cortical myoclonus may be measured with time-locked potentials, giant SEPs and a long latency response. However, in cases where subcortical pathways are more affected, these features can be absent. EEG abnormalities include isolated spikes at the vertex or in the contralateral cortical motor area. When reflex reticular myoclonus is present, either in isolation or associated with cortical myoclonus, the phenotype is usually more severe [8, 13, 17, 18].

Myoclonus in LAS may be cortical, subcortical, or both forms may be present in the same patient. Back-averaging is not widely available, requiring clinical examination to try to help define the myoclonus phenomenology.

The prognosis of patients with LAS is very different from acute PHM. Indeed, LAS implies a recovery of consciousness, residual cognitive impairment is usually mild, and myoclonus typically improves over time. A study of a large cohort of patients with LAS after cardiac arrest showed that preserved brainstem reflexes and a reactive EEG were more suggestive of LAS, and associated with better outcomes [29]. Pediatric cases of LAS are rare. Of two patients reported in the literature, one was a neonatal case secondary to extensive brain lesions, and involuntary movements disappeared after 1 year [12, 13]. In rare situations, acute and chronic PHM can present as focal myoclonus. There have been reports of myoclonus affecting one isolated limb, the trunk, facial muscles, platysma, or manifesting as inspiratory myoclonus, abdominal status myoclonus, periodic eye opening, upward eye deviation, as well as ocular bobbing [15, 30–40].

EEG signals in PHM have been extensively reported in the literature, although variability in presentation hinders outcome prediction, especially in the setting of acute PHM [41]. EEG abnormalities can help discriminate between myoclonic events where subcortical pathways are also activated, versus pure epileptic and Jacksonian seizures associated with cortical epileptic discharges [42]. This distinction helps to guide treatment since not all antiepileptic drugs are equally effective in treating myoclonus. In acute PHM, the EEG usually manifests burst suppression, spike-wave activity, status epilepticus, diffuse slow waves, as well as alpha-coma [27]. Some have attempted to correlate EEG patterns and outcomes in acute PHM, to help guide prognosis and therapeutic decision-making in comatose patients who survive a cardiopulmonary arrest [43]. However, the reliability of these approaches has been challenged by the introduction of therapeutic hypothermia that may either mask myoclonus or affect EEG signals themselves [44–46].

In LAS, back-averaging is suggestive of cortical myoclonus in the majority of cases with spikes or polyspikes that may precede jerks and that are usually localized at the vertex [27]. EEG recording during sleep in a patient with LAS reported fast spikes and polyspikes even in the absence of clinical epileptic syndromes [47]. Interestingly, one report of a case of LAS showed that cortical spikes at the vertex, recorded with EEG, were activated even when the patient only imagined moving an extremity [48]. Brain MRI in subjects with PHM, when available, showed various abnormalities including cortical and cerebellar atrophy, as well as cortical and cerebellar hemisphere infarcts [8, 9, 49]. Interestingly, in one case of LAS, serial brain MRIs performed shortly after the acute hypoxic event [50] showed transient hypoperfusion in the cerebellum and thalamic nuclei with no structural abnormalities, which resolved on follow-up imaging study 2 weeks later [50]. Consistent with these findings, positron emission tomography (PET) scans from seven patients with LAS showed increased glucose metabolism in the pontine tegmentum, mesencephalon, and ventrolateral nucleus of the thalamus [51]. These findings are consistent with increased thalamocortical firing due to impaired connectivity, given the role of the VL nuclei of the thalamus and the pontine nuclei as relay hubs for projections to cerebellar and cortical motor areas. In other case of LAS, PET and single-photon emission computed tomography (SPECT) showed decreased perfusion and glucose metabolism in the frontal lobe [52]. Cortical abnormalities have also been shown in one report, where resting-state functional MRI (rs-fMRI) in a patient with PHM documented increased functional connectivity between the primary and supplementary motor cortex mostly with the somatosensory areas [53].

Pathogenic Mechanisms

The pathogenic mechanisms underlying PHM are incompletely defined. As previously described, PHM can present with cortical, multifocal, or subcortical myoclonus. Most neuropathological studies, especially those in patients with acute PHM after cardiopulmonary arrest, found neuronal cell loss in the cerebral and cerebellar cortex, as well as in the hippocampus, thalamus, and brainstem, suggesting that damage of one or a combination of these systems may be responsible for PHM [2]. Another study assessed autopsy specimens in 15 cases of acute PHM, showing classical severe anoxic brain damage with neuronal loss in the cortical lamina and Purkinje cells [54]. There are few neuropathological studies of LAS. The ones that are available show either a neuronal loss in subcortical structures (mostly striatum, thalamus, mammillary bodies, and raphe nuclei), or astrocytic reaction in the midbrain, and in the cuneiform and subcuneiform nuclei with no prominent neuronal degeneration [55, 56].

Cortical involvement may explain both multifocal or generalized cortical myoclonus, the latter due to seizures spreading ipsilateral and contralaterally in the cortex [41]. In the context of subcortical acute PHM, loss of neurons in the reticular formation of the medulla oblongata has been correlated with "reticular reflex myoclonus" [17]. Diffuse projections from subcortical structures would explain the presentation of this entity as a symmetric and proximal myoclonus, with major involvement of the flexor muscles and with cranial nerves activated in ascending order starting from the lower medulla [14]. Interestingly, although LAS is considered to arise from a combination of cortical and subcortical involvement, a study analyzing stereotaxic EEG in patients with LAS noticed that spikes from the thalamus actually precede the cortical spikes, suggesting the hypothesis that cortical myoclonus may be generated by discharge from the VL nucleus of the thalamus to the cortex through the corticothalamic projections [57]. However, given the limited number of neuropathological studies, it is difficult to draw definitive conclusions.

Animal models of posthypoxic myoclonus recapitulate some of the EEG abnormalities observed in PHM, particularly the susceptibility of thalamic nuclei. The thalamic reticular nucleus (TRN) (part of the projection system from the thalamus to the cortex) may be involved, as well as injury to pyramidal neurons, CA1 and CA2 layers of the hippocampus, and cerebellar neuronal loss due to NMDA-mediated glutamatergic toxicity [58–60]. Disruption of Purkinje cells may be responsible for the cerebellar impairment observed in patients with LAS. Understanding the specific mechanisms and structures involved in this condition may guide management. For example, hypothermia, now used in prolonged

CPA, has been shown to limit cerebellar neuron loss in animal models thus possibly addressing one of the pathogenic events involved in PHM [61].

Impairments in specific neurotransmitters and their receptors have been reported as well, especially serotonin and GABA-mediated pathways. A general observation from multiple studies and case reports is that GABA, homovanillic acid (HVA), and 5-hydroxyindoleacetic acid (5-HIAA)—a serotonin metabolite—are decreased in the cerebrospinal fluid of subjects with PHM [62]. In animal models, injections of a $GABA_A$ agonist, but not of $GABA_A$ blockers, are able to induce contralateral (when injected intracerebroventricularly or in the caudate) or ipsilateral (when injected in the nucleus reticularis of the thalamus) myoclonus [63, 64]. Epileptic manifestations and EEG patterns are triggered only by intrastriatal injections [63]. The very beneficial effect of treatments that bind GABA receptors, such as clonazepam and valproic acid, and the attenuation of myoclonus in rat models of postanoxic conditions upon inhibition of GABA re-uptake, supports the idea of a central role of GABA in the pathogenesis of PHM [65]. Indeed, the nucleus reticularis of the thalamus, an important connection between the thalamus and the cortex, is enriched in GABAergic neurons whose impairment could result in myoclonus. Interestingly, the delayed response observed in animal models from the time of injection of $GABA_A$ agonist in this area and the development of myoclonic jerks suggests that activation of thalamic connections ends in a progressive recruitment of cortical neurons for the generation of myoclonic jerks [63].

Conversely, serotonin (5-hydroxytryptamine, 5-HT) decreases myoclonus both in animal models as well as in reports from human subjects, particularly by targeting the serotonin receptors 5-HT1B, 5-HT2A/2B, and possibly 5-HT1D [17, 57, 66, 67]. Treatment with the serotonin precursor 5-hydroxytryptophan (5-HTP) was reported to help in reducing myoclonus in posthypoxic conditions [17, 57, 67, 68]. Since neuropathological data did not show neuronal loss in the serotoninergic system, the deficit may be related to a neurotransmitter imbalance rather than to an actual loss of neurons or receptors [66]. In the context of myoclonus, impaired serotonin can cause loss of inhibition on the olivocerebellar rhythmicity ending in an oscillatory pathway via the thalamus [69]. The central role of thalamic neurons as an important relay station in the generation of myoclonus is supported also by the finding in the brain of rat models of cardiac-arrest induced posthypoxic myoclonus of increased levels of c-Fos (a marker of neuronal hyperactivation) in discrete thalamic nuclei, such as the reticular thalamic nucleus, the medial longitudinal fasciculus, and in the locus coeruleus and the periventricular gray substance [70]. Finally, a possible correlation between the causative event of the cardiopulmonary arrest and the subtype of PHM (acute vs chronic) has been postulated. Indeed, cases of LAS are more frequently associated with respiratory than cardiac arrests [6]. The period of hypoxia preceding CPA caused by a gradual respiratory insufficiency might generate preconditioning in different brain neurons through activation of specific metabolic pathways, resulting in different brain lesions compared to CPA caused by a sudden arrhythmia [71–73].

Therapeutic Approaches

Management of acute and chronic PHM lacks specific guidelines due to the paucity of controlled trials available in the literature [74]. Appropriate treatment reduces distress in comatose patients in the ICU, as well as improves function and quality of life in subjects who develop LAS.

For the treatment of acute PHM, antiepileptic medications are usually first-line treatments, especially when seizures coexist (Fig. 11.1). Benzodiazepines (mostly diazepam, clonazepam, lorazepam), phenytoin, phenobarbital, and valproic acid have been used in this setting following the dosages normally used for convulsive status epilepticus [2, 75]. Phenytoin should be used with caution since it can paradoxically worsen subcortical myoclonus [5]. In severe cases of acute PHM where generalized myoclonus does not respond to antiepileptics, propofol has been utilized to control the symptoms, although with no change in the outcome of these patients [75–77]. In one case of refractory myoclonic status epilepticus, isoflurane was used with success, possibly because of its modulatory effect on the GABAergic system [78]. The introduction of targeted temperature management (TTM, i.e., normothermia at 36 °C for 24 h, or therapeutic hypothermia at 32 °C) has improved the outcomes for patients with posthypoxic or postanoxic conditions. However, after discontinuation of hypothermia and sedation, myoclonus can still be observed in about one out of six subjects and the presence of status myoclonus within 72 h is

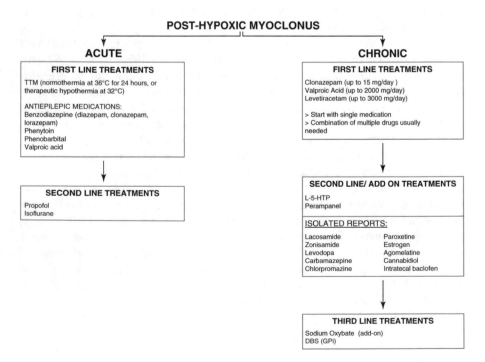

Fig. 11.1 Flowchart of therapeutic approaches for acute and chronic posthypoxic myoclonus

still associated with a poorer outcome [4, 6, 79–82]. On the other hand, some reports have suggested a beneficial effect of this treatment on the outcome of patients with early massive myoclonus after cardiac arrest [83, 84].

After the acute episodes, PHM can improve spontaneously in a number of cases [8]. While acute PHM usually resolves after the acute event (usually within 24 h), in LAS myoclonus is persistent although it can improve over time. However, while symptoms are present and in those cases in which they persist long after the acute event, symptomatic treatments are required to control these invalidating symptoms. The literature encompassing therapeutic approaches for LAS mostly consists of cohort studies or single case reports (see Fig. 11.1). First-line treatments consist of antiepileptic drugs, especially clonazepam (up to 15 mg/day), levetiracetam (up to 3000 mg/day), and valproic acid (up to 2000 mg/day) [9, 29, 85–88]. In the literature, the beneficial effects of clonazepam, valproic acid, and piracetam have been reported in about 50% of the cases [9]. Levetiracetam has been extensively used for the treatment of PHM [88–91]. Levetiracetam is an antiepileptic medication that modulates neurotransmitter release via SV2A binding. In PHM, doses ranging from 500 to 1500 mg twice daily have been reported [88, 90]. After its introduction, levetiracetam has gradually replaced piracetam, previously prescribed in these cases because of its beneficial effect in PHM [9]. However, piracetam is not approved in the USA, thus limiting its use when compared to levetiracetam. Brivaracetam, another molecule that is structurally related to levetiracetam, has been shown to be even more potent (about tenfold more) than levetiracetam, and useful in controlling myoclonus in a rat model of PHM [92]. However, this medication has not been approved for the treatment of myoclonus so far.

Because of the reduced levels of 5-HT and its metabolite 5-HIAA in the CSF of numerous patients with PHM, 5-HT and L-5-HTP have been used in patients who were not responsive to first-line treatments. The first report was in 1973, followed by a number of other cases in the literature [57, 67, 93]. Possible side effects such as nausea, vomiting, and diarrhea need to be taken into consideration, although they can be attenuated by the concomitant administration of carbidopa. Perampanel, an alpha-amino-3-hydroxy-5-methyl-4-isoxazolepropionic acid (AMPA) receptor antagonist, has been used as an add-on for the treatment of LAS as well, but few reports are available [94–98]. Doses are usually 2 to 4 mg daily although higher doses, up to 10 mg, have been reported [96]. In one case, perampanel was utilized also for posthypoxic myoclonic status, after all the other treatments failed to control myoclonus, at a dose up to 8 mg [99].

Numerous other medications have been attempted in patients with PHM. Isolated successes have been reported with intrathecal baclofen, lacosamide, levodopa, carbamazepine, chlorpromazine, paroxetine, estrogen, agomelatine, zonisamide, and cannabidiol [9, 100–107]. On the contrary, no clear benefits or only inconsistent results have been shown with phenobarbital, phenytoin, primidone or nitrazepam, amantadine, tetrabenazine, nortriptyline, and vasopressin [9]. Among benzodiazepines, diazepam does not seem to be as effective as clonazepam [27].

In the majority of the cases of PHM and LAS, a multidrug regimen is required to achieve satisfactory control of symptoms (see Fig. 11.1). In cases of LAS, it is usually recommended to start with first-line options (clonazepam, valproic acid, and levetiracetam) and then gradually add other available treatments until symptoms are controlled (see Fig. 11.1). Nevertheless, despite all the available treatment options, multidrug-resistant cases of LAS are not infrequent. For these refractory cases, additional approaches may be considered. Although not approved in the US for the treatment of this condition, sodium oxybate (SXB) has shown positive results in PHM as an add-on medication. PHM, similarly to other hyperkinetic movement disorders, positively responds to alcohol ingestion [108, 109]. SXB is a sodium salt of γ-hydroxybutyrate that can easily cross the blood-brain barrier and was proven to be effective in alcohol-responsive movement disorders such as essential and vocal tremor, myoclonus-dystonia, and spasmodic dysphonia [110]. Eight cases have been reported in the literature where SXB was utilized in patients with LAS [110–114]. Improvements of action and stimulus-induced myoclonus, as well as myoclonus at rest were documented upon using SXB as an add-on treatment to various combinations of first-line medications for PHM [110]. SXB is usually started at a low dose of 1 g twice daily and slowly increased to the final target dose, which can be different between subjects, but usually below 4 g twice per day. The effect of the medication usually lasts between 3 and 4 h. Possible serious side effects, such as respiratory suppression, depression, and amnesia, should always be monitored when administering this medication and may limit tolerability.

Many patients with LAS experience improvement of their myoclonus with alcohol, which suggests treatment with sodium oxybate if other medications are ineffective.

In severe and nonresponsive cases, surgical approaches with deep brain stimulation have been attempted as well. There are only four single case reports documenting the use of DBS in patients with LAS [38, 115–117]. In three of these cases, DBS was implanted in the globus pallidus internus (GPi), bilaterally in two patients (stimulation setting: amplitude 2–2.8 V, frequency 125–130 Hz, pulse width 60–90 ms) and unilaterally in one case because of a residual hemiparesis on the other side (stimulation setting: amplitude 1.8 V, frequency 130 Hz, pulse width 450μsec). These were all adult cases (of 26, 54, and 71 year of age), presenting with generalized and/or multifocal myoclonus at rest and with action that started within 24 h and 2 days after CPA. Surgery was performed between 1 and 3 years after the initial insult. Previous treatments with clonazepam, valproic acid, levetiracetam, gabapentin, and intrathecal baclofen were attempted in various combinations with only partial benefit. GPi-DBS showed various degrees of sustained improvement at follow-up visits between 6 and 10 months after surgery, of both action and intention myoclonus as well as myoclonic jerks at rest [38, 115, 117]. In one case, a prominent improvement of the myoclonus of the lower limbs, and thus of gait, was documented [115]. Few additional DBS targets have been considered. In one of the described cases, before targeting the GPi, stimulation of the posterior subthalamic area (PSA) and the ventral intermediate nucleus (Vim) were attempted during the surgery while the patient was awake [115]. However, stimulation in these areas failed to improve the myoclonus when the subject was attempting to write [115]. In one additional case, the ventralis oralis (Vo) and ventralis intermedius (Vim) nuclei of the thalamus were targeted (frequency 135 Hz, pulse width of 0.21 ms) [116]. This was an adult case (36 years of age) with a history of perinatal hypoxia who started experiencing proximal myoclonus of the upper limbs, at rest and with action, at the age of 4 with significant worsening after the age of 13 years [116]. The improvements were persistent at 24-month follow-up after DBS [116].

Together with pharmacological and surgical approaches, rehabilitation and occupational therapy are also very important in patients with severe sequela of LAS, particularly to maximize independence in daily activities and gait, increase safety and prevent falls.

Prognosis

Prognostic features in PHM are an important element to guide treatment and the management of these patients. In particular, PHM can present very different outcomes between acute and chronic cases. Onset of myoclonus after CPR has been noted as a prognostic factor for patients in the ICU. Studies considering survival and disability rates after CPA before targeted temperature management reported a survival rate of 0–11% at discharge in patients who manifested PHM during coma after CPR [2, 3, 30, 43, 76, 118, 119]. It is important to consider that these numbers may underestimate poor outcome, as some survivals progressed to a vegetative state [27]. In the same patients, good neurological outcomes were reported in 12% of cases after 6 months, and only 9–14% of patients who developed PHM after an anoxic event survive with only mild cognitive sequelae [3, 8, 41, 118]. In some studies, the type of myoclonus (i.e., cortical vs subcortical) does not affect the rate of positive neurological outcome, while in others focal and multifocal acute PHM myoclonus, thus suggesting a cortical origin, showed better survival compared to subcortical generalized myoclonus (17% vs. 3%, respectively) [3, 5, 118]. Time of onset and duration of the myoclonus do not seem to influence outcomes [1]. The American Academy of Neurology's 2006 guidelines regarding neurological outcomes in patients with CPA indicate the onset of acute myoclonus status epilepticus within the first 24 h as a negative prognostic feature [7]. This is particularly relevant in the context of patients in the ICU since it can influence the decision to continue or suspend treatments in critical patients. However, after the introduction of TTM in patients with cardiopulmonary arrest, the sensitivity of PHM after CPA has been reconsidered [19, 83]. Indeed, according to the updated AAN report from 2017, studies about myoclonus as a sequela of post-CPR are still too small to draw guidelines for the management of these patients [74]. Concerns have been raised around the fact that sedation and use of muscle relaxants post-CPR can mask the presence of myoclonus and thus confound prognostic data relative to this condition [44–46]. At the same time, even if after the introduction of TTM early myoclonus is still present and associated with poor outcome, there are also some reports showing a possible positive trend in patients with PHM undergoing this treatment [5, 82–84].

Acute PHM, and especially myoclonus status epilepticus, usually resolves within 24 h. If myoclonus persists upon regaining consciousness, this suggests

LAS. Different from acute PHM, the prognosis of patients with LAS is more benign [15]. Indeed, in these cases, the neurological sequela, other than myoclonus, can be very limited [8]. Myoclonus itself can improve over time, although in some cases it remains prominent and limits patients' recovery. Myoclonus affects patient's gait and stability, speech, and autonomy in daily living [8]. No clear features have been identified to explain when symptoms will resolve or persist in LAS. In particular, no correlation was found between the duration of coma and the outcome of myoclonus [8]. In one case, relapses of myoclonus were reported 8 years after the initial event in a patient who developed PHM after a cardiac arrest due to a myocardial infarct. After the acute event as well as after this first relapse, myoclonus resolved. However, after this second episode, the patient presented again with a similar pattern of myoclonus responsive to clonazepam triggered by a new respiratory infection [120].

Conclusion

Because of the significant differences in outcome between acute PHM and LAS, distinguishing between these two entities is critical for patients, families, and treating physicians in order to adequately manage these conditions. However, the differences are not always clear-cut as described above [121]. Expert clinical evaluation, supported by ancillary tests and attentive assessment of the progression of the symptoms, is still important for the diagnosis and correct management of posthypoxic myoclonus.

References

1. Snyder BD, Hauser WA, Loewenson RB, Leppik IE, Ramirez-Lassepas M, Gumnit RJ. Neurologic prognosis after cardiopulmonary arrest: III. Seizure activity. Neurology. 1980;30:1292–7.
2. Wijdicks EFM, Parisi JE, Sharbrough FW. Prognostic value of myoclonus status in comatose survivors of cardiac arrest. Ann Neurol. 1994;35:239–43.
3. Bouwes A, van Poppelen D, Koelman JH, Kuiper MA, Zandstra DF, Weinstein HC, et al. Acute posthypoxic myoclonus after cardiopulmonary resuscitation. BMC Neurol. 2012;12:63.
4. Oddo M, Rossetti AO. Early multimodal outcome prediction after cardiac arrest in patients treated with hypothermia. Crit Care Med. 2014;42:1340–7.
5. Reynolds AS, Rohaut B, Holmes MG, Robinson D, Roth W, Velazquez A, et al. Early myoclonus following anoxic brain injury. Neurol Clin Pract. 2018;8(3):249–56.
6. Freund B, Sutter R, Kaplan PW. Lance-adams syndrome in the pretargeted temperature management era. Clin EEG Neurosci. 2017;48(2):130–8.
7. Wijdicks EFM, Hijdra A, Young GB, Bassetti CL, Wiebe S. Practice parameter: prediction of outcome in comatose survivors after cardiopulmonary resuscitation (an evidence-based review). Report of the Quality Standards Subcommittee of the American Academy of Neurology. Neurology. 2006;67:203–10.
8. Werhahn KJ, Brown P, Thompson PD, Marsden CD. The clinical features and prognosis of chronic posthypoxic myoclonus. Mov Disord. 1997;12:216–20.
9. Frucht S, Fahn S. The clinical spectrum of posthypoxic myoclonus. Mov Disord. 2000;15:2–7.

10. Sugama S, Kusano K. A case of dyskinetic cerebral palsy resembling post-anoxic action myoclonus. Brain and Development. 1995;17:210–2.
11. Obeso JA, Lang AE, Rothwell JC, Marsden CD. Postanoxic symptomatic oscillatory myoclonus. Neurology. 1983;33:240–3.
12. Kakisaka Y, Haginoya K, Togashi N, Kitamiura T, Uematsu M, Hino-Fukuyo N, et al. Neonatal-onset brainstem reticular reflex myoclonus following a prenatal brain insult: generalized myoclonic jerk and a brainstem lesion. Tohoku J Exp Med. 2007;211:303–8.
13. Ong MT, Sarrigiannis PG, Baxter PS. Post-anoxic reticular reflex myoclonus in a child and proposed classification of post-anoxic myoclonus. Pediatr Neurol. 2020;68:68–72.
14. Hallett M. Physiology of human posthypoxic myoclonus. Mov Disord. 2000;15:8–13.
15. Lance JW, Adams RD. The syndrome of intention or action myoclonus as a sequel to hypoxic encephalopathy. Brain. 1963;86:111–36.
16. Mikhaeil-Demo Y, Gavvala JR, Bellinski II, Macken MP, Narechania A, Templer JW, et al. Clinical classification of post anoxic myoclonic status. Resuscitation. 2017;119:76–80.
17. Hallett M, Chadwick D, Adam J, Marsden CD. Reticular reflex myoclonus: a physiological type of human post hypoxic myoclonus. J Neurol Neurosurg Psychiatry. 1977;40:253–64.
18. Brown P, Thompson PD, Rothwell JC, Day BL, Marsden CD. A case of postanoxic encephalopathy with cortical action and brainstem reticular reflex myoclonus. Mov Disord. 1991;6:139–44.
19. Sandroni C, Cariou A, Cavallaro F, Cronberg T, Friberg H, Hoedemaekers C, et al. Prognostication in comatose survivors of cardiac arrest: an advisory statement from the European Resuscitation Council and the European Society of Intensive Care Medicine. Resuscitation. 2014;85:1779–89.
20. Fernandez-Torre JL, González-Rato J, Martínez-Martínez M. Acute stimulus-sensitive post-anoxic myoclonus: description of a case. Clin EEG Neurosci. 2005;36:199–201.
21. Fernández-Torre JL, Hernández-Hernández MA. Acute stimulus-sensitive postanoxic myoclonus: the importance of sensory stimulation in comatose patients. Clin EEG Neurosci. 2012;43:312–4.
22. Niedermeyer E, Bauer G, Burnite R, Reichenbach D. Selective stimulus-sensitive myoclonus in acute cerebral anoxia: a case report. Arch Neurol. 1977;34:365–8.
23. Zivkovic SA, Brenner RP. A case of area-specific stimulus-sensitive postanoxic myoclonus. J Clin Neurophysiol. 2003;20:111–6.
24. Bruno MK, Lee HY, Auburger GWJ, Friedman A, Nielsen JE, Lang AE, et al. Genotype-phenotype correlation of paroxysmal nonkinesigenic dyskinesia. Neurology. 2007;68:1782–9.
25. Cott AC, Blatt I, Brenner RP. Stimulus-sensitive seizures in postanoxic coma. Epilepsia. 1996;37:868–74.
26. Harper SJ, Wilkes RG. Posthypoxic myoclonus (the Lance-Adams syndrome) in the intensive care unit. Anaesthesia. 1991;46:199–201.
27. Gupta HV, Caviness JN. Post-hypoxic myoclonus: current concepts, neurophysiology, and treatment. Tremor Other Hyperkinet Mov (N Y). 2016;6:409.
28. Fahn S. Posthypoxic action myoclonus: literature review update. Adv Neurol. 1986;43:157–69.
29. Aicua Rapun I, Novy J, Solari D, Oddo M, Rossetti AO. Early Lance–Adams syndrome after cardiac arrest: prevalence, time to return to awareness, and outcome in a large cohort. Resuscitation. 2017;115:169–72.
30. Young GB, Gilbert JJ, Zochodne DW. The significance of myoclonic status epilepticus in postanoxic coma. Neurology. 1990;40:1843–8.
31. Budhram A, Lipson D, Nesathurai S, Harvey D, Rathbone MP. Postanoxic myoclonus: two case presentations and review of medical management. Arch Phys Med Rehabil. 2014;95:588–90.
32. Dekker MCJ, Kilonzo KG, Howlett WP, Guttman M, Cubo E. Inspiratory myoclonus. Tremor Other Hyperkinet Mov (N Y). 2019;9:625.
33. Gasca-Salas C, Lang AE. Focal predominant forms of posthypoxic action myoclonus. Mov Disord Clin Pract. 2016;3:417–20.

34. Chee YC, Poh SC. Myoclonus following severe asthma: clonazepam relieves. Aust NZ J Med. 1983;13:285–6.
35. Magnussen I, Dupont E, Engbaek F, De Fine Olivarius B. Post-hypoxic intention myoclonus treated with 5-hydroxytryptophan and an extracerebral decarboxylase inhibitor. Acta Neurol Scand. 1978;57:289–94.
36. Magnussen I, Mondrup K, Engbék F, Lademann A, de Fine Olivarius B. Treatment of myoclonic syndromes with paroxetine alone or combined with 5-HTP. Acta Neurol Scand. 1982;66:276–82.
37. Huang HC, Chen JC, Lu MK, Chen JM, Tsai CH. Post-hypoxic cortical myoclonus mimicking spinal myoclonus – electrophysiological and functional MRI manifestations. Eur J Neurol. 2011;18(1):e4–5.
38. Yamada K, Sakurama T, Soyama N, Kuratsu JI. GPi Pallidal stimulation for Lance-Adams syndrome. Neurology. 2011;76:1270–2.
39. Legriel S, Le Stang MB, Merceron S, Cronier P, Troche G. Ongoing abdominal status myoclonus in postanoxic coma. Neurocrit Care. 2012;16:136–8.
40. Cho AR, Kwon JY, Kim JY, Kim ES, Kim HY. Acute onset Lance-Adams syndrome following brief exposure to severe hypoxia without cardiac arrest – a case report. Korean J Anesthesiol. 2013;65:341–4.
41. van Zijl JC, Beudel M, Elting JJ, de Jong BM, van der Naalt J, van den Bergh WM, et al. The inter-rater variability of clinical assessment in post-anoxic myoclonus. Tremor Other Hyperkinet Mov (N Y). 2017;7:470.
42. Kanemoto K, Ozawa K. A case of post-anoxic encephalopathy with initial massive myoclonic status followed by alternating Jacksonian seizures. Seizure. 2000;9:352–5.
43. Elmer J, Rittenberger JC, Faro J, Molyneaux BJ, Popescu A, Callaway CW, et al. Clinically distinct electroencephalographic phenotypes of early myoclonus after cardiac arrest. Ann Neurol. 2016;80:175–84.
44. Sandroni C, Cavallaro F, Callaway CW, Sanna T, D'Arrigo S, Kuiper M, et al. Predictors of poor neurological outcome in adult comatose survivors of cardiac arrest: a systematic review and meta-analysis. Part 1: patients not treated with therapeutic hypothermia. Resuscitation. 2013;84(10):1310–23.
45. Sandroni C, Cavallaro F, Callaway CW, D'Arrigo S, Sanna T, Kuiper MA, et al. Predictors of poor neurological outcome in adult comatose survivors of cardiac arrest: a systematic review and meta-analysis. Part 2: patients treated with therapeutic hypothermia. Resuscitation. 2013;84(10):1324–38.
46. Rossetti AO, Oddo M, Logroscino G, Kaplan PW. Prognostication after cardiac arrest and hypothermia: a prospective study. Ann Neurol. 2010;67:301–7.
47. Tassinari CA, Coccagna G, Mantovani M, Dalla Bernardina B, Roger J. Polygraphic study of dyssynergia cerebellaris myoclonica (Ramsay-Hunt syndrome) and of the intention myoclonus (lance-adams syndrome) during sleep. Eur Neurol. 1973;9:105–20.
48. Witte OW, Niedermeyer E, Arendt G, Freund HJ. Post-hypoxic action (intention) myoclonus: a clinico-electroencephalographic study. J Neurol. 1988;235:214–8.
49. Waddell A, Dirweesh A, Ordonez F, Kososky C, Reddy Peddareddygari L, Grewal RP. Lance–Adams syndrome associated with cerebellar pathology. J Community Hosp Intern Med Perspect. 2017;7:182–4.
50. Ferlazzo E, Gasparini S, Cianci V, Cherubini A, Aguglia U. Serial MRI findings in brain anoxia leading to Lance-Adams syndrome: a case report. Neurol Sci. 2013;34:2047–50.
51. Frucht SJ, Trošt M, Ma Y, Eidelberg D. The metabolic topography of posthypoxic myoclonus. Neurology. 2004;62:1879–81.
52. Zhang YX, Liu JR, Jiang B, Liu HQ, Ding MP, Song SJ, et al. Lance-Adams syndrome: a report of two cases. J Zhejiang Univ Sci B. 2007;8(10):715–20.
53. Park KM, Han YH, Kim TH, Mun CW, Shin KJ, Ha SY, et al. Increased functional connectivity between motor and sensory cortex in a patient with Lance-Adams syndrome. Clin Neurol Neurosurg. 2015;139:241–3.
54. Wolf P. Periodic synchronous and stereotyped myoclonus with postanoxic coma. J Neurol. 1977;215:39–47.

55. De Léan J, Richardson JC, Rewcastle NB. Pathological findings in a case of hypoxic myoclonus treated with 5-hydroxytryptophan and a decarboxylase inhibitor. Adv Neurol. 1986;43:215–23.
56. Hauw JJ, Escourolle R, Baulac M, Morel-Maroger A, Goulon M, Castaigne P. Postmortem studies on posthypoxic and post-methyl bromide intoxication: case reports. Adv Neurol. 1986;43:201–14.
57. Lhermitte F, Talairach J, Buser P, Gautier JC, Bancaud J, Gras R, et al. Myoclonies d'intention et d'acton post-anoxiques. Etude stéréotaxique et destruction du noyau ventral latéral du thalamus [Postanoxic-action and intention myoclonus. Stereotaxic study and destruction of the lateral ventral nucleus of the thalamus]. Rev Neurol (Paris). 1971;124(1):5–20. French
58. Quillinan N, Grewal H, Deng G, Shimizu K, Yonchek JC, Strnad F, et al. Region-specific role for GluN2B-containing NMDA receptors in injury to Purkinje cells and CA1 neurons following global cerebral ischemia. Neuroscience. 2015;284:555–65,
59. Geocadin RG, Muthuswamy J, Sherman DL, Thakor NV, Hanley DF. Early electrophysiological and histologic changes after global cerebral ischemia in rats. Mov Disord. 2000;15:14–21.
60. Tai KK, Bhidayasiri R, Truong DD. Post-hypoxic animal model of myoclonus. Parkinsonism Relat Disord. 2007;13(7):377–81.
61. Paine MG, Che D, Li L, Neumar RW. Cerebellar Purkinje cell neurodegeneration after cardiac arrest: effect of therapeutic hypothermia. Resuscitation. 2012;83:1511–6.
62. Guilleminault C, Tharp BR, Cousin D. HVA and 5HIAA CSF measurements and 5HTP trials in some patients with involuntary movements. J Neurol Sci. 1973;18:435–41.
63. Matsumoto RR, Truong DD, Nguyen KD, Dang AT, Hoang TT, Vo PQ, et al. Involvement of GABAA receptors in myoclonus. Mov Disord. 2000;15:47–52.
64. Tarsy D, Pycock CJ, Meldrum BS, Marsden CD. Focal contralateral myoclonus produced by inhibition of GABA action in the caudate nucleus of rats. Brain. 1978;101(1):143–62.
65. Jaw SP, Nguyen B, Vuong QTV, Trinh TA, Nguyen M, Truong DD. Effects of GABA uptake inhibitors on posthypoxic myoclonus in rats. Brain Res Bull. 1996;39:189–92.
66. Pappert EJ, Goetz CG, Vu TQ, Ling ZD, Leurgans S, Raman R, et al. Animal model of post-hypoxic myoclonus: effects of serotonergic antagonists. Neurology. 1999;52:16–21.
67. Carroll WM, Walsh PJ. Functional independence in post-anoxic myoclonus: contribution of L-5-HTP sodium valproate and clonazepam. Br Med J. 1978;2(6152):1612.
68. Van Woert and myoclonus – Search Results – PubMed [Internet]. [cited 2020 May 31]. Available from: https://pubmed.ncbi.nlm.nih.gov/?term=VanWoert and myoclonus&sort=date
69. Welsh JP, Placantonakis DG, Warsetsky SI, Marquez RG, Bernstein L, Aicher SA. The serotonin hypothesis of myoclonus from the perspective of neuronal rhythmicity. Adv Neurol. 2002;89:307–29.
70. Tai KK, Truong DD. Post-hypoxic myoclonus induces Fos expression in the reticular thalamic nucleus and neurons in the brainstem. Brain Res. 2005;1059:122–8.
71. English WA, Giffin NJ, Nolan JP. Myoclonus after cardiac arrest: pitfalls in diagnosis and prognosis. Anaesthesia. 2009;64(8):908–11.
72. Simon RP. Hypoxia versus ischemia. Neurology. 1999;52(1):7–8.
73. Obrenovitch TP. Molecular physiology of preconditioning-induced brain tolerance to ischemia. Physiol Rev. 2008;88(1):211–47.
74. Geocadin RG, Wijdicks E, Armstrong MJ, Damian M, Mayer SA, Ornato JP, et al. Practice guideline summary: reducing brain injury following cardiopulmonary resuscitation: report of the Guideline Development, Dissemination, and Implementation Subcommittee of the American Academy of Neurology. Neurology. 2017;88:2141–9.
75. Thömke F, Weilemann SL. Poor prognosis despite successful treatment of postanoxic generalized myoclonus. Neurology. 2010;74(17):1392–4.
76. Thömke F, Marx JJ, Sauer O, Hundsberger T, Hägele S, Wiechelt J, et al. Observations on comatose survivors of cardiopulmonary resuscitation with generalized myoclonus. BMC Neurol. 2005;5:14.
77. Wijdicks EFM. Propofol in myoclonus status epilepticus in comatose patients following cardiac resuscitation. J Neurol Neurosurg Psychiatry. 2002;73(1):94–5.

78. Rayadurg V, Muthuchellappan R, Rao U. Volatile anesthetic for the control of posthypoxic refractory myoclonic status. Indian J Crit Care Med. 2016;20:485–8.
79. Samaniego EA, Mlynash M, Caulfield AF, Eyngorn I, Wijman CAC. Sedation confounds outcome prediction in cardiac arrest survivors treated with hypothermia. Neurocrit Care. 2011;15:113–9.
80. Al Thenayan E, Savard M, Sharpe M, Norton L, Young B. Predictors of poor neurologic outcome after induced mild hypothermia following cardiac arrest. Neurology. 2008;71:1535–7.
81. Kim YM, Youn CS, Kim SH, Lee BK, Cho IS, Cho GC, et al. Adverse events associated with poor neurological outcome during targeted temperature management and advanced critical care after out-of-hospital cardiac arrest. Crit Care. 2015;19(1):283.
82. Fugate JE, Wijdicks EFM, Mandrekar J, Claassen DO, Manno EM, White RD, et al. Predictors of neurologic outcome in hypothermia after cardiac arrest. Ann Neurol. 2010;68:907–14.
83. Lucas JM, Cocchi MN, Salciccioli J, Stanbridge JA, Geocadin RG, Herman ST, et al. Neurologic recovery after therapeutic hypothermia in patients with post-cardiac arrest myoclonus. Resuscitation. 2012;83:265–9.
84. Rossetti AO, Oddo M, Liaudet L, Kaplan PW. Predictors of awakening from postanoxic status epilepticus after therapeutic hypothermia. Neurology. 2009;72:744–9.
85. Rollinson RD, Gilligan BS. Postanoxic action myoclonus (Lance-Adams syndrome) responding to valproate. Arch Neurol. 1979;36(1):44–5.
86. Bruni J, Willmore LJ, Wilder BJ. Treatment of postanoxic intention myoclonus with valproic acid. Can J Neurol Sci. 1979;6:39–42.
87. Fahn S. Post-anoxic action myoclonus: improvement with valproic acid. N Engl J Med. 1978;299(6):313–4.
88. Frucht SJ, Louis ED, Chuang C, Fahn S. A pilot tolerability and efficacy study of Levetiracetam in patients with chronic myoclonus. Neurology. 2001;57:1112–4.
89. Krauss GL, Bergin A, Kramer RE, Cho YW, Reich SG. Suppression of posthypoxic and postencephalitic myoclonus with levetiracetam. Neurology. 2001;56:411–2.
90. Genton P, Gelisse P. Suppression of post-hypoxic and post-encephalitic myoclonus with levetiracetam. Neurology. 2001;57(6):1144–5.
91. Venot M, Weiss N, Espinoza S, Imbert A, Tadie JM, Fagon JY, et al. Improvement of early diagnosed post-anoxic myoclonus with levetiracetam. Intensive Care Med. 2011;37(1):177–9.
92. Tai KK, Truong DD. Brivaracetam is superior to levetiracetam in a rat model of post-hypoxic myoclonus. J Neural Transm (Vienna). 2007;114(12):1547–51. [cited 2020 May 29]. Available from: http://www.ncbi.nlm.nih.gov/pubmed/17690949
93. Chadwick D, Hallett M, Harris R, Jenner P, Reynolds EH, Marsden CD. Clinical, biochemical, and physiological features distinguishing myoclonus responsive to 5-hydroxytryptophan, tryptophan with a monoamine oxidase inhibitor, and clonazepam. Brain. 1977;100(3):455–87.
94. Lim S-Y, Jasti DB, Tan AH. Improvement of "Bouncy Gait" in Lance-Adams syndrome with perampanel. Cureus. 2020;12(1):e6773.
95. Steinhoff BJ, Bacher M, Kurth C, Staack AM, Kornmeier R. Add-on perampanel in Lance-Adams syndrome. Epilepsy Behav Case Rep. 2016;6:28–9.
96. Oi K, Neshige S, Hitomi T, Kobayashi K, Tojima M, Matsuhashi M, et al. Low-dose perampanel improves refractory cortical myoclonus by the dispersed and suppressed paroxysmal depolarization shifts in the sensorimotor cortex. Clin Neurophysiol. 2019;130:1804–12.
97. Gil-López FJ, Montoya J, Falip M, Aparicio J, López-González FJ, Toledano R, et al. Retrospective study of perampanel efficacy and tolerability in myoclonic seizures. Acta Neurol Scand. 2018;138:122–9.
98. Kamel WA, Al-Hashel JY, Abdulsalam AJ, Arabi M. Perampanel in refractory post-hypoxic myoclonus: see the difference! Acta Neurol Belg. 2020;120(3):741–2.
99. Santamarina E, Sueiras M, Lidón RM, Guzmán L, Bañeras J, González M, et al. Use of perampanel in one case of super-refractory hypoxic myoclonic status: case report. Epilepsy Behav Case Rep. 2015;4:56–9.
100. Birthi P, Walters C, Vargas OO, Karandikar N. The use of intrathecal baclofen therapy for myoclonus in a patient with Lance Adams syndrome. PM R. 2011;3:671–3.

101. Wicklein EM, Schwendemann G. Use of clonazepam and valproate in patients with Lance Adams syndrome. J R Soc Med. 1993;86(10):618.
102. Galldiks N, Timmermann L, Fink GR, Burghaus L. Posthypoxic myoclonus (Lance-Adams Syndrome) treated with lacosamide. Clin Neuropharmacol. 2010;33(4):216–7.
103. De La Aleja JG, Saiz-Díaz RA, De La Peña P. Relief of intractable posthypoxic myoclonus after administration of agomelatine. Clin Neuropharmacol. 2012;35:258–9.
104. Polesin A, Stern M. Post-anoxic myoclonus: a case presentation and review of management in the rehabilitation setting. Brain Inj. 2006;20(2):213–7.
105. Zöllner JP, Noda AH, Rosenow F, Strzelczyk A. Improving post-hypoxic myoclonus using cannabidiol. Seizure. 2019;67:38–9.
106. Coletti A, Mandelli A, Minoli G, Tredici G. Post-anoxic action myoclonus (Lance-Adams syndrome) treated with levodopa and gabaergic drugs. J Neurol. 1980;223:67–70.
107. Whitlock JA Jr, Dumigan RW. Treatment of postanoxic action myoclonus with intrathecal baclofen: a case report. PM R. 2018,10(8).870–2.
108. Genton P, Guerrini R. Effect of alcohol on action myoclonus in Lance Adams syndrome and progressive myoclonus epilepsy. Mov Disord. 1992;7(1):92.
109. Jain S, Jain M. Action myoclonus (Lance-Adam syndrome) secondary to strangulation with dramatic response to alcohol. Mov Disord. 1991;6(2):183.
110. Riboldi GM, Frucht SJ. Increasing evidence for the use of sodium oxybate in multi-drug-resistant Lance–Adams syndrome. Tremor Other Hyperkinet Mov (N Y). 2019;9 https://doi.org/10.7916/d8-rnsh-c024.
111. Frucht SJ, Bordelon Y, Houghton WH, Reardan D. A pilot tolerability and efficacy trial of sodium oxybate in ethanol-responsive movement disorders. Mov Disord. 2005;20(10):1330–7.
112. Frucht SJ, Bordelon Y, Houghton WH. Marked amelioration of alcohol-responsive posthypoxic myoclonus by gamma-hydroxybutyric acid (Xyrem). Mov Disord. 2005;20(6):745–51.
113. Frucht SJ, Houghton WC, Bordelon Y, Greene PE, Louis ED. A single-blind, open-label trial of sodium oxybate for myoclonus and essential tremor. Neurology. 2005;65(12):1967–9.
114. Arpesella R, Dallocchio C, Arbasino C, Imberti R, Martinotti R, Frucht SJ. A patient with intractable posthypoxic myoclonus (Lance-Adams syndrome) treated with sodium oxybate. Anaesth Intensive Care. 2009;37:314–8.
115. Asahi T, Kashiwazaki D, Dougu N, Oyama G, Takashima S, Tanaka K, et al. Alleviation of myoclonus after bilateral pallidal deep brain stimulation for Lance–Adams syndrome. J Neurol. 2015;262(6):1581–3.
116. Kobayashi K, Katayama Y, Otaka T, Obuchi T, Kano T, Nagaoka T, et al. Thalamic deep brain stimulation for the treatment of action myoclonus caused by perinatal anoxia. Stereotact Funct Neurosurg. 2010;88:259–63.
117. Ramdhani RA, Frucht SJ, Kopell BH. Improvement of post-hypoxic myoclonus with bilateral pallidal deep brain stimulation: a case report and review of the literature. Tremor Other Hyperkinet Mov (N Y). 2017;7:461.
118. Seder DB, Sunde K, Rubertsson S, Mooney M, Stammet P, Riker RR, et al. Neurologic outcomes and postresuscitation care of patients with myoclonus following cardiac arrest. Crit Care Med. 2015;43:965–72.
119. Hui ACF, Cheng C, Lam A, Mok V, Joynt GM. Prognosis following postanoxic myoclonus status epilepticus. Eur Neurol. 2005;54:10–3.
120. Lagrand T, Winogrodzka A. Late relapse myoclonus in a case of Lance-Adams syndrome. BMJ Case Rep. 2013;2013:bcr2013201543. https://doi.org/10.1136/bcr-2013-201543.
121. van Zijl JC, Beudel M, de Jong BM, van der Naalt J, Zutt R, Lange F, et al. The interrelation between clinical presentation and neurophysiology of posthypoxic myoclonus. Ann Clin Transl Neurol. 2018;5:386–96.

Part III

Acute Movement Disorder Emergencies

Tic Emergencies

12

Vanessa K. Hinson and Christopher G. Goetz

Patient Vignettes

Patient 1

Natural exacerbation of fluctuations in chronic tics with the emergence of falls and near falls from tics. An adult woman with a 20-year history of tics had been under recent stress and her tics became severe enough for her to seek additional care. Whereas her usual tics involved eye and neck movements, over 3 months their severity increased to include flailing arm jerks and truncal movements that caused her to stumble and, in some instances, fall to the ground. She became cautious about taking public transportation and standing on train platforms because of fears that she would stumble and fall onto the train tracks.

Patient 2

Compressive neuropathy from tics: An adult with over 40 years of tics was concerned about muscle wasting and numbness in one leg. He had an array of fluctuating tics that included loud vocalizations, bruxism, and nasal and facial movements that waxed and waned. Over the last year, he developed leg tics that involved knee

Supplementary Information The online version of this chapter (https://doi.org/10.1007/978-3-030-75898-1_12) contains supplementary material, which is available to authorized users.

V. K. Hinson (✉)
Department of Neurology, Medical University of South Carolina, Charleston, SC, USA
e-mail: hinsonvk@musc.edu

C. G. Goetz
Department of Neurological Sciences, Rush University Medical Center, Chicago, IL, USA

© Springer Nature Switzerland AG 2022
S. J. Frucht (ed.), *Movement Disorder Emergencies*, Current Clinical Neurology,
https://doi.org/10.1007/978-3-030-75898-1_12

221

banging and unusual rotational movements of one leg. When he performed these leg tics, he had a tingling sensation in the involved leg that was uncomfortable but "strangely satisfying." On examination, tics were observed, but also wasting of muscles supplied by the sciatic nerve. Electromyography confirmed a sciatic neuropathy at the level of the sciatic notch.

Patient 3

Sydenham's disease with chorea and tics (no video) A 9-year-old girl with no prior history of tics presented with a 3-week history of facial grimacing, abdominal flexion, and finger curling. She described a sensation in her abdomen preceding the involuntary movements, and she was able to temporarily suppress the facial and abdominal movements. Simultaneously, she developed mild confusion and headaches. Laboratory workup through the pediatrician's office revealed a positive strep throat culture and elevated antistreptolysin O titer. On examination, there were fine, random choreic movements of hands and fingers but in addition, there were distinct, repetitive eye blinks, stereotypic neck jerks, and abdominal thrusting tics.

Patient 4

Neuroleptic-induced akathisia, initially diagnosed as a new tic: A patient with a 10-year history of Tourette syndrome presented with a complaint of worsening leg and truncal tics. He had been started on pimozide 3 weeks prior because of facial and neck tics. One week later, his family physician further increased the pimozide because of his complaint of new leg movements and truncal rocking. On examination by a neurologist, multifocal motor tics affecting eyes, face, neck, and shoulder were present, as well as complex phonic tics. In addition, marked rhythmic leg movements and rocking motions were accompanied by a subjective sense of inner restlessness and an inability to sit still. When asked if the leg and truncal movements seemed different than his familiar tics, he affirmed that they were. Whereas he could suppress his eye, face, and neck movements for several minutes, he could not keep his legs or trunk still for even a few seconds.

Patient 5

Acute worsening of chronic depression with the initiation of vesicular monoamine transporter-2 (VMAT-2) inhibitor therapy for tic disorder (no video) A 50-year-old man with a long-standing history of Tourette syndrome complicated by coexisting anxiety and depression called urgently into his psychiatrist's office with suicidal thoughts. His mood had been worsening over the past 4 weeks despite compliance with his antidepressant drug regimen. When asked about other medication changes, he reported that his neurologist had added tetrabenazine 6 weeks ago because of worsening tics. He had titrated up slowly and was now taking tetrabenazine 25 mg twice a day.

Introduction

Tics are sudden involuntary stereotypic movements or sounds that emerge out of a normal background. Tic disorders usually start in childhood and typically wax and wane over many years. In our tertiary care centers, only one-third of subjects evaluated for tics require medical therapy. For most subjects, education of the patients, their families, and school and work personnel with or without targeted behavioral therapy are sufficient. When medications are needed, tics can be controlled in most patients, although side effects may arise. The identification of comorbid conditions such as attention deficit hyperactivity disorder (ADHD) or obsessive-compulsive disorder (OCD) is important because these disorders often cause more impairment than the tics themselves. Because the long-term history of tics is generally benign, the primary aim of treatment is to maintain a patient in the school or work environment so that normal or near-normal socialization and school achievement occur.

In rare instances, tics are severe enough to cause a neurologic emergency, and these fall into several categories (Table 12.1). First, intense exacerbations may occur in the normal context of waxing and waning. On occasion, these fluctuations are exacerbated by medication or stress (patient vignette 1), can frighten patients and their families, and limit social or academic integration. Second, tics can cause secondary neurological impairment that may result in new disability, as seen in patient vignette 2 with sciatic nerve damage due to marked leg tics. Third, sudden and unusual tics can emerge in the context of acute neurological disorders other than Tourette syndrome (such as Sydenham's disease, patient vignette 3), and therapies aimed at the primary disorder need to be started promptly. Finally, the pharmacological treatment of tics can cause sudden adverse events, as seen in patient vignette 4 with emerging akathisia caused by neuroleptic therapy, or patient vignette 5 with acute worsening of chronic depression with VMAT-2 inhibitor therapy. In this chapter, each of these tic emergencies is discussed, and the diagnosis and treatment are reviewed.

Table 12.1 Tic emergencies

Tic exacerbations
Neurological impairment secondary to tics
Pain syndromes caused by tics
Sudden and unusual tics in the context of global neurological injury
New abnormal movements caused by pharmacotherapy for tics
Mood disturbance caused by pharmacotherapy for tics

Tic Exacerbations

The natural history of chronic childhood-onset tic disorders is well described. Typically, symptoms start at around 5 or 6 years of age, often with simple motor tics such as frequent eye blinking. Tics tend to peak in severity between 7 and 15 years of age, followed by a steady decline [1, 2]. Tics wax and wane in frequency and severity, and the tic repertoire varies. Simple motor tics (only affecting one muscle group) may migrate or become more complex (coordinated, sequenced movements). Complex tics often resemble normal movements or gestures, but they occur at an inappropriate time or with exaggerated intensity. Gestures may be obscene or provocative and are often socially embarrassing. Phonic tics might appear in the form of simple noises (e.g., throat clearing, sniffing, and humming), or complex words or phrases. Complex phonic tics containing profanities are referred to as *coprolalia*, repetitions of someone else's words *echolalia*, and repetitions of the subject's own words *palilalia*. Tics are temporarily suppressible, often preceded by a premonitory sensation or urge to perform them, and usually produce a sense of relief. Tics can persist in adulthood [2], but are usually mild or well suppressed and do not cause disability.

Because tics occur in bouts, and the course of chronic tic disorders waxes and wanes, exacerbations are common. Factors that influence tic severity and may trigger exacerbations can be divided into *internal* and *external* factors (Table 12.2). An individual's susceptibility to these factors varies greatly. Internal factors include fatigue, hormone status, and levels of perceived stress. Children commonly experience exacerbations of tics at the beginning of the school year and at the time of return from school holidays. Tics also may increase during relaxation after a period of stress. Lack of sleep has been well documented to cause tic exacerbations [3]. Late or night-shift work may not be advisable in a professional with problematic tics. Hormonal fluctuations during teenage years have been implicated in worsening tics. Some patients also report fluctuations with their monthly menstrual cycles [4].

External factors that may exacerbate tics are diet, drugs, and concurrent infections. Even though there is no proven link between dietary products and tic severity, some patients report symptom exacerbations associated with the consumption of certain foods. Numerous drugs have been reported to exacerbate tics (Table 12.3). The most commonly encountered scenario occurs with stimulant drugs for the treatment of comorbid ADHD [5, 6] or performance-enhancing stimulants used by some

Table 12.2 Tics: exacerbating factors	
	Internal
	Fatigue
	Hormone status
	Level of perceived stress
	External
	Diet
	Drugs
	Infections

students during exam time. Over-the-counter drugs for common colds [7], anticonvulsants [8], tricyclic antidepressants [9], selective serotonin reuptake inhibitors [10], and certain illicit drugs [11] have also been reported to exacerbate tics. A patient suffering from a concurrent infection may experience a tic exacerbation related either to the drugs used to treat the infection or to compromised general health.

During these periods, tics may become disabling, requiring urgent management, as illustrated by patient vignette 1. In the case of an external provoking factor, the elimination of the latter (e.g., discontinuation of the offending drug) may solve the problem. If there is no reversible causative agent, drugs for tic suppression may be warranted (Table 12.4). At present, the only agents approved for the treatment of tics by the US Food and Drug Administration are haloperidol, pimozide, and aripiprazole [12, 13, 14]. Other neuroleptics commonly used to treat tics are fluphenazine, risperidone, and ziprasidone [15]. Because of the potential side effects of neuroleptics (parkinsonism, tardive dyskinesia, sedation, weight gain, and cardiac arrhythmias), the lowest possible dose should be used, and the need for treatment

Table 12.3 Drugs implicated in tic exacerbations

Methylphenidate
Pemoline
Dexedrine
Decongestants
Levodopa
Phenytoin
Carbamazepine
Lamotrigine
Phenobarbital
Imipramine
Clomipramine
Fluoxetine
Sertraline
Fluvoxamine
Bupropion
Amphetamine
Cocaine

Table 12.4 Selected drugs to treat tics

Drug	Usual adult starting dose	Usual maximum dose/day
Pimozide	1 mg at bedtime	10 mg
Haloperidol	0.25 mg at bedtime	20 mg
Aripiprazole	5 mg once daily	20 mg
Fluphenazine	0.5 mg at bedtime	5 mg
Risperidone	0.25 mg at bedtime	4 mg
Tetrabenazine	12.5 mg at bedtime	200 mg
Deutetrabenazine	6 mg once daily	48 mg
Valbenazine	40 mg once daily	80 mg
Clonidine	0.05 mg at bedtime	0.8 mg
Guanfacine	0.5 mg at bedtime	3 mg
Botulinum toxin	Varies with injected muscle	Varies with injected muscle

critically reviewed on a regular basis. The dopamine depletors tetrabenazine, valbenazine, and deutetrabenazine have the advantage of not causing tardive dyskinesia and can be effective anti-tic agents [16–18]. With this class of drugs, inhibitors of the vesicular monoamine transporter-2 (VMAT-2), the patient needs to be carefully watched for signs of depression and parkinsonism. In the case of tic exacerbations associated with prominent restlessness or ADHD, the alpha-adrenergic receptor agonists clonidine and guanfacine are useful, although less potent. Selected patients with prominent, disabling focal tics may benefit from botulinum toxin injections. This form of treatment is best suited for patients whose tics can be readily targeted for treatment with the toxin. Eye blinking tics, facial grimacing tics, and neck jerks can be particularly well suited for such injections. Several case series and one double-blind, placebo-controlled trial demonstrate reduction of motor tics and the premonitory urge [19, 20]. The double-blind trial studied relatively mild patients with multifocal tics and failed to show a change in the indices of overall patient well-being. Other case reports have described the improvement of disruptive vocal tics with intralaryngeal botulinum toxin injections [21, 22]. In rare situations, patients with disabling tic disorders will be referred for deep brain stimulation [23]. Education is an important arm of intervention, and the Tourette Syndrome Association (www.tsa-usa.org) has special programs that can be organized to inform teachers and students about tic disorders. These programs aim to defuse misunderstanding and stigmatization related to tic exacerbations.

In the case of patient vignette 1, the exacerbating influences included recent stress resulting in poor sleep. The patient was counseled about stress management techniques, but given the dramatic character of her new tics including falls and near falling episodes, the decision was made to start medication. The neurologist opted to start 2 mg of pimozide each evening after checking an electrocardiogram and verifying that the QT interval was normal. The pimozide was helpful in promoting sleep the first night and tics improved slightly. Over a 2-week period, the tics improved substantially and although they were still present, the emergency situation was considered to have passed.

Neurological Complications from Tics

Occasionally, violent motor tics can result in secondary neurologic injury, particularly radiculopathy or compressive neuropathy. In a previous report of two cases of secondary compressive neuropathies in patients with Tourette syndrome, both patients developed peripheral nerve or radicular injury within the area involved by violent tics [24]. In patient vignette 2, a hip-thrusting tic led to a compressive neuropathy at the sciatic notch. Severe motor tics have also been reported to cause cervical myelopathy [25]. Rapid recognition and treatment of the tic disorder are essential to prevent permanent neurological deficits. The tics should be treated according to the treatment principles outlined in the previous section. Botulinum toxin injections can be particularly useful for the treatment of severe cervical tics. In addition, physical therapy can often facilitate recovery from the neurologic injury. Patient 2 was taking haloperidol (1 mg/day) at the time of his presentation. The dose was gradually increased to 4 mg/day, with the improvement of the leg tics. He was also referred to the physical therapy department for rehabilitation of his leg weakness.

Pain Related to Tics

Tic disorders can cause acute pain syndromes that require urgent management. Riley and Lang reviewed pain in tic disorders [26] and classified these conditions into four categories: (1) pain resulting from the actual performance of the tic (such as neck pain caused by sudden neck movements); (2) pain resulting from a traumatic injury from being struck by a body part involved in a tic, or pain to a body part striking against nearby objects; (3) pain caused by the effort of tic suppression (excessive isometric muscle contraction), or self-inflicted pain in order to reduce tic expression; and (4) pain caused by behavioral abnormalities accompanying the tic disorder such as self-mutilating compulsions. Pain caused by tic disorders may be a source of significant disability for patients, and the same treatment principles discussed in the management of tic exacerbations apply.

Abrupt Onset of Tics Secondary to Central Nervous System Disorders

The abrupt onset of new tics in a patient with other neurological signs, particularly at an atypical age for the first presentation of tics, warrants the careful search for an underlying cause. Numerous acquired and genetic conditions as well as exposure to various drugs and toxins may cause secondary tics [27, 28]. Central nervous system infections, autoimmune disorders, metabolic and toxic encephalopathies, stroke, head trauma, and psychogenic disorders all have been implicated in triggering tics. During the pandemic of encephalitis lethargica (1926–1927), tics were frequently observed as one of a variety of different movement disorders secondary to the infection [29]. This disorder is now rarely seen, but tics have been described in encephalitis secondary to other infectious agents such as herpes simplex virus [30, 31] and human immunodeficiency virus [32]. Given the emergence of the 2020 COVID-19 pandemic, movement disorder specialists need to be vigilant to detect any possible postinfectious tic sequelae of similar character to the above-referenced viral epidemics.

The other infection-related phenomenon is that of tic disorders caused by an autoimmune response triggered by an underlying infection. Sydenham's chorea is the prototype example, following beta-hemolytic streptococcal infection. Tics have been reported to occur at the onset, or following Sydenham's chorea [33, 34], as in the case of patient vignette 3, a clinical presentation showing encephalopathy and chorea along with motor tics. There is also an ongoing debate whether streptococcal infection and rheumatic fever can lead not only to Sydenham's chorea, but also trigger pediatric autoimmune neuropsychiatric disorders associated with strepto-coccal infection (PANDAS) [35]. Treatment of these cases includes antibiotics and appropriate tic treatment as necessary. Patient 3 was started on amoxicillin by the infectious disease specialists, and clonidine by the treating neurologist with a good response of her movements and behavioral disturbances. Concerns that the serious morbidity of COVID-19 involves an immunological cytokine storm evokes similar pathophysiological issues and again warrants vigilance among treating physicians who will want to consider this possibility in patients with new or unusual tics after COVID-19 recovery [36, 37].

⊶ Sydenham's chorea should be considered in a child with an acute onset of new involuntary movements.

Cases of tics occurring after carbon monoxide poisoning have also been described [38]. The documentation of tics attributable to metabolic disturbances such as hypoglycemia is questionable. Strokes can cause the abrupt onset of a tic disorder. Most documented cases describe multifocal or facial tics following cere-bral infarction, but unilateral tics in the distribution of the accompanying neuro-logical deficit have also been reported [39]. In one instance, magnetic resonance imaging findings linked an anatomic region to a case of post-stroke tics [40]: An 8-year-old boy suffered a left hemiparesis, followed by the development of hemi-dystonia and facial tics. The MRI scan demonstrated a lesion in the right middle cerebral artery territory including the head of the caudate nucleus. A few cases of tics following or exacerbated by head trauma have also been described [41]. Even though it is conceivable that traumatic brain injury induces tics, pathophysiologic mechanisms remain unknown, and neuroimaging studies of affected patients have been unrevealing.

Psychogenic tics can be seen in somatoform disorders, factitious disorders, and malingering [27]. They can be hard to diagnose because they share common char-acteristics with organic tics, namely, suppressibility, distractibility, and variabil-ity. Certain atypical features evoke a diagnosis of psychogenic tics: abrupt onset in the context of a life-stressor, entrainment of tics with synkinetic hand move-ments, lack of response to antidopaminergic therapy, resolution with suggestion, placebo, psychotherapy or financial settlement, association with other false neu-rological signs (such as give-way weakness), and psychiatric comorbidity. In these cases, the underlying psychiatric disorder needs to be treated in order to ameliorate the tics.

These examples underscore the importance of a careful differential diagnosis in the evaluation of a tic disorder. When tics occur in a typical pattern and con-text, follow the expected waxing and waning natural history, are not associated with other neurological signs, and a family history of tics is clear, additional workup is not generally required. In other instances, further evaluation is required, because a treatable neurologic condition may underlie the tics, and standard tic treatment, although potentially beneficial in controlling the tics, misses the etiological source.

New Involuntary Movements from Tic Drugs

The chronic tic patient may present for an urgent consultation because of the onset of new abnormal movements. In this context, it is important to differentiate tic exacerbations from new movement disorders secondary to anti-tic medications. Kompoliti and Goetz [42] reported on 12 tic patients with treatment-induced movement disorders. Both acute (akathisia, acute dystonia) and tardive (tardive dystonia, tardive chorea, withdrawal-emergent chorea) phenomena were observed during treatment with typical neuroleptics (pimozide, haloperidol, and fluphenazine). All patients had been misdiagnosed as having tic exacerbations by the referring physicians. Akathisia was the most common phenomenon in this series. Akathisia affects trunk and leg muscles, is associated with an inner feeling of restlessness, and typically starts after neuroleptic initiation or dose increase as seen in patient vignette 4. Usually, a significant decrease in neuroleptic medication is required to achieve relief of akathisia. If the neuroleptic dose cannot be reduced, the addition of anticholinergics, amantadine, beta-blockers, or mirtazapine may be helpful. In the case of patient 4, the neuroleptic dose could not be decreased because of severe complex vocal tics, and the patient was treated successfully with benztropine.

Acute dystonia, especially oculogyric crisis, can also occur in association with the start of a neuroleptic or an increase in dosage. This frightening and often painful disorder requires the addition of an anticholinergic agent to the neuroleptic, usually in the form of an intramuscular or intravenous dose followed by oral anticholinergic, often for the duration of neuroleptic therapy. Reports of tardive syndromes in tic patients are few [43–45], but the phenomenon needs to be recognized and appropriately managed. As opposed to tics that are generally perceived as "voluntary" and suppressible, patients usually perceive tardive dystonic or choreic movements as "involuntary" and not suppressible [46]. Unlike tics, dystonic, or choreic movements usually remain unchanged or even increase during distraction or the performance of skilled tasks. The first step in the management of these tardive syndromes consists of withdrawal of the neuroleptic if possible. Should the tardive symptoms persist and are primarily dystonic, oral anticholinergic drugs can be used, but these drugs often increase choreic movements. VMAT-2 inhibitors are considered particularly useful in this context as deutetrabenazine and valbenazine are FDA approved for tardive dyskinesia, and have also shown to treat tics [47, 48]. In addition, tardive dystonia may be amenable to treatment with botulinum toxin if specific problematic muscle groups are targeted.

Mood Disturbance Caused by Pharmacotherapy for Tics

Mood disturbances, especially anxiety and depression, are common comorbidities in patients with tic disorders [49]. Tic patients treated with one of the VMAT-2 inhibitors might present with new-onset depressive symptoms, acute exacerbation of pre-existing depression, or even suicidality. Tetrabenazine, originally developed in the late 1950s to treat psychosis, was the first VMAT-2 inhibitor used to treat hyperkinetic movement disorders, including tic disorders [50]. In addition to depression, drawbacks to tetrabenazine treatment include fluctuating response, the need for frequent intake due to its rapid metabolism, as well as the risk for parkinsonism, akathisia, and somnolence. This has led to the development of two tetrabenazine analogs, valbenazine, and deutetrabenazine with the goal of improved tolerability. Both tetrabenazine and deutetrabenazine carry a Black Box Warning for depression and suicidality in their drug label, mandated by the US Food and Drug Administration. Retrospective chart review studies suggest that the risk for depression with these agents is especially high for patients with pre-existing depression, such as seen in patient vignette 5 [51, 52]. Review of data from three double-blind, placebo-controlled trials indicates that valbenazine treatment does not seem to be associated with worsening depression or an increased risk of suicidal ideation [53]. In case of mood exacerbation from treatment with one of these agents, the VMAT-2 inhibitor should be discontinued and psychiatric consultation obtained. For the patient in vignette 5, the psychiatrist stopped the tetrabenazine in consultation with the prescribing neurologist immediately, hospitalized the patient for 5 days for observation, and once suicidal thoughts cleared, the patient returned home safely.

Depression may occur suddenly in patients treated with VMAT-2 inhibitors and requires immediate evaluation and management.

References

1. Leckman JF, Zhang H, Vitale A, Lahnin F, Lynch K, Bondi C, et al. Course of tic severity in Tourette's syndrome: the first two decades. Pediatrics. 1998;102:14–9.
2. Goetz CG, Tanner CM, Stebbins GT, Leipzig G, Carr WC. Adult tics in Gilles de la Tourette's syndrome: description and risk factors. Neurology. 1992;42:784–8.
3. Rothenberger A, Kostanecka T, Kinkelbur J, Cohrs S, Woerner W, Hajak G. Sleep and Tourette syndrome. Adv Neurol. 2001;85:245–59.
4. Kompoliti K, Goetz CG, Leurgans S, Raman R, Comella CL. Estrogen, progesterone, and tic severity in women with Gilles de la Tourette syndrome. Neurology. 2001;57:1519.
5. Erenberg G, Cruse RP, Rothner AD. Gilles de la Tourette's syndrome: effect of stimulant drugs. Neurology. 1985;35:1346–8.
6. Price RA, Leckman JF, Pauls DL, Cohen DJ, Kidd KK. Gilles de la Tourette syndrome: tics and central nervous system stimulants in twins and non-twins. Neurology. 1986;36:232–7.
7. Shafii M. The effects of sympathomimetic and antihistaminic agents on chronic motor tics and Tourette's disorder. N Engl J Med. 1986;315:1228–9.
8. Burd L, Kerbeshian J, Fisher W, Gascon G. Anticonvulsant medications: an iatrogenic cause of tic disorders. Can J Psychiatr. 1986;31:419–23.
9. Fras I. Gilles de la Tourette's syndrome: effects of tricyclic antidepressants. N Y State J Med. 1978;78:1230–2.
10. Gatto E, Pikielny R, Micheli F. Fluoxetine in Tourette's syndrome. Am J Psychiatry. 1994;151:946–7.
11. Mesulam M. Cocaine and Tourette's syndrome. N Engl J Med. 1986;315:389.

12. Sallee FR, Nesbitt L, Jackson C, Sine L, Sethuraman G. Relative efficacy of haloperidol and pimozide in children and adolescents with Tourette's disorder. Am J Psychiatry. 1997;154:1057–62.
13. Lyon GJ, Samar S, Jummani R, Hirsch S, Spirgel A, Goldman R, et al. Aripiprazole in children and adolescents with Tourette disorder with and without explosive outbursts. J Child Adolesc Psychopharmacol. 2009;19:623–33.
14. Janik P, Szeiko N. Aripiprazole in treatment of Gilles de la Tourette syndrome–new therapeutic option. Neurol Neurochir Pol. 2018;52:84–7.
15. Budman CL. The role of atypical antipsychotics for treatment of Tourette's syndrome: an overview. Drugs. 2014;74:1177–93.
16. Kenney C, Hunter CB, Mejia NI, Jankovic J. Tetrabenazine in the treatment of Tourette syndrome. J Pediatr Neurol. 2007;5:9–13.
17. Jankovic J, Jimenez-Shahed J, Budman C, Coffey B, Murphy T, Shprecher D, et al. Deutetrabenazine in tics associated with Tourette syndrome. Tremor Other Hyperkinet Mov (NY). 2016;6:422.
18. Niemann N, Jankovic J. Real-World Experience with VMAT2 Inhibitors. Clin Neuropharmacol. 2019;42(2):37–41.
19. Jankovic J. Botulinum toxin in the treatment of dystonic tics. Mov Disord. 1994;9:347–9.
20. Marras C, Andrews D, Sime E, Lang AE. Botulinum toxin for simple motor tics: a randomized, double blind, controlled clinical trial. Neurology. 2001;56:605–10.
21. Scott BL, Jankovic J, Donovan DT. Botulinum toxin injection into vocal cord in the treatment of malignant coprolalia associated with Tourette's syndrome. Mov Disord. 1996;11:431–3.
22. Salloway S, Stewart CF, Israeli L, Morales X, Rasmussen S, Blitzer A, et al. Botulinum toxin for refractory vocal tics. Mov Disord. 1996;11:746–8.
23. Casagrande SCB, Cury RG, Alho EJL, Fonoff ET. Deep brain stimulation in Tourette's syndrome: evidence to date. Neuropsychiatr Dis Treat. 2019;15:1061–75.
24. Goetz CG, Klawans HL. Gilles de la Tourette syndrome and compressive neuropathies. Ann Neurol. 1980;8:453.
25. Krauss JK, Jankovic J. Severe motor tics causing cervical myelopathy in Tourette's syndrome. Mov Disord. 1996;11:563–6.
26. Riley DE, Lang AE. Pain in Gilles de la Tourette syndrome and related tic disorders. Can J Neurol Sci. 1989;16:439–41.
27. Kumar R, Lang AE. Secondary tic disorders. Neurol Clin. 1997;15:309–31.
28. Chouinard S, Ford B. Adult onset tic disorders. J Neurol Neurosurg Psychiatry. 2000;68:738–43.
29. von Economo C. Encephalitis lethargica: its sequelae and treatment. London: Oxford University Press; 1931.
30. Turley JM. Tourette-like disorder after herpes simplex encephalitis. Am J Psychiatry. 1988;145:1604–5.
31. Northam RS, Singer HS. Postencephalitic Tourette-like syndrome in a child. Neurology. 1991;4:592–3.
32. McDaniel JS, Summerville MB. Tic disorder associated with encephalopathy in advanced HIV disease. Gen Hosp Psychiatry. 1974;125:593–4.
33. Behan P, Geschwind N, Quadfase FA. Coprolalia in Sydenham's chorea. Abstract. First International Gilles de la Tourette Syndrome Meeting, New York; 1981.
34. Lees AJ. Tics occurring in association with neurological disorders. In: Lees AJ, editor. Tics and related disorders. New York: Churchill Livingstone; 1985. p. 70–82.
35. Swedo SE. Sydenham's chorea: a model for childhood autoimmune psychiatric disorders. JAMA. 1994;272:1788–91.
36. Mehta P, McAuley DF, Brown M, Sanchez E, Tattersall RS, Manson JJ. COVID-19: consider cytokine storm syndromes and immunosuppression. Lancet. 2020;395(10229):1033–4.
37. Liu K, Pan M, Xiao Z, Xu X. Neurological manifestations of the coronavirus (SARS-CoV-2) pandemic 2019–2020. J Neurol Neurosurg Psychiatry. 2020 Apr 20. pii: jnnp-2020-323177. https://doi.org/10.1136/jnnp-2020-323177. [Epub ahead of print].

38. Pulst S, Walshe TM, Romero JA. Carbon monoxide poisoning with features of Gilles de la Tourette's syndrome. Arch Neurol. 1983;40:443–4.
39. Sacks OW. Tourettism in strokes. Tourette Syndrome Association Newsletter. 1980;(VII:4:7).
40. Jankovic J. Tics in other neurologic disorders. In: Kurlan R, editor. Handbook of Tourette's syndrome and related tic and behavioral disorders. New York: Marcell Dekker, Inc; 1993. p. 167–82.
41. Krauss JK, Jankovic J. Tics secondary to craniocerebral trauma. Mov Disord. 1997;12:776–82.
42. Kompoliti K, Goetz CG. Hyperkinetic movement disorders misdiagnosed as tics in Gilles de la Tourette syndrome. Mov Disord. 1998;13:477–80.
43. Bruun RD. Subtle and underrecognized side effects of neuroleptic treatment in children with Tourette's disorder. Am J Psychiatry. 1988;145:621–4.
44. Shapiro E, Shapiro AK. Tardive dyskinesia and chronic neuroleptic treatment of Tourette patients. Adv Neurol. 1982;35:413.
45. Thomas N, Swamidhas P, Russell S, Angothu H. Tardive dyskinesia following risperidone treatment in Tourette's syndrome. Neurol India. 2009;57:94–5.
46. Lang A. Patient perception of tics and other movement disorders. Neurology. 1991;41:223–8.
47. Hauser RA, Factor SA, Marder SR, Knesevich MA, Ramirez PM, Jimenez R, et al. KINECT 3: a phase 3 randomized, double-blind, placebo-controlled trial of valbenazine for tardive dyskinesia. Am J Psychiatry. 2017;174:476–84.
48. Anderson KE, Stamler D, Davis MD, Factor SA, Hauser RA, Isojärvi J, et al. Deutetrabenazine for treatment of involuntary movements in patients with tardive dyskinesia (AIM-TD): a double-blind, randomized, placebo-controlled, Phase III trial. Lancet Psychiatry. 2017;4(8):595–604.
49. Srour M, Lespérance P, Richer F, Chouinard S. Psychopharmacology of tic disorders. J Can Acad Child Adolesc Psychiatry. 2008;17(3):150–9.
50. Ondo WG, Hanna PA, Jankovic J. Tetrabenazine treatment for tardive dyskinesia: assessment by randomized videotape protocol. Am J Psychiatry. 1999;156:1279–81.
51. Kenney C, Hunter C, Jankovic J. Long-term tolerability of tetrabenazine in the treatment of hyperkinetic movement disorders. Mov Disord. 2007;22(2):193–7.
52. Kenney C, Hunter C, Mejia N, Jankovic J. Is history of depression a contraindication to treatment with tetrabenazine? Clin Neuropharmacol. 2006;29(5):259–64.
53. Remington G, Thai-Cuarto D, Burke J, Siegert S, Liang G. 132 effects of Valbenazine on depression and suicidality in adults with tardive dyskinesia: pooled results of 3 double-blind, placebo-controlled trials. CNS Spectrum. 2018;23(1):82–3.

Coprolalia and Malignant Phonic Tics 13

Joseph Jankovic

Introduction

Understanding the phenomenology and associated symptoms of tic disorders facilitates prompt diagnosis and treatment [1]. Often misconstrued as a disorder of psychological origin, partly because of its peculiar behavioral, motor, and phonic manifestations and fluctuating course, Tourette syndrome (TS) has been frequently misdiagnosed as a "mental illness" and affected patients were often confined to psychiatric institutions. The discovery in the 1960s that dopamine receptor-blocking drugs (neuroleptics) markedly improve tics helped change the image of TS from a bizarre psychiatric disorder to a neurobiological and neurobehavioral condition.

Motor tics are among the most common childhood-onset genetic movement disorders, affecting about 20% of all school children, 1% of whom have persistent tics and satisfy the diagnostic criteria for TS [1, 2]. Tics, the clinical hallmark of TS, are relatively brief, intermittent movements (motor tics), or sounds (vocal or phonic tics) [3–5]. Motor tics typically consist of sudden, abrupt, transient, often repetitive, and coordinated (stereotypic) movements that may resemble gestures and mimic fragments of normal behavior. They typically vary in intensity, are often exacerbated by stress, and are repeated at irregular intervals. Although the diagnostic criteria for definite TS require the presence of "vocal tics" [6], we believe that because the sounds that patients with TS make do not always involve the vocal cords, the term "phonic tic" is preferable and will be used in this review. Actually, phonic tics

Supplementary Information The online version of this chapter (https://doi.org/10.1007/978-3-030-75898-1_13) contains supplementary material, which is available to authorized users.

J. Jankovic (✉)
Parkinson's Disease Center and Movement Disorders Clinic, Department of Neurology, Baylor College of Medicine, Houston, TX, USA
e-mail: josephj@bcm.edu

© Springer Nature Switzerland AG 2022
S. J. Frucht (ed.), *Movement Disorder Emergencies*, Current Clinical Neurology,
https://doi.org/10.1007/978-3-030-75898-1_13

are motor tics involving respiratory, laryngeal, pharyngeal, oral, or nasal musculature. Contractions of these muscles may produce sounds such as barking, excessive throat clearing, grunting, inhaling, sniffing, yelping, clicking of the teeth, and other noises. Phonic tics are often the most distressing and debilitating symptoms of TS. The severity of phonic tics may be measured by the volume of voice projection, effect on respiration, frequency of tics, and their social impact. Assessment of phonic tics is also incorporated in the Yale Global Tic Severity Scale (YGTSS), considered the "gold standard" instrument in evaluating the severity and impact of TS [5]. Complex vocal phenomena include echolalia (repetition of others' words), palilalia (repetition of one's own words), and coprolalia (socially inappropriate words or phrases, obscene utterances, and shouting of profanities) [7]. The latter phenomenon usually leads to the most troublesome social and sometimes legal problems [8].

⊙━━━ Severe phonic tics can exert an extraordinarily negative impact on patients and their families, preventing participation in school, social activities, and daily life. The stigma and shame associated with these tics can exert a profound negative influence on patient's and family's quality of life.

Clinical Symptoms

Patients with TS rarely present with an emergency as a complication of their disease. Nevertheless, we have seen patients who sustained life-threatening injuries such as avulsing their own cornea or the entire eye, or evisceration by cutting an abdominal wall with a razor in response to an inner obsession and the need to satisfy a sexual urge [9]. Rare patients have become quadriparetic as a result of compressive myelopathy caused by repetitive, violent "whiplash" tics of the neck [10]. Others may present because of severe scratches, hematomas, or other serious outcomes of self-injurious behaviors [11]. Some TS patients may present to the emergency room or clinic with loud uncontrollable barking, yelping, shouting of obscenities, or other vocal utterances. Of 332 TS patients evaluated at Baylor College of Medicine Movement Disorders Clinic over a 3-year period, 17 (5.1%) met the criteria for "malignant TS," defined as ≥2 emergency room (ER) visits or ≥ 1 hospitalization for TS symptoms or its associated behavioral comorbidities [9]. The patients exhibited tic-related injuries, self-injurious behavior, uncontrollable violence and temper, and suicidal ideation/attempts. Compared to patients with nonmalignant TS, those with malignant TS were significantly more likely to have a personal history of obsessive-compulsive behavior/disorder (OCB/OCD), complex phonic tics, coprolalia, copropraxia, self-injurious behavior (SIB), mood disorder, suicidal ideation, and poor response to medications.

⊙━━━ Patients with malignant TS are more likely to have significant mood disorders and suicidal ideation.

Coprolalia, derived from the Greek "kopros," which means "dung, feces" and "lalein," meaning "to babble," is one of the most notorious and recognizable symptoms of TS. There are many misperceptions about coprolalia and some clinicians even insist on this symptom to be present in order to make a diagnosis. However, in a study of 597 individuals with TS from seven countries, coprolalia occurred at some point in the course of the disease in only 19.3% of males and 14.6% of females (copropraxia in 5.9% of males and 4.9% of females) [7]. Coprolalia is difficult to study because many patients deny having this phenomenon and others try to "hide" it by uttering only parts of the words, such as four-letter words, by shortening them to "sh," "f," etc. Coprolalia associated with TS is usually in the form of uttering (swearing) obscenities (foul, repulsive, language often with sexual or scatological meaning), rather than profanity (cursing or cussing with religious meaning), although some have racist, sexist, or vulgar (coarse or crude) meaning.

Although relatively uncommon in patients with TS, in some cases coprolalia can be the main or most disabling manifestation of the disease. Scott et al. [12] described a TS patient who exhibited severe coprolalia with racial slurs, sniffing, and grunting refractory to treatment with fluoxetine, fluphenazine, guanfacine, pimozide, and tetrabenazine. He blurted out obscenities and profanities while riding the school bus, resulting in school absences owing to embarrassment. A stranger in a public bathroom also attacked him after he blurted out a racial slur. He expressed a need to repeat his vocal utterances until they seemed "just right." There have been many other reports of coprolalia and other complex severe (malignant) phonic tics [13, 14]. Furthermore, it is important to recognize that there are many other disorders besides TS associated with involuntary vocalizations including coprolalia, such as various neurodevelopmental disorders, stereotypies, tardive dyskinesia, and a variety of neurodegenerative disorders such as progressive supranuclear palsy, multiple system atrophy, Alzheimer's disease, and Huntington's disease [15].

Striatal and cortical disinhibition resulting from a dysfunction of the cortico-striato-thalamo-cortical circuits and GABAergic alterations have been implicated in the pathophysiology of motor and phonic tics, as well as comorbid hyperactivity in TS [16]. The limbic system and ventral basal ganglia may be involved in generating aberrant impulses to the motor cortex. Motor and phonic tics have been categorized as "unvoluntary" movements, with a semivolitional component and underlying sensory phenomenon. Indeed, many patients report that they perform the movements voluntarily in response to an involuntary sensory urge [3, 17, 18]. One of the most prominent sensory aspects of TS is the premonitory sensation typically present before the tics and relieved after their execution [19, 20].

Treatment

Several behavioral and pharmacological treatments have been used to treat severe phonic tics (Fig. 13.1) [1, 21–23]. Dopamine receptor-blocking drugs are often tried first for moderate to severe motor tics, but these are often associated with a variety of adverse effects including sedation, weight gain, and risk of development of

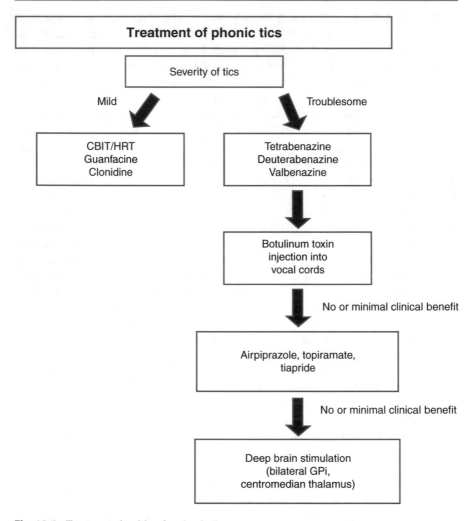

Fig. 13.1 Treatment algorithm for phonic tics

tardive dyskinesia. Haloperidol and pimozide are the two medications currently approved for the treatment of tics by the US Food and Drug Administration (FDA). We prefer fluphenazine and risperidone, although the atypical neuroleptics aripiprazole, olanzapine, quetiapine, ziprasidone, and other third-generation neuroleptics may also be helpful; all can cause tardive dyskinesia [24]. Tetrabenazine, a synthetic benzoquinoline that presynaptically depletes monoamines by blocking vesicular membrane transporter type 2 (VMAT2) has also shown to reduce tic severity without incurring the risk of tardive dyskinesia. Other VMAT2 inhibitors have been investigated and found to be safe and effective in the treatment of motor and phonic tics [22, 23, 25–27], but none of them have been approved yet by the FDA for the treatment of TS. Nevertheless, VMAT2 inhibitors are considered among the most effective and safest drugs in the treatment of TS and are used by many experienced clinicians as first-line therapy (see Fig. 13.1). Adrenergic drugs such as clonidine and guanfacine possess a moderate benefit for tics [28, 29].

All atypical neuroleptics, with the exception of clozapine, carry a risk of engendering tardive syndromes. Before committing a patient to treatment, a complete discussion of the risk/benefit ratio should occur, and this discussion must be documented in the medical record.

Behavioral techniques utilizing habit-reversal training and distraction tasks may provide some benefit, but few studies have systematically examined these approaches in patients with severe phonic tics. Many reports are hampered by small sample size and limited follow-up [30]. Overall, case studies using behavior reinforcement-based interventions are disappointing in reducing tic severity.

BoNT injections have shown to be particularly useful in treating focal motor and phonic tics [12–14, 31–35]. Scott et al. [12] were the first to report a patient with TS whose severe coprolalia markedly improved with unilateral vocal cord injection of BoNT. After injection of 30 mouse U of BoNTA into the left vocal cord under electromyographic guidance, the patient reported a reduction of coprolalia by "at least 75%," with only moderate hoarseness and hypophonia. The premonitory urge to shout was also markedly decreased. A repeat injection of 25 U produced similar benefit, and the patient was able to return to school. Salloway also reported a refractory case of phonic tics responsive to BoNT type A (OnabotulinumtoxinA) injections [31]. Trimble [32] described a TS patient with coprolalia refractory to behavioral therapy, clonidine, and neuroleptics. The patient's coprolalia was so severe that he was threatened with eviction from his residence. The patient also reported strong premonitory "feelings in the brain," rather than in the throat. Selective serotonin reuptake inhibitors, neuroleptics, and behavior therapy failed to improve his severe coprolalia, echolalia, and vocalizations of birdlike noises. Both thyroarytenoid muscles were injected under local anesthesia and electromyogram with 3.75 mouse U of BoNTA (AbobotulinumtoxinA). He reported an excellent response, with a reduction in the intensity of obscene outbursts. Mild side effects included a breathy, weak voice (hypophonia) and slight aspiration of liquids. The severity of the premonitory sensation remained unchanged after the injection [32]. Kwak et al. [33] reported four patients with phonic tics in a large series of various motor tics treated with BoNT. The mean dose given to the vocal cords was 17.8 ± 6.5 mouse U (range 10–23.8). Transient side effects included mild dysphagia and hypophonia. The study reported a global response score of 2.7 ± 1.5 in 35 patients injected with BoNT in various muscle sites. BoNT injections have thus become an effective treatment option for patients with severe, loud, and disabling involuntary vocalizations. One of the interesting observations has been the remarkable improvement of not only the volume and frequency of vocalizations but also the premonitory sensation and urge in nearly all cases. Unfortunately, except for one study [34] all other reports of BoNT in the treatment of motor or phonic tics have been based on open-label observations [35–37].

⌒━━▼ Botulinum toxin injections offer an important therapeutic option for patients with intractable vocal tics.

If all pharmacologic therapy and BoNT therapies fail and the patient continues to be disabled by tics, then deep brain stimulation (DBS) may be considered as an option, although this procedure has not been specifically evaluated in the treatment of phonic tics [38].

Conclusion

Coprolalia and malignant phonic tics may lead to a severe or even incapacitating movement disorder emergency. With appropriate interventions including the careful application of antidopaminergic drugs and skilled injections of vocal cords with BoNT, patients can be effectively managed. Rarely, neurosurgical intervention such as deep brain stimulation is required to control disabling vocalizations.

References

1. Jankovic J, Kurlan R. Tourette syndrome: evolving concepts. Mov Disord. 2011;26(6):1149–56.
2. Scharf JM, Miller LL, Gauvin CA, Alabiso J, Mathews CA, Ben-Shlomo Y. Population prevalence of Tourette syndrome: a systematic review and meta-analysis. Mov Disord. 2015;30(2):221–8.
3. Jankovic J. Tourette's syndrome. N Engl J Med. 2001;345:1184–92.
4. Thenganatt MA, Jankovic J. Recent advances in understanding and managing Tourette syndrome. F1000Res. 2016;5:F1000.
5. Robertson MM, Eapen V, Singer HS, Martino D, Scharf JM, Paschou P, et al. Gilles de la Tourette syndrome. Nat Rev Dis Primers. 2017;3:16097.
6. Deeb W, Malaty IA, Mathews CA. Tourette disorder and other tic disorders. Handb Clin Neurol. 2019;165:123–53.
7. Freeman RD, Zinner SH, Müller-Vahl K, Fast DK, Burd LJ, Kano Y, et al. Coprophenomena in Tourette syndrome. Dev Med Child Neurol. 2009;51:218–27.
8. Jankovic J, Kwak C, Frankoff R. Tourette syndrome and the law. J Neuropsychiatry Clin Neurosci. 2006;18:86–95.
9. Cheung MY, Shahed J, Jankovic J. Malignant Tourette syndrome. Mov Disord. 2007;22:1743–50.
10. Krauss JK, Jankovic J. Severe motor tics causing cervical myelopathy in Tourette's syndrome. Mov Disord. 1996;11:563–6.
11. Fischer JF, Mainka T, Worbe Y, Pringsheim T, Bhatia K, Ganos C. Self-injurious behaviour in movement disorders: systematic review. J Neurol Neurosurg Psychiatry. 2020;91(7):712–9.
12. Scott B, Jankovic J, Donovan D. Botulinum toxin into vocal cord in the treatment of malignant coprolalia associated with Tourette's syndrome. Mov Disord. 1996;11:431–3.
13. Eddy CM, Cavanna AE. 'It's a curse!': Coprolalia in Tourette syndrome. Eur J Neurol. 2013;20(11):1467–70.
14. Kobierska M, Sitek M, Gocyła K, Janik P. Coprolalia and copropraxia in patients with Gilles de la Tourette syndrome. Neurol Neurochir Pol. 2014;48(1):1–7.
15. Mainka T, Balint B, Gövert F, Kurvits L, van Riesen C, Kühn AA, et al. The spectrum of involuntary vocalizations in humans: a video atlas. Mov Disord. 2019;34(12):1774–91.
16. Israelashvili M, Yael D, Vinner E, Belelovsky K, Bar-Gad I. Common neuronal mechanisms underlying tics and hyperactivity. Cortex. 2020;127:231–47.

17. Patel N, Jankovic J, Hallett M. Sensory aspects of movement disorders. Lancet Neurol. 2014;13(1):100–12.
18. Isaacs D, Riordan H. Sensory hypersensitivity in Tourette syndrome: a review. Brain Dev. 2020;42(9):627–38.
19. Kwak C, Vuong KD, Jankovic J. Premonitory sensory phenomenon in Tourette's syndrome. Mov Disord. 2003;18:1530–3.
20. Prado HS, Rosario MC, Lee J, Hounie AG, Shavitt RG, Miguel EC. Sensory phenomena in obsessive–compulsive disorder and tic disorders: a review of the literature. CNS Spectr. 2008;13:425–32.
21. Pringsheim T, Holler-Managan Y, Okun MS, Jankovic J, Piacentini J, Cavanna AE, et al. Comprehensive systematic review summary: treatment of tics in people with Tourette syndrome and chronic tic disorders [published correction appears in Neurology. 2019 Aug 27;93(9):415]. Neurology. 92(19):907–15.
22. Jankovic J. Treatment of tics associated with Tourette syndrome. J Neural Transm (Vienna). 2020;127(5):843–50.
23. Billnitzer A, Jankovic J. Current management of tics and Tourette syndrome: behavioral, pharmacologic, and surgical treatments. Neurotherapeutics. 2020;17(4):1681–93.
24. Peña MS, Yaltho TC, Jankovic J. Tardive dyskinesia and other movement disorders secondary to aripiprazole. Mov Disord. 2011;26:147–52.
25. Kenney C, Hunter C, Mejia N, Jankovic J. Tetrabenazine in the treatment of Tourette syndrome. J Pediatr Neurol. 2007;5:9–13.
26. Jankovic J, Jimenez-Shahed J, Budman C, Coffey B, Murphy T, Shprecher D, Stamler D. Deutetrabenazine in tics associated with Tourette syndrome. Tremor Other Hyperkinet Mov (N Y). 2016;6:422.
27. Niemann N, Jankovic J. Real-world experience with VMAT2 inhibitors. Clin Neuropharmacol. 2019;42(2):37–41.
28. Scahill L, Chappell P, Kim Y, Schultz RT, Katsovich L, Shepherd E, et al. A placebo-controlled study of guanfacine in the treatment of children with tic disorders and attention deficit hyperactivity disorder. Am J Psychiatry. 2001;158:1067–74.
29. Gaffney G, Perry P, Lund B, Bever-Stille K, Arndt S, Kuperman S. Risperidone versus clonidine in the treatment of children and adolescents with Tourette's syndrome. J Am Acad Child Adolesc Psychiatry. 2002;41:330–6.
30. McGuire JF, Piacentini J, Brennan EA, Lewin AB, Murphy TK, Small BJ, Storch EA. A meta-analysis of behavior therapy for Tourette syndrome. J Psychiatr Res. 2014;50:106–12.
31. Salloway S, Stewart C, Israeli L. Botulinum toxin for refractory vocal tics. Mov Disord. 1996;11:746–8.
32. Trimble M, Whurr R, Brookes F, Robertson M. Vocal tics in Gilles de la Tourette syndrome treated with botulinum toxin injections. Mov Disord. 1998;13:617–9.
33. Kwak C, Hanna P, Jankovic J. Botulinum toxin in the treatment of tics. Arch Neurol. 2000;57:1190–3.
34. Marras C, Andrews D, Sime E, Lang A. Botulinum toxin for simple motor tics: a randomized, double-blind, controlled clinical trial. Neurology. 2001;56:605–10.
35. Aguirregomozcorta M, Pagonabarraga J, Diaz-Manera J, Pascual-Sedano B, Gironell A, Kulisevsky J. Efficacy of botulinum toxin in severe Tourette syndrome with dystonic tics involving the neck. Parkinsonism Relat Disord. 2008;14:443–5.
36. Pandey S, Srivanitchapoom P, Kirubakaran R, Berman BD. Botulinum toxin for motor and phonic tics in Tourette's syndrome. Cochrane Database Syst Rev. 2018;1(1):CD012285. https://doi.org/10.1002/14651858.CD012285.pub2.
37. Lotia M, Jankovic J. Botulinum toxin for the treatment of tremor and tics. Semin Neurol. 2016;36:54–63.
38. Xu W, Zhang C, Deeb W, Patel B, Wu Y, Voon V, et al. Deep brain stimulation for Tourette's syndrome. Transl Neurodegener. 2020;9:4.

Hemiballism-Hemichorea

14

Blas Couto, Ronald B. Postuma, and Anthony E. T. Lang

Patient Vignettes

Patient 1

A 69-year-old man was followed at the Toronto Western Hospital with a 7-year history of Parkinson's disease. Other past medical history included diabetes, coronary artery disease, and a previous stroke involving the right frontal lobe. Two weeks before presentation he noticed the acute onset of involuntary movements of the left side, predominantly affecting the arm but also involving the leg and face. They tended to worsen soon after taking his levodopa. Clinical examination showed choreic movements of the left arm. Interestingly, the bradykinesia and rigidity were significantly ameliorated on the left side. Magnetic resonance imaging (MRI) examination demonstrated an infarction of the posterior putamen and globus pallidus, extending upwards into the periventricular white matter (Fig. 14.1). Dopaminergic medications were decreased, resulting in improvement of his symptoms. During his admission, he began to have a spontaneous improvement in symptoms and did not require therapy.

This case illustrates several points. The first is that although stroke is the commonest single cause of hemiballism, lesions are often outside of the subthalamic

Supplementary Information The online version of this chapter (https://doi.org/10.1007/978-3-030-75898-1_14) contains supplementary material, which is available to authorized users.

B. Couto (✉) · A. E. T. Lang
Toronto Western Hospital, Morton and Gloria Shulman Movement Disorders Center and the Edmond J. Safra Program in Parkinson's Disease, Toronto, ON, Canada
e-mail: BLAS.COUTO@UHNRESEARCH.CA

R. B. Postuma
Department of Neurology, McGill University, Montreal General Hospital, Montreal, QC, Canada

Fig. 14.1 Axial FLAIR
and high-resolution
coronal T2-weighted
imaging. (Reprinted with
permission from Riley and
Lang [37])

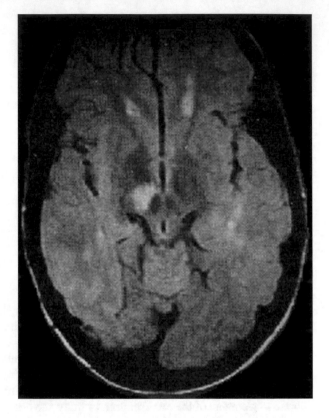

nucleus. The second is that prognosis is often benign. The third is that dopaminergic medications (in this case levodopa) worsen hemiballism, just as dopamine antagonists treat it. Finally, we note the fortuitous effect of his stroke upon his Parkinson's disease, perhaps due to infarction of the motor GPi.

Patient 2

This 24-year-old woman had a 5-year history of multiple sclerosis with frequent relapses. She presented with paresthesias and left-sided incoordination associated with mild involuntary movements. As her sensory symptoms and coordination improved, involuntary movements increased in amplitude and became more violent, predominantly in the left arm and leg. Over time, smaller amplitude movements became evident on the right side, and these also progressed over time. MRI examination demonstrated numerous white matter lesions, including a large plaque in the area of the right subthalamic nucleus. The ballismus persisted despite trials of pimozide, trifluoperazine, haloperidol, tetrabenazine, bromocriptine, sodium valproate, diazepam, and carbamazepine. A stereotactic thalamotomy (performed many years before the potential beneficial effect of GPi appellate autonomy was recognized) provided no benefit and was complicated by transient hemiparesis and postoperative epilepsy. Over the next 5 years, she developed severe dystonia and athetosis of the left side. As the dystonia developed, the ballistic movements diminished. This patient illustrates the more severe end of the spectrum of hemiballismus, with complete resistance to treatment. Hemiballism can be caused by any type of focal basal ganglia lesion, in this case a demyelinating plaque.

Patient 3

A 30-year-old woman with a history of pulmonary hypertension secondary to chronic pulmonary thrombosis and atrial septal defect (ASD) underwent pulmonary endarterectomy and ASD closure, a procedure requiring hypothermia, cardiopulmonary bypass, and three circulatory arrests. After 6 days postoperation, she developed involuntary movements involving the face, flinging of the right arm, which then spread to the contralateral arm and evolved to generalized chorea. Examination showed normal cranial nerve function, mild motor impersistence in the tongue, ballistic movements of both arms with choreoathetotic movements of the fingers, and less frequent hip flexion and abduction movements in the legs. A brain MRI done on day 8 post-operation showed DWI restriction in the bilateral STN and globus pallidus. Laboratory investigations were negative for rheumatologic markers/antibodies (warranted given her medical history), serology for syphilis and Lyme were negative, and vitamin B12 and TSH were within the normal range. She received a diagnosis of post-pump/hypoxic-ischemic choreoballism. She was first treated with olanzapine 5 mg TID without benefit. After consultation with us tetrabenazine 50 mg TID was added with remission of ballistic movements. At 3 months follow-up on tetrabenazine 25 mg TID she had only mild distal chorea interfering with fine motor tasks with no difficulty in gait or speech.

Clinical Description and Etiology

Hemiballism is one of the most dramatic disorders in neurology. Because of its acute onset, it is frequently seen in the emergency room. Typically, the patient presents with an acute or subacute onset of flinging movements of one side of the body. These tend to occur both in the arm and leg, with variable involvement of the face. Movements often have a rotatory component and usually predominantly affect proximal muscles. They can be severe enough to cause the patient to strike walls and bedrails, causing bruising and lacerations of the limb. Movements increase with action and with stress. They are rarely suppressible for more than a few seconds and generally disappear in sleep. Hemichorea refers to movements that are similar in character but lower in amplitude. There is probably little pathophysiologic difference between the two movement disorders, as they share common etiologies, prognosis, and treatment. In fact, they can often be present in the same patient, with hemiballism more prominent early and lower-amplitude hemichorea emerging as the disorder resolves. Therefore, for the purposes of this chapter, we will consider them to be the same disorder (i.e., on a spectrum) and will use the terms interchangeably. Bilateral ballistic movement ("bi-ballism," or "para-ballism" if lower limbs are predominantly involved) is very uncommon and occurs with bilateral central nervous system (CNS) lesions.

Hemiballism is an uncommon disorder, and most general neurologists would not expect to see more than a handful of cases in their careers. Dewey and Jankovic reported 21 patients with hemiballism out of 3084 patients evaluated in a specialty movement disorder clinic [1]. Of 2000 strokes in the Lausanne stroke registry, 550 involved basal ganglia structures but only 11 caused hemiballism [2]. A population-based study in Serbia found an incidence of vascular hemiballism of 0.45 per 100,000 [3]. Pareés et al. [4] described 15 patients with vascular chorea (0.2%) out of 7780 consecutive patients seen in a neurologic referral center in Barcelona; only three of these had hemiballism. In most series, the mean onset age is 55 to 75; however, these data are derived from subspecialty clinics, probably biasing toward younger, more atypical patients. This is supported by the older median age of 78 (range: 29–85) in the Barcelona series [4]. There is no clear gender predominance.

O━━🔑 Although dramatic, hemiballism is an uncommon movement disorder, typically seen only in the hospital or in the emergency room.

Classical neurological teaching has localized hemiballism to lesions of the subthalamic nucleus (STN). This belief originated in the early pathological and animal lesion studies which suggested that hemiballism was reliably evoked by ablation of at least 20% of the subthalamic nucleus (see below). However, a review of the more recent stroke literature suggests that the subthalamic nucleus is not the site of the lesion in most cases. Stroke is without question the single most common cause of hemiballism. Hemiballism can be caused by infarcts or hemorrhages in a variety of locations both inside and outside the basal ganglia, including some cortical regions.

Stroke causing hemiballism was localized to the subthalamic nucleus in only 4 of 27 cases with neuroimaging reported by Ristic et al., 4 of 27 reported by Chung, 4 of 22 reported by Vidakovic, 4 of 21 reported by Dewey and Jankovic, 4 of 11 in the Lausanne stroke registry, 1 of 15 reported by Pareé, and 2 of 15 in our series at the Toronto Western Hospital [1, 2, 4–8]. However, since only CT imaging was performed in some, STN lesions could have been missed. Langaniere et al. described 39 poststroke hemichorea/hemiballism-causing lesions from a literature review, 11 of which located to the STN, 7 to the caudate nucleus, and 6 in the contralateral posterior putamen [9]. There is some evidence that hemiballism is more severe and persistent when due to subthalamic nucleus lesions [6]; this may have skewed early pathologic studies. Therefore, while stroke is the commonest cause of hemiballism, the minority of these infarcts involve the STN directly.

More recently, attention has been drawn to hemiballism associated with nonketotic hyperglycemia. With more than 100 cases reported to date, it is the second most common cause of hemiballism. The condition has been described most commonly in Asian populations. Classic patients are older females, presenting with hemiballism and severe nonketotic hyperosmolar hyperglycemia [10]. As the blood glucose is corrected the disorder usually resolves in days to weeks, although in 20% of the patients milder symptoms persist for more than 3 months. Some series have shown persistence for up to 69 months [11]. Delayed onset after the hyperglycemic episode, treatment resistance and recurrence either on the same side or contralateral side have all been reported [11–14]. Neuroimaging findings in these patients are striking. In all reported cases, the high signal is seen on T1-weighted images in the putamen, with a similar signal occasionally found in the globus pallidus and remainder of the striatum [10]. The signal abnormalities on T2-weighted sequences vary between hyper and hypointensity, and the corresponding increased signal on diffusion-weighted imaging with the decreased signal on gradient-echo has been reported [10, 15, 16]. PET scanning has demonstrated decreased glucose uptake, suggestive of metabolic failure/infarction [17]. Pathologic studies in two patients several months after symptoms resolved demonstrated significant gliosis, with microglial activation and presence of gemistocytic astrocytes [18, 19]. This might represent a reaction to microinfarction or incomplete infarction, although no blood vessel abnormalities were visualized. Two other pathological cases have revealed more classic signs of infarction, and isolated activation of microglia in the subthalamic nucleus with no other signs of infarction [20, 21]. Therefore, the cause of this striking condition remains uncertain. Dynamic changes in perfusion and reperfusion might also cause hemichorea [22]. For example, we have reported a patient with transient ischemic attacks manifesting as hemiballism [23]. Reports of resolution of hemichorea in three patients with carotid endarterectomy for severe stenosis, as well a case of transient hemichorea after tissue-plasminogen activator (tPA) revascularization in a parietal stroke [24] are further support for this etiology.

🔑 Acute hemiballism should immediately prompt consideration of a new diagnosis of diabetes.

Numerous other causes of hemiballism have been reported (Table 14.1). These include mass lesions involving the basal ganglia or STN (often in association with HIV infection), medications, and medical diseases that predispose to infarction or hemorrhage. A variety of autoimmune disorders should be considered, including Sydenham's chorea and systemic lupus erythematosus (often associated with anticardiolipin antibodies) as well as many more recently described autoimmune encephalitides associated with specific antibodies reacting against basal-ganglia neurons (such as anti-Hu [25], DR2, CRMP-5, CASPR2, LGI-1, NMDA-R, IgLON5, GABA A/B-R; for a review see [26]).

Pathophysiology

Much of our understanding of the pathophysiology of hemiballism derives from classic animal models of lesions of the subthalamic nucleus. The original experiments were carried out by Whittier, Mettler, and Carpenter in 1949 and 1950 [27], in which lesions of the basal ganglia were created in primates and their behavioral

Table 14.1 Causes of hemiballism

Common
   Stroke (ischemic or hemorrhagic) in basal ganglia structures
   Nonketotic hyperglycemia
Uncommon or single case reports
Focal lesions in basal ganglia
   Neoplastic
Metastases
Other primary CNS tumors
   Infectious
      Cryptococcal granuloma
      Toxoplasmosis
      Tuberculoma
   Vascular
      Cavernous angioma
      Postsurgical complications
   Inflammatory
      Multiple sclerosis
      Iatrogenic
      Subthalmotomy
      Thalamotomy
   Other mass lesions
   Cerebellar metastases
   Strokes in nonbasal ganglia areas
   Subcortical white matter
   Middle cerebral artery territory
Immunologic disorders/vasculitis
SLE—Often with anticardiolipin antibodies
Scleroderma
Bechet's disease
Hypoglycemia
Meningitis/encephalitis
   Cryptococcal
   Tuberculous
Sydenham's chorea
Head injury
Medications (usually if superimposed on pre-existing basal ganglia lesion)
   Anticonvulsants
   Oral contraceptives
   Levodopa
   Ibuprofen

effects monitored. Contralateral hemiballism could be reliably produced only by lesions that destroyed more than 20% of the STN. Lesions in some areas of the globus pallidus occasionally caused hemiballism, and it was postulated that these were due to disruption of connections to the STN. A second lesion to some areas of the globus pallidus interna (GPi) could abolish the movements. Crossman injected GABA antagonists, which affect neuronal cell bodies but not axons, into basal ganglia locations in alert monkeys, and again, only STN injections reliably caused hemiballism [28]. This confirms that the effects are due to lesions of neuronal cell bodies and not to passing white matter tracts. Injections in the lateral globus pallidus occasionally caused slower hemichoreic/hemiathetoid movements. This may be analogous to hyperglycemic hemichorea, in which the areas predominantly affected are the putamen and GPi, and movements tend to be slower than those after a lesion of the STN.

The classic basal ganglia model postulates that STN lesions interrupt the excitatory connections to the GPi, resulting in hypoactivity of the GPi. This disinhibits the motor thalamus, which in turn drives the motor cortex, resulting in excessive movement [29]. However, this simple model based predominantly on neuronal firing rate does not explain many aspects of hemiballism including its association with lesions outside of the STN, why movements are ballistic and intermittent, and why lesioning of the apparently hypoactive GPi is capable of abolishing hemiballism. Nor does it adequately explain why dopamine antagonists, which target the striatum, are especially effective in treating hemiballism (see management section). Finally, it does not explain why subthalamotomy and subthalamic nucleus stimulation for Parkinson's disease are only very uncommonly complicated by hemiballism [30].

Despite the clear involvement of BG circuits, the fact that cortical lesions can rarely cause hemiballismus points to a more widespread neural network involved in HC/HB with the participation of the supplementary motor area and bilateral motor/premotor cortex, thalamus, and posterior putamen. This has been shown by means of a recently validated technique termed lesion network mapping whereby connectome data from 98 healthy adults were used to identify a network associated with the basal ganglia site of overlap of lesions causing HC/HB (posterior putamen) in 39 cases [9]. Some additional pathophysiological insights have come from electrophysiologic studies of patients undergoing pallidotomy for hemiballism, in which microrecording of individual neurons was obtained. The most recent report involving a patient with medication-resistant posthyperglycemic hemichorea who required pallidotomy showed GPi neuronal discharge with high frequency ($n = 14$; mean firing rate 79 Hz) resembling the firing rate of Parkinson's disease patients in OFF-medication status; and GP externus neurons with the previously described slow firing rate ($n = 3$, mean firing rate 48 Hz) [14]. In contrast, an earlier study of three patients with HB due to cerebral infarcts (2 in the STN and one more extensive [31–33]) reported firing rates of GPi neurons that were lower than expected normal values in the two cases with STN lesions, whereas the third had a rate within the normal range. However, all three demonstrated an altered firing *pattern* with intermittent bursts followed by pauses and EMG examination demonstrated that ballistic movements correlated with pauses in firing of some individual GPi neurons. This suggests that the temporal pattern of GPi neuronal activity rather than the overall rate of firing is important in hemiballism and that brief pauses in GPi firing may be responsible for the generation of ballistic movements. In line with this (and with the network hypothesis involving cortical sites), Li and Chen found that the long interval intracortical inhibition and the silent period are increased in the motor cortex contralateral to the hemichorea in hyperglycemic HC-HB, but only during muscle activation. This suggests that hemichorea-hemiballism may be associated with increased GABA-B receptor-mediated inhibitory activity in the motor cortex [34].

Prognosis

In the early literature, hemiballism was thought to carry a grave prognosis. Exhaustion and self-injury could cause significant morbidity, and at a time when medical therapy was unavailable, measures as extreme as limb amputation were sometimes considered. However, it has become clear that the natural history of hemiballism is much more benign than previously thought, and numerous effective treatments are now available. Since most cases are treated medically, the natural history of hemiballism is unknown. Most cases will resolve spontaneously, usually in a few months to a year. Hyland and Foreman presented 14 patients with hemiballism, 12 of whom had spontaneous resolution within 3 months [35] and in 11 out of 15 vascular chorea symptoms subsided in the first 2 months, sometimes as fast as 2 weeks in a more recent series [4, 16]. Similarly, 15 of 16 patients reported by Vidakovic had successful withdrawal of medication without recurrence [8] and in a series by Klawans, only 3 of 11 patients required long-term perphenazine therapy [17, 18, 36]. Ryan reported that 4/6 patients treated with neuroleptics had persistent mild chorea on treatment. They argued that our understanding of the natural history is biased by previous reports emphasizing spontaneous resolution of symptoms that failed to specify attempts to wean neuroleptic treatment [12]. Nevertheless, and as mentioned above, hemiballism associated with hyperglycemia usually improves over days. The tendency for hemiballism to spontaneously improve should be considered when planning treatment and when interpreting reports of responses to treatment in the literature.

Management

An algorithm for treating hemiballism is presented in Fig. 14.2. Given its rarity, there are no specific guidelines, and management is derived mainly from reviews of the topic and expert opinion [37]. The first priority in the management of hemiballism is to look for reversible causes. Hyperglycemia, infectious and neoplastic lesions of the basal ganglia should be excluded. Treatment of the underlying cause may reverse the hemiballism, although severely affected patients may still require concomitant pharmacologic therapy. If stroke is the cause, standard stroke management such as antiplatelet therapy and secondary preventive measures such as blood pressure control and normalization of blood sugar must be implemented. The next step is to decide whether hemiballism is severe enough to warrant therapy. As mentioned previously, many cases will be mild and the majority of these will improve spontaneously. If therapy is required, nonpharmacologic therapy, such as padding of the affected limb should be considered. In severe cases, attention should be paid to systemic complications such as exhaustion, dehydration, and rhabdomyolysis. In the very rare case of extremely severe hemiballism causing dangerous complications, patients may require sedation or even intubation with neuromuscular blockade as a temporary bridge until effective pharmacologic therapy is instituted.

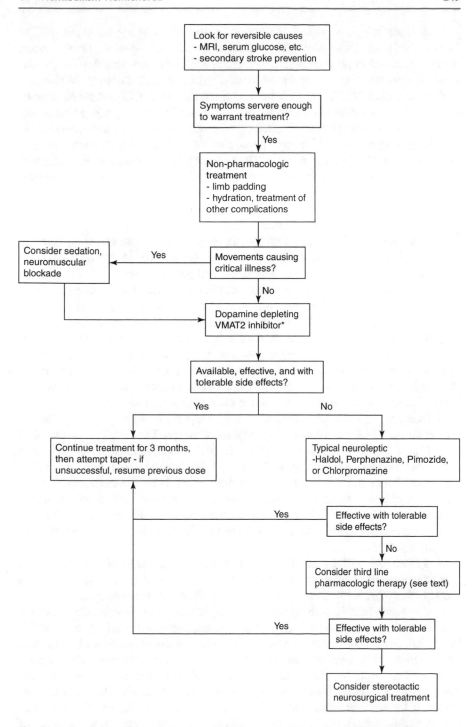

Fig. 14.2 Treatment algorithm. (Reprinted with permission from Riley and Lang [37])

Antidopaminergic therapy is the mainstay of treatment for hemiballism. The best-studied medications are typical neuroleptics such as haloperidol, perphenazine, pimozide, and chlorpromazine [36, 38]. However, dopamine-depleting drugs, particularly tetrabenazine, can also produce marked benefits similar to those obtained with neuroleptics [7, 20, 39]. Given the minimal risk of tardive dyskinesia or acute dystonic reactions associated with its use, tetrabenazine is our preferred treatment for patients with persistent hemiballism who require ongoing dopaminergic blockade. Dosage can start at 12.5 mg TID and be titrated upwards to a maximum of approximately 150–200 mg per day. The speed of the titration and the maximum dose depend on the severity of symptoms and the initial response to therapy. Clinicians should remain vigilant for the side effects of depression, orthostatic hypotension, parkinsonism, and akathisia. Blood pressure reduction may be a dose-limiting side effect if rapid titration is required for severe hemiballism. Newer dopamine-depleting drugs (i.e., VMAT-2 blockers such as valbenazine or deutetra-benazine) have also been reported beneficial in hemichorea [40], with potentially less side effects such as sedation, depression, and parkinsonism.

If dopamine depletors such as tetrabenazine are unavailable, ineffective, cause severe side effects, or if the patient has a history of severe depression, typical neuroleptics should be tried. Although there is a wide variety of neuroleptics that may work, we favor haloperidol, starting at a dose of 0.5 to 1 mg BID, and titrating upwards as needed. In emergency situations, this can be given as an intramuscular dose of 1 mg, and if ineffective, 2 mg can be given 4 hours later. If there is still no improvement, 4 mg q4 hours or even higher doses can be used, with subsequent attempts at downward titration if movements are successfully suppressed [41]. In urgent situations, tetrabenazine and haloperidol can be given together, to take advantage of their different mechanisms of action. The side effects of typical neuroleptics are well known and will not be elaborated on further. However, one somewhat unique, but not uncommon, problem encountered with dopamine antagonists in hemiballism, especially in the elderly, is the development of drug-induced parkinsonism on the nonhemiballistic side. When this problem occurs before substantial benefit to the hyperkinetic movements, one may see an impressive combination of persistent hemiballism and contralateral parkinsonism, both causing disability.

Response rates to dopamine-antagonist drugs are on the order of 90%, with quite dramatic reductions often achieved [2, 36, 38]. If typical neuroleptics fail, it is unlikely that other medications will have a dramatic effect. However, positive results have also been obtained with atypical neuroleptics such as risperidone, olanzapine, and clozapine, and with other presynaptic dopamine-depletors such as reserpine [7, 8, 19, 20]. In addition, there have been reports of effective treatment with clonazepam, valproic acid, levetiracetam, topiramate, gabapentin, trihexyphenidyl, citalopram, and amitriptyline [7, 42–45]. Although the use of amantadine has not been documented in hemiballism, its utility in chorea associated with Huntington's disease and levodopa-induced dyskinesia suggests that it may be helpful. As noted above, carotid endarterectomy may be effective for hemichorea in some cases of severe carotid stenosis [22].

If effective, treatment should be maintained for a period of approximately 3 months after which the medication should be gradually withdrawn. It is likely that the majority of patients will not have a significant recurrence. If pharmacologic therapy is ineffective and patients have severe unremitting hemiballism for at least 3 months (or shorter, if symptoms have life-threatening consequences), surgical intervention may be appropriate. The procedure with the greatest reported experience (largely in the older literature) is ventrolateral nucleus thalamotomy, with just under 30 patients reported. Here the lesion is placed in the VA/VL thalamus (the region that receives basal ganglia (GPi, SNr) outflow) in contrast to the Vim thalamotomy used for tremor (which is directed more posteriorly to areas that receive cerebellar input). Krauss and Mundinger have reported the largest series, with 13 patients followed more than 3 years [46]. Eleven of these 13 patients had significant improvement in their hemiballism. Side effects were few, with one patient suffering a transient hemiparesis, and two with mild persistent dystonia. Another good option is GPi pallidotomy, with numerous case reports of successful treatment also for posthyperglycemia patients with persistent and medication refractory chorea [6, 12–14, 22, 31, 33, 46]. No large-scale series exist to thoroughly evaluate the efficacy of this approach. Finally, with the development of deep brain stimulation (DBS) of the pallidum or thalamus, this approach has become an option for the treatment of hemiballism. This is anticipated to have clinical effects similar to lesioning. However, many of the advantages of DBS, such as the greater safety of bilateral procedures (obviously irrelevant in hemiballism), and the ability to change stimulation parameters as the disease progresses (less crucial for static processes such as those that cause hemiballism) are less important than for other conditions such as Parkinson's disease. This, in addition to the potential for long-term DBS hardware complications such as infection, breakage, and battery failure may argue for lesioning as the surgical treatment of choice in those rare patients who require surgery. Although no studies comparing thalamotomy to pallidotomy have been performed (given the rarity of persistent hemiballism, it is very unlikely that they ever will be), based on our experience with modern pallidotomy for movement disorders, including its potential and sustained effect on levodopa-induced dyskinesia [47], we would favor pallidotomy directed at the sensorimotor ventroposterior medial pallidum as the surgical treatment of choice. To date, we are not aware of reports of pallidotomy performed for HB using MRI-guided focused ultrasound; however, practical methodological issues (e.g., the need to keep the patient awake and the subsequent impact of ongoing ballism) would probably make this approach unfeasible.

Conclusion

In summary, the view of hemiballism as a disorder localized to the STN carrying a grave prognosis is incorrect. Hemiballism has a variety of causes, most commonly basal ganglia stroke and hyperglycemia. While it has a dramatic presentation, it frequently resolves spontaneously and usually responds well to dopamine antagonist treatment. Treatment complications and drug-resistant cases do occur, representing important therapeutic challenges.

References

1. Dewey RB Jr, Jankovic J. Hemiballism-hemichorea. Clinical and pharmacologic findings in 21 patients. Arch Neurol. 1989;46(8):862–7. Epub 1989/08/01.
2. Ghika-Schmid F, Ghika J, Regli F, Bogousslavsky J. Hyperkinetic movement disorders during and after acute stroke: the Lausanne Stroke Registry. J Neurol Sci. 1997;146(2):109–16. Epub 1997/03/10.
3. Pekmezovic T, Svetel M, Ristic A, Raicevic R, Ivanovic N, Smiljkovic T, et al. Incidence of vascular hemiballism in the population of Belgrade. Mov Disord. 2004;19(12):1469–72. Epub 2004/09/25.
4. Parees I, Hernandez-Vara J, Alvarez-Sabin J. Post-stroke hemichorea: observation-based study of 15 cases. Revista de neurologia. 2010;51(8):460–4. Epub 2010/10/07. Hemicorea postictus: estudio observacional de 15 casos.
5. Ristic A, Marinkovic J, Dragasevic N, Stanisavljevic D, Kostic V. Long-term prognosis of vascular hemiballismus. Stroke. 2002;33(8):2109–11. Epub 2002/08/03.
6. Chung SJ, Im JH, Lee MC, Kim JS. Hemichorea after stroke: clinical-radiological correlation. J Neurol. 2004;251(6):725–9. Epub 2004/08/18.
7. Postuma RB, Lang AE. Hemiballism: revisiting a classic disorder. Lancet Neurol. 2003;2(11):661–8. Epub 2003/10/24.
8. Vidakovic A, Dragasevic N, Kostic VS. Hemiballism: report of 25 cases. J Neurol Neurosurg Psychiatry. 1994;57(8):945–9. Epub 1994/08/01.
9. Laganiere S, Boes AD, Fox MD. Network localization of hemichorea-hemiballismus. Neurology. 2016;86(23):2187–95. Epub 2016/05/14.
10. Oh SH, Lee KY, Im JH, Lee MS. Chorea associated with non-ketotic hyperglycemia and hyperintensity basal ganglia lesion on T1-weighted brain MRI study: a meta-analysis of 53 cases including four present cases. J Neurol Sci. 2002;200(1–2):57–62. Epub 2002/07/20.
11. Su CS, Chang YY, Liu KT, Lan MY, Liu JS. Risk factors for prolonged hemichorea-hemiballism caused by hyperglycemia. Parkinsonism Relat Disord. 2012;18(1):96–8. Epub 2011/07/12.
12. Ryan C, Ahlskog JE, Savica R. Hyperglycemic chorea/ballism ascertained over 15 years at a referral medical center. Parkinsonism Relat Disord. 2018;48:97–100. Epub 2018/01/07.
13. Cosentino C, Torres L, Nunez Y, Suarez R, Velez M, Flores M. Hemichorea/Hemiballism associated with hyperglycemia: report of 20 cases. Tremor Other Hyperkinet Mov (NY). 2016;6:402. Epub 2016/08/19.
14. De Vloo P, Breen DP, Milosevic L, Lee DJ, Dallapiazza RF, Hutchison WD, et al. Successful pallidotomy for post-hyperglycemic hemichorea-ballism. Parkinsonism Relat Disord. 2019;61:228–30. Epub 2018/12/06.
15. Cherian A, Thomas B, Baheti NN, Chemmanam T, Kesavadas C. Concepts and controversies in nonketotic hyperglycemia-induced hemichorea: further evidence from susceptibility-weighted MR imaging. J Magn Reson Imaging. 2009;29(3):699–703. Epub 2009/02/27.
16. Yu F, Steven A, Birnbaum L, Altmeyer W. T2*-based MR imaging of hyperglycemia-induced hemichorea-hemiballism. J Neuroradiol. 2017;44(1):24–30. Epub 2016/11/12.
17. Hsu JL, Wang HC, Hsu WC. Hyperglycemia-induced unilateral basal ganglion lesions with and without hemichorea. A PET study. J Neurol. 2004;251(12):1486–90. Epub 2005/01/13.
18. Shan DE. Hemichorea-hemiballism associated with hyperintense putamen on T1-weighted MR images: an update and a hypothesis. Acta Neurol Taiwanica. 2004;13(4):170–7. Epub 2005/01/26.
19. Ohara S, Nakagawa S, Tabata K, Hashimoto T. Hemiballism with hyperglycemia and striatal T1-MRI hyperintensity: an autopsy report. Mov Disord. 2001;16(3):521–5. Epub 2001/06/08.

20. Maeda K, Katayama Y, Sugimoto T, Somura M, Kajino Y, Ogasawara K, et al. Activated microglia in the subthalamic nucleus in hyperglycaemic hemiballism: a case report. J Neurol Neurosurg Psychiatry. 2010;81(10):1175–7. Epub 2010/06/16.
21. Nath J, Jambhekar K, Rao C, Armitano E. Radiological and pathological changes in hemiballism-hemichorea with striatal hyperintensity. J Magn Reson Imaging. 2006;23(4):564–8. Epub 2006/03/04.
22. Galea I, Norwood F, Phillips MJ, Shearman C, McMonagle P, Gibb WR. Pearls & Oy-sters: resolution of hemichorea following endarterectomy for severe carotid stenosis. Neurology. 2008;71(24):e80–2. Epub 2008/12/10.
23. Gasca-Salas C, Lang AE. Paroxysmal Hemiballism/Hemichorea resulting from transient ischemic attacks. Mov Disord Clin Pract. 2016;3(3):303–5. Epub 2015/12/09.
24. Murakami T, Wada T, Sasaki I, Yoshida K, Segawa M, Kadowaki S, et al. Hemichorea-Hemiballism in a patient with temporal-parietal lobe infarction appearing after reperfusion by recombinant tissue plasminogen activator. Mov Disord Clin Pract. 2015;2(4):426–8. Epub 2015/07/20
25. Kujawa KA, Niemi VR, Tomasi MA, Mayer NW, Cochran E, Goetz CG. Ballistic-choreic movements as the presenting feature of renal cancer. Arch Neurol. 2001;58(7):1133–5. Epub 2001/08/02.
26. Damato V, Balint B, Kienzler AK, Irani SR. The clinical features, underlying immunology, and treatment of autoantibody-mediated movement disorders. Mov Disord. 2018;33(9):1376–89. Epub 2018/09/16.
27. Carpenter MB, Whittier JR, Mettler FA. Analysis of choroid hyperkinesia in the rhesus monkey: surgical and pharmacological analysis of hyperkinesia resulting from lesions in the subthalamic nucleus of Luys. J Comp Neurol. 1950;92:293–331.
28. Crossman AR, Sambrook MA, Jackson A. Experimental hemichorea/hemiballismus in the monkey. Studies on the intracerebral site of action in a drug-induced dyskinesia. Brain. 1984;107(Pt 2):579–96. Epub 1984/06/01.
29. DeLong MR. Primate models of movement disorders of basal ganglia origin. Trend Neurosci. 1990;13(7):281–5. Epub 1990/07/01.
30. Guridi J, Obeso JA. The subthalamic nucleus, hemiballismus and Parkinson's disease: reappraisal of a neurosurgical dogma. Brain. 2001;124(Pt 1):5–19. Epub 2001/01/03.
31. Lenz FA, Suarez JI, Metman LV, Reich SG, Karp BI, Hallett M, et al. Pallidal activity during dystonia: somatosensory reorganisation and changes with severity. J Neurol Neurosurg Psychiatry. 1998;65(5):767–70. Epub 1998/11/12.
32. Suarez JI, Metman LV, Reich SG, Dougherty PM, Hallett M, Lenz FA. Pallidotomy for hemiballismus: efficacy and characteristics of neuronal activity. Ann Neurol. 1997;42(5):807–11. Epub 1997/12/10.
33. Vitek JL, Chockkan V, Zhang JY, Kaneoke Y, Evatt M, DeLong MR, et al. Neuronal activity in the basal ganglia in patients with generalized dystonia and hemiballismus. Ann Neurol. 1999;46(1):22–35. Epub 1999/07/13.
34. Li JY, Chen R. Increased intracortical inhibition in hyperglycemic hemichorea-hemiballism. Mov Disord. 2015;30(2):198–205. Epub 2014/06/13.
35. Hyland HF, Forman D. Prognosis in hemiballismus. Neurology. 1957;7:381–91.
36. Klawans HL, Moses H 3rd, Nausieda PA, Bergen D, Weiner WJ. Treatment and prognosis of hemiballismus. N Engl J Med. 1976;295(24):1348–50. Epub 1976/12/09.
37. Riley D, Lang AE. Hemiballism in multiple sclerosis. Mov Disord. 1988;3(1):88–94. Epub 1988/01/01.
38. Johnson WG, Fahn S. Treatment of vascular hemichorea and hemiballismus with perphenazine. Trans Am Neurol Assoc. 1974;99:222–4. Epub 1974/01/01.
39. Sitburana O, Ondo WG. Tetrabenazine for hyperglycemic-induced hemichorea-hemiballismus. Mov Disord. 2006;21(11):2023–5. Epub 2006/09/21.
40. Fiedler E, Biller J. Hemichorea in a woman with diabetes. Pract Neurol. 2019;2019:44–6.
41. Ranawaya R, Lang AE. Neurological emergences in movement disorders. In: Weiner WJ, editor. Emergent and urgent neurology. 1st ed. Philadelphia: JB Lippincott; 1992. p. 277–319.

42. Marchione P, Vento C, Marianetti M, Romeo T, Amabile GA, Giacomini P. Hemiballismus in subthalamic haemorrhage: efficacy of levetiracetam. Eur J Neurol. 2009;16(6):e112–3. Epub 2009/05/21.
43. Obeso JA, Marti-Masso JF, Astudillo W, de la Puente E, Carrera N. Treatment with hemiballism with reserpine. Ann Neurol. 1978;4(6):581. Epub 1978/12/01.
44. Driver-Dunckley E, Evidente VG. Hemichorea-hemiballismus may respond to topiramate. Clin Neuropharmacol. 2005;28(3):142–4. Epub 2005/06/21.
45. Kothare SV, Pollack P, Kulberg AG, Ravin PD. Gabapentin treatment in a child with delayed-onset hemichorea/hemiballismus. Pediatr Neurol. 2000;22(1):68–71. Epub 2000/02/11.
46. Krauss JK, Pohle T, Borremans JJ. Hemichorea and hemiballism associated with contralateral hemiparesis and ipsilateral basal ganglia lesions. Mov Disord. 1999;14(3):497–501. Epub 1999/05/29.
47. Kleiner-Fisman G, Lozano A, Moro E, Poon YY, Lang AE. Long-term effect of unilateral pallidotomy on levodopa-induced dyskinesia. Mov Disord. 2010;25(10):1496–8. Epub 2010/06/23.

Sydenham's Chorea, PANDAS, and Other Post-streptococcal Neurological Disorders

15

Roser Pons

Patient Vignette

A 12-year-old boy developed hyperthyroidism secondary to Grave's disease, which was successfully treated with I-131 treatment. Several months later, pharyngeal infection with group A β-hemolytic *Streptococcus* was documented by throat culture and subsequent rise in antistreptolysin O titer. He was treated with oral antibiotics, and 2 weeks later developed insidious, progressive chorea, incoordination of the right hemibody, and imbalance. Examination revealed moderate chorea affecting the eyes, arms, and legs, incoordination of fine hand movements, motor impersistence on hand grip and tongue protrusion, and near inability to walk. He was treated with valproic acid, and his symptoms resolved within 3 weeks.

Introduction

In 1686, Thomas Sydenham described the entity that bears his name as a syndrome of involuntary, purposeless, rapid movements of the limbs accompanied by muscular weakness and emotional lability. Bouteille in 1810 and Bright in 1831 recognized the association of chorea with rheumatic fever (RF) [1]. In 1889, Cheadle described the full rheumatic syndrome of carditis, polyarthritis, chorea, subcutaneous nodules, and erythema marginatum. Subsequent epidemiological and microbiological studies

Supplementary Information The online version of this chapter (https://doi.org/10.1007/978-3-030-75898-1_15) contains supplementary material, which is available to authorized users.

R. Pons (✉)
First Department of Pediatrics, National and Kapodistrian University of Athens, Agia Sofia, Athens, Greece
e-mail: roserpons@med.uoa.gr

confirmed the link between *Streptococcus*, Sydenham's chorea, and RF. Since 1944, chorea has been included as one of the major criteria in the diagnosis of RF and its presence alone is sufficient to make the diagnosis of RF [2].

During the second half of the twentieth century, behavioral and emotional difficulties in patients with Sydenham's chorea were increasingly recognized [3]. In the 1980s, in the setting of an outbreak of group A streptococcal infection, a group of patients with acute, explosive tics and psychiatric disorders were recognized. The clinical phenotype of postinfectious immune-mediated neurobehavioral syndromes mimicking Tourette's syndrome was termed pediatric autoimmune neuropsychiatric disorders associated with streptococcal infections (PANDAS) [4].

More recently, although in a small number of patients, other post-streptococcal diseases have been reported, suggesting that the spectrum of post-streptococcal central nervous system (CNS) diseases is broader, and include a subgroup of patients with acute disseminated encephalomyelitis with basal ganglia lesions [5], acute myoclonus [6], striatal necrosis [7, 8], paroxysmal dystonic choreoathetosis [23], acute parkinsonism [1, 25], and opsoclonus myoclonus [3, 27] (Table 15.1).

In a number of patients with post-streptococcal CNS manifestations, antineuronal antibodies have been detected, supporting the hypothesis of an autoimmune pathophysiological mechanism [9, 10]. These conditions are now considered within the group of autoimmune basal ganglia disorders that are defined as autoimmune or immune-mediated conditions with predominant involvement of the basal ganglia, manifesting with movement and neuropsychiatric disturbances [9].

Clinical Features and Diagnosis

Sydenham's Chorea

Sydenham's chorea is the neurological manifestation of RF and it is a major criterion for the diagnosis of RF. When chorea occurs in isolation it is sufficient to make the diagnosis of RF [2]. Up to a quarter of acute rheumatic fever cases develop Sydenham's chorea, though this proportion varies according to temporal and geographic factors [11–14]. Usually, Sydenham's chorea begins after a prolonged latent period following group A streptococcal infection. Generally, patients develop chorea 4–8 weeks after an episode of streptococcal pharyngitis, but a delay of several months has also been described [15–17]. Chorea may begin acutely or subacutely. The age of presentation ranges from 5 to 15 years, and there is a female preponderance [6, 15–17] (see Table 15.1). The main features of Sydenham's chorea are involuntary, random, purposeless, nonrhythmic, sudden, brief movements. They flow from one body part to another, and patients often appear restless. Chorea spreads rapidly, although in 20–30% of cases it remains unilateral [11, 15, 17]. Chorea is often severe enough to be disabling, and in rare cases may prevent the patient from walking [11, 17]. Patients display motor impersistence, noticeable during tongue protrusion or with sustaining muscle contraction. Muscle tone is usually decreased. In rare cases, symptoms are so severe that the patient becomes bedridden (so-called

Table 15.1 Clinical spectrum of post-streptococcal movement disorders

	Sydenham's chorea	PANDAS	Post-streptococcal acute disseminated encephalomyelitis [5]	Post-streptococcal myoclonus [6]	Post-streptococcal isolated bilateral striatal necrosis [7, 8]	Post-streptococcal paroxysmal dystonic choreoathetosis [23]	Post-streptococcal parkinsonism [24, 25]	Post-streptococcal opsoclonus myoclonus syndrome [26, 27]
Age	5–15 years	3–8 years	3–14 years	5–12 years	1–4 years	8 years	7–17 years	10–22 years
Gender	F > M	M > F	M > F	M	M	M	M	F
Onset	Acute/subacute	Acute	Acute	Acute	Acute	Acute paroxysmal	Acute	Acute
Movement disorders	Chorea tics	Tics Choreiform Movements	Dystonia tremor Rigidity paroxysmal dystonia	Myoclonus	Dystonia rigidity Tremor chorea	Chorea dystonia	Akinetic-rigid syndrome Tremor rigidity dystonia	Opsoclonus myoclonus Ataxia
Psychiatric disorders	Emotional lability, anger OCD, anxiety, depression, ADHD	OCD, anxiety, major depression, ADHD	Emotional lability, disinhibition, perseverations, inattention, separation anxiety, confusion	Aggression, hyperactivity	Emotional lability	Immature behavior, separation anxiety, depression	NR	Insomnia, auditory hallucinations, disinhibition, anxiety, low mood
↓Level of consciousness	–	–	50%	–	25%	–	–	–
Exacerbations/recurrences	20–60%	100%	20%	33%	–	+	–	–
Heart involvement	+(up to 48%)	–	–	–	–	–	–	–
↑ASO	±	+	+	+	+	+	+	+

(continued)

Table 15.1 (continued)

	Sydenham's chorea	PANDAS	Post-streptococcal acute disseminated encephalomyelitis [5]	Post-streptococcal myoclonus [6]	Post-streptococcal isolated bilateral striatal necrosis [7, 8]	Post-streptococcal paroxysmal dystonic choreoathetosis [23]	Post-streptococcal parkinsonism [24, 25]	Post-streptococcal cpsoclonus rnyoclonus syndrome [26, 27]
Antineuronal antibodies[a]	+	+	+	NR	+	+	+	+
Brain MRI	Normal Increased BG signal Enlarged BG	Normal Enlarged BG	Basal ganglia demyelinating lesions	Normal	Striatal abnormalities	Normal	Increased BG signal Enlarged BG	Normal

PANDAS pediatric autoimmune neuropsychiatric disorder associated with streptococcal infections, *F* female, *M* male, *OCD* obsessive compulsive symptoms, *ADHD* attention deficit hyperactivity disorder, *ASO* antistreptolysin, *O* titers, *NR* not reported, *BG* basal ganglia, *MRI* magnetic resonance imaging

[a]Antineuronal antibodies reported in some patients +

paralytic chorea). Other neurological features include dysarthria, weakness, clumsy gait, hypometric saccades, and hung-up reflexes [11, 16]. Motor and vocal tics can also occur, and oculogyric crises have been reported [11].

O━━🔑 Sydenham's chorea and other post-streptococcal CNS disorders are immune-mediated conditions characterized by predominant involvement of the basal ganglia; their clinical manifestations can evolve rapidly, requiring prompt intervention.

Psychiatric symptoms are common in Sydenham's chorea. These include emotional lability, anger, distractibility, obsessive-compulsive symptoms, depression, and separation anxiety [3, 9, 18]. Clinical features of RF accompanying chorea, such as cardiac involvement, have been reported in 10–84% of patients [11, 12]. Arthritis is seen in up to 30% [11]. Sydenham's chorea is a self-limited condition, usually spontaneously remitting after 2–6 months [16, 17]. In some patients it may last up to 2 years, and in rare cases it may persist [12, 19]. Chorea may recur, and the incidence of recurrence may be as high as 20–60% [12, 17] (see Table 15.1). Recurrence may be induced by reinfection with *Streptococcus*, birth control pills, and pregnancy ("chorea gravidarum").

Diagnosis relies on clinical findings of acute chorea with a history of prior *Streptococcus* infection. Because chorea is generally a late manifestation of RF, it is unusual to find clinical evidence of acute streptococcal infection and a throat culture is positive in only a minority of cases [2, 17]. Elevated acute-phase reactants and antistreptococcal antibodies (antistreptolysin O, antiDNAse-B antibodies) are found in 15–80% of cases. CSF analysis is usually normal [17]. Cardiologic assessment is mandatory to rule out asymptomatic carditis [9]. Brain magnetic resonance imaging (MRI) is usually normal, although reversible hyperintensities in the basal ganglia have been reported, and volumetric studies have shown enlargement of the basal ganglia volume [9, 17, 18, 20, 21] (see Table 15.1). A diagnosis of Sydenham's chorea is largely presumptive in some cases based merely on the clinical manifestations of chorea in a young patient, and by the exclusion of conditions such as systemic lupus erythematosus, drug intoxication, Wilson's disease, benign hereditary chorea, and hyperthyroidism [17].

Pandas

PANDAS is a contested diagnostic entity applied to children with tics and/or obsessive-compulsive symptoms temporally linked to prior streptococcal infection. These patients show a relapsing–remitting course, often with significant psychiatric comorbidity. Clinical criteria for this condition include (1) presence of tics and/or obsessive-compulsive disorder, (2) prepubertal symptom onset, (3) episodic course of symptom severity, (4) association with group A streptococcal infections, and (5) association with neurological abnormalities [4]. In 1998, Swedo [4] reported clinical features of the first 50 patients diagnosed with PANDAS. The age of presentation ranged from 3 to 10 years, with a male preponderance. Forty-eight percent of the patients presented with acute obsessive-compulsive symptoms, and 52% presented primarily with motor and vocal tics. The severity of obsessive-compulsive symptoms and tics was moderate on average, and comorbid psychiatric symptoms were common. Patients typically presented abruptly, often in significant distress. The most prevalent psychiatric diagnoses were ADHD, affective disorders, and anxiety disorders. Choreiform movements described as small, jerky movements occurring irregularly and arrhythmically in different muscles were noted in half of the patients. No child had overt chorea [4]. The clinical course was episodic, characterized by a waxing and waning course and abrupt onset of symptoms. Symptom onset and exacerbations were temporally related to preceding streptococcal infection. Such infection was not always proven, although each child had at least one symptom exacerbation that was preceded by a documented streptococcal infection within the prior 6 weeks [4] (see Table 15.1). The diagnosis of PANDAS is based on the five inclusion criteria mentioned above. In order to prove the temporal association with *Streptococcus*, diagnostic criteria required elevation of antistreptococcal titers with onset and exacerbations, and falling titers with symptom remission [4].

Post-streptococcal Acute Disseminated Encephalomyelitis

Acute disseminated encephalomyelitis is a postinfectious or postvaccination inflammatory disease of the CNS. The pathological hallmark is scattered foci of demyelination throughout the brain and spinal cord. Various viral and bacterial pathogens have been associated with this condition [28]. A subgroup of patients with acute disseminated encephalomyelitis associated with streptococcal infections has been reported [5]. Recently, Dale [5] presented ten patients with post-streptococcal acute disseminated encephalomyelitis. Extrapyramidal manifestations were present in 50% of the patients: four had dystonia, three had axial and limb rigidity, and two had resting tremor. Behavioral problems were seen in seven patients. Streptococcal serologies were significantly elevated in all patients, and 80% showed basal ganglia lesions on neuroimaging. Thalamus, subthalamus, and substantia nigra were also involved in 60%, 30%, and 50% of the cases, respectively (see Table 15.1).

Post-streptococcal Acute Myoclonus

In 1998, three patients with acute-onset myoclonus following streptococcal infection were reported [6]. Myoclonus was generalized in two patients and segmental in another. In one patient, myoclonus was associated with behavioral change, including aggression and hyperactivity. Streptococcal serologies were elevated in all patients (see Table 15.1).

Post-streptococcal Autoimmune Dystonia with Isolated Striatal Necrosis

Bilateral striatal necrosis is an acute-onset extrapyramidal disorder that may occur following a variety of infections. Neuroimaging shows symmetric lesions in the striatum [29]. Two patients with isolated striatal necrosis occurring shortly after a streptococcal pharyngitis were reported [7]. One patient presented with an acute neurological illness with weakness, ataxia and dystonic posturing followed by rigidity and tremor, oropharyngeal incoordination and generalized chorea. The second patient presented with lethargy, episodic dystonic posturing, ataxia, and emotional lability. Cerebrospinal fluid protein concentration was elevated in both patients. Brain MRI showed selective striatal abnormalities. Streptococcal serologies were elevated and convalescent serology showed a reduction in titers (see Table 15.1). More recently, a new patient with post-streptococcal striatal necrosis has been reported. In this case the patient, a 7-year-old boy, had been previously diagnosed with Sydenham's chorea; he was managed with haloperidol and reached full remission after 10 days. He was asymptomatic for 20 days and then presented with generalized dystonia-chorea, and brain imaging showed evidence of bilateral striatal necrosis. Streptococcal serologies were elevated. CSF analysis was normal [8] (see Table 15.1).

Post-Streptococcal Paroxysmal Dystonic Choreoathetosis

There is one reported case of paroxysmal dystonic choreoathetosis occurring 1 week after a streptococcal pharyngitis [23]. This patient presented with acute onset of paroxysmal episodes of dystonic posturing, choreoathetosis, visual hallucinations, and immature behavior lasting minutes to hours. The episodes occurred several times per day, and symptoms fluctuated, lasting 6 months. Streptococcal serologies were elevated, and convalescent serologies showed a reduction in titers (see Table 15.1).

Post-streptococcal Parkinsonism

There have been two reports of acute parkinsonism precipitated by streptococcal pharyngitis. One patient was a 17-year-old boy who presented with a severe acute akinetic-rigid disorder 2 weeks after an episode of pharyngitis; anti-basal ganglia antibodies were found in the serum [24]. The second patient was a 7-year-old boy diagnosed with a streptococcal pharyngitis who presented with acute parkinsonism-dystonia, mutism, dysphagia, and incontinence. Both patients had serological evidence of a recent streptococcal infection and brain MRI showed abnormal signal and enlargement of the basal ganglia [24, 25] (see Table 15.1).

Post-streptococcal Opsoclonus-Myoclonus Syndrome

Opsoclonus-myoclonus syndrome is a rare neuroinflammatory disease of paraneo-plastic, postinfectious or idiopathic origin characterized by opsoclonus, myoclonus, ataxia, and behavioral disturbance. Two cases of post-streptococcal opsoclonus-myoclonus syndrome have also been described [26]. Both patients experienced a prodromal upper respiratory tract illness with elevated antistreptolysin O. In addi-tion to the opsoclonus-myoclonus syndrome they both presented with psychiatric disturbances. Both had evidence of anti-neuroleukin antibodies [26]. More recently, a 22-year-old girl presented with opsoclonus-myoclonus syndrome in the setting of a positive throat culture to *Streptococcus pyogenes* and elevated antistreptococcal antibodies (antistreptolysin O). In all patients, brain MRI was normal and there was no evidence of an underlying tumor [27] (see Table 15.1).

Pathophysiology

The basal ganglia are believed to be the source of the problem in Sydenham's cho-rea and other post-streptococcal movement disorders. This is supported by the known role of the basal ganglia in motor and behavior control, and by postmortem and neuroimaging studies in patients with Sydenham's chorea. Early pathological reports of Sydenham's chorea showed inflammatory changes involving the basal ganglia, and to a lesser extent, the cortex [1]. MRI has shown signal abnormalities in the striatum in some patients with Sydenham's chorea [20, 21]. Abnormal striatal spectra consistent with neuronal damage have been reported in one patient with Sydenham's chorea [21]. Volumetric studies have demonstrated enlargement of the caudate, putamen, and pallidum in patients with Sydenham's chorea and PANDAS [20, 30]. Single-photon emission computed tomography studies have revealed hyper- or hypometabolism in the basal ganglia in some patients with Sydenham's chorea [9]. Furthermore, patients with post-streptococcal acute disseminated encephalomyelitis showed basal ganglia lesions in 80% of the cases [5] and bilateral striatal lesions were noted in the patients with post-streptococcal autoimmune dys-tonia with isolated striatal necrosis [7, 8], and in the patients with acute parkinson-ism [24, 25].

Sydenham's chorea is considered the prototype autoimmune disease of CNS triggered by a streptococcal infection. Serotypes of the group A β-hemolytic *Streptococcus* are involved in RF and post-streptococcal disorders. The likely mech-anism in Sydenham's chorea involves induction of auto-antibodies against *Streptococcus* that cross-react with neuronal antigens. This is supported by the induction of such antibodies when rats are immunized with the major virulence fac-tor of group A *Streptococcus* (surface M protein) [22]. Anti-basal ganglia antibodies have been found in 45–100% of patients with Sydenham's chorea, and their levels correlate with disease activity [31, 32]. Anti-basal ganglia antibodies have also been reported in other post-streptococcal disorders, including PANDAS, acute dissemi-nated encephalomyelitis, paroxysmal dyskinesias, striatal necrosis, and acute parkinsonism [5, 7–24, 33]. Cross-reactive antibodies against brain tubulin and lysoganglioside altering cell signaling have also been identified in Sydenham's chorea [9, 10]; however, their pathogenicity has been questioned because they are not neuronal cell surface antigens [9]. More recently, dopamine receptor autoantibodies have been detected in Sydenham's chorea and their levels correlate with clinical symptoms [34]. On the other hand, the autoantibody data in PANDAS has been conflicting [9, 10], and unlike Sydenham's chorea, no correlation between the production of autoantibodies and severity of symptoms has been demonstrated, and no features of RF have been reported to date [9, 10].

Given the fact that RF and Sydenham's chorea are more common in first-degree relatives of affected patients [22], and the fact that obsessive-compulsive disorder and tics are more common in family members of PANDAS patients [4], an underlying genetic predisposition has been proposed. The B-lymphocyte marker D8/D17 has been detected in high levels in patients with RF, Sydenham's chorea, and PANDAS supporting this concept [35, 36]. The biological function of this marker remains undefined. In fact, it is fair to say that the relationship of streptococcal infection with post-streptococcal CNS syndromes other than Sydenham's is controversial. Evidence of current or recent streptococcal infection in school children in winter is common, and symptom exacerbations related to streptococcal or other infections may represent a nonspecific response to stress [7].

Treatment

The symptoms of Sydenham's chorea, PANDAS, and other post-streptococcal CNS disorders can evolve rapidly, often requiring prompt intervention. Management of post-streptococcal CNS disorders is discussed in these settings (Table 15.2): (1) symptomatic treatment of the acute movement disorder and/or psychiatric problem, (2) antibiotic therapy, and (3) immunotherapy.

Sydenham's Chorea

Symptomatic Treatment

Sedatives, anticonvulsants, and neuroleptics have been used in the symptomatic management of Sydenham's chorea [37]. Valproic acid is the anticonvulsant most widely used for the treatment of Sydenham's chorea. Several reports have shown that valproic acid is effective, at doses of 10 to 25 mg/kg/day. Patients who respond to valproic acid may show a marked reduction of involuntary movements within 1 week of treatment, although slower onset of action has also been reported [37]. Treatment is usually given for 4 to 8 weeks, although in cases where symptoms recur, patients may need to be treated for a longer period. Carbamazepine at doses of 4–15 mg/kg/day has also been reported as a successful treatment for Sydenham's chorea [37]. Neither carbamazepine nor valproic acid has been assessed in controlled trials with significant numbers of patients [37]. Because of the potential risk

Table 15.2 Treatment options reported in post-streptococcal movement disorders[a]

	Sydenham's chorea	PANDAS	Post-streptococcal acute disseminated encephalomyelitis [5]	Post-streptococcal myoclonus [6]	Post-streptococcal isolated bilateral striatal necrosis [7, 8]	Post-streptococcal paroxysmal dystonic choreoathetosis [23]	Post-streptococcal parkinsonism [24, 25]	Post-streptococcal opsoclonus myoclonus syndrome [26, 27]
Symptomatic treatment	First line: Valproic acid Carbamazepine Second line: Pimozide Haloperidol	Serotonin reuptake inhibitors Clonidine Neuroleptics	NR	NR	NR	Carbamazepine	None	None
Antibiotic therapy for streptococcal acute infection	+	+		+	+		+	+
Antibiotic therapy for prophylaxis	+	−	+	−	+	+	−	−
Immunotherapy	Steroids Immunoglobulin Plasma exchange	Plasma exchange Immunoglobulin	Steroids	NR	Steroids	NR	Steroids Immunoglobulin	Steroids

NR not reported, + antibiotic treatment was not specified in these reports, PANDAS pediatric autoimmune neuropsychiatric disorder associated with streptococcal infections

[a]Except for antibiotic prophylaxis in Sydenham's chorea, there are not routine treatment guidelines for the management of poststreptococcal movement disorders

of tardive dyskinesias, dopamine receptor blockers are typically reserved for situations when chorea is severe and refractory to other treatments. Pimozide (1–2 mg twice a day) has been very effective, often controlling chorea within a few days [37]. Haloperidol (0.025–0.05 mg/kg/day) has also been used successfully [37], although a recent study comparing valproic acid, carbamazepine, and haloperidol suggested that haloperidol was the least effective of the three agents [38]. Tetrabenazine, a dopamine receptor blocker and monoaminergic depletor, may also be useful, and has the advantage of carrying little to no risk of engendering tardive syndromes.

Antibiotic Treatment

Prevention of rheumatic recurrences against further streptococcal infections is of great importance, since up to 60% of patients with Sydenham's chorea will later develop rheumatic heart disease [37]. Penicillin is the antibiotic of choice. Monthly injections of 1.2 million U of benzathine penicillin G are recommended, although in populations where the prevalence of rheumatic fever is high, injections every 3 weeks are indicated. In areas where RF is no longer prevalent, 600,000 U of oral penicillin V twice a day or 0.5 g of sulfadiazine twice a day will suffice. Treatment is maintained for several years, generally until the age of 21 years [9]. The decision to discontinue depends on the community's rheumatogenic characteristics [37, 39].

The use of antibiotic prophylaxis in post-streptococcal CNS disorders other than Sydenham's chorea is generally not indicated.

Immunotherapy

Although immunomodulatory treatment is not routinely used in patients with Sydenham's chorea, there is evidence that this type of treatment can shorten the duration of symptoms. Corticosteroids, intravenous immunoglobulins, and plasma exchange have been used [9, 37]. Corticosteroids are the modality of immunomodulatory treatment that is more frequently used, mainly in severe cases. Variable regimen strategies have been proposed, such as prednisone 1 to 2 mg/kg/day for 10 days to 1 month, and pulses of methylprednisolone followed by steroid tapper [37]. In some patients, recurrence of chorea after discontinuation of treatment occurs and longer periods of steroid therapy are then required [40]. Although there are no guidelines for immunotherapy in Sydenham's chorea, it is considered reasonable to try a short course of steroids in severe cases in which symptoms fail to respond to conventional treatment [17]. The role of intravenous immunoglobulin for the treatment of Sydenham's chorea has been investigated. A randomized controlled study was designed to determine if intravenous immunoglobulin or plasma exchange would be superior to prednisone in decreasing the severity of chorea [41]. Although the differences between groups were not statistically significant due to small patient numbers, clinical improvements were more rapid and robust in the intravenous immunoglobulin and plasma exchange groups than in the prednisone group. So, although further studies are needed, it appears that intravenous immunoglobulin may become an alternative to steroids in the treatment of severe Sydenham's chorea [41].

Although there are no guidelines for immunotherapy in Sydenham's chorea, a course of steroids or IVIG in severe cases should be considered.

Pandas

Symptomatic Treatment

The neuropsychiatric symptoms of PANDAS at onset or during acute exacerbations may be severe. Symptomatic treatments include serotonin-specific reuptake inhibitors for obsessive-compulsive symptoms, and clonidine or neuroleptics for tics. However, often patients are refractory to treatment with standard agents [9, 42].

Antibiotic Treatment

A recent, prospective study of patients with new-onset PANDAS and documented Streptococcal infection showed that the use of penicillins or cephalosporins produced improvement of the neuropsychiatric symptoms within 5 to 21 days [42]. A double-blind crossover study comparing penicillin prophylaxis to placebo in patients with PANDAS failed, however, to show any change in symptom severity. The authors raised the possibility that failure to achieve acceptable antibiotic prophylaxis may have explained the negative results [43].

Immunotherapy

Currently, despite the debatable origin of PANDAS, an immune-mediated mechanism remains possible and consequently immunomodulatory therapy is considered in severe, impaired patients who are unresponsive to conventional neuropsychiatric approaches [9]. A double blind, randomized, placebo-controlled study compared either plasma exchange or intravenous immunoglobulins with placebo in a group of 30 patients with severe neuropsychiatric symptoms meeting criteria for PANDAS [44]. One month after treatment, patients who received plasma exchange or intravenous immunoglobulins showed significant improvement in obsessive-compulsive symptoms and psychosocial functioning. The plasma exchange group showed significant improvements in tic severity, whereas the intravenous immunoglobulin group did not. The beneficial effect was noted at the end of the first week in patients who received plasma exchange and at 3 weeks in the patients receiving intravenous immunoglobulins. Benefits of treatment were maintained at 1 year in both groups. Based on this single study, it appears that immunotherapy may be beneficial in select cases. The authors were careful to stress that their study did not provide support for generalized routine use. The decision to use immunomodulatory therapy in children is difficult, and must be balanced with the potential immediate and long-term risks of treatment.

Post-streptococcal Acute Disseminated Encephalomyelitis

Of the ten reported patients with post-streptococcal acute disseminated encephalo-myelitis, nine were treated with intravenous methylprednisolone for 3 days [5]. This was followed by rapid clinical improvement in all treated patients, and subsequent relapse in two patients several months after presentation. Patients who relapsed were given penicillin prophylaxis to minimize the occurrence of further relapses [5].

Post-streptococcal Acute Myoclonus

Two reported patients with post-streptococcal myoclonus showed resolution of their symptoms within several weeks of administration of antibiotics for streptococcal pharyngitis. A third patient did not respond to antistreptococcal antibiotic therapy or conventional treatment for myoclonus [6].

Post-streptococcal Autoimmune Dystonia with Isolated Striatal Necrosis

Of the first two reported patients with post-streptococcal striatal necrosis, one was treated with antibiotic prophylaxis and oral prednisolone with significant improvement over several weeks. The second patient was treated with antibiotics, with improvement of symptoms within a few days [7]. The more recently reported patient was treated with antibiotics and immunomodulatory treatment. He failed treatment with intravenous immunoglobulins but showed considerable improvement with pulse methylprednisolone [8].

Post-streptococcal Paroxysmal Dystonic Choreoathetosis

In the reported patient with paroxysmal dystonic choreoathetosis associated with streptococcal infection, there was no response to antibiotic prophylaxis. Chlorpromazine also failed, whereas carbamazepine decreased the number of attacks [23].

Post-streptococcal Parkinsonism

The first reported case of post-streptococcal parkinsonism was treated with high doses of intravenous steroids and immunoglobulins. He improved steadily over the following weeks and made a full recovery [24]. The second reported case was treated with antibiotics and dexamethasone, which did not prevent further deterioration. After the acute phase he improved considerably within the following 12 months [25].

Post-streptococcal Opsoclonus-Myoclonus Syndrome

The first reported cases of post-streptococcal opsoclonus-myoclonus syndrome were treated with antibiotics and steroids. One case improved steadily, while the other was resistant to the initial treatment and required prolonged steroid treatment [26]. The more recently reported patient was managed with antibiotics and monthly intravenous immunoglobulin with a favorable response [27].

○━━━▼ Management of post-streptococcal CNS disorders includes symptomatic treatment of the acute movement disorder and/or psychiatric problem, antibiotic therapy and immunotherapy.

Conclusion

Post-streptococcal movement disorders are phenomenologically varied. These illnesses often present suddenly, and it is not uncommon for them to cause significant disability. With proper management, including pharmacological intervention and immunologic modulation if needed, most patients can be effectively treated.

References

1. Jummani R, Okun M. Sydenham chorea. Neurology. 2001;58:311–3.
2. Shiffman RN. Guideline maintenance and revision; 50 years of the Jones criteria for diagnosis of rheumatic fever. Arch Pediatr Adolesc Med. 1995;149:727–32.
3. Swedo SE, Rapoport JL, Cheslow DL, Leonard HL, Ayoub EM, Hosier DM, et al. High prevalence of obsessive-compulsive symptoms in patients with Sydenham's chorea. Am J Psychiatry. 1989;146:246–9.
4. Swedo SE, Leonard HL, Garvey M, Mittleman B, Allen AJ, Perlmutter S, et al. Pediatric autoimmune neuropsychiatric disorders associated with streptococcal infections: clinical description of the first 50 cases. Am J Psychiatry. 1998;155:264–71.
5. Dale RC, Church AJ, Cardoso F, Goddard E, Cox TC, Chong WK, et al. Poststreptococcal acute disseminated encephalomyelitis with basal ganglia involvement and auto-reactive antibasal ganglia antibodies. Ann Neurol. 2001;50:588–95.
6. DiFazio MP, Morales J, Davis R. Acute myoclonus secondary to group A beta-hemolytic streptococcus infection: a PANDAS variant. J Child Neurol. 1998;13:516–8.
7. Dale RC, Church AJ, Benton S, Surtees RA, Lees A, Thompson EJ, et al. Post-streptococcal autoimmune dystonia with isolated bilateral striatal necrosis. Dev Med Child Neurol. 2002;44:485–9.

8. Canavese C, Davico C, Casabianca M, Olivieri C, Mancini S, Migliore G, et al. Bilateral stria-tal necrosis after Sydenham's chorea in a 7-year-old boy: a 2-year follow-up. Neuropediatrics. 2018;49:209–12.

9. Dale RC, Brilot F. Autoimmune basal ganglia disorders. J Child Neurol. 2012;27:1470–81.

10. Singer HS, Mascaro-Blanco A, Alvarez K, Morris-Berry C, Kawikova I, Ben-Pazi H, et al. Neuronal antibody biomarkers for Sydenham's chorea identify a new group of children with chronic recurrent episodic acute exacerbations of tic and obsessive compulsive symptoms fol-lowing a streptococcal infection. PLoS One. 2015;10:e0120499.

11. Cardoso F, Eduardo C, Silva AP, Mota CC. Chorea in fifty consecutive patients with rheumatic fever. Mov Disord. 1997;12:701–3.

12. Carapetis JR, Currie BJ. Rheumatic fever in a high incidence population: the importance of monoarthritis and low-grade fever. Arch Dis Child. 2001;85:223–7.

13. Terreri MT, Roja SC, Len CA, Faustino PC, Roberto AM, Hilario MO. Sydenham's chorea clinical and evolutive characteristics. Sao Paulo Med J. 2002;120:16–9.

14. Crealey M, Allen NM, Webb D, Bouldin A, Mc Sweeney N, Peake D, et al. Sydenham's cho-rea: not gone but perhaps forgotten. Arch Dis Child. 2015;100:1160–2.

15. Ghram N, Allani C, Oudali B, Fitouri Z, Ben BS. Sydenham's chorea in children. Arch Pediatr. 1999;6:1048–52.

16. Nausieda PA, Grossman BJ, Koller WC, Weiner WJ, Klawans HL. Sydenham chorea: an update. Neurology. 1980;30:331–4.

17. Oosterveer DM, Overweg-Plandsoen WC, Roos RA. Sydenham's chorea: a practical overview of the current literature. Pediatr Neurol. 2010;43:1–6.

18. Mercadante MT, Busatto GF, Lombroso PJ, Prado L, Rosário-Campos MC, do Valle R, et al. The psychiatric symptoms of rheumatic fever. Am J Psychiatry. 2000;157:2036–8.

19. Cardoso F, Vargas AP, Oliveira LD, Guerra AA, Amaral SV. Persistent Sydenham's chorea. Mov Disord. 1999;14:805–7.

20. Giedd JN, Rapoport JL, Kruesi MJ, et al. Sydenham's chorea: magnetic resonance imaging of the basal ganglia. Neurology. 1995;45:2199–202.

21. Castillo M, Kwock L, Arbelaez A. Sydenham's chorea: MRI and proton spectroscopy. Neuroradiology. 1999;41:943–5.

22. Dale RC. Autoimmunity and the basal ganglia: new insights into old diseases. QJM. 2003;96:183–91.

23. Dale RC, Church AJ, Surtees RA, Thompson EJ, Giovannoni G, Neville BGR. Post-streptococcal autoimmune neuropsychiatric disease presenting as paroxysmal dystonic cho-reoathetosis. Mov Disord. 2002;17:817–20.

24. McKee DH, Sussman JD. Case report: severe acute parkinsonism associated with streptococ-cal infection and antibasal ganglia antibodies. Mov Disord. 2005;20:1661–3.

25. Karagulle Kendi AT, Krenzel C, Ott FW, Brace JR, Norberg SK, Kieffer SA. Poststreptococcal dystonia with bilateral striatal enlargement: MR imaging and spectroscopic findings. AJNR Am J Neuroradiol. 2008;29:1276–8.

26. Candler PM, Dale RC, Griffin S, Church AJ, Wait R, Chapman MD, et al. Post-streptococcal opsoclonus-myoclonus syndrome associated with anti-neuroleukin antibodies. J Neurol Neurosurg Psychiatry. 2006;77:507–12.

27. Radic B, Cajic I, Petelin Gadze Z, Sulentic V, Nankovic S. A case of adult-onset poststrepto-coccal opsoclonus-myoclonus syndrome. Acta Neurol Belg. 2018;118:541–2.

28. Dale RC, de Sousa C, Chong WK, Cox TC, Harding B, Neville BG. Acute disseminated encephalomyelitis, multiphasic disseminated encephalomyelitis and multiple sclerosis in chil-dren. Brain. 2000;123:2407–22.

29. Leuzzi V, Bertini E, De Negri AM, Gallucci M, Garavaglia B. Bilateral striatal necrosis, dys-tonia and optic atrophy in two siblings. J Neurol Neurosurg Psychiatry. 1992;55:16–9.

30. Giedd JN, Rapoport JL, Garvey MA, Perlmutter S, Swedo SE. MRI assessment of children with obsessive-compulsive disorder or tics associated with streptococcal infection. Am J Psychiatry. 2000;157:281–3.

31. Husby G, van de Rijn I, Zabriskie JB, Abdin ZH, Williams RC Jr. Antibodies reacting with cytoplasm of subthalamic and caudate nuclei neurons in chorea and acute rheumatic fever. J Exp Med. 1976;144:1094–110.
32. Kotby AA, El Badawy N, El Sokkary S, Moawad H, El Shawarby M. Antineuronal antibodies in rheumatic chorea. Clin Diagn Lab Immunol. 1998;5:836–9.
33. Church AJ, Dale RC, Lees AJ, Giovannoni G, Robertson MM. Tourette's syndrome: a cross sectional study to examine the PANDAS hypothesis. J Neurol Neurosurg Psychiatry. 2003;74:602–7.
34. Ben-Pazi H, Stoner JA, Cunningham MW. Dopamine receptor autoantibodies correlate with symptoms in Sydenham's chorea. PLoS One. 2013;8(9):e73516.
35. Khanna AK, Buskirk DR, Williams RC Jr, Gibofsky A, Crow MK, Menon A, et al. Presence of a non-HLA B cell antigen in rheumatic fever patients and their families as defined by a monoclonal antibody. J Clin Invest. 1989;83:1710–6.
36. Swedo SE, Leonard HL, Mittleman BB, Allen AJ, Rapoport JL, Dow SP, et al. Identification of children with pediatric autoimmune neuropsychiatric disorders associated with streptococcal infections by a marker associated with rheumatic fever. Am J Psychiatry. 1997;154:110–2.
37. Walker KG, Wilmshurst JM. An update on the treatment of Sydenham's chorea: the evidence for established and evolving interventions. Ther Adv Neurol Disord. 2010;3:301–9.
38. Pena J, Mora E, Cardozo J, Molina O, Montiel C. Comparison of the efficacy of carbamazepine, haloperidol and valproic acid in the treatment of children with Sydenham's chorea: clinical follow-up of 18 patients. Arq Neuropsiquiatr. 2002;60:374–7.
39. Stollerman GH. Rheumatic fever in the 21st century. Clin Infect Dis. 2001;33:806–14.
40. Green LN. Corticosteroids in the treatment of Sydenham's chorea. Arch Neurol. 1978;35:53–4.
41. Garvey MA, Snider LA, Leitman SF, Werden R, Swedo SE. Treatment of Sydenham's chorea with intravenous immunoglobulin, plasma exchange, or prednisone. J Child Neurol. 2005;20:424–9.
42. Murphy ML, Pichichero ME. Prospective identification and treatment of children with pediatric autoimmune neuropsychiatric disorder associated with group A streptococcal infection (PANDAS). Arch Pediatr Adolesc Med. 2002;156:356–61.
43. Garvey MA, Perlmutter SJ, Allen AJ, Hamburger S, Lougee L, Leonard HL, et al. A pilot study of penicillin prophylaxis for neuropsychiatric exacerbations triggered by streptococcal infections. Biol Psychiatry. 1999;45:1564–71.
44. Perlmutter SJ, Leitman SF, Garvey MA, Hamburger S, Feldman E, Leonard HL, et al. Therapeutic plasma exchange and intravenous immunoglobulin for obsessive-compulsive disorder and tic disorders in childhood. Lancet. 1999;354:1153–8.

Anti-NMDA Receptor Encephalitis and Other Autoimmune and Paraneoplastic Movement Disorders

16

Jessica Panzer, Josep Dalmau, and Russell C. Dale

Patient Vignette

A 22-year-old woman, previously in excellent health, developed a subacute deterioration over several weeks characterized by progressive obtundation, decreased responsiveness, autonomic instability, and eventual respiratory insufficiency leading to ventilator support. Diffuse myoclonus and orobuccal-lingual dyskinesias were noted. Due to the recognition of the NMDA receptor antibody association with ovarian teratoma, a search for a teratoma was initiated and confirmed, with high titers of antibodies. Her hospital course was marked by months of intensive care treatment, with a persistent state of wakeful inattention, multiple medical complications, and slow improvement despite treatment with intravenous immunoglobulin (IVIG), plasmapheresis, and steroids. She was treated with rituximab, with eventual good long-term recovery.

Supplementary Information The online version of this chapter (https://doi.org/10.1007/978-3-030-75898-1_16) contains supplementary material, which is available to authorized users.

J. Panzer (Deceased)

J. Dalmau
Hospital Clinic, University Barcelona, Barcelona, Spain

University Pennsylvania, Philadelphia, PA, USA

R. C. Dale (✉)
The Children's Hospital at Westmead, University of Sydney Specialty of Child & Adolescent Health, Westmead, NSW, Australia
e-mail: Russell.dale@health.nsw.gov.au

© Springer Nature Switzerland AG 2022
S. J. Frucht (ed.), *Movement Disorder Emergencies*, Current Clinical Neurology,
https://doi.org/10.1007/978-3-030-75898-1_16

Introduction

Paraneoplastic and autoimmune mechanisms may result in movement disorders [1] and can present acutely or subacutely in previously well individuals. Paraneoplastic disorders (PNDs) occur in patients with cancer and can affect any part of the nervous system, including the basal ganglia and brainstem, causing abnormal movements. Many PNDs are immune-mediated; the patient's immune response against the cancer is misdirected against neurons, causing the syndrome. Other immune-mediated movement disorders may be post-infectious, likely triggered by molecular mimicry or other, as yet unknown, mechanisms. The etiology of many immune-mediated movement disorders however remains idiopathic, with no clear oncologic or infectious trigger [2]. There is an expanding group of syndromes that are associated with antibodies against cell surface or synaptic proteins that may cause early and prominent movement disorders [3]. Anti-NMDA receptor encephalitis is the most frequent of these disorders that may occur with or without tumor association, and although severe, may respond robustly to treatment. Because the presentation and clinical course of immune-mediated syndromes often develop quickly, and failure to diagnose can be lethal, we classify these disorders as movement disorder emergencies. This chapter focuses on anti-NMDA receptor encephalitis and other autoimmune or paraneoplastic movement disorders, with emphasis on their clinical presentations, differential diagnoses, immunological associations and antigens, and treatment strategies. Although autoantibody testing has changed the face of neurology, some neuroinflammatory syndromes with dominant movement disorders lack diagnostic biomarkers and are still recognized by their clinico-radiological syndrome, such as opsoclonus–myoclonus–ataxia syndrome and Sydenham's chorea.

General Concepts

With a few exceptions, such as the opsoclonus–myoclonus–ataxia syndrome in children with neuroblastoma, the majority of classic paraneoplastic syndromes resulting in movement disorders were until recently considered to affect adults or older individuals. This concept has changed with the discovery of several syndromes associated with antibodies against cell surface or synaptic proteins, such as NMDAR, which often affects children and young individuals. Moreover, while the patients with classical paraneoplastic antibodies to intracellular antigens (e.g., anti-Hu or CRMP5) often have limited benefit from immunotherapy or treatment of the tumor, patients with antibodies to cell surface or synaptic proteins may show dramatic responses to immunotherapy even before the tumor is identified or treated [3]. This, however, should not discourage physicians from searching for an underlying neoplasm, because if identified, removal of the tumor along with instituting immunotherapy usually expedites recovery and reduces relapses.

For most of these autoimmune encephalitic disorders (paraneoplastic or not), there is usually early evidence of cerebrospinal fluid (CSF) inflammatory changes, including lymphocytic pleocytosis and a variable increase in CSF protein concentration, IgG index, and oligoclonal bands [4]. This CSF inflammation fades over time and these parameters normalize. Therefore, CSF abnormalities and identification of antineuronal antibodies in serum or CSF are important early clues for diagnosis and treatment. Some antibodies, usually targeting intracellular antigens (Hu, CRMP5, Ma2, amphiphysin) almost always associate with cancer, and the associated neurological disorders are likely mediated by cytotoxic T-cell responses [5]. Other antibodies directed against cell surface antigens (NMDAR, LGI1) are excellent diagnostic markers of characteristic syndromes that can occur with or without tumor association, and probably result from a direct pathogenic effect of the antibodies. Of these, the most common and best studied is anti-NMDAR encephalitis [6].

General Classification

It is possible to separate the entities as follows:

Autoimmune encephalitis These disorders can be paraneoplastic but are often idiopathic or infection-provoked. Autoimmune encephalitis typically has autoantibodies which bind to the cell surface of receptors or synaptic proteins involved in neuronal function [3]. These "cell surface" autoantibodies have proven or suspected pathogenic function, and the clinical syndrome is typically reversible with immunotherapy. Examples of autoimmune encephalitis are anti-NMDAR encephalitis and LGI1 encephalitis.

Paraneoplastic encephalitis or degeneration These disorders are always paraneoplastic and associated with tumors, typically affect older people, and have autoantibody biomarkers that bind to intracellular antigens. Although these intracellular "onconeuronal" antibodies are very specific diagnostic biomarkers, they are not typically pathogenic. Instead, the neurological disease process is thought to be T-cell mediated, and these disorders are less reversible with immunotherapy. Examples include anti-Hu and anti-Yo antibody paraneoplastic disease [5].

Suspected autoimmune clinico-radiological central nervous system (CNS) syndromes Some neuroinflammatory diseases have highly specific clinical and radiological phenotypes, which support the presence of a specific adaptive autoreactive immune response against the CNS. However, no diagnostic autoantibody biomarker has been defined or proven to be pathogenic. In these syndromes, there is either an unidentified pathogenic autoantibody, or a T-cell mediated or other immune process. The diagnosis is dependent on recognition of the clinical syndrome, such as opsoclonus–myoclonus–ataxia syndrome or Sydenham's chorea. These disorders respond to immune therapy, and early treatment often improves outcomes.

In order to organize our approach, we present the syndromes in a clinical way, separating the clinical syndromes by movement disorder phenomenology:

Table 16.1 Clinical syndromes plus autoantibody associations are presented by dominant movement disorder. The autoantibodies in bold are most strongly associated with the clinical scenario

Ataxia	Chorea	Dystonia	Myoclonus	Parkinsonism	Stiff-person syndrome
Paraneoplastic cerebellar degeneration (*Yo, -Hu, −Tr, DNER, Ri*)	Autoimmune encephalitis (*NMDAR,* Neurexin3, LGI1, CASPR2, IgLON5)	Autoimmune encephalitis (*NMDAR*)	Opsoclonus myoclonus ataxia syndrome	Basal ganglia encephalitis (children)	Stiff person syndrome (*GAD65, Glycine receptor, Amphiphysin*)
Autoimmune ataxia (*GAD65,* CASPR2, GluR1)	Post-HSV autoimmune encephalitis (*NMDAR,* D2R)	Paraneoplastic dystonia (−Ri, IgLON5)	Autoimmune encephalitis (CASPR2, LGI1, glycine receptor, DPPX, IgLON5)	Paraneoplastic parkinsonism (*CRMP5,* −*Ma*)	Progressive encephalomyelitis and rigidity myoclonus (PERM) (*Glycine receptor, GAD65,* DPPX)
	Paraneoplastic chorea (*CRMP5*, Hu)			Autoimmune encephalitis (NMDAR, D2R, DPPX glycine receptor, GAD6S, LGI1, CASPR2, IgLON5)	

hyperkinetic (excess of movements) first, then hypokinetic (paucity of movements) and stiff movements second. Table 16.1 outlines this approach, including the autoantibody associations.

Anti-NMDAR Encephalitis and Other Disorders Resulting in an Excess of Movements

Anti-NMDAR Encephalitis

This disorder usually affects young women and children of both sexes [7]. This is a multistage illness that progresses from psychosis, memory deficits, seizures, and language disintegration to a state of unresponsiveness with catatonic features and autonomic and breathing instability [8]. Abnormal movements are prominent at this stage [9]. Dyskinesias are the most frequent and are observed in 80% of patients. While they may involve any part of the body, orobuccolingual dyskinesias are particularly prominent. They manifest as pouting, grimacing, tongue protrusion and rolling, palatal elevation, nares flaring, smiling-like motions, frowning, bruxism, oculogyric crisis, and forceful jaw opening and closing severe enough to cause tongue, teeth, and lip injuries [7–10]. Less commonly, chorea, ballismus, or opisthotonic postures may occur [11–13]. In adults the movement disorder is often orobuccal, whereas in children the movement disorder is more likely to be generalized. A study of the movement phenomenology in children noted that although chorea and dystonia were common, more characteristic and distinguishing features were the presence of perseverative, repetitive and stereotypical movements such as semi-purposeful touching, posturing or vocalizations [14, 15]. Likewise, vocalizations can be repetitive such as echolalia or palilalia. These hyperkinetic movements may alternate and evolve over time, with catatonia, catalepsy, dystonia, and rigidity [14–16]. Due to the initial neuropsychiatric disturbance, patients may be given antipsychotic medications and the orobuccolingual dyskinesias may be misinterpreted as tardive dyskinesias, while hyperthermia, rigidity and elevated creatinine kinase or rhabdomyolysis that can occur even in the absence of antipsychotic medication may falsely be ascribed to neuroleptic malignant syndrome [17, 18]. There is increasing evidence that antipsychotics can exacerbate rigidity or even neuroleptic malignant syndrome [18], and although antipsychotics still have a symptomatic role in the treatment of anti-NMDAR encephalitis, caution and extra monitoring is required [19]. Motor or complex seizures can occur at any time during the disease. The overlap of abnormal movements and epileptic seizures may confound recognition of the seizures, or lead to unnecessary escalation of antiepileptics for movements that are misinterpreted as seizures [7, 20].

The association of anti-NMDAR encephalitis with an underlying tumor is related to the gender and age of the patient. In adult women, over 50% have an ovarian teratoma, while only one-third of teenage girls have a proven teratoma. Girls and boys under age 14 and adult men only rarely are found to have a tumor [6, 21]. The diagnosis can be made by recognition of the characteristic and progressive clinical syndrome. Half of patients will have MRI findings that may include mild or transient T2/FLAIR signal hyperintensity in the hippocampi, cerebellum, cerebral cortex, subcortical regions, basal ganglia, or brainstem [8, 10]. The finding of CSF pleocytosis and mild fever at presentation can lead to an initial diagnosis of viral encephalitis; however, viral studies will be negative and the progression of the clinical syndrome usually points to synaptic autoimmunity as the cause [22]. Other diagnoses that may be considered include encephalitis lethargica, late-onset autism, and childhood disintegrative disorders [23]. Primary inherited dystonias, such as DYT1 dystonia or dopa-responsive dystonia, can be excluded by the typically acute-onset of symptoms in anti-NMDA receptor encephalitis, the presence of MRI changes, CSF inflammatory changes, and other associated symptoms such as encephalopathy and seizures [24]. In children with possible anti-NMDA receptor encephalitis and chorea, Sydenham's chorea (SC) may be considered. However, while patients with SC may have neuropsychiatric symptoms such as obsessive–compulsive disorder (OCD), anxiety, and paranoia [25], frank psychosis or encephalopathy is rare. SC often results in pure chorea, whereas the movement disorder of anti-NMDAR encephalitis is complex and stereotypical [14, 26]. Further, the MRI in SC is most often normal or shows only subtle basal ganglia changes [27]. As anti-NMDAR encephalitis progresses, the onset of autonomic instability and seizures also helps distinguish it.

○━━━☞ Anti-NMDAR encephalitis is associated with ovarian teratoma in half of adult women, but rarely associated with tumor in men or children.

Treatment is successful in 75% of cases and is centered on removal of any associated tumor, and immunotherapy (usually corticosteroids, IVIG, and/or plasmapheresis). Refractory patients may respond to cyclophosphamide or rituximab [6, 28, 29]. Increasingly rituximab is favored over cyclophosphamide. Less than a quarter of patients may experience relapses, particularly those without a tumor or those who receive suboptimal immunotherapy. The rate of relapses has reduced since the initial descriptions, possibly related to increasing use of immunotherapy including rituximab. Relapse may occur months or years after initial recovery [8, 10]. Relapse presentations are typically more limited, with isolated symptoms or with partial aspects of the full-blown syndrome. Treatment of the first episode with immunotherapy reduces the risk of relapse [29, 30, 31]. Since the descriptions of anti-NMDAR encephalitis, there have been a number of other much rarer autoantibodies associated with anti-NMDAR-like encephalitis (see Table 16.1) [32].

Anti-NMDAR Encephalitis After Herpes Simplex Encephalitis

It has been recognized for decades that during the recovery phase after herpes simplex encephalitis, some patients appear to go into a "deteriorating second phase," often approximately 2–4 weeks after the herpes simplex encephalitis [33]. Rather than being typical of the first phase (seizures, encephalopathy with radiological cortical often temporal lobe encephalitis), the second phase is often characterized by evolving movement disorders often with worsening encephalopathy, psychiatric features, and often a "leukoencephalopathy" on MRI [34]. The movement disorder is similar to the movement disorder described in "idiopathic and paraneoplastic" anti-NMDAR encephalitis, with chorea and dystonia in young children being typical. In the first phase, there is evidence of herpes simplex virus (HSV) replication in CSF, but in the second phase instead there is production of NMDAR antibodies in CSF (and serum). Termed post-HSV chorea, and suspected to be autoimmune for some time, only recently have reports confirmed that the second phase is an autoimmune complication of HSV encephalitis, and in most instances the autoantibodies are NMDAR antibodies [35–38]. A recent study from Spain showed that autoimmune encephalitis complicates 27% of HSV encephalitis [38]. The discovery of autoimmune encephalitis after infectious encephalitis is important for two reasons. First, this description recognizes that a destructive inflammatory encephalitis can induce a secondary autoimmune process, and therefore increases our understanding about the origins of autoimmunity. Second, this syndrome is treatable with immunotherapy. Although there remain some concerns about treating a complication of an infectious encephalitis with immune suppression, the literature seems to demonstrate that immunotherapy including with rituximab and cyclophosphamide is needed to treat post-HSV anti-NMDAR encephalitis, similar to idiopathic and paraneoplastic anti-NMDAR encephalitis [34].

Paraneoplastic Chorea and CRMP5 Antibodies

Choreic movements can occur in association with antibodies to collapsin response mediator protein 5 (CRMP5, also termed CV2). When these antibodies are found, the disorder is almost always paraneoplastic and the chorea is part of a diffuse encephalomyelitis that may include limbic encephalitis, cerebellar ataxia, peripheral neuropathy, uveitis, optic neuritis, or retinitis [39–41]. The most commonly associated tumors are small cell lung cancer and thymoma [42]. In these patients, brain MRI often shows abnormal FLAIR hyperintensities involving limbic regions, striatum, basal ganglia, brainstem, or white matter, which may resemble a leukoencephalopathy [43]. The associated neurological symptoms and MRI findings help to exclude many of the genetic causes of chorea such as Huntington's disease, neuroacanthocytosis, and Wilson's disease. Inflammatory causes of chorea such as systemic lupus erythematosus (SLE) or antiphospholipid antibody syndrome (APS) should be considered and might prove more difficult to exclude, since these disorders may present with chorea and other neuropsychiatric symptoms prior to any other systemic manifestations [2]. Discovery of the underlying tumor or appropriate serologic testing to screen for SLE/APS should clarify the diagnosis.

CRMP5 is an intracellular antigen that regulates neurite outgrowth, neuronal polarity, and dendritic branching in the developing brain [44, 45]. CRMP5 expression is seen within almost all high-grade neuroendocrine lung tumors, including SCLC, but not in other lung tumors [46]. Exposure to this tumor antigen likely results in an immune response against CRMP5 expressed in brain. The management of paraneoplastic chorea focuses on treatment of the tumor and, since the autoantigen is intracellular, immunotherapy targeting T-cell-mediated mechanisms. Antibodies against CRMP5 may modify progression of the underlying oncologic disease; median survival is longer in patients with SCLC and anti-CRMP5 related encephalitis as compared to those patients with SCLC and anti-Hu related encephalitis, independent of the severity of the neurologic disease [47].

Pseudoathetoid Movements in Paraneoplastic Sensory Neuronopathy

Paraneoplastic sensory neuronopathy (PSN) may develop in isolation but is most often a fragment of paraneoplastic encephalomyelitis. Patients typically develop asymmetric pain and paresthesias that progress to involve other extremities, and sometimes the trunk or cranial nerves. Eventually the severe involvement of all modalities of sensation results in dystonic or pseudoathetotic postures as well as a debilitating sensory ataxia [4]. Although not a "subcortical movement disorder," PSN can result in a movement disorder due to peripheral nerve sensory dysfunction and should be considered in the diagnostic workup of acquired movement disorders.

Patients who develop PSN alone or as a component of paraneoplastic encephalomyelitis often have anti-Hu antibodies, and the associated cancer is almost always a SCLC, although other cancers (e.g., non-SCLC or breast carcinomas) may be found especially in those patients with PSN without anti-Hu antibodies [48, 49]. The pathological substrate is an immune-mediated degeneration of the neurons of the dorsal root ganglia, likely caused by cytotoxic T-cells. The sensory neuronopathy may mimic disorders such as Guillain–Barré syndrome, particularly if there is also involvement of lower motor neurons and peripheral nerves [50]. PSN is poorly responsive to treatment and at best, patients will stabilize or have mild improvement after oncologic and immunologic therapies [51]. In some patients, rituximab has been effective [52].

Opsoclonus–Myoclonus–Ataxia Syndrome

Opsoclonus is characterized by involuntary, arrhythmic, chaotic, multidirectional saccades without intersaccadic intervals. When paraneoplastic, opsoclonus is variably associated with encephalitis, myoclonus, and ataxia of the trunk and limbs (opsoclonus–myoclonus–ataxia syndrome, OMAS) and most commonly occurs in children between 6 months and 6 years of age [53, 54]. Half of these children will be found to have an associated neuroblastoma. In adults, the tumors more frequently associated include SCLC and breast or ovarian cancer. Other than a small subset of patients with breast or ovarian cancer who develop Ri antibodies [55], OMAS has not been consistently associated with any specific antineuronal antibody. Recent studies have suggested possible association with glutamate receptor delta 2 autoantibodies [56], but these findings have not been reproduced [57], and most patients do not have antibodies binding to the cell surface of neurons [58]. The differential diagnosis includes post-infectious cerebellitis, toxic ingestions, and posterior fossa tumors [59]. OMAS can be distinguished from cerebellitis by the presence of opsoclonus and the lack of symptomatic improvement within the expected time-frame. Early recognition of OMAS in children is important, because delay in the initiation of immunomodulatory treatment has been shown to increase long-term neurological deficits [60]. In adults, other degenerative or inflammatory causes of ataxia should be considered, but the presence of opsoclonus is relatively specific for this disease.

Treatment of OMAS in children involves resection of the neuroblastoma, if present, and immunotherapy, including corticosteroids, ACTH, IVIG, plasmapheresis, rituximab, or cyclophosphamide [61, 62]. Several case series suggest that high-dose pulsed dexamethasone therapy may be beneficial [62, 63]. Although the opsoclonus and ataxia often improve or resolve, children are frequently left with motor, speech, behavioral, and sleep disorders. Relapses are frequent, usually during intercurrent illnesses or attempts to reduce immunotherapy; few children have a monophasic disease course [64]. In general, the therapeutic aims should be to induce a complete remission and avoid relapses, as ongoing symptoms suggest ongoing brain injury including cognitive decline (an insidious dementia) [65]. In adults with idiopathic OMAS, corticosteroids or IVIG can accelerate improvement, but those with paraneoplastic disease only benefit from immunotherapy if the tumor is controlled [66].

⚬━━▼ Half of children presenting with OMAS will be found to have an underlying neuroblastoma.

Sydenham's Chorea

Despite Sydenham's chorea being described four centuries ago, there is still a paucity of understanding about the precise immune mechanism. Sydenham's chorea is the prototypic autoimmune chorea syndrome and is part of the post-streptococcal rheumatic fever spectrum. Unlike anti-NMDAR encephalitis which has an extremely complex and often evolving movement phenotype, Sydenham's chorea results in a pure chorea, usually bilateral but sometimes unilateral [14]. Orobuccal involvement with dysarthria is typical, and emotional plus behavioral phenotypes are expected. By contrast, frank encephalopathy and seizures do not occur and suggest alternative diagnoses such as anti-NMDAR encephalitis. Investigation for streptococcal infection is often positive, and another organ involvement (cardiac) is mandatory. CSF and MRI are typically non-contributory. Despite the fact that rheumatic fever is clearly a post-infectious autoimmune multi-organ disorder, there is no convincing diagnostic biomarker for Sydenham's chorea. Although many autoantibodies have been described, none fulfill pathogenic criteria [67]. Although the clinical course is often one of the improvements within a few months, 50% of patients will have minor residual chorea at 2 year follow-up [68], neuropsychiatric sequelae are common and estrogen-induced chorea (chorea gravidarum or triggered by oral contraceptive pill) suggests that Sydenham's chorea results in permanent alteration to the brain in many patients [69]. Therefore, it is some clinicians' practice to use a pulse of corticosteroids or intravenous immunoglobulin, which empirically certainly improves symptoms in the short term, and may improve outcomes at 1 year. Long-term outcomes are lacking for this to be a standard of care at this time [70, 71].

Myoclonic-Like Movements in Patients with LGI1 Antibodies

LGI1 antibodies have been found to be one of the main autoantigens associated with limbic encephalitis previously attributed to VGKC antibodies. Patients with these antibodies develop limbic encephalitis that at least in 40% of cases is preceded or accompanied by myoclonic-like movements [72]. These movements are brief, short-lasting and repetitive, and can involve face, arm, or leg, often predominating in face and arm. They can occur many times per day (in some patients 80–100 times) and have been described as "twitches," "myoclonus," or "stereotyped brief monomorphic movements" [73]. These movements are highly stereotypical and "shock-like" and have been described as "faciobrachiodystonic" seizures, which describes the facial and limb posture, which is repetitive and stereotypical and short-lived (mycolonic/dystonic) [74]. The exact etiology of these episodes has been discussed—whether they represent movement disorders or seizures has been argued, but their stereotypical nature makes seizure the best description. Studies using continuous video EEG recordings have demonstrated that these movements are preceded by approximately 500 ms of electrodecremental events, typical of epileptic tonic seizures [75]. Using functional brain imaging, basal ganglia dysfunction was demonstrated in five of eight patients [76]. Recognition of the epileptic origin of these "myoclonic-like" movements is important because they usually precede the development of a full-blown limbic encephalitis associated with LGI1 antibodies, and usually respond to immunotherapy. Therefore, early identification and treatment with immunotherapy can prevent cognitive decline. Although FBDS and LGI1 encephalitis appears to be a steroid-responsive and sometimes steroid-dependent condition, other immune therapy such as rituximab appears to also have effect and utility [77].

LGI1 encephalitis presenting with fasciobrachiodystonic seizures is a pathognomic entity that warrants immediate immunosuppressive treatment.

Tremor and Ataxia in Paraneoplastic Cerebellar Degeneration

Paraneoplastic cerebellar degeneration (PCD) is characterized by the acute to subacute development of severe pancerebellar dysfunction. In adults the rapidity of onset distinguishes PCD from inherited or neurodegenerative causes of cerebellar ataxia [78]. The disorder usually develops over days or weeks, but in some instances, it has developed overnight, clinically suggesting a stroke. PCD has mostly been reported in association with gynecologic tumors, breast cancer, lung cancer (particularly SCLC), and Hodgkin's lymphoma. While almost all known paraneoplastic antibodies have been found in association with PCD, the most commonly associated are anti-Yo (also called PCA-1) in patients with breast or ovarian cancer [79], anti-Tr in patients with Hodgkin's lymphoma [80], and antibodies to voltage-gated calcium channels (VGCC) in patients with SCLC [81]. Patients with Hodgkin's lymphoma can also develop cerebellar degeneration in association with antibodies against mGluR1 [82].

As with all paraneoplastic neurologic disorders, the best approach to treatment of PCD is identification and treatment of the underlying cancer and possibly immunotherapy. Except for some patients with Hodgkin's lymphoma and Tr or mGluR1 antibodies who may respond to treatment, most patients with PCD are refractory to treatment, suggesting that there is early and irreversible neuronal cell death [83, 84]. This is supported by autopsy studies demonstrating extensive loss of Purkinje neurons with relative preservation of other cerebellar neurons.

Disorders Resulting in a Paucity of Movement or Stiffness

Anti-Ma2 Encephalitis and Hypokinesis

Anti-Ma2 encephalitis is paraneoplastic and commonly occurs in young men with testicular tumors [85]. A few cases have been described in older men and women with lung or breast cancer [86]. In addition to short-term memory loss from limbic encephalitis, these patients also have involvement of the hypothalamus and brainstem leading to disorders of sleep and wakefulness such as hypersomnia or narcolepsy-cataplexy, hyperthermia, hyperphagia, and hypothalamic–pituitary dysfunction [86]. Parkinsonian features are prominent, including bradykinesia, masked facies, hypophonia, and rigidity; less frequently, tremor is present. Dyskinesias may also occur, including forceful jaw opening and closure, and oculogyric crisis [87]. Rostrocaudal brainstem involvement often leads to progressive ophthalmoparesis, cranial neuropathies, and ataxia. Early eye movement deficits include vertical gaze paresis predominantly involving saccades, with relative preservation of pursuit and oculocephalic movements [88]. The facial and eye movement abnormalities can be confused with progressive supranuclear palsy or Whipple's disease [89]. Neuroimaging can be helpful, as half of patients with anti-Ma2 encephalitis will have FLAIR/T2 hyperintensities in the medial temporal lobes, hypothalamus, thalamus, or upper brainstem, at times with contrast enhancement [86, 87]. The parkinsonian features may respond to carbidopa/levodopa, and the facial dystonia usually improves with muscle relaxants or botulinum toxin injections [90]. However, all efforts should be made to identify and treat the underlying tumor, as this is critical to improving outcome. Case series have shown that 35% of patients will improve after tumor treatment and immunotherapy, while immunotherapy in the absence of tumor treatment is ineffective [86, 91].

⚷ Consider anti-Ma encephalitis and testicular tumor in a young man with subacute parkinsonism.

Basal Ganglia Encephalitis

An important but rare syndrome that appears to affect children and young adults is an acute onset inflammatory syndrome selectively affecting the striatum, best called basal ganglia encephalitis. In contrast to acute disseminated encephalomyelitis, which results in encephalopathy, motor deficits and disseminated inflammatory lesions affecting the white matter and gray matter, basal ganglia encephalitis results in a specific dystonic-akinetic syndrome and selective basal ganglia inflammatory lesions [92]. The clinical syndrome is characterized by an acute onset dystonia or akinesia, with associated behavioral change. MRI imaging in more than 50% of patients shows bilateral inflammatory lesions of the caudate and putamen, without involvement of the thalamus or white matter (Fig. 16.1). This symmetrical striatal inflammation associated with dystonia-akinesia is an important clinico-radiological syndrome as early use of high-dose corticosteroids can reduce inflammation and prevent cellular loss and striatal atrophy with associated cognitive and inattentive deficits on follow-up [93]. Intravenous immunoglobulin and plasma exchange should be used if corticosteroids do not produce benefit in the first days of treatment. CSF demonstrates pleocytosis or oligoclonal bands in some patients. Suspicion of the autoimmune nature of this entity is supported by the presence of dopamine-2 receptor autoantibodies in the serum of some patients [92].

Fig. 16.1 A 4-year-old boy with acute onset dystonia, rigidity, and akinesia. Axial T2-weighted MRI shows a specific localized inflammation of the caudate and putamen. High-dose methylprednisolone resulted in improvement within 2 weeks. He has been left with some residual mild upper limb dystonia

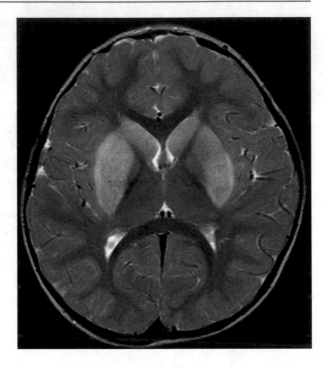

Acute-onset akinesia or dystonia in a young child with striatal lesions warrants immunomodulatory treatment of basal ganglia encephalitis.

Stiff-Person Syndrome

Progressive muscle stiffness, aching, muscle spasms, and rigidity characterize this syndrome. Symptoms develop over months and are most prominent in the paraspinal muscles and lower limbs. The majority of cases (about 85%) are idiopathic and not associated with cancer [94]. These patients usually have antibodies against glutamic acid decarboxylase 65 (GAD65). GAD65 antibodies can occur also in patients with cerebellar ataxia and refractory epilepsy, which may overlap with SPS and rarely, are found in patients with paraneoplastic SPS, most often in association with thymoma [95]. Additionally, patients with SPS and anti-GAD65 antibodies may also have antibodies against GABA$_A$-receptor-associated protein (GABARAP), suggesting that both antibodies may play a role in the disorder [96].

When SPS is paraneoplastic the tumors more frequently found are SCLC and breast cancer. These patients will often have antibodies to amphiphysin. Compared to the idiopathic form of SPS, patients with paraneoplastic SPS are older and more likely to have asymmetric and distal symptoms [97, 98]. SPS and mediastinal cancer can also have antibodies against gephyrin, a cytosolic protein associated with

GABA$_A$ and glycine receptors [99]. Progressive encephalomyelitis with rigidity and myoclonus (PERM) is likely related to SPS and is characterized by diffuse rigidity, painful spasms, and myoclonus. Antibodies against the α1 subunit of the glycine receptor have been reported in some of these patients as well as in patients with hyperekplexia, and atypical stiff-person or stiff-limb syndrome without GAD65 antibodies [100, 101]. Subsequent studies have found the spectrum of neurological disease associated with glycine receptor antibodies to be broad, beyond PERM, including optic neuritis and epilepsy, questioning the pathogenic and specific nature of these antibodies [102–104].

For the non-paraneoplastic disorder, IVIG has been shown to be beneficial [105], but this remains unproven for the paraneoplastic syndrome. Paraneoplastic SPS should be managed by treatment of the underlying cancer and corticosteroids. Additional immunotherapy such as IVIG or cyclophosphamide can be considered in refractory cases, given that similar immunotherapies are used for other autoimmune encephalomyelitis [106]. Symptomatic improvement is provided by drugs that enhance GABAergic transmission such as diazepam, baclofen, sodium valproate, tiagabine, and vigabatrin [107].

Peripheral Nerve Hyperexcitability

Peripheral nerve hyperexcitability (PNH, also called acquired neuromyotonia or Isaacs' syndrome) results from spontaneous and continuous muscle fiber activity due to peripheral nerve dysfunction [108]. Patients develop muscle cramps, stiffness, muscle twitching, and pseudomyotonia. Other related symptoms include hyperhidrosis, fatigue, and exercise intolerance. Symptoms are most prominent in the calves, legs, and trunk, but can also affect other body parts including the face and neck. At least a third of those affected also experience paresthesias. Approximately 25% of patients with PNH have CNS symptoms (Morvan's syndrome) including confusion, mood changes, sleep disruption, and hallucinations [109].

In most cases, PNH has a non-paraneoplastic etiology. In addition to idiopathic cases, there are inherited causes of neuromyotonia such as that associated with voltage-gated potassium-channel (KCNA1) gene mutations. Multiple toxins, including gold, oxaliplatin, penicillamine, herbicides, insecticides, and toluene may also cause neuromyotonia [110]. Patients with non-paraneoplastic PNH may have other autoimmune disorders, including myasthenia gravis, diabetes mellitus, chronic inflammatory demyelinating neuropathy, rheumatoid disease, systemic lupus erythematosus, and vitiligo [110, 111]. When paraneoplastic, the most commonly associated cancers are thymoma and SCLC [112]. In one series, patients with paraneoplastic PNH tended to be older and have more weakness and myokymia but less cramping and dysautonomia than those with non-paraneoplastic PNH [113].

Antibodies in PNH and Morvan's syndrome target the autoantigen contactin-associated protein-like 2 (CASPR2) [72, 114, 115]. The remaining cases are considered antibody negative at this time, although further studies may identify specific antibody associations. Recognition of this disorder is important because patients respond to immunotherapy. LGI1 and CASPR2 antibodies are the main autoantibodies previously attributed to VGKC antibodies [116]. LGI1 antibodies are most strongly associated with the "central" limbic encephalitis syndrome with FBDS, whereas CASPR2 antibodies are more strongly associated with peripheral neuromyotonia and Morvan's syndrome, although there is significant overlap and both are now recognized as important causes of autoimmune pain and seizures, in addition to the PNH [116].

Other than oncologic therapy when appropriate, treatment recommendations for PNH have reported response to plasmapheresis, IVIG, and prednisolone with or without steroid-sparing agents [116]. Some patients have had symptomatic improvement with carbamazepine or phenytoin [117].

General Management Considerations

When a paraneoplastic movement disorder is suspected the first concern should be the diagnosis and treatment of the underlying tumor, as this offers the best chance for stabilization or improvement of the neurologic disorder [118]. For some disorders associated with antibodies to intracellular antigens (Hu, CRMP5, Ma2, amphiphysin), the search for a tumor should be aggressive and tumor screenings should be repeated regularly, every 6 months for at least 2 years. Moreover, the immunotherapy strategy for these disorders should consider that they are mediated by T-cells (amphiphysin may be an exception). Therefore, IVIG and plasma exchange usually fail in the treatment of the associated syndromes, and more aggressive immunotherapies, including rituximab (to reduce antigen presentation by B-cells) or cyclophosphamide should be promptly considered. Except for Ma2-associated encephalitis, which associates with improvement in ~30% of the patients [86], the other disorders have limited response to treatments. Although GAD65 is an intracellular antigen, the related symptoms of the stiff-person syndrome (but less frequently cerebellar ataxia) may respond to IVIG [105]. Antibodies to amphiphysin may have a direct effect on the target antigen [119], but in many patients the response to plasma exchange or IVIG is unsatisfactory. The titers of most antibodies against intracellular antigens (except GAD65 and amphiphysin, which are located close to the cell surface) do not correlate well with the outcome of the disease.

In contrast, the disorders associated with antibodies against cell surface or synaptic extracellular epitopes (e.g., anti-NMDAR encephalitis or LGI1 encephalitis) are more responsive to immunotherapy. Patients who do not improve with first-line immunotherapies such as corticosteroids, IVIG or plasma exchange, often improve with rituximab or cyclophosphamide [31]. For anti-NMDAR encephalitis there is evidence of a rapid and robust intrathecal synthesis of antibodies and intracerebral infiltrates of plasma cells, which probably explain the failure of plasma exchange, IVIG, and corticosteroids in some of these patients, particularly those with delayed diagnosis and treatment [29, 31]. Nevertheless, these patients often improve with cyclophosphamide and rituximab [29, 31]. Overall, 75–80% of patients with syndromes related to cell surface antigens (NMDAR, LGI1, Caspr2) substantially improve or fully recover with immunotherapy and treatment of the tumor when appropriate [3, 6, 31, 116]. As expected for antibodies with a potential pathogenic effect, the change of titers of these antibodies correlates well with the course of the disease; in some disorders, such as anti-NMDAR encephalitis, the CSF titers have better clinical correlation than serum titers.

Other than immunotherapy, symptomatic therapy should also be considered. For example, symptomatic management of movement disorders in anti-NMDAR encephalitis can be challenging, and conventional movement disorder drugs such as L-dopa, antipsychotics, tetrabenazine, and anticholinergics are often unhelpful. Instead prioritizing inducing sleep and sedating agents are often more successful such as alpha-agonists, benzodiazepines, or sedating anti-histamines [19]. Muscle stiffness and rigidity may respond to pharmacologic treatment with GABAergic drugs, while muscle cramps and pseudomyotonia may respond to anticonvulsants that block sodium channels [107]. Although there is limited experience, some patients with anti-Ma2 or NMDA receptor encephalitis with involuntary forceful movements of the jaw that precluded feeding or carried the risk of tongue and mouth injuries benefited from local application of botulinum toxin [120].

Acknowledgments The first edition of this chapter was drafted by the late Jessica Panzer, with co-authorship by Josep Dalmau; the second edition of this chapter was updated by Russell Dale in 2021.

References

1. Grant R, Graus F. Paraneoplastic movement disorders. Mov Disord. 2009;24:1715–24.
2. Panzer J, Dalmau J. Movement disorders in paraneoplastic and autoimmune disease. Curr Opin Neurol. 2011;24(4):346–53.
3. Lancaster E, Martinez-Hernandez E, Dalmau J. Encephalitis and antibodies to synaptic and neuronal cell surface proteins. Neurology. 2011;77:179–89.
4. Psimaras D, Carpentier AF, Rossi C. Cerebrospinal fluid study in paraneoplastic syndromes. J Neurol Neurosurg Psychiatry. 2010;81:42–5.
5. Tuzun E, Dalmau J. Limbic encephalitis and variants: classification, diagnosis and treatment. Neurologist. 2007;13:261–71.
6. Dalmau J, Lancaster E, Martinez-Hernandez E, Rosenfeld MR, Balice-Gordon R. Clinical experience and laboratory investigations in patients with anti-NMDAR encephalitis. Lancet Neurol. 2011;10:63–74.
7. Florance-Ryan N, Dalmau J. Update on anti-*N*-methyl-d-aspartate receptor encephalitis in children and adolescents. Curr Opin Pediatr. 2010;22:739–44.
8. Dalmau J, Gleichman AJ, Hughes EG, Rossi JE, Peng X, Lai M, et al. Anti-NMDA-receptor encephalitis: case series and analysis of the effects of antibodies. Lancet Neurol. 2008;7:1091–8.
9. Kleinig TJ, Thompson PD, Matar W, Duggins A, Kimber TE, Morris JG, et al. The distinctive movement disorder of ovarian teratoma-associated encephalitis. Mov Disord. 2008;23:1256–61.
10. Irani SR, Bera K, Waters P, Zuliani L, Maxwell S, Zandi MS, et al. *N*-methyl-d-aspartate antibody encephalitis: temporal progression of clinical and paraclinical observations in a predominantly non-paraneoplastic disorder of both sexes. Brain. 2010;133:1655–67.

11. Iizuka T, Sakai F, Ide T, Monzen T, Yoshii S, Iigaya M, et al. Anti-NMDA receptor encephalitis in Japan: long-term outcome without tumor removal. Neurology. 2008;70:504–11.
12. Tonomura Y, Kataoka H, Hara Y, Takamure M, Naba I, Kitauti T, et al. Clinical analysis of paraneoplastic encephalitis associated with ovarian teratoma. J Neuro-Oncol. 2007;84:287–92.
13. Koide R, Shimizu T, Koike K, Dalmau J. EFA6A-like antibodies in paraneoplastic encephalitis associated with immature ovarian teratoma: a case report. J Neuro-Oncol. 2007;81:71–4.
14. Mohammad SS, Fung VS, Grattan-Smith P, Gill D, Pillai S, Ramanathan S, et al. Movement disorders in children with anti-NMDAR encephalitis and other autoimmune encephalopathies. Mov Disord. 2014;29(12):1539–42.
15. Baizabal-Carvallo JF, Stocco A, Muscal E, Jankovic J. The spectrum of movement disorders in children with anti-NMDA receptor encephalitis. Mov Disord. 2013;28(4):543–7.
16. Rubio-Agusti I, Dalmau J, Sevilla T, Burgal M, Beltran E, Bataller L. Isolated hemidystonia associated with NMDA receptor antibodies. Mov Disord. 2011;26:351–2.
17. Sansing LH, Tuzun E, Ko MW, Baccon J, Lynch DR, Dalmau J. A patient with encephalitis associated with NMDA receptor antibodies. Nat Clin Pract Neurol. 2007;3:291–6.
18. Lejuste F, Thomas L, Picard G, Desestret V, Ducray F, Rogemond V, et al. Neuroleptic intolerance in patients with anti-NMDAR encephalitis. Neurol Neuroimmunol Neuroinflamm. 2016;3(5):e280.
19. Mohammad SS, Jones H, Hong M, Nosadini M, Sharpe C, Pillai SC, et al. Symptomatic treatment of children with anti-NMDAR encephalitis. Dev Med Child Neurol. 2016;58(4):376–84.
20. Bayreuther C, Bourg V, Dellamonica J, Borg M, Bernardin G, Thomas P. Complex partial status epilepticus revealing anti-NMDA receptor encephalitis. Epileptic Disord. 2009;11:261–5.
21. Florance NR, Davis RL, Lam C, Szperka C, Zhou L, Ahmad S, et al. Anti-N-methyl-d-aspartate receptor (NMDAR) encephalitis in children and adolescents. Ann Neurol. 2009;66:11–8.
22. Gable MS, Gavali S, Radner A, Tilley DH, Lee B, Dyner L, et al. Anti-NMDA receptor encephalitis: report of ten cases and comparison with viral encephalitis. Eur J Clin Microbiol Infect Dis. 2009;28:1421–9.
23. Dale RC, Irani SR, Brilot F, Pillai S, Webster R, Gill D, et al. N-methyl-d-aspartate receptor antibodies in pediatric dyskinetic encephalitis lethargica. Ann Neurol. 2009;66:704–9.
24. Ozelius LJ, Lubarr N, Bressman SB. Milestones in dystonia. Mov Disord. 2011;26:1106–26.
25. Ridel KR, Lipps TD, Gilbert DL. The prevalence of neuropsychiatric disorders in Sydenham's chorea. Pediatr Neurol. 2010;42:243–8.
26. Varley JA, Webb AJS, Balint B, Fung VSC, Sethi KD, Tijssen MAJ, et al. The movement disorder associated with NMDAR antibody-encephalitis is complex and characteristic: an expert video-rating study. J Neurol Neurosurg Psychiatry. 2019;90(6):724–6.
27. Cardoso F, Eduardo C, Silva AP, Mota CC. Chorea in fifty consecutive patients with rheumatic fever. Mov Disord. 1997;12:701–3.
28. Ishiura H, Matsuda S, Higashihara M, Hasegawa M, Hida A, Hanajima R, et al. Response of anti-NMDA receptor encephalitis without tumor to immunotherapy including rituximab. Neurology. 2008;71:1921–3.
29. Titulaer MJ, McCracken L, Gabilondo I, Armangue T, Glaser C, Iizuka T, et al. Treatment and prognostic factors for long-term outcome in patients with anti-NMDA receptor encephalitis: an observational cohort study. Lancet Neurol. 2013;12(2):157–65.
30. Gabilondo I, Saiz A, Galán L, González V, Jadraque R, Sabater L, et al. Analysis of relapses in anti-NMDA receptor encephalitis. Neurology. 2011;77:996–9.
31. Nosadini M, Mohammad SS, Ramanathan S, Brilot F, Dale RC. Immune therapy in autoimmune encephalitis: a systematic review. Expert Rev Neurother. 2015;15(12):1391–419.
32. Govert F, Leypoldt F, Junker R, Wandinger KP, Deuschl G, Bhatia KP, et al. Antibody-related movement disorders – a comprehensive review of phenotype-autoantibody correlations and a guide to testing. Neurol Res Pract. 2020;2:6.
33. Pike MG, Kennedy CR, Neville BG, Levin M. Herpes simplex encephalitis with relapse. Arch Dis Child. 1991;66(10):1242–4.

34. Nosadini M, Mohammad SS, Corazza F, Ruga EM, Kothur K, Perilongo G, et al. Herpes simplex virus-induced anti-N-methyl-d-aspartate receptor encephalitis: a systematic literature review with analysis of 43 cases. Dev Med Child Neurol. 2017;59(8):796–805.
35. Armangue T, Titulaer MJ, Malaga I, Bataller L, Gabilondo I, Graus F, et al. Pediatric anti-N-methyl-D-aspartate receptor encephalitis-clinical analysis and novel findings in a series of 20 patients. J Pediatr. 2013;162(4):850–6. e2
36. Mohammad SS, Sinclair K, Pillai S, Merheb V, Aumann TD, Gill D, et al. Herpes simplex encephalitis relapse with chorea is associated with autoantibodies to N-methyl-D-aspartate receptor or dopamine-2 receptor. Mov Disord. 2014;29(1):117–22.
37. Hacohen Y, Deiva K, Pettingill P, Waters P, Siddiqui A, Chretien P, et al. N-methyl-D-aspartate receptor antibodies in post-herpes simplex virus encephalitis neurological relapse. Mov Disord. 2014;29(1):90–6.
38. Armangue T, Spatola M, Vlagea A, Mattozzi S, Carceles-Cordon M, Martinez-Heras E, et al. Frequency, symptoms, risk factors, and outcomes of autoimmune encephalitis after herpes simplex encephalitis: a prospective observational study and retrospective analysis. Lancet Neurol. 2018;17(9):760–72.
39. Vernino S, Tuite P, Adler CH, Meschia JF, Boeve BF, Boasberg P, et al. Paraneoplastic chorea associated with CRMP-5 neuronal antibody and lung carcinoma. Ann Neurol. 2002;51:625–30.
40. Samii A, Dahlen DD, Spence AM, Maronian NC, Kraus EE, Lennon VA. Paraneoplastic movement disorder in a patient with non-Hodgkin's lymphoma and CRMP-5 autoantibody. Mov Disord. 2003;18:1556–8.
41. Yu Z, Kryzer TJ, Griesmann GE, Kim K, Benarroch EE, Lennon VA. CRMP-5 neuronal autoantibody: marker of lung cancer and thymoma-related autoimmunity. Ann Neurol. 2001;49:146–54.
42. Moss HE, Liu GT, Dalmau J. Glazed (vision) and confused. Surv Ophthalmol. 2010;55:169–73.
43. Muehlschlegel S, Okun MS, Foote KD, Coco D, Yachnis AT, Fernandez HH. Paraneoplastic chorea with leukoencephalopathy presenting with obsessive-compulsive and behavioral disorder. Mov Disord. 2005;20:1523–7.
44. Yamashita N, Mosinger B, Roy A, Miyazaki M, Ugajin K, Nakamura F, et al. CRMP5 (collapsin response mediator protein 5) regulates dendritic development and synaptic plasticity in the cerebellar Purkinje cells. J Neurosci. 2011;31:1773–9.
45. Brot S, Rogemond V, Perrot V, Chounlamountri N, Auger C, Honnorat J, et al. CRMP5 interacts with tubulin to inhibit neurite outgrowth, thereby modulating the function of CRMP2. J Neurosci. 2010;30:10639–54.
46. Meyronet D, Massoma P, Thivolet F, Chalabreysse L, Rogemond V, Schlama A, et al. Extensive expression of collapsin response mediator protein 5 (CRMP5) is a specific marker of high-grade lung neuroendocrine carcinoma. Am J Surg Pathol. 2008;32:1699–708.
47. Honnorat J, Cartalat-Carel S, Ricard D, Camdessanche JP, Carpentier AF, Rogemond V, et al. Onco-neural antibodies and tumour type determine survival and neurological symptoms in paraneoplastic neurological syndromes with Hu or CV2/CRMP5 antibodies. J Neurol Neurosurg Psychiatry. 2009;80:412–6.
48. Dalmau J, Graus F, Rosenblum MK, Posner JB. Anti-Hu-associated paraneoplastic encephalomyelitis/sensory neuronopathy. A clinical study of 71 patients. Medicine. 1992;71:59–72.
49. Molinuevo JL, Graus F, Serrano C, Rene R, Guerrero A, Illa I. Utility of anti-Hu antibodies in the diagnosis of paraneoplastic sensory neuropathy. Ann Neurol. 1998;44:976–80.
50. Nokura K, Nagamatsu M, Inagaki T, Yamamoto H, Koga H, Sugimura K, et al. Acute motor and sensory neuronopathy associated with small-cell lung cancer: a clinicopathological study. Neuropathology. 2006;26:329–37.
51. Graus F, Keime-Guibert F, Reñe R, Benyahia B, Ribalta T, Ascaso C, et al. Anti-Hu-associated paraneoplastic encephalomyelitis: analysis of 200 patients. Brain. 2001;124:1138–48.
52. Coret F, Bosca I, Fratalia L, Perez-Griera J, Pascual A, Casanova B. Long-lasting remission after rituximab treatment in a case of anti-Hu-associated sensory neuronopathy and gastric pseudo obstruction. J Neuro-Oncol. 2009;93:421–3.

53. Tate ED, Allison TJ, Pranzatelli MR, Verhulst SJ. Neuroepidemiologic trends in 105 US cases of pediatric opsoclonus-myoclonus syndrome. J Pediatr Oncol Nurs. 2005;22:8–19.
54. Bataller L, Graus F, Saiz A, Vilchez JJ. Clinical outcome in adult onset idiopathic or paraneoplastic opsoclonus-myoclonus. Brain. 2001;124:437–43.
55. Luque FA, Furneaux HM, Ferziger R, Rosenblum MK, Wray SH, Schold SC Jr, et al. Anti-Ri: an antibody associated with paraneoplastic opsoclonus and breast cancer. Ann Neurol. 1991;29:241–51.
56. Berridge G, Menassa DA, Moloney T, Waters PJ, Welding I, Thomsen S, et al. Glutamate receptor delta2 serum antibodies in pediatric opsoclonus myoclonus ataxia syndrome. Neurology. 2018;91(8):e714–e23.
57. Petit-Pedrol M, Guasp M, Armangue T, Lavarino C, Morales La Madrid A, Saiz A, et al. Absence of GluD2 antibodies in patients with opsoclonus-myoclonus syndrome. Neurology. 2020. https://doi.org/10.1212/WNL.0000000000011410.
58. Panzer JA, Anand R, Dalmau J, Lynch DR. Antibodies to dendritic neuronal surface antigens in opsoclonus myoclonus ataxia syndrome. J Neuroimmunol. 2015;286:86–92.
59. Wong A. An update on opsoclonus. Curr Opin Neurol. 2007;20:25–31.
60. Gorman MP. Update on diagnosis, treatment, and prognosis in opsoclonus-myoclonus-ataxia syndrome. Curr Opin Pediatr. 2010;22:745–50.
61. Pranzatelli MR, Tate ED, Swan JA, Travelstead AL, Colliver JA, Verhulst SJ, et al. B cell depletion therapy for new-onset opsoclonus-myoclonus. Mov Disord. 2010;25:238–42.
62. Rostásy K, Wilken B, Baumann M, Müller-Deile K, Bieber I, et al. High dose pulsatile dexamethasone therapy in children with opsoclonus-myoclonus syndrome. Neuropediatrics. 2006;37:291–5.
63. Wilken B, Baumann M, Bien CG, Hero B, Rostasy K, Hanefeld F. Chronic relapsing opsoclonus-myoclonus syndrome: combination of cyclophosphamide and dexamethasone pulses. Eur J Paediatr Neurol. 2008;12:51–5.
64. Mitchell WG, Brumm VL, Azen CG, Patterson KE, Aller SK, Rodriguez J. Longitudinal neurodevelopmental evaluation of children with opsoclonus-ataxia. Pediatrics. 2005;116:901–7.
65. Pranzatelli MR, Tate ED. Trends and tenets in relapsing and progressive opsoclonus-myoclonus syndrome. Brain and Development. 2016;38(5):439–48.
66. Erlich R, Morrison C, Kim B, Gilbert MR, Alrajab S. ANNA-2: an antibody associated with paraneoplastic opsoclonus in a patient with large-cell carcinoma of the lung with neuroendocrine features–correlation of clinical improvement with tumor response. Cancer Investig. 2004;22:257–61.
67. Mohammad SS, Ramanathan S, Brilot F, Dale RC. Autoantibody-associated movement disorders. Neuropediatrics. 2013;44(6):336–45.
68. Cardoso F, Vargas AP, Oliveira LD, Guerra AA, Amaral SV. Persistent Sydenham's chorea. Mov Disord. 1999;14(5):805–7.
69. Punukollu M, Mushet N, Linney M, Hennessy C, Morton M. Neuropsychiatric manifestations of Sydenham's chorea: a systematic review. Dev Med Child Neurol. 2016;58(1):16–28.
70. Mohammad SS, Nosadini M, Grattan-Smith P, Dale RC. Intravenous immunoglobulin in acute Sydenham's chorea: a systematic review. J Paediatr Child Health. 2015;51(12):1235–8.
71. Walker KG, Wilmshurst JM. An update on the treatment of Sydenham's chorea: the evidence for established and evolving interventions. Ther Adv Neurol Disord. 2010;3(5):301–9.
72. Lai M, Huijbers MG, Lancaster E, Graus F, Bataller L, Balice-Gordon R, et al. Investigation of LGI1 as the antigen in limbic encephalitis previously attributed to potassium channels: a case series. Lancet Neurol. 2010;9:776–85.
73. Andrade DM, Tai P, Dalmau J, Wennberg R. Tonic seizures: a diagnostic clue of anti-LGI1 encephalitis? Neurology. 2011;76:1355–7.
74. Irani SR, Michell AW, Lang B, Pettingill P, Waters P, Johnson MR, et al. Faciobrachial dystonic seizures precede Lgi1 antibody limbic encephalitis. Ann Neurol. 2011;69:892–900.
75. Barajas RF, Collins DE, Cha S, Geschwind MD. Adult-onset drug-refractory seizure disorder associated with anti-voltage-gated potassium-channel antibody. Epilepsia. 2010;51:473–7.

76. Irani SR, Buckley C, Vincent A, Cockerell OC, Rudge P, Johnson MR, et al. Immunotherapy-responsive seizure-like episodes with potassium channel antibodies. Neurology. 2008;71:1647–8.
77. Irani SR, Gelfand JM, Bettcher BM, Singhal NS, Geschwind MD. Effect of rituximab in patients with leucine-rich, glioma-inactivated 1 antibody-associated encephalopathy. JAMA Neurol. 2014;71(7):896–900.
78. Dalmau J, Gonzalez RG, Lerwill MF. Case records of the Massachusetts General Hospital. Case 4–2007. A 56-year-old woman with rapidly progressive vertigo and ataxia. N Engl J Med. 2007;356:612–20.
79. Rojas I, Graus F, Keime-Guibert F, Reñé R, Delattre JY, Ramón JM, et al. Long-term clinical outcome of paraneoplastic cerebellar degeneration and anti-Yo antibodies. Neurology. 2000;55:713–5.
80. Bernal F, Shams'ili S, Rojas I, Sanchez-Valle R, Saiz A, Dalmau J, et al. Anti-Tr antibodies as markers of paraneoplastic cerebellar degeneration and Hodgkin's disease. Neurology. 2003;60:230–4.
81. Graus F, Lang B, Pozo Rosich P, Saiz A, Casamitjana R, Vincent A. P/Q type calcium-channel antibodies in paraneoplastic cerebellar degeneration with lung cancer. Neurology. 2002;59:764–6.
82. Sillevis SP, Kinoshita A, De Leeuw B, Moll W, Coesmans M, Jaarsma D, et al. Paraneoplastic cerebellar ataxia due to autoantibodies against a glutamate receptor. N Engl J Med. 2000;342:21–7.
83. Graus F, Dalmau J, Valldeoriola F, Ferrer I, Reñe R, Marin C, et al. Immunological characterization of a neuronal antibody (anti-Tr) associated with paraneoplastic cerebellar degeneration and Hodgkin's disease. J Neuroimmunol. 1997;74:55–61.
84. Voltz R, Gultekin SH, Rosenfeld MR, Gerstner E, Eichen J, Posner JB, et al. A serologic marker of paraneoplastic limbic and brain-stem encephalitis in patients with testicular cancer [see comments]. N Engl J Med. 1999;340:1788–95.
85. Rosenfeld MR, Eichen JG, Wade DF, Posner JB, Dalmau J. Molecular and clinical diversity in paraneoplastic immunity to Ma proteins. Ann Neurol. 2001;50:339–48.
86. Dalmau J, Graus F, Villarejo A, Posner JB, Blumenthal D, Thiessen B, et al. Clinical analysis of anti-Ma2-associated encephalitis. Brain. 2004;127:1831–44.
87. Bennett JL, Galetta SL, Frohman LP, Mourelatos Z, Gultekin SH, Dalmau JO, et al. Neuro-ophthalmologic manifestations of a paraneoplastic syndrome and testicular carcinoma. Neurology. 1999;52:864–7.
88. Hoffmann LA, Jarius S, Pellkofer HL, Schueller M, Krumbholz M, Koenig F, et al. Anti-Ma and anti-Ta associated paraneoplastic neurological syndromes: twenty-two newly diagnosed patients and review of previous cases. J Neurol Neurosurg Psychiatry. 2008;79:767–73.
89. Castle J, Sakonju A, Dalmau J, Newman-Toker DE. Anti-Ma2-associated encephalitis with normal FDG-PET: a case of pseudo-Whipple's disease. Nat Clin Pract Neurol. 2006;2:566–72.
90. Kraker J. Treatment of anti-Ma2/Ta paraneoplastic syndrome. Curr Treat Options Neurol. 2009;11:46–51.
91. de Beukelaar JW, Sillevis Smitt PA. Managing paraneoplastic neurological disorders. Oncologist. 2006;11:292–305.
92. Dale RC, Merheb V, Pillai S, Wang D, Cantrill L, Murphy TK, et al. Antibodies to surface dopamine-2 receptor in autoimmune movement and psychiatric disorders. Brain. 2012;135(Pt 11):3453–68.
93. Pawela C, Brunsdon RK, Williams TA, Porter M, Dale RC, Mohammad SS. The neuropsychological profile of children with basal ganglia encephalitis: a case series. Dev Med Child Neurol. 2017;59(4):445–8.
94. Alexopoulos H, Dalakas MC. A critical update on the immunopathogenesis of Stiff Person Syndrome. Eur J Clin Investig. 2010;40:1018–25.
95. Saiz A, Blanco Y, Sabater L, González F, Bataller L, Casamitjana R, et al. Spectrum of neurological syndromes associated with glutamic acid decarboxylase antibodies: diagnostic clues for this association. Brain. 2008;131:2553–63.

96. Raju R, Rakocevic G, Chen Z, Hoehn G, Semino-Mora C, Shi W, et al. Autoimmunity to GABAA-receptor-associated protein in stiff-person syndrome. Brain. 2006;129:3270–6.
97. Pittock SJ, Lucchinetti CF, Parisi JE, Benarroch EE, Mokri B, Stephan CL, et al. Amphiphysin autoimmunity: paraneoplastic accompaniments. Ann Neurol. 2005;58:96–107.
98. Murinson BB, Guarnaccia JB. Stiff-person syndrome with amphiphysin antibodies: distinctive features of a rare disease. Neurology. 2008;71:1955–8.
99. Butler MH, Hayashi A, Ohkoshi N, Villmann C, Becker CM, Feng G, et al. Autoimmunity to gephyrin in Stiff-Man syndrome. Neuron. 2000;26:307–12.
100. Mas N, Saiz A, Leite MI, Waters P, Baron M, Castaño D, et al. Antiglycine-receptor encephalomyelitis with rigidity. J Neurol Neurosurg Psychiatry. 2011;82:1399–401.
101. Hutchinson M, Waters P, McHugh J, Gorman G, O'Riordan S, Connolly S, et al. Progressive encephalomyelitis, rigidity, and myoclonus: a novel glycine receptor antibody. Neurology. 2008;71:1291–2.
102. Carvajal-Gonzalez A, Leite MI, Waters P, Woodhall M, Coutinho E, Balint B, et al. Glycine receptor antibodies in PERM and related syndromes: characteristics, clinical features and outcomes. Brain. 2014;137(Pt 8):2178–92.
103. Martinez-Hernandez E, Sepulveda M, Rostasy K, Hoftberger R, Graus F, Harvey RJ, et al. Antibodies to aquaporin 4, myelin-oligodendrocyte glycoprotein, and the glycine receptor alpha1 subunit in patients with isolated optic neuritis. JAMA Neurol. 2015;72(2):187–93.
104. Swayne A, Tjoa L, Broadley S, Dionisio S, Gillis D, Jacobson L, et al. Antiglycine receptor antibody related disease: a case series and literature review. Eur J Neurol. 2018;25(10):1290–8.
105. Dalakas MC, Fujii M, Li M, Lutfi B, Kyhos J, McElroy B. High-dose intravenous immune globulin for stiff-person syndrome. N Engl J Med. 2001;345:1870–6.
106. Schmierer K, Valdueza JM, Bender A, DeCamilli P, David C, Solimena M, et al. Atypical stiff-person syndrome with spinal MRI findings, amphiphysin autoantibodies, and immunosuppression. Neurology. 1998;51:250–2.
107. Vasconcelos OM, Dalakas MC. Stiff-person syndrome. Curr Treat Options Neurol. 2003;5:79–90.
108. Isaacs H. A syndrome of continuous muscle-fibre activity. J Neurol Neurosurg Psychiatry. 1961;24:319–25.
109. Liguori R, Vincent A, Clover L, Avoni P, Plazzi G, Cortelli P, et al. Morvan's syndrome: peripheral and central nervous system and cardiac involvement with antibodies to voltage-gated potassium channels. Brain. 2001;124:2417–26.
110. Maddison P. Neuromyotonia. Clin Neurophysiol. 2006;117:2118–27.
111. Hart IK, Maddison P, Newsom-Davis J, Vincent A, Mills KR. Phenotypic variants of autoimmune peripheral nerve hyperexcitability. Brain. 2002;125:1887–95.
112. Lahrmann H, Albrecht G, Drlicek M, Oberndorfer S, Urbanits S, Wanschitz J, et al. Acquired neuromyotonia and peripheral neuropathy in a patient with Hodgkin's disease. Muscle Nerve. 2001;24:834–8.
113. Rubio-Agustí I, Perez-Miralles F, Sevilla T, Muelas N, Chumillas MJ, Mayordomo F, et al. Peripheral nerve hyperexcitability. A clinical and immunologic study of 38 patients. Neurology. 2011;76:172–8.
114. Lancaster E, Huijbers MG, Bar V, Boronat A, Wong A, Martinez-Hernandez E, et al. Investigations of caspr2, an autoantigen of encephalitis and neuromyotonia. Ann Neurol. 2011;69:303–11.
115. Irani SR, Alexander S, Waters P, Kleopa KA, Pettingill P, Zuliani L, et al. Antibodies to Kv1 potassium channel-complex proteins leucine-rich, glioma inactivated 1 protein and contactin-associated protein-2 in limbic encephalitis, Morvan's syndrome and acquired neuromyotonia. Brain. 2010;133:2734–48.
116. Binks SNM, Klein CJ, Waters P, Pittock SJ, Irani SR. LGI1, CASPR2 and related antibodies: a molecular evolution of the phenotypes. J Neurol Neurosurg Psychiatry. 2018;89(5):526–34.
117. Newsom-Davis J, Buckley C, Clover L, Hart I, Maddison P, Tüzüm E, et al. Autoimmune disorders of neuronal potassium channels. Ann N Y Acad Sci. 2003;998:202–10.

118. Dalmau J, Rosenfeld MR. Paraneoplastic syndromes of the CNS. Lancet Neurol. 2008;7:327–40.
119. Geis C, Weishaupt A, Hallermann S, Grünewald B, Wessig C, Wultsch T, et al. Stiff person syndrome-associated autoantibodies to amphiphysin mediate reduced GABAergic inhibition. Brain. 2010;133(11):3166–80.
120. Gallego J, Dalmau J. Classic paraneoplastic syndromes: diagnostic and treatment approach. Neurologia. 2008;23(7):441–8.

Psychosis and Parkinson's Disease

Christina L. Vaughan and Jennifer G. Goldman

Patient Vignettes

Patient 1

A 67-year-old bus driver with a 7-year history of Parkinson's disease (PD) presented to the emergency department with agitation. For the past 2 weeks he had accused his wife of having an affair with the neighbor, believed that strangers were living in his house, and insisted that the dog gates were installed to prevent him from leaving the house. He had threatened family members, and finally his wife called the paramedics to bring him to the hospital. His medications included the following: carbidopa/levodopa 25/100 mg—two tablets every 4 h (total eight tablets daily) along with entacapone 200 mg with each dose, carbidopa/levodopa CR 50/200 mg nightly, amitriptyline 25 mg nightly, and aspirin. His medical history revealed frequent urinary tract infections. On examination, he was confused and exhibited typical motor features of PD including bradykinesia, rigidity, and rest tremor. He was afebrile, and laboratory tests revealed normal blood counts and electrolytes. Urinalysis was suspicious for infection with positive leukocyte esterase and increased white cells. Neuroimaging did not reveal intracranial hemorrhage or evidence of acute stroke. He was admitted to the psychiatric ward for further management of his psychosis.

C. L. Vaughan (✉)
Departments of Neurology and Medicine, University of Colorado,
Anschutz Medical Center, Aurora, CO, USA
e-mail: christina.vaughan@cuanschutz.edu

J. G. Goldman
Shirley Ryan AbilityLab, Northwestern University Feinberg School of Medicine,
Chicago, IL, USA

© Springer Nature Switzerland AG 2022
S. J. Frucht (ed.), *Movement Disorder Emergencies*, Current Clinical Neurology,
https://doi.org/10.1007/978-3-030-75898-1_17

Patient 2

A 70-year-old retired professor with a 15-year history of akinetic-rigid PD presented to the emergency department after lighting his bedspread on fire to kill the insects that he thought were infesting his bed. En route, he called the police claiming that the ambulance driver had kidnapped him against his will. Over the past year, he was reported to spend most of the day in his bedroom obsessing about "bugs" on his skin. He had arranged an elaborate system of locks and alarms to protect his belongings from intruders and believed that his wife was an imposter. His nightly sleep was poor, and he took frequent short naps throughout the day. His medication regimen included carbidopa/levodopa 48.75/195 mg four capsules three times daily (total 12 capsules daily). A prior trial of quetiapine up to 200 mg daily failed to improve his psychosis. On examination, he was agitated with persistent lateral bending of the trunk and marked generalized dyskinesias. He repeatedly insisted that he had been kidnapped against his will although he was alert and fully oriented, with no evidence of dementia. Vital signs and basic laboratory studies including toxicology screen were unremarkable.

Introduction

Psychiatric symptoms are among the most common reasons for emergency department visits by Parkinson's disease (PD) patients. The disorders most likely to result in a visit are psychosis, acute confusion, and panic attacks [1]. Psychosis is a frequent and troublesome complication in PD, often associated with increased morbidity, mortality, nursing home placement [2], caregiver stress [3, 4], and worsened quality of life [5]. Revised criteria for PD psychosis were proposed by a NINDS-NIMH working group: these include illusions, a false sense of presence, hallucinations, and delusions occurring chronically and in the setting of a clear sensorium [6]. While illusions and a sense of presence may be part of the PD psychosis spectrum, in this chapter we will focus on hallucinations and delusions as they may present an emergency situation for patients and their caregivers. Hallucinations can be very frightening and distressing to both the patient and caregiver, though in some cases they may be "benign" or even pleasant. Delusions, or idiosyncratic false and fixed beliefs, are often paranoid in nature and can be especially disruptive. When psychosis develops acutely or suddenly worsens, becomes troublesome or frightening, or poses a safety risk, urgent attention is required.

Hallucinations and delusions in PD may be acute or chronic, occur with clear or clouded sensorium, or retained or absent insight. Dopaminergic medications influence these scenarios, but other factors play a role as well. We will review the phenomenology, epidemiology, and pathophysiology of PD psychosis, and then discuss its evaluation in the emergency setting.

Phenomenology

The clinical spectrum of PD psychosis ranges from mild illusions to formed hallucinations or even frank delusions. Illusions and benign hallucinations (passage or presence, defined below) are often grouped together and called "minor" hallucinations [7]. *Illusions* are misperceptions of real stimuli, including phenomena such as interpreting inanimate objects as living beings (e.g., a chair mistaken for a dog, a lamppost mistaken for a tree). *"Passage" hallucinations* involve the sensation of a person or animal passing in the person's peripheral visual field, and *"presence" hallucinations* involve the sense that someone is present close by when no one is really there. These "minor" hallucinations are usually not troublesome for the patient or caregiver, and are unlikely to constitute a movement disorder emergency.

Hallucinations are spontaneously fabricated perceptions occurring while the patient is awake. Most hallucinations in PD are visual in nature, although other sensory modalities may be involved [6]. Hallucinations in PD may be categorized as simple or complex. Simple hallucinations lack form and frequently include photopsias such as flashes of light or color, while complex hallucinations include visions that are clearly defined, taking the shape of animals, humans, or objects [8]. Examples of complex visual hallucinations in PD include mice scurrying on the floor or children playing in the house, but they can be frightening including distorted, grotesque, or bizarre figures. Hallucinations in PD usually are not threatening, occurring with a clear sensorium [9, 10]. They are typically brief, lasting seconds to minutes, and may occur or increase at night. By their recurrent and stereotyped character, the hallucinatory figures may become familiar to the patient, who may even observe them with sympathy [11]. These seemingly benign hallucinations however often progress into more elaborate hallucinations, particularly in the setting of a clouded sensorium or when accompanied by delusions [12]. Not all hallucinations are benign, and as insight decreases their content may become frightening. The phenomenology of hallucinations also may change with advancing disease, becoming "malignant," disabling, and intermingled with paranoid thoughts of suspiciousness, sexual accusations, and contamination [13]. In general, hallucinations tend to occur when the patient is in a low sensory environment, and thus can be more dependent on sensory state than dopaminergic drug dose [14]. Visual hallucinations frequently manifest in dim light, when vision is compromised [15]. Visual hallucinations are more common in PD, whereas auditory hallucinations are more common in schizophrenia [16].

Hallucinations in nonvisual modalities also occur, but they generally accompany visual hallucinations [11]. When they begin, older patients more frequently experience nonvisual or mixed hallucinations rather than purely visual ones, suggesting that age may influence their phenomenology [17]. Unlike visual hallucinations, auditory hallucinations are often vague; for example, auditory hallucinations commonly feature the din of a party heard coming from another room, people talking indistinguishably outside, or music of various types [7]. Rarely do auditory hallucinations interact with the patient or involve back and forth conversation [13]. Auditory hallucinations in PD thus differ from those of schizophrenia. Auditory hallucinations in PD are not usually threatening and are less likely to be the sole modality of hallucinations present. Tactile or olfactory hallucinations are less common in PD, but they may occur. Tactile hallucinations often involve a feeling of contact with small animals or being touched by someone else [18]. Olfactory hallucinations may be pleasant or unpleasant in smell, even involving one nostril more than the other [15, 19].

Delusions are less common than hallucinations, affecting about 5–10% of medication-treated PD patients [20]. In PD, delusions often consist of well-systematized ideas focused on a single theme. Common delusional themes include the following: jealousy or spousal infidelity; paranoia; fears of being poisoned, injured, or filmed; elaborate schemes about conspiracies; stealing; abandonment; or somatic illnesses [15]. In a small cohort of PD patients with psychosis, systematized paranoid delusions (i.e., a single delusion with multiple elaborations or a group of delusions related to a single event or theme) were more common than nonspecific paranoid ideation (56% vs. 44%) [21]. A persistent suspicion may evolve into a fixed delusion, which may escalate causing injury or hospitalization. While delusions of persecution are common in both schizophrenia and PD, delusions in schizophrenia more frequently encompass themes of grandiosity, reference, and bizarre beliefs such as thought broadcasting, thought withdrawal, and thought insertion [22].

Misidentification syndromes are a specific type of delusion that present a particularly challenging situation for the patient and caregiver. Two common misidentification syndromes include the following: *Capgras syndrome*, in which the patient thinks that his recognizable spouse is an imposter, [23] and *Fregoli syndrome*, in which the patient believes that familiar people are, often malevolently, disguised as strangers [24]. These misidentification syndromes have been reported in PD, particularly in the setting of PD dementia (PDD). In one report of a PD patient with Fregoli syndrome, symptoms completely resolved with reduction in levodopa dose [24]. In a prospective study of demented PD patients, Pagonabarraga reported a prevalence of delusional misidentification syndromes of 16.7% [25]. Roane described three cases of misidentification associated with parkinsonism, all of whom were demented [26]. In addition to PDD, delusions may accompany other Parkinsonian disorders. Delusions have been reported in about 80% of patients with dementia with Lewy bodies (DLB) [27].

🔑 Misidentification syndromes are common in advanced Parkinson's disease, and can be extremely upsetting to the spouse and family.

Epidemiology

Methodological differences among studies complicate attempts to estimate the frequency of PD psychosis. These differences include the following: the population source (community vs. movement disorder clinic-based), design (retrospective vs. prospective), types of prevalence values (point, period, or lifetime), symptoms included (illusions, hallucinations and/or delusions), and measurements or rating scales used. Further, reliance on the subjective accounts of the patient and/or caregiver makes identifying and rating psychosis challenging. As a result, prevalence estimates of PD psychosis in the literature vary greatly, ranging from approximately 20–60% [7, 10, 20, 28–30, 31]. Many studies are clinic-based and cross-sectional thereby providing point prevalence rates in PD patients on dopaminergic treatment [20]. In a clinic-based cross-sectional study of 116 consecutively seen PD patients, 60% met NINDS-NIMH criteria [6] for PD psychosis [32]. In an earlier cross-sectional study of 129 patients, Graham established a prevalence of 25% [10]. Several studies provide longitudinal information on the development of hallucinations. In a prospective, longitudinal cohort study, 60% of PD patients developed hallucinations or delusions at 12 years, and 42% of the cohort developed new psychosis during the study, occurring at a mean of 13 years after motor symptom onset [33]. In a long-term follow-up study of PD patients initially free of hallucinations, Goetz found that at 10 years, 93% of the original 60 non-hallucinating PD patients had hallucinations on at least one interview. The prevalence of hallucinations increased from 33% at baseline to 63% at 10 years, and the odds of having hallucinations increased annually by a factor of 1.26 [34]. In the Sydney Multicenter Study that followed a cohort of initially levodopa-naïve PD patients, at 15 years follow-up, 50% of patients had formed visual hallucinations, with a mean time to onset of hallucinations of 10.7 years [35]. Among the survivors of the same cohort, 74% experienced visual hallucinations at 20-year follow-up, requiring reduction of dopaminergic medication in all, and initiation of an atypical antipsychotic in ten patients [36].

Factors That Influence Development of PD Psychosis

Several factors may influence the development of PD psychosis. In general, risk factors for developing hallucinations include older age, concomitant depression, and coexistent cognitive impairment [7, 28], and visual perceptive disturbances [30, 37–40]. Other studies have reported greater axial rigidity, increased dopaminergic medication doses, sleep disturbances, and multiple medical problems in affected individuals [7, 8, 10, 31, 33, 41–44] (Table 17.1). While hallucinations occur more

Table 17.1 Risk factors for PD psychosis

Older age
Older age at PD onset
Worse motor function, particularly axial function
Higher baseline levodopa equivalent dose
Advanced disease
Lower cognitive status
Concomitant dementia
Concomitant depression
Sleep disturbances (e.g., REM sleep behavior disorder)
Multiple medical problems
Visual perceptive disorders

often in PD patients with dementia, they may occur in up to 17% of non-demented PD patients, as demonstrated in a large prospective study of 1351 patients [45]. In a 10-year longitudinal study, Goetz found that time influenced their development, while sleep fragmentation, overall sleep function, total daily levodopa dose, Unified Parkinson's Disease Rating Scale (UPDRS) motor score, and Mini-mental State Examination score did not [34]. In another long-duration longitudinal study, Forsaa found that baseline levodopa equivalent dose, age at PD onset, and probable rapid-eye movement (REM) sleep behavior disorder independently increased the risk of hallucinations. A secondary analysis of data from the CALM-PD study revealed that older age and the existence of multiple medical problems were associated with the development of hallucinations [46].

Pathophysiology

PD psychosis may be caused by extrinsic (i.e., pharmacological treatment) and/or intrinsic (i.e., disease-related) factors. It is well known that dopaminergic medications can induce psychosis in PD by stimulating or inducing hypersensitivity of mesocorticolimbic dopamine receptors [47]. Virtually all classes of anti-Parkinsonian medications may produce psychosis. Some studies suggest that dopamine agonists are more likely culprits than levodopa [46, 48–50], and anticholinergics are a frequent trigger especially in elderly PD patients [51]. While dopaminergic medications contribute to PD psychosis, several intrinsic factors also play a role [46–53].

Investigations of PD psychosis have focused on three primary areas: primary visual system, brainstem, and cortex [12]. Dysregulation in these areas often manifests as visual disturbances, sleep or mood disorders, or cognitive impairment—suggesting abnormalities in "top-down" and/or "bottom-up" processing. The visual system may be affected in PD patients at multiple levels, and hallucinations are associated with ocular and retinal dysfunction in addition to central processing deficits [4, 54–55]. Dopaminergic innervation around the fovea is reduced in PD, and this contributes to altered visual processing at the level of the receptive fields of ganglion cells [56]. Retinal dopaminergic dysfunction reduces meaningful information for central visual processing such that finer details of visual stimuli are blurred, and contrast and color discrimination are reduced [57]. Compared to PD patients without hallucinations, PD hallucinators have reduced visual acuity [30, 58] and impaired contrast sensitivity [57].

Cortical abnormalities and dysregulation have been suggested on the basis of neuroimaging studies. In a structural magnetic resonance imaging (MRI) study, Goldman et al. demonstrated gray matter atrophy in occipital areas involved in the "what" and "where" visuoperceptive pathways in PD visual hallucinators compared to PD non-hallucinators, who were matched for cognitive status and other potential confounders [59]. Functional and metabolic neuroimaging studies reveal different responses to visual stimuli or perfusion patterns in PD hallucinators compared to PD non-hallucinators. In a functional magnetic resonance imaging (fMRI) study, Holroyd and Wooten showed that PD hallucinators demonstrated increased activation in the visual association cortex and deficits in the primary visual cortex [60]. Stebbins found that hallucinating PD patients had more frontal and subcortical activation and less posterior cortical activation than non-hallucinating PD patients [61]. These studies suggest that retinal dopamine deficiency or decreased visual input (afferent abnormalities), or disruptions in the pathways mediating visual attention may alter how the visual cortex processes stimuli. Significantly reduced occipital–inferior temporal–parietal perfusion patterns have been shown in PD patients with visual hallucinations using n-isopropyl-p-[^{123}I] iodoamphetamine single photon emission computed tomography (^{123}I-IMP SPECT) [58] and ^{18}F-deoxyglucose positron emission technology (^{18}F-FDG PET) [62]. In a study using ([^{123}I]IMP) SPECT, Matsui found that PD hallucinators had significant perfusion reductions in the bilateral inferior parietal lobule, inferior temporal gyrus, precuneus gyrus, and occipital cortex compared to PD non-hallucinators. Using ^{18}F-FDG PET, Boecker found significant metabolic abnormalities in regions of the dorsal and ventral visual streams, but not in primary visual cortex in PD hallucinators compared to PD non-hallucinators; they did not find increased glucose metabolism in frontal regions, although this has been demonstrated in some studies. The two principal visual processing routes may be especially relevant to PD hallucinations as the ventral stream is involved in object and form vision ("what"), and the dorsal stream in spatial location and motion vision ("where") [62].

While the loss of substantia nigra pars compacta dopaminergic neurons is a neuropathologic hallmark of PD, it is well recognized that PD pathology extends well beyond the nigrostriatal system [63]. Postmortem studies have shown increased extranigral Lewy body burden in PD patients with visual hallucinations, including the ventral temporal lobe [64]. PD cases with well-formed visual hallucinations contained high densities of Lewy bodies in the amygdala and parahippocampus, with early hallucinations associated with higher densities in parahippocampal and inferior temporal cortices [65]. Brainstem changes with loss of noradrenergic neurons of the locus ceruleus, serotonergic neurons of the raphe nuclei, and the cholinergic parabrachial and pedunculopontine nuclei may also play a role in PD hallucinations [16, 63].

The relationship between hallucinations, sleep, and brainstem dysfunction has been based on observations that hallucinations can occur as rapid-eye movement

(REM) intrusions, and that hallucinating PD patients have altered sleep-wake patterns [12]. Visual hallucinations in PD may represent intrusions of REM sleep into wakefulness, and the hypothesis of visual hallucinations as overflow dream phenomena has been supported by several studies [66, 67]. This concept has focused anatomic attention on the reticular activating system and the parapontine nucleus [34]. Also hypothesized is a link between hallucinations and REM sleep behavior disorder (RBD) [68]. In a prospective study of PD patients, RBD significantly correlated with hallucinations independently of age, gender, PD duration or PD stage, and also correlated with dopaminergic dose [41]. The underlying mechanisms of RBD may relate to brainstem alterations of cholinergic [67] or noradrenergic activity [41].

PD psychosis is closely linked to cognitive impairment and dementia. Neuroimaging studies comparing hallucinating PD and non-hallucinating PD patients demonstrate greater volume loss in temporal and parietal lobes as well as limbic regions in PD hallucinators [69, 70]. In addition, postmortem studies reveal Lewy body pathology in temporal and limbic regions, areas associated with memory function, in PD hallucinators [64, 65]. Clinically, many PD patients may lose insight into their psychosis when they develop cognitive impairment [7]. Cognitive deficits in PD hallucinators frequently affect visual and verbal memory, executive function, and visuoperceptive–visuospatial tasks [71]. In demented PD patients, hallucinations may be more complex, more frequent, and are more likely to be perceived as unpleasant [72]. In a prospective study of PD patients with and without visual hallucinations, Llebaria showed that PD patients with hallucinations without insight were impaired in cognitive tasks reflecting posterior cortical dysfunction [73]. PD patients with major hallucinations and intact insight, however, had frontal-subcortical impairment reflecting executive dysfunction. Posterior cortical dysfunction may be a risk factor for both PD dementia [74] and hallucinations [62, 73]. Thus, the close relationship of hallucinations and cognitive impairment in PD may reflect shared neuroanatomical substrates.

Evaluation

When a PD patient presents with acute psychosis, several medical and neurological conditions may be entertained in the differential diagnosis. A toxic-metabolic encephalopathy may occur in patients who are medically ill, infected, or acutely overmedicated. In these cases, delirium is frequently present, and hallucinations may be associated with confusion, agitation, or myoclonus. The medication regimen must be carefully reviewed, with attention to recent changes in drugs or doses, or drug–drug interactions (e.g., serotonin syndrome). In cases of anticholinergic toxicity, psychosis may be accompanied by dry skin, urinary retention, and mydriasis [11]. Early identification and treatment of delirium is essential. Frequently, delirium or an acute change in mental status indicates a "medical" explanation (Table 17.2). Particularly with concomitant delirium, evaluation for acute psychosis requires basic laboratory studies, workup for infection, toxicology screens, and

Table 17.2 Evaluation of acute PD psychosis

Differential diagnosis
P—Parkinson's disease medications
SY—Systemic illness
C—Centrally acting medication
H—Hepatic, renal, or other metabolic dysfunction
O—Overdose of medications or intoxication
S—Sensory deprivation (hearing, visual impairment)
I—Infection (urinary tract infection, pneumonia)
S—Structural lesions (stroke, subdural hematoma, intracranial hemorrhage, trauma)
Proposed tests, depending on scenario:
  Labs: complete blood count, comprehensive metabolic profile, thyroid function, toxicology
  screen, urinalysis, urine culture, cerebrospinal fluid analysis
  Imaging: head computed tomography or magnetic resonance imaging, chest X-ray
  Other: electroencephalogram

neuroimaging for evaluation of intracranial hemorrhage or infarct. It is helpful to learn if the patient has previously experienced similar presentations, particularly urinary tract infections or noncompliance with medications.

For those PD patients with new-onset psychosis, hallucinations early in the course of parkinsonism (e.g., within the first 12 months or even before dopaminergic drugs are introduced) may indicate DLB [11]; this "1-year rule" has been used to separate DLB from PDD [13]. This distinction has treatment implications as DLB patients may have marked neuroleptic sensitivity and, in rare cases, develop a neuroleptic malignant-like syndrome [75]. Psychosis in DLB patients also may respond to cholinesterase inhibitors [76].

For those PD patients with an acute exacerbation of chronic psychosis, in addition to excluding "medical" etiologies, medication changes, or medication interactions, several other points merit attention. Underlying sensory deficits (i.e., visual or hearing impairment) may contribute to psychosis. For example, visual impairment can lead to hallucinations; in the Charles-Bonnet syndrome, elderly people with low visual acuity may experience benign visual hallucinations as "release" phenomena [14]. One should also inquire about primary psychiatric conditions such as depression, schizophrenia, schizoaffective disorder, or bipolar disorder. Depression in PD approaches 30–40% [77], and psychosis occasionally accompanies moderate-to-severe depression [78]. Previous studies suggest that psychosis due to comorbid psychiatric conditions differs from PD psychosis; PD psychosis does not usually include thought broadcasting, delusions of grandeur, voices talking about the patient, mind reading, being controlled by foreign forces, or hyper-religiosity [14].

🔑   Hallucinations present within the first year of diagnosis suggests a diagnosis of dementia with Lewy bodies.

Regardless of whether a PD patient presents with first-time psychosis or an acute exacerbation of chronic psychosis, the psychosis may be a consequence of PD medications, especially when there is no "medical" cause or other explanation. The initial workup for acute PD psychosis frequently occurs in the emergency department or outpatient clinic. From there, patients are usually admitted to the hospital for further evaluation and management, particularly when the psychosis cannot be managed effectively in an outpatient setting. Of all PD patient admissions to a community hospital during a 6-year period, 24% were due to psychosis, and drug-induced psychosis was the cause of repeated and prolonged admissions in 29% of patients [79]. The best setting for acutely psychotic PD patients is a well-controlled, calm environment where people are equipped to manage psychotic patients; this type of environment may be in a psychiatry unit but other settings also may be appropriate. Neurological consultation should be obtained early in the hospital course as there are often multiple considerations for hospitalized PD patients, such as the appropriate dose and timing of PD medications and the avoidance of medications that can worsen PD.

Treatment

In the setting of acute psychosis, patients may be very agitated. In this situation, low-dose benzodiazepines (intramuscular or oral) may be necessary to calm them [15]. Typical antipsychotics with dopamine blocking properties should be avoided as they can trigger a significant deterioration of motor symptoms, and a neuroleptic malignant syndrome [80]. If a specific etiology for the acute psychosis is determined, this should be addressed (e.g., antibiotics for an infection, correction of metabolic derangements) (Fig. 17.1).

Once the patient is no longer agitated, the next step is to reduce non-PD medications that may have psychoactive properties. Common medications in this category include anticholinergics for bladder hyperactivity, tricyclics for depression, benzodiazepines for anxiety or sleep, hypnotics for sleep, and opioids for pain. If there is no timely improvement, then PD medications should be gradually reduced. In reducing PD medications, the general consensus is to taper and stop the medications with the highest risk-to-benefit ratio first [81]. One proposed order of reduction or discontinuation includes the following: anticholinergics first, followed by amantadine (especially to note if a patient has impaired renal clearance), selegiline or rasagiline, dopamine agonists, COMT-inhibitors, and then levodopa [82]. The reduction or discontinuation of PD medications should be done under close observation by the neurologist as motor symptoms may worsen. A point, however, may be reached at which the PD medications cannot be reduced without compromising motor function, at which time antipsychotic medications are frequently added [81].

Despite the high prevalence of psychosis in PD, there are few randomized, double-blind, placebo-controlled trials of the atypical antipsychotics in PD. Atypical antipsychotics include (in order of arrival in the United States) the following: clozapine, risperidone, olanzapine, quetiapine, ziprasidone, aripiprazole [78], and pimavanserin that was given accelerated approval by the FDA in 2016. The American Academy of Neurology (AAN) practice parameter on treatment of PD psychosis (2006) considered only three atypical antipsychotics and recommended that clozapine should be considered (Level B), quetiapine *may* be considered (Level C), and

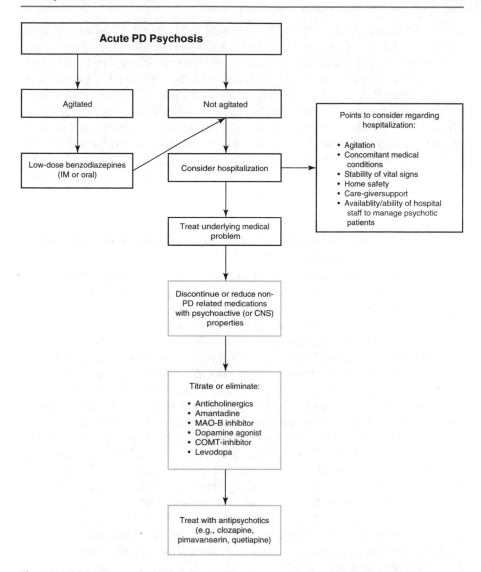

Fig. 17.1 Management of acute PD psychosis

olanzapine should not be considered (Level B) [83]. This practice parameter has since been retired (as of February 23, 2018) and an updated evidence-based medicine review commissioned by the International Parkinson and Movement Disorder Society (MDS) reviewed the latest studies to include pimavanserin [84].

Clozapine has been studied in several double-blind, placebo-controlled trials that have shown improvement in psychosis with negligible motor worsening [85–87]. In a double-blind study by Pollak, low-dose clozapine (mean dose 35.8 mg/day) improved PD psychosis as early as a few days after initiation [88]. Furthermore, more than one-third of patients were able to benefit from increased doses of levodopa or from the introduction of a dopaminergic agonist, without significant changes in clozapine dose and without recurrence of psychiatric symptoms [88]. In PD psychosis, the effective dose of clozapine is relatively low—6.25–75 mg daily compared with 300–900 mg daily in adult patients with schizophrenia [87, 88]. One commonly used regimen is to begin clozapine at 6.25 mg at bedtime and increase by the same amount every 4–7 days until psychosis remits or side effects occur [81]. The biggest drawback to its use is the risk of agranulocytosis, which is idiosyncratic rather than dose dependent and requires close monitoring. The incidence of agranulocytosis was found to be 0.38% in a sample of 99,502 patients with schizophrenia [89]. White blood cell counts should be monitored weekly for the first 6 months. If the white blood cell counts are normal, the patient can be monitored every 2 weeks for an additional 6 months. Afterwards, the patient may qualify for every 4-week monitoring with physician authorization. Other side effects of clozapine include sedation, orthostatic hypotension, confusion, and sialorrhea [88].

O⎯⎯🔑 Clozapine requires careful monitoring and is labor-intensive for the treating physician. However, clozapine is a remarkable drug, and can keep patients out of nursing homes. Delusions are especially responsive to clozapine.

Although open-label reports of quetiapine demonstrated improvements in PD psychosis, double-blind, placebo-controlled trials have failed to establish this. A review of several open-label reports of quetiapine revealed approximately 80% subjective improvement of psychosis in PD patients, all with doses less than 100 mg per day [90]. Two rater-blinded studies suggested efficacy, one by lack of inferiority to clozapine [91] and the other by showing that clozapine had greater efficacy in reducing the frequency of hallucinations and delusions [92]. Three double-blind trials, however, did not show efficacy for psychosis [93–95] though all showed no change in motor function. The practice implication remains "possibly useful" for the treatment of psychosis in PD [84] though it is often initiated first due to its ease of use. Quetiapine doses used to treat PD psychosis are also relatively low, typically 12.5 mg at bedtime, then increasing by 12.5 mg every 4–7 days until on 25 mg twice a day or 50 mg at night [81], but many physicians use up to 100–200 mg per night. Drawbacks of quetiapine include some reports of mild motor worsening [96], particularly among demented patients [90], and side effects including excessive sedation, orthostasis, or confusion [96].

Pimavanserin, a selective serotonin 5-HT2A inverse agonist without dopaminergic, adrenergic, histaminergic, or muscarinic affinity, is the first medication specifically developed for hallucinations and delusions associated with PD psychosis, and has been evaluated in two level I studies [97, 98]. The larger trial enrolled 199 participants from 52 centers in North America with primary outcome measure of the PD-adapted scale for assessment of positive symptoms (SAPS-PD). Although the study did not provide safety data or evidence regarding durability of response beyond 6 weeks, it concluded pimavanserin was well tolerated and the drug "may benefit patients with PD psychosis for whom few other treatment options exist" [98, 99]. The other trial was a double-blind, randomized multicenter 28-day study of 60 participants in which efficacy of antipsychotic response was measured by the SAPS total domain score, and only showed a trend [97]. The pimavanserin-treated patients showed significantly greater improvement in some (not all) measures of psychosis, including SAPS global measures of hallucinations and delusions, persecutory delusions, and the UPDRS measure of delusions and hallucinations [97]. The FDA completed a review of all post-marketing reports of deaths and serious adverse events reported with the use of pimavanserin and did not identify any new or unexpected safety findings (2018) [100]. Thus, pimavanserin is considered *clinically useful* for the treatment of psychosis in PD in the recent MDS review [84]. Current dosing is 34 mg once daily; a 10 mg tablet is also available.

Other atypical antipsychotics have shown even fewer promise for treating PD psychosis and importantly, increased motor side effects. Olanzapine was evaluated in a 4-week, double-blind, placebo-controlled, parallel group, fixed-dose trial (0, 2.5, or 5 mg) in 23 PD patients with psychosis and found to be ineffective with motor worsening in many [101]. In two double-blind, placebo-controlled studies, low-dose olanzapine again did not significantly improve psychosis and worsened motor function [102, 103]. Two open label studies using aripiprazole had discouraging results [104, 105], with one study demonstrating significant motor worsening. Two small prospective open label trials of ziprasidone showed improvement in psychosis without motor compromise [106, 107]. In a series of four PD cases, one patient had an increase in off-periods and two patients developed pathological laughing [106]. In a review of these two trials and 11 case reports or series, Younce et al. [108] found ziprasidone to be generally effective for treatment of psychosis and with few adverse events reported, but there remain no randomized controlled trials or other blinded studies of ziprasidone. One double-blind study of risperidone versus clozapine showed similar improvement of psychosis to clozapine, but worsened motor function with risperidone [109]. Furthermore, treatment of PD psychosis is complicated by the "black box" warning by the FDA regarding increased risk of death in elderly, demented patients treated with antipsychotics, and there are reports of increased risk of pneumonia in patients with PD in nursing homes who are treated with inappropriate antipsychotics [110]. One study reported a 1.53-fold increased risk of ventricular arrhythmia and/or sudden cardiac death with antipsychotic drug use [111], and as such a baseline electrocardiogram should be performed to ensure normal QTc interval.

Other medications have been used to treat PD psychosis with variable success. Several reports suggest that cholinesterase inhibitors might improve neuropsychiatric features and behavioral problems associated with PDD and DLB [112–115]. Based on data from a double-blind, placebo-controlled study of rivastigmine in PDD, rivastigmine was found to be mildly more effective in PD hallucinators compared to non-hallucinators, but did not significantly reduce the visual hallucinations [14, 116]. While cholinesterase inhibitors may provide a treatment option for the management of psychosis in demented PD patients, these medications take longer to work and thus are not useful in acute psychosis, particularly in the emergency setting. At present, there is not enough evidence to suggest cholinesterase inhibitors for psychosis in non-demented PD patients. Electroconvulsive therapy, a treatment used for refractory depression with or without psychosis, has been found to be helpful in case reports of PD psychosis [117, 118]. While epidemiological and clinical studies have implicated regular cannabis use as a risk factor for the development of psychosis, some evidence suggests that cannabidiol (CBD) can have beneficial effects on psychotic symptoms [119]. One open label 4-week trial of CBD in six patients with PD psychosis showed a significant decrease in psychosis as measured by the Brief Psychiatric Rating Scale and the Parkinson Psychosis Questionnaire [120]. Overall, these other therapies for PD psychosis require additional study and rigorous evaluation before they can be definitively included in treatment algorithms.

Follow-Up of Patient Vignettes

The patient in the first vignette was treated with ciprofloxacin for a presumed urinary tract infection. Within 24 hours, his delirium cleared but vivid hallucinations and paranoia persisted. His amitriptyline was also discontinued, and subsequently his entacapone doses were reduced and discontinued. His psychosis slowly improved, and he was discharged from the psychiatric unit after 10 days. In this case, the acute presentation of somnolence and confusion were indicative of a "medical" explanation (i.e., urinary tract infection). The exacerbation of his psychosis, however, occurred in the context of mild baseline hallucinations, advanced PD, and use of medications that could aggravate psychosis (i.e., amitriptyline, nighttime levodopa, and high doses of levodopa). Treatment of the underlying cause of his acute exacerbation of his psychosis and modifying his PD medication regimen led to a satisfactory outcome; in his case, antipsychotic medications were not needed, and his family was educated about recurrent urinary tract infections and psychosis exacerbations.

The second vignette illustrates a patient with delusions occurring in the context of long-standing PD with motor fluctuations. He did not exhibit features of delirium or dementia but had marked sleep fragmentation, which may have contributed to his psychosis. His psychosis had escalated to a dangerous point, and previous treatment with quetiapine had not been effective. This patient required admission to the psychiatry unit where clozapine was started, and his carbidopa/levodopa dose reduced. Although his motor function was somewhat compromised on the lower levodopa dose, he had less dyskinesia and improved psychosis, although mild delusions persisted. After several weeks of hospitalization and rehabilitation therapy, he was able to return home on a reduced dopaminergic medication regimen and a maintenance dose of clozapine.

Conclusion

Acute psychosis is one of the most common reasons for emergency department visits in PD patients. When evaluation is approached in a timely, stepwise fashion with close monitoring of the patient, psychosis in most PD patients can be effectively managed and major morbidity can be avoided.

References

1. Factor SA, Molho ES. Emergency department presentations of patients with Parkinson's disease. Am J Emerg Med. 2000;18:209–15.
2. Goetz CG, Stebbins GT. Risk factors for nursing home placement in advanced Parkinson's disease. Neurology. 1993;43:2227–9.
3. Stella F, Banzato CE, Quagliato EM, Viana MA, Christofoletti G. Psychopathological features in patients with Parkinson's disease and related caregivers' burden. Int J Geriatr Psychiatry. 2009;24:1158–65.
4. Melamed E, Friedberg G, Zoldan J. Psychosis: impact on the patient and family. Neurology. 1999;52:S14–6.
5. McKinlay A, Grace RC, Dalrymple-Alford JC, Anderson T, Fink J, Roger D. A profile of neuropsychiatric problems and their relationship to quality of life for Parkinson's disease patients without dementia. Parkinsonism Relat Disord. 2008;14:37–42.
6. Ravina B, Marder K, Fernandez HH, Friedman JH, Friedman JH, McDonald W, Murphy D, et al. Diagnostic criteria for psychosis in Parkinson's disease: report of an NINDS, NIMH work group. Mov Disord. 2007;22:1061–8.
7. Fenelon G, Mahieux F, Huon R, Ziegler M. Hallucinations in Parkinson's disease: prevalence, phenomenology, and risk factors. Brain. 2000;123(4):733–45.
8. Barnes J, David AS. Visual hallucinations in Parkinson's disease: a review and phenomenological survey. J Neurol Neurosurg Psychiatry. 2001;70:727–33.
9. Goetz CG, Tanner CM, Klawans HL. Pharmacology of hallucinations induced by long-term drug therapy. Am J Psychiatry. 1982;139:494–7.
10. Graham JM, Grunewald RA, Sagar HJ. Hallucinosis in idiopathic Parkinson's disease. J Neurol Neurosurg Psychiatry. 1997;63:434–40.
11. Rabey J. Hallucinations and psychosis in Parkinson's disease. Parkinsonism Relat Disord. 2009;15S:S105–10.
12. Goetz C. New developments in depression, anxiety, compulsiveness, and hallucinations in Parkinson's disease. Mov Disord. 2010;25:S104–9.
13. Papapetropoulos S, Mash DC. Psychotic symptoms in Parkinson's disease: from description to etiology. J Neurol. 2005;252:753–64.
14. Friedman J. Parkinson's disease psychosis 2010: a review article. Parkinsonism Relat Disord. 2010;16(9):1–8.
15. Marsh L. Psychosis in Parkinson's disease. Prim Psychiatry. 2005;12:56–62.
16. Diederich NJ, Goetz CG, Stebbins GT. Repeated visual hallucinations in Parkinson's disease as disturbed external/internal perceptions: focused review and a new integrative model. Mov Disord. 2005;20:130–40.
17. Goetz CG, Wuu J, Curgian L, Leurgans S. Age-related influences on the clinical characteristics of new-onset hallucinations in Parkinson's disease patients. Mov Disord. 2005;21:267–70.
18. Fenelon G, Thobois S, Bonnet AM, Broussolle E, Tison F. Tactile hallucinations in Parkinson's disease. J Neurol. 2002;249:1699–703.
19. Tousi B, Frankel M. Olfactory and visual hallucinations in Parkinson's disease. Parkinsonism Relat Disord. 2004;10:253–4.

20. Fénelon G. Epidemiology of psychosis in Parkinson's disease. J Neurol Sci. 2010;289:12–7.
21. Marsh L, Williams JR, Rocco M, Grill S, Munro C, Dawson TM. Psychiatric comorbidities in patients with Parkinson disease and psychosis. Neurology. 2004;63:293–300.
22. Black DW, Boffeli TJ. Simple schizophrenia: past, present, and future. Am J Psychiatry. 1989;146:1267–73.
23. Aarsland DML, Schrag A. Neuropsychiatric symptoms in Parkinson's disease. Mov Disord. 2009;24:2175–86.
24. Stewart JT. Fregoli syndrome associated with levodopa treatment. Mov Disord. 2008;23:308–9.
25. Pagonabarraga J, Llebaria G, Garcia-Sanchez C, Pascual-Sedano B, Gironell A, Kulisevsky J. A prospective study of delusional misidentification syndromes in Parkinson's disease with dementia. Mov Disord. 2008;23:443–8.
26. Roane DM, Rogers JD, Robinson JH, Feinberg TE. Delusional misidentification in association with parkinsonism. J Neuropsychiatry Clin Neurosci. 1998;10:194–8.
27. McKeith IG, Fairbairn AF, Bothwell RA, Moore PB, Ferrier IN, Thompson P, et al. An evaluation of the predictive validity and inter-rater reliability of clinical diagnostic criteria for senile dementia of Lewy body type. Neurology. 1994;44:872–7.
28. Sanchez-Ramos JR, Ortoll R, Paulson GW. Visual hallucinations associated with Parkinson disease. Arch Neurol. 1996;53:1265–8.
29. Inzelberg R, Kipervasser S, Korczyn AD. Auditory hallucinations in Parkinson's disease. J Neurol Neurosurg Psychiatry. 1998;64:533–5.
30. Holroyd S, Currie L, Wooten GF. Prospective study of hallucinations and delusions in Parkinson's disease. J Neurol Neurosurg Psychiatry. 2001;70:734–8.
31. Aarsland D, Larsen JP, Cummins JL, Laake K. Prevalence and clinical correlates of psychotic symptoms in Parkinson disease: a community-based study. Arch Neurol. 1999;56:595–601.
32. Fenelon G, Soulas T, Zenasni F, de Langavant LC. The changing face of Parkinson's disease-associated psychosis: a cross-sectional study based on the new NINDS-NIMH criteria. Mov Disord. 2010;25:755–9.
33. Forsaa EB, Larsen J, Wentzel-Larsen T, Goetz CG, Stebbins GT, Aarsland D, et al. A 12-year population-based study of psychosis in Parkinson disease. Arch Neurol. 2010;67:996–1001.
34. Goetz CG, Ouyang B, Negron A, Stebbins GT. Hallucinations and sleep disorders in PD: ten-year prospective longitudinal study. Neurology. 2010;75:1773–9.
35. Hely MA, Morris JG, Reid WG, Trafficante R. Sydney multicenter study of Parkinson's disease: non-L-dopa-responsive problems dominate at 15 years. Mov Disord. 2005;20:190–9.
36. Hely MA, Reid WG, Adena MA, Halliday GM, Morris JG. eThe Sydney multicenter study of Parkinson's disease: the inevitability of dementia at 20 years. Mov Disord. 2008;23:837–44.
37. Archibald NK, Clarke MP, Mosimann UP, Burn DJ. Visual symptoms in Parkinson's disease and Parkinson's disease dementia. Mov Disord. 2011;26(13):2387–95.
38. Matsui H, Udaka F, Tamura A, Oda M, Kubori T, Nishinaka K, et al. Impaired visual acuity as a risk factor for visual hallucinations in Parkinson's disease. J Geriatr Psychiatry Neurol. 2006;19(1):36–40.
39. Diederich NJ, Pappert EJ, Leurgans S, Piery V. Poor visual discrimination and visual hallucinations in Parkinson's disease. Clin Neuropharmacol. 1998;21(5):289–95.
40. Lee JY, Kim JM, Ahn J, Kim HJ, Jeon BS, Kim TW. Retinal nerve fiber layer thickness and visual hallucinations in Parkinson's disease. Mov Disord. 2014;29(1):61–7.
41. Onofrj M, Bonanni L, Albani G, Mauro A, Bulla D, Thomas A. Visual hallucinations in Parkinson's disease: clues to separate origins. J Neurol Sci. 2006;248:143–50.
42. Weintraub D, Morales KH, Duda JE, Moberg PJ, Stern MB. Frequency and correlates of co-morbid psychosis and depression in Parkinson's disease. Parkinsonism Relat Disord. 2006;12:427–31.
43. Papapetropoulos S, Argyriou AA, Ellul J. Factors associated with drug-induced visual hallucinations in Parkinson's disease. J Neurol. 2005;252:1223–8.

44. Aarsland D, Ballard C, Larsen JP, McKeith I. A comparative study of psychiatric symptoms in dementia with Lewy bodies and Parkinson's disease with and without dementia. Int J Geriatr Psychiatry. 2001;16:528–36.
45. Kulisevsky J, Pagonabarraga J, Pascual-Sedano B, Garcia-Sanchez C, Gironell A. Trapecio Group Study. Prevalence and correlates of neuropsychiatric symptoms in Parkinson's disease without dementia. Mov Disord. 2008;23:1889–96.
46. Biglan KM, Holloway RG Jr, McDermott MP, Richard IH. Risk factors for somnolence, edema, and hallucinations in early Parkinson disease. Neurology. 2007;69:187–95.
47. Wolters E. PD-related psychosis: pathophysiology with therapeutical strategies. J Neural Transm Suppl. 2006;71:31–7.
48. LeWitt PA, Lyons KE, Pahwa R. Advanced Parkinson disease treated with rotigotine transdermal system: PREFER study. Neurology. 2007;68:1262–7.
49. Rascol O, Brooks DJ, Korczyn AD, De Deyn PP, Clarke CE, Lang AE. A five-year study of the incidence of dyskinesia in patients with early Parkinson's disease who were treated with ropinirole or levodopa; 056 study group. N Engl J Med. 2000;342:1484–91.
50. Group TPS. Pramipexole vs. levodopa as initial treatment for Parkinson disease: a randomized controlled trial; Parkinson study group. JAMA. 2000;284:1931–8.
51. de Smet Y, Ruberg M, Serdaru M, Dubois B, Lhermitte F, Agid Y. Confusion, dementia and anticholinergics in Parkinson's disease. J Neurol Neurosurg Psychiatry. 1982;45:1161–4.
52. Wolters EC. Intrinsic and extrinsic psychosis in Parkinson's disease. J Neurol. 2001;248 Suppl 3:III/22–7.
53. Rinne UK, Bracco F, Chouza C, Dupont E, Gershanik O, Marti Masso JF, et al. Early treatment of Parkinson's disease with cabergoline delays the onset of motor complications; results of a double-blind levodopa controlled trial; the PKDS009 study group. Drugs. 1998;55(Suppl 1):23–30.
54. Biousse V, Skibell BC, Watts RL, et al. Ophthalmologic features of Parkinson's disease. Neurology. 2004;62:177–80.
55. de Maindreville AD, Fenelon G, Mahieux F. Hallucinations in Parkinson's disease: a follow-up study. Mov Disord. 2005;20:212–7.
56. Djamgoz MB, Hankins MW, Hirano J, Archer SN. Neurobiology of retinal dopamine in relation to degenerative states of the tissue. Vis Res. 1997;37:3509–29.
57. Pieri V, Diederich NJ, Raman R, Goetz CG. Decreased color discrimination and contrast sensitivity in Parkinson's disease. J Neurol Sci. 2000;172:7–11.
58. Diederich H, Nishinaka K, Oda M, Hara N, Komatsu K, Kubori T, et al. Hypoperfusion of the visual pathway in parkinsonian patients with visual hallucinations. Mov Disord. 2006;21:2140–4.
59. Goldman JG, Stebbins GT, Dinh V, Bernard B, Merkitch D. deToledo-Morrell L, Goetz CG. Visuoperceptive region atrophy independent of cognitive status in patients with Parkinson's disease with hallucinations. Brain. 2014;137(3):849–59.
60. Holroyd S, Wooten GF. Preliminary FMRI evidence of visual system dysfunction in Parkinson's disease patients with visual hallucinations. J Neuropsychiatry Clin Neurosci. 2006;18:402–4.
61. Stebbins GT, Goetz CG, Carrillo MC, Bangen KJ, Turner DA, Glover GH, et al. Altered cortical visual processing in PD with hallucinations: an fMRI study. Neurology. 2004;63:1409–16.
62. Boecker H, Ceballos-Baumann AO, Volk D, Conrad B, Forstl H, Haussermann P. Metabolic alterations in patients with Parkinson disease and visual hallucinations. Arch Neurol. 2007;64:984–8.
63. Braak H, Del Tredici K, Bratzke H, Hamm-Clement J, Sandmann-Keil D, Rüb U. Staging of the intracerebral inclusion body pathology associated with idiopathic Parkinson's disease (preclinical and clinical stages). J Neurol. 2002;249 Suppl 3:III/1–5.
64. Papapetropoulos S, McCorquodale DS, Gonzalez J, Jean-Gilles L, Mash DC. Cortical and amygdalar Lewy body burden in Parkinson's disease patients with visual hallucinations. Parkinsonism Relat Disord. 2006;12:253–6.

65. Harding AJ, Broe GA, Halliday GM. Visual hallucinations in Lewy body disease relate to Lewy bodies in the temporal lobe. Brain. 2002;125:391–403.
66. Comella CL, Tanner CM, Ristanovic RK. Polysomnographic sleep measures in Parkinson's disease patients with treatment-induced hallucinations. Ann Neurol. 1993;34:710–4.
67. Arnulf I, Bonnet AM, Damier P, Bejjani BP, Seilhean D, Derenne JP, et al. Hallucinations, REM sleep, and Parkinson's disease: a medical hypothesis. Neurology. 2000;55:281–8.
68. Pappert EJ, Goetz CG, Niederman FG, Raman R, Leurgans S. Hallucinations, sleep fragmentation, and altered dream phenomena in Parkinson's disease. Mov Disord. 1999;14:117–21.
69. Ramirez-Ruiz B, Marti MJ, Tolosa E, Giménez M, Bargalló N, Valldeoriola F, et al. Cerebral atrophy in Parkinson's disease patients with visual hallucinations. Eur J Neurol. 2007;14:750–6.
70. Ibarretxe-Bilbao N, Ramirez-Ruiz B, Tolosa E, Martí MJ, Valldeoriola F, Bargalló N, et al. Hippocampal head atrophy predominance in Parkinson's disease with hallucinations and with dementia. J Neurol. 2008;255:1324–31.
71. Ramirez-Ruiz B, Junque C, Marti MJ, Valldeoriola F, Tolosa E. Neuropsychological deficits in Parkinson's disease patients with visual hallucinations. Mov Disord. 2006;21:1483–7.
72. Mosimann UP, Rowan EN, Partington CE, Collerton D, Littlewood E, O'Brien JT, et al. Characteristics of visual hallucinations in Parkinson disease dementia and dementia with Lewy bodies. Am J Geriatr Psychiatry. 2006;14:153–60.
73. Llebaria G, Pagonabarraga J, Martinez-Corral M, García-Sánchez C, Pascual-Sedano B, Gironell A, et al. Neuropsychological correlates of mild to severe hallucinations in Parkinson's disease. Mov Disord. 2010;25:2785–91.
74. Williams-Gray CH, Foltynie T, Brayne CE, Robbins TW, Barker RA. Evolution of cognitive dysfunction in an incident Parkinson's disease cohort. Brain. 2007;130:1787–98.
75. McKeith I, Fairbairn A, Perry R, Thompson P, Perry E. Neuroleptic sensitivity in patients with senile dementia of Lewy body type. BMJ. 1992;305:673–8.
76. McKeith I, Del Ser T, Spano P, Emre M, Wesnes K, Anand R, et al. Efficacy of rivastigmine in dementia with Lewy bodies: a randomized, double blind, placebo-controlled international study. Lancet. 2000;356:2031–6.
77. Schrag A. Quality of life and depression in Parkinson's disease. J Neurol Sci. 2006;248:151–7.
78. Hasnain M, Vieweg WV, Baron MS, Beatty-Brooks M, Fernandez A, Pandurangi AK. Pharmacological management of psychosis in elderly patients with parkinsonism. Am J Med. 2009;122:614–22.
79. Klein C, Prokhorov T, Miniovitz A, Dobronevsky E, Rabey JM. Admission of parkinsonian patients to a neurological ward in a community hospital. J Neural Transm. 2009;116:1509–12.
80. Munhoz RP, Moscovich M, Araujo PD, Teive HA. Movement disorders emergencies: a review. Arq Neuropsiquiatr. 2012;70(6):453–61.
81. Friedman JH, Factor SA. Atypical antipsychotics in the treatment of drug-induced psychosis in Parkinson's disease. Mov Disord. 2000;15:201–11.
82. Olanow CW, Watts RL, Koller WC. An algorithm (decision tree) for the management of Parkinson's disease (2001): treatment guidelines. Neurology. 2001;56:S1–88.
83. Miyasaki JM, Shannon K, Voon V, Ravina B, Kleiner-Fisman G, Anderson K, et al. Practice parameter: evaluation and treatment of depression, psychosis, and dementia in Parkinson disease (an evidence-based review); report of the quality standards subcommittee of the American Academy of Neurology. Neurology. 2006;66:996–1002.
84. Seppi K, Ray Chaudhuri K, Coelho M, Fox SH, Katzenschlager R, Perez Lloret S, et al. Update on treatments for nonmotor symptoms of Parkinson's disease-an evidence-based medicine review. Mov Disord. 2019;34(2):180–98.
85. Wolters EC, Hurwitz TA, Mak E, Teal P, Peppard FR, Remick R, et al. Clozapine in the treatment of parkinsonian patients with dopaminomimetic psychosis. Neurology. 1990;40:832–4.
86. Group TFCPS. Clozapine in drug-induced psychosis in Parkinson's disease. Lancet. 1999;353:2041–2.
87. Group TPS. Low-dose clozapine for the treatment of drug-induced psychosis in Parkinson's disease. N Engl J Med. 1999;340:757–63.

88. Pollak P, Tison F, Rascol O, Destee A. on behalf of the French clozapine Parkinson study group, et al. Clozapine in drug-induced psychosis in Parkinson's disease; a randomized, placebo controlled study with open follow up. J Neurol Neurosurg Psychiatry. 2004;75:689–95.
89. Honigfeld G, Arellano F, Sethi J, Bianchini A, Schein J. Reducing clozapine-related morbidity and mortality: 5 years of experience with the Clozaril National Registry. J Clin Psychiatry. 1998;59(Suppl 3):3–7.
90. Reddy SFS, Molho ES, Feustel PJ. The effect of quetiapine on psychosis and motor function in parkinsonian patients with and without dementia. Mov Disord. 2002;17:676–81.
91. Morgante L, Epifanio A, Spina E, Zappia M, Di Rosa AE, Marconi R, et al. Quetiapine and clozapine in parkinsonian patients with dopaminergic psychosis. Clin Neuropharmacol. 2004;27:153–6.
92. Merims BM, Peretz C, Shabtai H, Giladi N. Rater-blinded, prospective comparison: quetiapine versus clozapine for Parkinson's disease psychosis. Clin Neuropharmacol. 2006;26:331–7.
93. Ondo WG, Tintner R, Voung KD, Lai D, Ringholz G. Double blind, placebo-controlled, unforced titration parallel trial of quetiapine for dopaminergic-induced hallucinations in Parkinson's disease. Mov Disord. 2005;20:958–63.
94. Rabey PT, Miniovitz A, Dobronevsky E, Klein C. Effect of quetiapine in psychotic Parkinson's disease patients: a double-blind labeled study of 3 months' duration. Mov Disord. 2007;22:313–8.
95. Shotbolt SM, Fox C, David AS. A randomized controlled trial of quetiapine for psychosis in Parkinson's disease. Neuropsychiatr Dis Treat. 2009;5:327–32.
96. Fernandez HH, Trieschmann M, Burke MA, Jacques C, Friedman JH. Long-term outcome of quetiapine use for psychosis among parkinsonian patients. Mov Disord. 2003;18:510–4.
97. Meltzer HY, Mills R, Revell S, Williams H, Johnson A, Bahr D, et al. Pimavanserin, a serotonin(2A) receptor inverse agonist, for the treatment of Parkinson's disease psychosis. Neuropsychopharmacology. 2010;35(4):881–92.
98. Cummings J, Isaacson S, Mills R, Williams H, Chi-Burris K, Corbett A, et al. Pimavanserin for patients with Parkinson's disease psychosis: a randomized, placebo-controlled phase 3 trial. Lancet. 2014;383(9916):533–40.
99. Webster P. Pimavanserin evaluated by the FDA. Lancet. 2018;391(10132):1762.
100. U.S. Food and Drug Administration. FDA analysis finds no new or unexpected safety risks associated with Nuplazid (pimavanserin), a medication to treat the hallucinations and delusions of Parkinson's disease psychosis. https://www.fda.gov/Drugs/DrugSafety/ucm621160.htm. Accessed 1 Aug 2020.
101. Nichols MJ, Hartlein JM, Eicken MG, Racette BA, Black KJ. A fixed-dose randomized controlled trial of olanzapine for psychosis in Parkinson disease. F1000Res. 2013;2:150.
102. Ondo WG, Vuong KD, Hunter C, Jankovic J. Olanzapine treatment for dopaminergic-induced hallucinations. Mov Disord. 2002;17:1031–5.
103. Breier SV, Feldman PD, Kadam DL, Ferchland I, Wright P, Friedman JH. Olanzapine in the treatment of dopamimetic-induced psychosis in patients with Parkinson's disease. Biol Psychiatry. 2002;52:438–45.
104. Friedman JH, Berman RM, Goetz CG, Factor SA, Ondo WG, Wojcieszek J, et al. Open-label flexible-dose pilot study to evaluate the safety and tolerability of aripiprazole in patients with psychosis associated with Parkinson's disease. Mov Disord. 2006;21:2078–81.
105. Fernandez HHTM, Friedman JH. Aripiprazole for drug-induced psychosis in Parkinson disease: preliminary experience. Clin Neuropharmacol. 2004;27:4–5.
106. Schindehutte TC. Treatment of drug-induced psychosis in Parkinson's disease with ziprasidone can induce severe dose-dependent off-periods and pathological laughing. Clin Neurol Neurosurg. 2007;109:188–91.
107. Gómez-Esteban JC, Zarranz JJ, Velasco F, Lezcano E, Lachen MC, Rouco I, et al. Use of ziprasidone in parkinsonian patients with psychosis. Clin Neuropharmacol. 2005;28:111–4.
108. Younce JR, Davis AA, Black KJ. A systematic review and case series of ziprasidone for psychosis in Parkinson's disease. J Parkinsons Dis. 2019;9(1):63–71.

109. Ellis T, Cudkowicz ME, Sexton PM, Growdon JH. Clozapine and risperidone treatment of psychosis in Parkinson's disease. J Neuropsychiatry Clin Neurosci. 2000;12:364–9.
110. Chekani F, Holmes HM, Johnson ML, Chen H, Sherer JT, Aparasu RR. Risk of pneumonia associated with atypical antipsychotic use in nursing home residents with Parkinson's disease. J Psychiatr Res. 2019;117:116–21.
111. Wu CS, Tsai YT, Tsai HJ. Antipsychotic drugs and the risk of ventricular arrhythmia and/or sudden cardiac death: a nation-wide case crossover study. J Am Heart Assoc. 2015;4(2):e001568.
112. Bhasin M, Rowan E, Edwards K, McKeith I. Cholinesterase inhibitors in dementia with Lewy bodies: a comparative analysis. Int J Geriatr Psychiatry. 2007;22:890–5.
113. Edwards KR, Hershey L, Wray L, Bednarczyk EM, Lichter D, Farlow M, et al. Efficacy and safety of galantamine in patients with dementia with Lewy bodies: a 24-week open-label study. Dement Geriatr Cogn Disord. 2007;23:401–5.
114. Rozzini L, Chilovi BV, Bertoletti E, Conti M, Delrio I, Trabucchi M, et al. Cognitive and psychopathologic response to rivastigmine in dementia with Lewy bodies compared to Alzheimer's disease: a case control study. Am J Alzheimers Dis Other Dement. 2007;22:42–7.
115. Thomas AJ, Burn DJ, Rowan EN, Littlewood E, Newby J, Cousins D, et al. A comparison of the efficacy of donepezil in Parkinson's disease with dementia and dementia with Lewy bodies. Int J Geriatr Psychiatry. 2005;20:938–44.
116. Burn D, Emre M, McKeith I, De Deyn PP, Aarsland D, Hsu C, et al. Effects of rivastigmine in patients with and without visual hallucinations in dementia associated with Parkinson's disease. Mov Disord. 2006;21:1899–907.
117. Factor SA, Molho ES, Brown DL. Combined clozapine and electroconvulsive therapy for the treatment of drug-induced psychosis in Parkinson's disease. J Neuropsychiatry Clin Neurosci. 1995;7:304–7.
118. Nishioka K, Tanaka R, Shimura H, Hirano K, Hatano T, Miyakawa K, et al. Quantitative evaluation of electroconvulsive therapy for Parkinson's disease with refractory psychiatric symptoms. J Neural Transm (Vienna). 2014;121(11):1405–10.
119. Bhattacharyya S, Wilson R, Appiah-Kusi E, O'Neill A, Brammer M, Perez J, et al. Effect of Cannabidiol on medial temporal, midbrain, and striatal dysfunction in people at clinical high risk of psychosis: a randomized clinical trial. JAMA Psychiat. 2018;75(11):1107–17.
120. Zuardi AW, Crippa JA, Hallak JE, Pinto JP, Chagas MH, Rodrigues GG, et al. Cannabidiol for the treatment of psychosis in Parkinson's disease. J Psychopharmacol. 2009;23(8):979–83.

Perioperative Emergencies Associated with Deep Brain Stimulation

18

Takashi Morishita, Adam P. Burdick, and Tooru Inoue

Patient Vignettes

We present 11 illustrative cases of perioperative emergencies associated with deep brain stimulation (DBS) from our experience and one case drawn from the literature [1]. The data and discussion for this chapter are also drawn from several recent publications [2–12].

Perioperative Emergencies

Patient 1: Intraventricular Hemorrhage

A 73-year-old man with a 16-year history of Parkinson's disease (PD) underwent unilateral subthalamic nucleus (STN) DBS. Following the procedure, he became somnolent, and a postoperative computed tomography (CT) scan revealed a hematoma in the left lateral ventricle (Fig. 18.1a). The hematoma involved the third ventricle and the Sylvian aqueduct, and the patient developed acute obstructive hydrocephalus. He required an emergent ventriculostomy on the same day. The management issues mandated 1 week of bed rest postoperatively, during which he then developed a deep venous thrombosis, aspiration pneumonia, atrial fibrillation, a urinary tract infection and sepsis. The total hospitalization was 40 postoperative days. Following 8 months of rehabilitation and anticoagulant therapy, implantation of an implantable pulse generator (IPG) was scheduled.

T. Morishita (✉) · T. Inoue
Department of Neurosurgery, Fukuoka University Faculty of Medicine, Fukuoka, Japan
e-mail: tmorishita@fukuoka-u.ac.jp

A. P. Burdick
Department of Neurosurgery, Scripps Clinic Medical Group, San Diego, CA, USA

© Springer Nature Switzerland AG 2022
S. J. Frucht (ed.), *Movement Disorder Emergencies*, Current Clinical Neurology,
https://doi.org/10.1007/978-3-030-75898-1_18

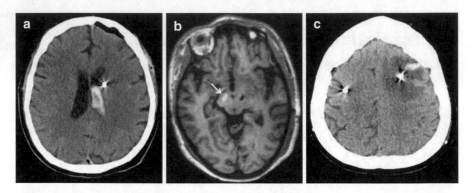

Fig. 18.1 Images of hemorrhagic complications. (**a**) A computed tomography (CT) scan shows left ventricular hemorrhage following the surgery (patient 1). (**b**) A T1-weighted image performed on the postoperative day 1 shows the microbleeding in the subthalamic nucleus (patient 2). (**c**) A CT scan image shows edematous lesion surrounding the left deep brain stimulation (DBS) lead with intracerebral hemorrhage (patient 4)

Patient 2: Intracerebral Hemorrhage

A 63-year-old woman with PD underwent simultaneous bilateral STN DBS. Following microelectrode recordings (MERs) on the right side, the patient developed a mild left hemiparesis intraoperatively. The DBS system was implanted only in the left hemisphere with IPG implanted on the same day. Postoperative magnetic resonance imaging (MRI) scan revealed microbleeding in the right STN (Fig. 18.1b).

Patient 3: Intraoperative Seizure

A 65-year-old man with PD underwent unilateral globus pallidus interna (GPi) DBS. Following MER macrostimulation to test the threshold levels of stimulation-induced side effects, it was noted that when the voltage was increased, a focal seizure was precipitated in the right arm transforming into a complex generalized subtype. Propofol was intravenously administered immediately and the seizure was terminated. The DBS procedure was completed and the postoperative CT scan revealed no lesions and no intracranial hemorrhage. The patient recovered without any neurological deficit.

Patient 4: Venous Infarct

A 67-year-old woman with PD underwent right STN DBS with good results; she requested contralateral stimulation. Six months after the right DBS implantation, a left STN DBS lead was implanted. She was discharged on postoperative day 1 after an uncomplicated hospital course, but that evening experienced word finding difficulties and an altered level of consciousness. When these symptoms persisted through the following morning, her husband brought her to the emergency room. On examination, except for a significant but incomplete expressive aphasia and disorientation, she was neurologically intact, including writing, repetition, and comprehension. A CT scan of the head demonstrated edema and hemorrhage surrounding the superficial aspect of the DBS lead (Fig. 18.1c). Her aphasia improved over the next several days, but some confusion persisted for several weeks. Her speech and cognition ultimately recovered completely, but she did report occasional slurring of her speech with fatigue.

Patient 5: Neuroleptic Malignant Syndrome (Parkinsonism-Hyperpyrexia Syndrome) [1]

A 54-year-old man with a 14-year history of PD underwent STN DBS. He was preoperatively treated with levodopa/carbidopa, entacapone and pramipexole, and all medications were discontinued 18 h prior to the procedure. DBS surgery was performed uneventfully; however, the patient developed tremor, muscle rigidity, and high fever 3 hours postoperatively. Laboratory investigation revealed extremely high creatinine kinase levels. The patient was intubated and admitted to the intensive care unit (ICU). Although treatment with dantrolene, levodopa, and apomorphine was immediately initiated, the hospital stay was extended to 4 months.

Patient 6: Myocardial Infarction

A 58-year-old male with PD underwent unilateral STN DBS placement. In addition to PD, his past medical history was significant for coronary artery disease (CAD) (previously treated with angioplasty), hypertension, diabetes mellitus (DM), and hyperlipidemia. An implantable pulse generator (IPG) was placed 4 weeks following the DBS lead under general anesthesia. Following IPG implantation the patient died of a myocardial infarction in his sleep on postoperative day 1.

Postoperative Emergencies

Patient 7: Superficial Wound Infection

A 62-year-old PD patient underwent a right DBS surgery uneventfully; however, he complained of inflammation of the left subclavian incisional site 4 months later (Fig. 18.2). He was then prescribed topical antibiotics, but the symptom progressed and redness and superficial hemorrhage developed. He came to the clinic and underwent an urgent wound revision without device explantation as the surgical site infection was superficial. The wound healed completely after wound revision.

Patient 8: Deep Infection

A 43-year-old man with a 9-year history of PD underwent unilateral STN DBS. He arrived for a routine clinic appointment and staple removal on postoperative day 17. Following the staple removal purulent drainage from the cranial incision site was noted, and the pectoral incision site was tender and erythematous. He was admitted to the hospital urgently, and both the IPG and the extension wire were removed. A course of intravenous antibiotics was administered and completed prior to reimplantation.

Patient 9: Intracerebral Infection

A 71-year-old man with a history of medically refractory essential tremor (ET) underwent a unilateral thalamic DBS implantation. Four weeks following surgery, the patient presented to clinic complaining of headache and progressive dysphagia. An emergent head CT revealed a brain abscess along the DBS lead tract. An edematous lesion surrounding the DBS lead enhanced with contrast media on CT scan (Fig. 18.3). An emergent craniotomy and DBS lead removal was performed.

Fig. 18.2 Photograph of superficial wound infection

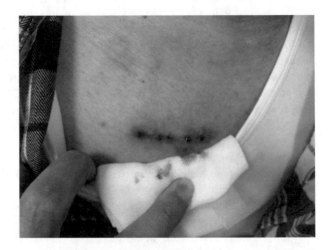

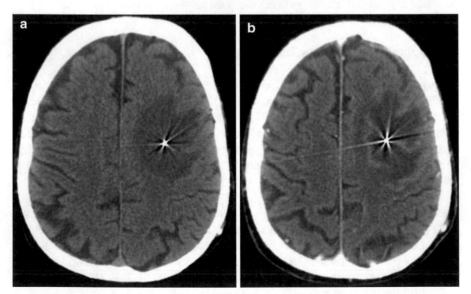

Fig. 18.3 Computed tomography (CT) scan images of a brain abscess following DBS lead implantation. A CT scan image without contrast (*left*) revealed a low-density edematous lesion surrounding the DBS lead. The lesion enhanced with contrast media (*right*). (Adapted with permission from Elsevier from Morishita et al. [2])

Patient 10: Lead Migration

A 40-year-old patient with DYT-1 dystonia underwent bilateral GPi DBS at age 26 at another institution. He was brought to the emergency department after a generalized tonic-clonic seizure. The seizure subsided immediately with administration of intravenous diazepam. The patient had no past medical history of epilepsy prior to the visit. His past medical history was complicated by removal of the left DBS system at age 35 due to severe infection following an IPG replacement. Although he underwent revision of the left DBS, his condition did not return to the same status as the first DBS surgery. A CT scan revealed that his bilateral DBS leads had migrated ventrally. We attributed his severe axial symptoms (head jerking) to migration of the DBS leads. The left electrode had completely migrated into the mesial temporal lobe, triggering his seizure. He therefore, underwent revision of the bilateral DBS leads in a staged fashion, and his dystonia symptoms improved (Fig. 18.4).

Patient 11: Hardware Malfunction

A 71-year-old woman underwent a left-sided unilateral GPi DBS for PD and was discharged uneventfully. She fell in her home 2 months after surgery with head trauma at the site of extension cable behind her ear. She then felt sudden loss of benefit of DBS, as her on/off motor fluctuations became aggravated. The impedance

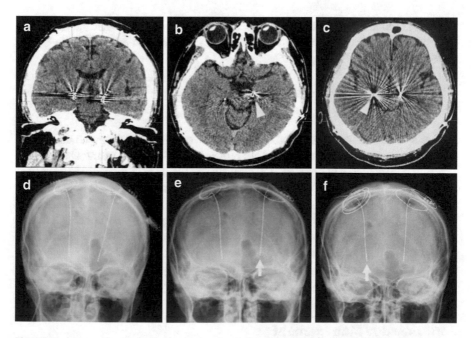

Fig. 18.4 A ventrally migrated deep brain stimulation (DBS) lead is shown on the coronal (**a**) and axial CT (**b, c**) images and a skull X-ray (**d**). Two preoperative axial CT images (**b, c**) show the tips of left and right DBS leads, respectively. The left and right leads were replaced with a new lead in a staged fashion (**e, f**). (Adapted from [12])

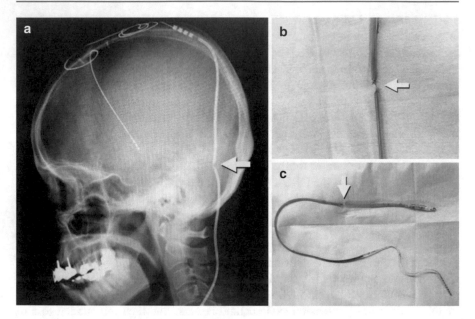

Fig. 18.5 Fractured lead shown on the skull X-ray (**a**), and intraoperative pictures (**b, c**). (Adapted from [12])

was extraordinarily high at all contacts, and an X-ray revealed that the cable was fractured. She underwent urgent replacement of the extension cable, which restored the benefits of the DBS (Fig. 18.5).

Introduction

DBS has become an established procedure for movement and neuropsychiatric disorders, and recent reports have revealed the efficacy of DBS for many indications [13–17]. With the increased use of DBS, DBS-related problems have emerged as important problems for management. When an adverse event occurs, clinicians should consider the most probable diagnoses and develop an appropriate treatment plan. DBS-related issues manifest in unusual forms, and the differential diagnoses vary widely [2, 4, 18]. We therefore separate the possible scenarios into: (1) perioperative (intra- and early postoperative) and (2) postoperative (following 2–4 weeks) scenarios. With the 11 clinical vignettes described above, we address how clinicians should appropriately detect and manage these "don't miss" emergent/urgent issues in DBS patients.

Perioperative Management

Intracranial Hemorrhage

Clinicians should maintain a high index of suspicion for intracranial hemorrhage, as this complication has a high propensity to result in neurological deficits. Damage to blood vessels by MER and/or macrostimulation passes can result in intracranial hemorrhage. Several authors argue that MER, especially multi-track MER, increases the risk of intracranial hemorrhage, but this topic remains controversial [19, 20]. The incidence of hemorrhage ranges from 0% to 5.3% [1, 7, 12, 21–27]. In the operative setting, intracerebral (ICH) and intraventricular hemorrhage (IVH) are the most frequent forms of serious bleeding encountered. Hemorrhage may manifest as an epileptic seizure, altered mental status (patient 1) or hemiparesis (patient 2) [1, 2]. When these symptoms emerge suddenly, clinicians should consider the possibility of ICH or IVH, and an immediate CT scan should be performed. Delay in identification and management of ICH may result in significant morbidity, and emergent care should be employed to prevent both primary and secondary complications. When an intracranial hemorrhage is diagnosed postoperatively, neurosurgical evaluation should be rapidly performed, preferably by the neurosurgeon who implanted the DBS system. Although most patients can be managed conservatively by optimizing blood pressure and with rest and neurorehabilitation, when the ICH is large, causes mass effect, and/or obstructive hydrocephalus, neurosurgical management such as craniotomy or intraventricular drainage may be necessary (Table 18.1).

Table 18.1 Management of DBS-related emergencies

Issues	Management
Intraoperative emergencies	
Intracerebral hemorrhage	If the hemorrhage is very large or has symptomatic mass effect, an emergent craniotomy may need to be performed
Intraventricular hemorrhage	Ventriculostomy, if necessary, for obstructive hydrocephalus
Subdural hematoma	Bur hole irrigation should be performed when the hematoma is symptomatic
Air embolus	Wax edges of the bur hole, occlude the bur hole with gel foam and saline, lower patient's head, jugular venous compression, administer oxygen
Dyskinetic storm	Sedative agents may be administered in select cases. Reducing the dopaminergic medication may help. In some cases, ICU care is necessary
Epileptic seizure	Sedative agents such as propofol or a benzodiazepine such as diazepam should be administered immediately
Early postoperative emergencies (<2–4 weeks)	
Venous infarction	Conservative supportive therapy is usually all that is necessary. An emergent craniotomy may be performed if hemorrhage is life-threatening
Myocardial infarction	Do not ignore chest pain in a patient who has just had a subclavicular IPG placed. Immediate diagnosis by 12-lead electrocardiogram and laboratory investigation, and cardiology consult should be performed
Neuroleptic malignant syndrome	IV fluid and L-dopa should be administered immediately. If necessary nasogastric tube should be placed for patients with difficulty in oral intake. ICU care is necessary. Administering dantrolene is an option

(continued)

Table 18.1 (continued)

Issues	Management
Behavioral/cognitive issues	Identify and treat the underlying issues (e.g., UTI and pneumonia). Selective dopamine blockers (e.g., clozapine, quetiapine) may be used, but nonselective blockers should be avoided if possible. Use a one to one sitter to avoid secondary injury, e.g., from falling
Infection-UTI/ pneumonia	Hydration and appropriate antibiotics. Care should be taken to adjust PD medications as levels may be altered by antibiotics. Surgical debridement or removal of hardware as necessary
Postoperative emergencies (≥2–4 weeks)	
Suicide ideation/ attempt	Admit the patient to the hospital for multi/interdisciplinary care, and treat underlying cause. May need both medication adjustment and programming. Check lead location
Severe depression	Behavioral therapy, counseling, medication adjustment, and/or stimulation adjustment. Check lead location. Consider admission for multi/interdisciplinary management
Superficial wound infection	Administration of antibiotics or surgical revision should be considered before development of deep infection
Infection-lead	The lead should be removed and appropriate antibiotics should be administered
Infection-IPG	The IPG and usually the extension cable should be removed and appropriate antibiotics should be administered
Lead migration	Lead replacement, or surgical alteration of lead position
Lead fracture	Lead replacement, if an appropriate candidate
Lead electrical short	Lead replacement, or potentially reprogramming at a different contact
IPG malfunction	IPG replacement, manage potential rebound symptoms
Accidental on/off	Turn on the IPG. Educate the patient and the family so they can use on/ off devices
Symptom rebound (motor and/or non-motor)	DBS hardware workup including impedance check, battery check, X-ray study, and assess for tolerance
Intracranial cyst	Steroids may be tried in mild cases but treatment usually requires removal of DBS lead

DBS deep brain stimulation, *ICU* intensive care unit, *UTI* urinary tract infection, *PD* Parkinson's disease, *IPG* implantable pulse generator

Intraoperative bleeding in DBS surgery may present as a seizure, change in mental status or hemiparesis.

Intracranial hemorrhage may also result from venous infarction as shown in patient 4, and in this case the symptoms emerged in delayed fashion [3, 20]. Patients with venous infarction may present to the emergency room complaining of altered mental status or hemiparesis, typically a few hours to days following DBS surgery. Venous infarction is associated with damage to the cortical veins and to venous lakes, and the damage may result in venous stasis and/or venous hypertension. In severe cases, the impaired venous circulation may result in ICH. Therefore, careful preoperative targeting utilizing a high-quality MRI (with contrast) to avoid superficial venous structures is helpful to prevent venous infarctions. Management of venous infarction is usually nonsurgical and includes optimizing venous return, appropriately managing blood pressure, and avoiding dehydration (see Table 18.1). A longer hospital stay following intracranial hemorrhage may result in secondary complications such as pneumonia and pulmonary embolism. Early initiation of rehabilitation may be useful to avoid secondary complications.

Subdural Hematoma

The burr hole opening for DBS, though small, can lead to the development of a subdural hematoma (SDH). A SDH forms with the accumulation of blood products in the space between the surface of the brain and the dura. The incidence of SDH after DBS has been estimated at 0.08–4.2% of leads [11, 28]. During DBS lead placement a burr hole and dural opening are created and left open for up to several hours. The exit of cerebrospinal fluid and entry of air can enlarge the subdural space, and combined with sagging or shift of the brain can lead to stretching of bridging veins. This brain sag and stretching of bridging veins can be exacerbated by atrophy, a finding not uncommon in the older population that is typically seen with DBS. Damage to bridging veins can lead to the development of a postoperative SDH. Furthermore, in this older DBS age group many patients take antiplatelet agents for cardiovascular health. They are also at an increased risk of falls due to their movement disorder diagnoses, although in one recent series of four SDHs after DBS there was no associated fall or trauma [11].

Subdural hematomas can enlarge to the point of herniation and neurologic deficits, brain damage, and death. An SDH in the setting of a patient with an implanted DBS lead presents a unique situation in that the operation to alleviate the pressure of the SDH (a straightforward burr hole or craniotomy) can lead to damage or removal of the DBS system, committing the patient to another procedure for reimplantation of the DBS lead if desired. Patients with chronic SDHs can undergo a simpler burr hole procedure to evacuate the blood products without sacrificing the lead. Care must be taken to avoid the DBS burr hole and locking mechanism, as well as the distal lead as it traverses the subgaleal plane toward the extension cable. Therefore, when a DBS patient presents with an SDH that needs surgical intervention, the first question is whether it can be treated with burr holes. If it is an acute SDH that does not look amenable to burr holes, can the patient wait a few weeks until the clot liquefies? Finally, if a large craniotomy is necessary to remove the acute solid-phase blood products, or if the SDH has organized membranes, fashioning a craniotomy that has a "plank" of bone that attaches the burr hole and locking mechanism to the rest of the patient's skull may save the lead. Care must be taken during the opening of larger scalp flaps that the lead, which can be scarred into the scalp flap, is not accidentally pulled or dislodged as the scalp flap is elevated. Some surgeons are concerned that with the removal of the SDH, the DBS lead will cause damage to the brain as it shifts back to its original position. In our experience, once the SDH has resolved, the DBS lead can regain efficacy and causes no new injury. There often is a significant delay (4–18 months) between the time of SDH evacuation and achievement of clinical efficacy of the DBS system, so providers must be patient to allow this to happen before prematurely repositioning the lead in the belief that it is ineffective [11].

In summary, for a SDH, the well-being of the patient must always come first even if it means sacrificing the lead. However, there are many strategies that can be used to salvage the DBS lead and still achieve clinical DBS efficacy while taking care of the SDH. The informed neurosurgeon must navigate these decisions by not damaging or removing the system whose implantation risks the patient has already endured.

Air Embolus

Air embolus is a relatively common complication of neurosurgical procedures, and neurosurgeons are cautious when a craniotomy is performed especially in a sitting position. Clinicians should be aware that DBS surgeries may result in a venous air embolus, and recent studies have shown that the incidence of air embolus during DBS surgery may be as high as 1.3–4.7% [6, 12, 29]. Entrainment of air into the venous system through diploic veins when fashioning a burr hole is the usual mechanism. Even though the clinical course is commonly benign, this complication can result in termination of the procedure [29]. It is therefore important to preoperatively adjust the head position of the patient to keep them as close to supine as possible. Waxing the edges of the burr hole, avoiding cortical veins and dural venous structures, keeping the burr hole filled with saline or occluded with a gel foam (or other material) plug are other ways of preventing the entry of air into the venous system.

DBS-related air embolus may manifest differently than in other neurosurgical procedures, since in DBS the patient is commonly awake rather than under general anesthesia [6, 12, 29, 30]. If a patient develops tachycardia, oxygen desaturation, and/or cough, clinicians should consider the possibility of a venous air embolus. In a recent series, the use of an external Doppler device was shown to aid in detection of an air embolus during DBS, although cough was the best predictive sign [6]. When an air embolus occurs, care should be taken to lower the head position, wax bone edges of the burr hole, vigorously irrigate the surgical field, and support the patient's cardiopulmonary status (see Table 18.1).

The triad of tachycardia, oxygen desaturation, and cough suggest an air embolus.

Dyskinetic Storm

Following MER and/or macrostimulation passes, immediate improvement of symptoms may be observed, and the improvement has been referred to as the "microlesion effect" or implantation effect. Microlesion effects have been considered to be a positive response, and may in some cases predict good prognosis [31–33]. Dyskinesias may be seen intraoperatively as a part of a microlesion effect in PD. Clinicians should be aware that intraoperative dyskinesia may develop into a severe situation referred to as "dyskinetic storm" [5, 32]. Dyskinetic storm may be an emergency as the head is usually fixed to the stereotactic frame during the operation. To secure the integrity of the head ring and to ensure the patient's respiratory condition, this situation should be quickly corrected. Emergent administration of sedative agents (e.g., intravenous (IV) propofol) may be required to stabilize the situation (see Table 18.1). If a dyskinetic storm persists or begins after the operation, judicious withdrawal of dopaminergic medications and/or the monitored administration of propofol can be used to dampen the dyskinesias.

Intraoperative Seizure

An intraoperative seizure can be induced by an intracranial hemorrhage, pneumocephalus, and intraoperative electrical stimulation (micro- and macrostimulation) as shown in patient 3 [1]. As the patient's head is fixed to the stereotactic frame, a generalized seizure may put the patient in a hazardous situation. When an intraoperative seizure is encountered, antiepileptics or sedative agents (e.g., IV propofol) should be immediately administered (see Table 18.1). Some authors recommend the use of IV lorazepam or thiopental in severe cases [1]. Intubation may be required in severe cases, although most cases are self-limited and can be managed conservatively [1]. If the patient recovers to be alert following the seizure, the procedure may in select cases be continued if the neurological examination is normal.

Neuroleptic Malignant Syndrome
(Parkinsonism-Hyperpyrexia Syndrome)

Discontinuation of PD medications for DBS surgery may result in NMS, or more appropriately named parkinsonism-hyperpyrexia syndrome (PHS) as shown in patient 5. PHS can occur as a postoperative emergency and is usually characterized by parkinsonism (rigidity, bradykinesia, and possibly tremor), fever, and in some cases rhabdomyolysis. PHS usually results either from exposure to dopamine blockers or from sudden withdrawal of dopamine (e.g., carbidopa/levodopa). It should be kept in mind that patients with PD usually undergo DBS in the off-medication condition, to allow physiology to be recorded in the abnormal state. Therefore, they are at theoretical risk for PHS, although usually PHS occurs after more than 24 hours of medication withdrawal [34]. Abrupt cessation of levodopa or dopamine agonists should be avoided postoperatively, and therapy restarted even if a nasogastric feeding tube is required. If PHS occurs, patients should be admitted to the ICU so that they can receive supportive care, fluids, and appropriate treatments. Administering dantrolene is an option [35]. PHS may innocently occur as postoperative hallucinations and/or behavioral anomalies that may prompt the clinical team to follow a course of dopamine cessation. In other cases, physicians may have stopped oral medications following surgery and forgotten to restart them. If PHS is encountered, we advocate restarting dopaminergic therapy as an urgent course of action.

Behavioral and Cognitive Problems

Behavioral and cognitive problems are often seen following DBS surgery, and the incidence of perioperative confusion and hallucinations were reported in a large single center study to be as high as 5.0% and 2.8% [18]. Early postoperative behavioral/cognitive problems were usually temporary; however, in some cases they required emergent/urgent management. If left unaddressed these problems may result in secondary complications such as falls and traumatic injury. Risk factors for mental status changes following DBS include advanced age and/or preexisting neurological compromise [36]. These issues are relatively common in the PD cohort [9]. The use of anticholinergics (including not only anti-parkinsonian medications but also medications for neurogenic bladder) can also be a risk factor, and discontinuation of these medications may be required in high risk cases [37]. In addition, previous reports have shown that STN DBS has a higher incidence of postoperative mental status change than GPi DBS (although this is not an absolute distinction) [16, 38–40]. Therefore, all patients should have neuropsychological testing preoperatively and the risks should be fully discussed. Tailoring approaches may be helpful to address these potential issues in the preoperative setting [2, 41]. When the estimated risk of behavioral and cognitive problems is high, GPi DBS and/or staged unilateral DBS implantation may be preferable. If patients become restless or violent postoperatively due to hallucinations/delusions, administering selective dopaminergic blockers such as quetiapine or clozapine may be useful (see Table 18.1) [42]. Nonselective dopaminergic blockers that lead to drug-induced parkinsonism as well as other movement disorders (e.g., olanzapine, risperidone, and haloperidol) are contraindicated [34, 35].

Myocardial Infarction

Several studies reported cases of myocardial infarction (MI) following DBS surgery [1, 9]. Although DBS has been considered to be a safe procedure even for patients with cardiac problems [43], medical comorbidities such as CAD may increase the risk of postoperative MI as seen in patient 6 [2, 36]. Medication lists should be also checked because specific medications such as meperidine, MAO-B inhibitors, bromocriptine, and tricyclic antidepressants (TCAs) may increase the risk of general anesthesia [44]. Although MI can be encountered following any surgical procedure under general anesthesia, clinicians should have a higher level of suspicion when a patient complains of chest pain following DBS so as not to confuse cardiac chest pain for postoperative chest pain. Chest pain is common in patients who have undergone DBS surgery as the battery packs (IPGs) are implanted in the chest wall in the majority of cases [9]. As MI is a life-threatening condition, the patient should be admitted to the ICU and a cardiology consultation should be performed (see Table 18.1).

ⓞ━━━☞   Chest pain in the postoperative period requires a rule out of myocardial infarction.

Postoperative Management

Suicide Attempt and Ideation

Suicidal ideation should be treated as an emergency as mortality rate can be high if suicide is attempted. A meta-analysis revealed that approximately 52% of cases with suicidal ideation and/or attempts were reported to complete suicide following DBS (data from 1996 to 2005) [45]. The same study revealed that most of the patients with suicidal ideation and/or attempts had undergone DBS for PD, and a recent multicenter study of an STN/DBS/PD cohort revealed several important risk factors for suicide: preoperative history of impulse control disorders or compulsive medication use, postoperative depression, postoperative apathy, and being single [46]. Previous suicide attempts, younger age of the patient, and younger onset of PD were also shown to be risk factors for suicide attempts. In addition, there have been several reports of suicide in patients with dystonia who underwent DBS, therefore clinicians should be aware that this issue is not limited to PD [47–49]. Preoperative neuropsychological and psychiatric evaluation is therefore highly recommended as a preventative measure for all patients who undergo DBS surgery [36, 50].

Appleby reported the mean time difference between implantation and the development of suicidality was 2.4 years, and other authors have reported even shorter durations [45]. Screening for suicidal ideation following DBS therefore should be routine, and if discovered, the issue should be treated as an emergency. Also of note is that stimulation of the limbic components of deep brain basal ganglia structures may result in acute depression [50–54]. Patients with suicide attempts and/or ideation should be admitted to the hospital for multi/interdisciplinary care including cognitive behavioral therapy, counseling, and/or medication/stimulation adjustment(s) (see Table 18.1).

Hardware Infection

Hardware-related infections are not rare in DBS. The incidence of infection and/or erosion following DBS surgery has been reported to range between 0% and 15.2% [1, 7, 12, 23, 55–61]. Even the most vigilant surgical technique cannot prevent all postoperative infectious complications. Although risk factors have not been clearly elucidated, medical comorbidities such as uncontrolled diabetes mellitus may increase the infection rate. Several authors have advocated the use of pre- and post-operative prophylactic antibiotics; however, the efficacy has not been clear [59]. One recent study did however report a reduction in infection rate by locally inject-ing anti-staphylococcal antibiotics (e.g., neomycin, polymyxin) directly into the operative wound [61]. Also, several studies showed the efficacy of intraoperative use of vancomycin in solution or powder form as an infection prophylaxis [62, 63].

The devices in an infectious scenario may require emergent removal, as shown in patients 8 and 9. Cultures should be sent anytime hardware is removed or a poten-tially infectious IPG pocket is aspirated. Several factors merit consideration when managing a DBS infection (1) whether the infection is deep or superficial, (2) whether the brain lead is involved or not, and (3) whether there are single or multi-ple sites of involvement [55]. Management of a hardware infection should be per-formed in an attempt to minimize hardware removal. In superficial infection, surgical revision of the wound may be an option, and patient education is important so that the problem can be found by clinicians before development of a deep infec-tion. Emergent hardware removal may be required in cases of deep infection; how-ever, select cases with a superficial infection may be managed with administration of antibiotics. When the brain leads and/or multiple sites are involved, most clini-cians remove all hardware including lead, extension, and IPG. However, in cases where only the IPG or extension cable appears infected, removing only the infected hardware in an attempt to preserve the brain lead is an option. In any cases with hardware removal following an infection, a course of 6–8 weeks of IV antibiotic therapy is required before device(s) reimplantation (see Table 18.1).

Lead Migration

Lead migration can be seen in patients complaining of loss of efficacy of their DBS device(s), and this issue can be the result of a malfunction of the anchoring devices, skull growth, vigorous head movements, or rarely from compulsive manipulation of the IPG referred to as "Twiddler's syndrome" [2, 4, 64, 65]. Yianni reported lead migration in 3 of 133 patients (2.3%), and all 3 underwent DBS for dystonia [64]. The authors hypothesized that axial movements contributed to lead migration, as seen in patient 10. When lead migration is noted, clinicians should be cautious as it may result in severe mood changes due to the spread of stimulation to other regions such as the amygdala [66]. Amygdala stimulation may also induce seizures as seen in patient 10 [12]. Skull growth in children is another cause of lead migration [2]. Twiddler's syndrome may also result in dorsal lead migration [65]. This adverse event highlights the importance of obtaining and reviewing postoperative imaging. When lead migration is noted, changing the active contact (deeper or shallower depending on the direction of migration) should be attempted prior to surgical revision [10].

Hardware Malfunction

When a DBS patient reports sudden loss of efficacy, the clinician should consider hardware malfunction [2, 4, 38]. Mechanical stress to the device may result in lead fracture, a break in the extension cable, or an IPG failure. A recent single center prospective study revealed that the incidence of hardware malfunction was 2.0% [8]. On the other hand, another study reported that 8 (6%) of 133 cases had lead fracture, and 7 of 8 broken electrodes in their cases were encountered in patients with ET [59]. They speculated that head tremor may have contributed to the adverse events [59]. Twiddler's syndrome has also been reported to result in lead and/or extension cable fractures [8, 65, 67, 68]. Head and neck trauma may also result in lead and/or cable fracture (patient 11), and it is theorized this may occur more commonly in dystonia. Clinicians should be aware that DBS patients complaining of a fall are relatively commonly encountered in the emergency room [9]. When clinicians encounter situations predisposing the patient to a hardware malfunction, skull X-rays and/or CT scan should be performed (see Fig. 18.5).

To confirm the diagnosis, the impedance and current drain for each of the four lead contacts should be measured with the DBS programming/interrogation device. High impedance along with a low current drain is consistent with a lead fracture or with an extension cable break. On the other hand, low impedance with possible high current drain may indicate a short circuit. In short circuits, palpating the IPG or the extension cable tract may cause a shock-like sensation. When any contacts with normal impedances/current drain values exist, reprogramming should be attempted (see Table 18.1). A plain film X-ray also yields useful information to identify a fracture along the course of the lead or extension wire. When the location of the problem cannot be precisely identified, replacement of the extension wire and retesting impedances in the operative setting is recommended. This procedure may save the intracranial lead replacement in select cases [4].

Accidental On/Off and Symptom Rebound

Clinicians should be aware that symptom rebound may include not only motor symptoms but also non-motor manifestations such as suicidal ideation (author observations) as well as severe depression. Several cases of severe symptom rebound following battery failure have been reported [69, 70]. The more beneficial

DBS proves for clinical symptoms, the more dramatic the rebound symptoms may be. Sudden worsening of symptoms should always prompt a battery status check by an experienced DBS programmer. If the device is on, hardware malfunction should be considered. The management includes checking impedances and current drain at each of the four DBS contacts and imaging studies as described above in the "Hardware Malfunction" section. If the device is off, resuming stimulation may be all that is necessary. When symptom rebound is seen following trauma, an X-ray film may be helpful to identify the cause such as DBS lead and/or extension cable fracture.

When the DBS device unpredictably turns off, the clinician must investigate potential environmental triggers (the device has a duty log to assist in documenting these occurrences). Exposure to magnetic forces (e.g., a magnetized ice freezer or store security devices) is the most commonly reported etiology [58]. Educating the patient to recheck the DBS device on a regular or semi-regular schedule may be useful. Additionally, documentation of daily activities and relevant environments that they frequent may help in identifying the source of the problem. Education is important so that the patients avoid strong magnetic fields, have their remote device with them at all times in order to recheck battery (on/off) status, and learn prevention strategies for accidental on/offs (see Table 18.1).

Aseptic Intraparenchymal Cyst

Intracranial cyst has been reported as a rare complication of DBS surgery for PD and ET [71–73]. The cyst gradually increases in size over months, and typically the patient visits the clinic or emergency department complaining of newly developed neurological symptoms such as dysarthria, gait disturbance, or hemiparesis. This complication has been considered to be due to autoimmune or inflammatory response to the DBS hardware, but the precise etiology remains unclear. Clinicians should examine the complete blood count (CBC), C-reactive protein (CRP), and cerebrospinal fluid (CSF) to rule out infectious etiologies. Treatment options include administration of steroids and intracranial lead explantation. In mild cases where the lead explantation is not necessary, higher intensity electrical stimulation may be required to control the symptoms of PD or ET.

Conclusion

Patient screening and standardized procedures may prevent avoidable complications. Preoperative evaluation by a multidisciplinary team assesses the detailed risks in each patient, and the DBS procedure and the perioperative management should be tailored for individual needs. Tailoring the approach in selecting the optimal target (e.g., GPi or STN), procedure (e.g., staged or simultaneous implantation of DBS leads), and perioperative medication adjustment may help in avoiding unnecessary complications. Development of DBS technologies will likely lead to new treatment options, but clinicians should remain vigilant that perioperative management is vital for managing patient-specific risks.

References

1. Boviatsis EJ, Stavrinou LC, Themistocleous M, Kouyialis AT, Sakas DE. Surgical and hardware complications of deep brain stimulation. A seven-year experience and review of the literature. Acta Neurochir. 2010;152(12):2053–62.
2. Morishita T, Foote KD, Burdick AP, Katayama Y, Yamamoto T, Frucht SJ, et al. Identification and management of deep brain stimulation intra- and postoperative urgencies and emergencies. Parkinsonism Relat Disord. 2010;16(3):153–62.
3. Morishita T, Okun MS, Burdick A, Jacobson CE 4th, Foote KD. Cerebral venous infarction: a potentially avoidable complication of deep brain stimulation surgery. Neuromodulation. 2013;16(5):407–13. discussion 413
4. Okun MS, Rodriguez RL, Foote KD, Sudhyadhom A, Bova F, Jacobson C, et al. A case-based review of troubleshooting deep brain stimulator issues in movement and neuropsychiatric disorders. Parkinsonism Relat Disord. 2008;14(7):532–8.
5. Hooper AK, Ellis TM, Foote KD, Zeilman P, Okun MS. Dyskinetic storm induced by intraoperative deep brain stimulator placement. Open Neurosurg J. 2009;2(3):1–3.
6. Hooper AK, Okun MS, Foote KD, Haq IU, Fernandez HH, Hegland D, et al. Venous air embolism in deep brain stimulation. Stereotact Funct Neurosurg. 2009;87(1):25–30.
7. Burdick AP, Fernandez HH, Okun MS, Chi YY, Jacobson C, Foote KD. Relationship between higher rates of adverse events in deep brain stimulation using standardized prospective recording and patient outcomes. Neurosurg Focus. 2010;29(2):E4.
8. Burdick AP, Okun MS, Haq IU, Ward HE, Bova F, Jacobson CE, et al. Prevalence of twiddler's syndrome as a cause of deep brain stimulation hardware failure. Stereotact Funct Neurosurg. 2010;88(6):353–9.
9. Resnick AS, Foote KD, Rodriguez RL, Malaty IA, Moll JL, Carden DL, et al. The number and nature of emergency department encounters in patients with deep brain stimulators. J Neurol. 2010;257(1):122–31.
10. Ellis TM, Foote KD, Fernandez HH, Sudhyadhom A, Rodriguez RL, Zeilman P, et al. Reoperation for suboptimal outcomes after deep brain stimulation surgery. Neurosurgery. 2008;63(4):754–60. discussion 60-1
11. Oyama G, Okun MS, Zeisevicz TA, Tamse T, Romrell J, Zeilman P, et al. Delayed clinical improvement after deep brain stimulation-related subdural hematoma. J Neurosurg. 2011;115:289.
12. Nonaka M, Morishita T, Yamada K, Fujioka S, Higuchi MA, Tsuboi Y, et al. Surgical management of adverse events associated with deep brain stimulation: a single-center experience. SAGE Open Med. 2020;8:2050312120913458.
13. Deuschl G, Schade-Brittinger C, Krack P, Volkmann J, Schafer H, Botzel K, et al. A randomized trial of deep-brain stimulation for Parkinson's disease. N Engl J Med. 2006;355(9):896–908.
14. Krack P, Batir A, Van Blercom N, Chabardes S, Fraix V, Ardouin C, et al. Five-year follow-up of bilateral stimulation of the subthalamic nucleus in advanced Parkinson's disease. N Engl J Med. 2003;349(20):1925–34.
15. Kupsch A, Benecke R, Müller J, Trottenberg T, Schneider GH, Poewe W, et al. Pallidal deep-brain stimulation in primary generalized or segmental dystonia. N Engl J Med. 2006;355(19):1978–90.

16. Okun MS, Fernandez HH, Wu SS, Kirsch-Darrow L, Bowers D, Bova F, et al. Cognition and mood in Parkinson's disease in subthalamic nucleus versus globus pallidus interna deep brain stimulation: the COMPARE trial. Ann Neurol. 2009;65(5):586–95.
17. Kiss ZH, Doig-Beyaert K, Eliasziw M, Tsui J, Haffenden A, Suchowersky O, et al. The Canadian multicentre study of deep brain stimulation for cervical dystonia. Brain. 2007;130(Pt 11):2879–86.
18. Kenney C, Simpson R, Hunter C, Ondo W, Almaguer M, Davidson A, et al. Short-term and long-term safety of deep brain stimulation in the treatment of movement disorders. J Neurosurg. 2007;106(4):621–5.
19. Hariz MI. Complications of deep brain stimulation surgery. Mov Disord. 2002;17(Suppl 3):S162–6.
20. Chang WS, Kim HY, Kim JP, Park YS, Chung SS, Chang JW. Bilateral subthalamic deep brain stimulation using single track microelectrode recording. Acta Neurochir. 2011;153:1087.
21. Binder DK, Rau GM, Starr PA. Risk factors for hemorrhage during microelectrode-guided deep brain stimulator implantation for movement disorders. Neurosurgery. 2005;56(4):722–32; discussion -32.
22. Sansur CA, Frysinger RC, Pouratian N, Fu KM, Bittl M, Oskouian RJ, et al. Incidence of symptomatic hemorrhage after stereotactic electrode placement. J Neurosurg. 2007;107(5):998–1003.
23. Beric A, Kelly PJ, Rezai A, Sterio D, Mogilner A, Zonenshayn M, et al. Complications of deep brain stimulation surgery. Stereotact Funct Neurosurg. 2001;77(1–4):73–8.
24. Lyons KE, Wilkinson SB, Overman J, Pahwa R. Surgical and hardware complications of subthalamic stimulation: a series of 160 procedures. Neurology. 2004;63(4):612–6.
25. Videnovic A, Metman LV. Deep brain stimulation for Parkinson's disease: prevalence of adverse events and need for standardized reporting. Mov Disord. 2008;23(3):343–9.
26. Voges J, Hilker R, Botzel K, Kiening KL, Kloss M, Kupsch A, et al. Thirty days complication rate following surgery performed for deep-brain-stimulation. Mov Disord. 2007;22(10):1486–9.
27. Gorgulho A, De Salles AA, Frighetto L, Behnke E. Incidence of hemorrhage associated with electrophysiological studies performed using macroelectrodes and microelectrodes in functional neurosurgery. J Neurosurg. 2005;102(5):888–96.
28. Simuni T, Jaggi JL, Mulholland H, Hurtig HI, Colcher A, Siderowf AD, et al. Bilateral stimulation of the subthalamic nucleus in patients with Parkinson disease: a study of efficacy and safety. J Neurosurg. 2002;96(4):666–72.
29. Chang EF, Cheng JS, Richardson RM, Lee C, Starr PA, Larson PS. Incidence and management of venous air embolisms during awake deep brain stimulation surgery in a large clinical series. Stereotact Funct Neurosurg. 2011;89(2):76–82.
30. Deogaonkar A, Avitsian R, Henderson JM, Schubert A. Venous air embolism during deep brain stimulation surgery in an awake supine patient. Stereotact Funct Neurosurg. 2005;83(1):32–5.
31. Mann JM, Foote KD, Garvan CW, Fernandez HH, Jacobson CE, Rodriguez RL, et al. Brain penetration effects of microelectrodes and DBS leads in STN or GPi. J Neurol Neurosurg Psychiatry. 2009;80(7):794–7.
32. Morishita T, Foote KD, Wu SS, Jacobson CE, Rodriguez RL, Haq IU, et al. Brain penetration effects of microelectrodes and deep brain stimulation leads in ventral intermediate nucleus stimulation for essential tremor. J Neurosurg. 2010;112(3):491–6.
33. Tasker RR. Deep brain stimulation is preferable to thalamotomy for tremor suppression. Surg Neurol. 1998;49(2):145–53. discussion 53-4
34. Frucht SJ. Movement disorder emergencies in the perioperative period. Neurol Clin. 2004;22(2):379–87.
35. Poston KL, Frucht SJ. Movement disorder emergencies. J Neurol. 2008;255(Suppl 4):2–13.
36. Rodriguez RL, Fernandez HH, Haq I, Okun MS. Pearls in patient selection for deep brain stimulation. Neurologist. 2007;13(5):253–60.
37. Tune LE, Damlouji NF, Holland A, Gardner TJ, Folstein MF, Coyle JT. Association of postoperative delirium with raised serum levels of anticholinergic drugs. Lancet. 1981;2(8248):651–3.

38. Deuschl G, Herzog J, Kleiner-Fisman G, Kubu C, Lozano AM, Lyons KE, et al. Deep brain stimulation: postoperative issues. Mov Disord. 2006;21(Suppl 14):S219–37.
39. Okun MS, Green J, Saben R, Gross R, Foote KD, Vitek JL. Mood changes with deep brain stimulation of STN and GPi: results of a pilot study. J Neurol Neurosurg Psychiatry. 2003;74(11):1584–6.
40. Hariz MI, Rehncrona S, Quinn NP, Speelman JD, Wensing C. Multicenter study on deep brain stimulation in Parkinson's disease: an independent assessment of reported adverse events at 4 years. Mov Disord. 2008;23(3):416–21.
41. Okun MS, Rodriguez RL, Mikos A, Miller K, Kellison I, Kirsch-Darrow L, et al. Deep brain stimulation and the role of the neuropsychologist. Clin Neuropsychol. 2007;21(1):162–89.
42. Poewe W. When a Parkinson's disease patient starts to hallucinate. Pract Neurol. 2008;8(4):238–41.
43. Capelle HH, Simpson RK Jr, Kronenbuerger M, Michaelsen J, Tronnier V, Krauss JK. Long-term deep brain stimulation in elderly patients with cardiac pacemakers. J Neurosurg. 2005;102(1):53–9.
44. Burton DA, Nicholson G, Hall GM. Anaesthesia in elderly patients with neurodegenerative disorders: special considerations. Drugs Aging. 2004;21(4):229–42.
45. Appleby BS, Duggan PS, Regenberg A, Rabins PV. Psychiatric and neuropsychiatric adverse events associated with deep brain stimulation: a meta-analysis of ten years' experience. Mov Disord. 2007;22(12):1722–8.
46. Voon V, Krack P, Lang AE, Lozano AM, Dujardin K, Schupbach M, et al. A multicentre study on suicide outcomes following subthalamic stimulation for Parkinson's disease. Brain. 2008;131(Pt 10):2720–8.
47. Foncke EM, Schuurman PR, Speelman JD. Suicide after deep brain stimulation of the internal globus pallidus for dystonia. Neurology. 2006;66(1):142–3.
48. Burkhard PR, Vingerhoets FJ, Berney A, Bogousslavsky J, Villemure JG, Ghika J. Suicide after successful deep brain stimulation for movement disorders. Neurology. 2004;63(11):2170–2.
49. Ghika J, Villemure JG, Miklossy J, Temperli P, Pralong E, Christen-Zaech S, et al. Postanoxic generalized dystonia improved by bilateral Voa thalamic deep brain stimulation. Neurology. 2002;58(2):311–3.
50. Doshi PK, Chhaya N, Bhatt MH. Depression leading to attempted suicide after bilateral sub-thalamic nucleus stimulation for Parkinson's disease. Mov Disord. 2002;17(5):1084–5.
51. Blomstedt P, Hariz MI, Lees A, Silberstein P, Limousin P, Yelnik J, et al. Acute severe depression induced by intraoperative stimulation of the substantia nigra: a case report. Parkinsonism Relat Disord. 2008;14(3):253–6.
52. Bejjani BP, Damier P, Arnulf I, Thivard L, Bonnet AM, Dormont D, et al. Transient acute depression induced by high-frequency deep-brain stimulation. N Engl J Med. 1999;340(19):1476–80.
53. Miyawaki E, Perlmutter JS, Troster AI, Videen TO, Koller WC. The behavioral complications of pallidal stimulation: a case report. Brain Cogn. 2000;42(3):417–34.
54. Romito LM, Raja M, Daniele A, Contarino MF, Bentivoglio AR, Barbier A, et al. Transient mania with hypersexuality after surgery for high frequency stimulation of the subthalamic nucleus in Parkinson's disease. Mov Disord. 2002;17(6):1371–4.
55. Sillay KA, Larson PS, Starr PA. Deep brain stimulator hardware-related infections: incidence and management in a large series. Neurosurgery. 2008;62(2):360–6. discussion 6-7
56. Joint C, Nandi D, Parkin S, Gregory R, Aziz T. Hardware-related problems of deep brain stimulation. Mov Disord. 2002;17(Suppl 3):S175–80.
57. Kondziolka D, Whiting D, Germanwala A, Oh M. Hardware-related complications after placement of thalamic deep brain stimulator systems. Stereotact Funct Neurosurg. 2002;79(3–4):228–33.
58. Oh MY, Abosch A, Kim SH, Lang AE, Lozano AM. Long-term hardware-related complications of deep brain stimulation. Neurosurgery. 2002;50(6):1268–74. discussion 74-6

59. Blomstedt P, Hariz MI. Hardware-related complications of deep brain stimulation: a ten year experience. Acta Neurochir. 2005;147(10):1061–4. discussion 4

60. Koller W, Pahwa R, Busenbark K, Hubble J, Wilkinson S, Lang A, et al. High-frequency unilateral thalamic stimulation in the treatment of essential and parkinsonian tremor. Ann Neurol. 1997;42(3):292–9.

61. Miller JP, Acar F, Burchiel KJ. Significant reduction in stereotactic and functional neurosurgical hardware infection after local neomycin/polymyxin application. J Neurosurg. 2009;110(2):247–50.

62. Pepper J, Meliak L, Akram H, Hyam J, Milabo C, Candelario J, et al. Changing of the guard: reducing infection when replacing neural pacemakers. J Neurosurg. 2017;126(4):1165–72.

63. Rasouli JJ, Kopell BH. The adjunctive use of vancomycin powder appears safe and may reduce the incidence of surgical-site infections after deep brain stimulation surgery. World Neurosurg. 2016;95:9–13.

64. Yianni J, Nandi D, Shad A, Bain P, Gregory R, Aziz T. Increased risk of lead fracture and migration in dystonia compared with other movement disorders following deep brain stimulation. J Clin Neurosci. 2004;11(3):243–5.

65. Gelabert-Gonzalez M, Relova-Quinteiro JL, Castro-Garcia A. "Twiddler syndrome" in two patients with deep brain stimulation. Acta Neurochir. 2010;152(3):489–91.

66. Piacentini S, Romito L, Franzini A, Granato A, Broggi G, Albanese A. Mood disorder following DBS of the left amygdaloid region in a dystonia patient with a dislodged electrode. Mov Disord. 2008;23(1):147–50.

67. Geissinger G, Neal JH. Spontaneous twiddler's syndrome in a patient with a deep brain stimulator. Surg Neurol. 2007;68(4):454–6. discussion 6

68. Machado AG, Hiremath GK, Salazar F, Rezai AR. Fracture of subthalamic nucleus deep brain stimulation hardware as a result of compulsive manipulation: case report. Neurosurgery. 2005;57(6):E1318; discussion E.

69. Hariz MI, Johansson F. Hardware failure in parkinsonian patients with chronic subthalamic nucleus stimulation is a medical emergency. Mov Disord. 2001;16(1):166–8.

70. Hariz MI, Shamsgovara P, Johansson F, Hariz G, Fodstad H. Tolerance and tremor rebound following long-term chronic thalamic stimulation for Parkinsonian and essential tremor. Stereotact Funct Neurosurg. 1999;72(2–4):208–18.

71. Ramirez-Zamora A, Levine D, Sommer DB, Dalfino J, Novak P, Pilitsis JG. Intraparenchymal cyst development after deep brain stimulator placement. Stereotact Funct Neurosurg. 2013;91(5):338–41.

72. Gupta HV, Lyons MK, Mehta SH. Teaching NeuroImages: noninfectious cyst as an unusual complication of deep brain stimulation. Neurology. 2016;87(18):e223–e4.

73. Sharma VD, Bona AR, Mantovani A, Miocinovic S, Khemani P, Goldberg MP, et al. Cystic lesions as a rare complication of deep brain stimulation. Mov Disord Clin Pract. 2016;3(1):87–90.

Part IV

Emergencies of Recognition: Pitfalls in Diagnosis

Startle Disorders

19

Christine M. Stahl

Patient Vignette

As the consultant neurologist in the hospital, you are called to the neonatal ICU to examine a full-term infant with hypertonia and jitteriness. On examination, the baby's tone is increased particularly in the axial muscles, and she is noted to have an exaggerated startle to noise and touch. She does not habituate to nose tapping and her Moro reflex is exaggerated and sustained. Otherwise, her neurologic examination is normal. The NICU team notes that the baby had a 30-second apneic spell after one particularly severe startle response, with prolonged body stiffening. After speaking with her parents, they report that she has an older brother who startles easily to sudden loud sounds. Based on her history and examination, you diagnose hyperekplexia and recommend starting clonazepam. Her exaggerated startle and increased tone improve significantly with the clonazepam and she is discharged home.

Introduction

The term "startle" describes a sudden, involuntary movement of the body in response to an unexpected stimulus. The startle reflex in humans is a normal physiologic symmetric flexor response present starting around 6 weeks of age and remaining for

Supplementary Information The online version of this chapter (https://doi.org/10.1007/978-3-030-75898-1_19) contains supplementary material, which is available to authorized users.

C. M. Stahl (✉)
Department of Neurology, NYU Langone Health, New York, NY, USA
e-mail: christine.stahl@nyulangone.org

© Springer Nature Switzerland AG 2022
S. J. Frucht (ed.), *Movement Disorder Emergencies*, Current Clinical Neurology,
https://doi.org/10.1007/978-3-030-75898-1_19

life [1]. Conditions with an abnormal or exaggerated startle are collectively referred to as startle syndromes, and are a rare, heterogeneous group of disorders. The startle syndromes are categorized into three broad groups: (1) hyperekplexia, (2) stimulus-induced disorders, and (3) neuropsychiatric startle disorders [2]. While startle syndromes are often relatively benign, medical emergencies can arise as complications from the abnormal startle. Most concerning is the increased morbidity and mortality from apneic episodes in patients with hyperekplexia, which can unfortunately lead to sudden death. Therefore, prompt recognition and treatment of this disorder is imperative. In this chapter, we review the normal human startle reflex and then provide an overview of the startle syndromes, with a particular focus on hyperekplexia given the movement disorder emergencies seen in this syndrome.

Normal Startle Reflex

The startle reflex in humans is a normal physiologic response to an unexpected stimulus, usually auditory, but can also be to somatosensory or visual stimuli. The motor response is characterized by bilateral synchronous, shock-like movements usually involving rapid closure of the eyes, elevating the arms over the head, and flexion of the neck, trunk, and limbs [1, 3]. The initial study of this reflex dates back to 1926 when Jacobsen recorded the movement of normal individuals in response to auditory stimuli by connecting a string between the subject's head and a drum [1, 4]. More recent and sophisticated neurophysiologic studies have since furthered our understanding of the normal startle reflex, particularly in response to auditory stimuli. It is now understood that the reflex is generated in the caudal brainstem, specifically the bulbopontine reticular formation. There is subsequent caudal and rostral propagation of the impulse with rapid activation of cranial nerve-innervated muscles starting with the orbicularis oculi (at 20–50 msec) followed by activation of the sternocleidomastoid and masseter. Activation of the trunk and limbs can occur, but is more variable [1, 5, 6]. There is marked habituation of the startle reflex within one to five trials of auditory stimulation, though the blink reflex often remains [1, 7]. Additionally, the magnitude and latency of the startle is affected by the intensity of the stimulus, as well as the individual's posture, focus, and emotional state at the time of the startle stimulus [1, 8].

Startle Syndromes

As previously mentioned, the startle syndromes are a group of heterogeneous disorders with abnormal or exaggerated startle responses. They are categorized into three main groups: (1) hyperekplexia, (2) stimulus-induced disorders, and (3) neuropsychiatric startle disorders (Table 19.1). In the case of hyperekplexia the movement disorder is characterized by an excessive startle reflex. With stimulus-induced disorders and neuropsychiatric startle disorders, there may or may not be an exaggerated startle; however, the startle triggers an additional abnormal response.

Table 19.1 Startle syndromes

Hyperekplexia	Startle-induced disorders	Neuropsychiatric startle disorders
Hereditary	*Epileptic*	Culture-specific
Genetic mutations: *GLRA1*, *GLRB*,	Startle epilepsy	syndromes
SLC6A6	Progressive	Latah (Southeast
Sporadic	myoclonic epilepsy	Asia)
Symptomatic (acquired cerebral or	*Non-epileptic*	Jumping Frenchmen
brainstem damage/dysfunction)	Paroxysmal	of Maine
Brainstem infarct/hemorrhage or	kinesigenic dyskinesia	Myriachit (Siberia)
compression	Episodic ataxia	Startle-induced tics
Cerebral palsy	Cataplexy	Functional startle
Encephalitis	Reflex myoclonus	syndromes
Multiple sclerosis	Stiff-person syndrome	Anxiety syndrome/
Neurodegenerative:		PTSD
Creutzfeldt-Jakob disease		
Tay-Sachs disease		
GM2 gangliosidosis		
Paraneoplastic Syndrome:		
Anti-glycine receptor antibody		
Post-hypoxic or post-traumatic		
encephalopathy		

Complications of hyperekplexia include sudden death from apnea, and are a true movement disorder emergency. We will focus the remainder of this chapter on the recognition, diagnosis, and treatment of this disorder. However, we will first briefly mention the other two categories of startle syndromes.

Stimulus-Induced Disorders

Stimulus-induced disorders show exaggerated responses to an unexpected stimulus. This diverse group is divided into non-epileptic disorders, such as paroxysmal kinesigenic dyskinesia, episodic ataxia, cataplexy, reflex myoclonus, stiff-person syndrome and epileptic disorders including startle epilepsy and progressive myoclonus epilepsy. Discussion of each of these disorders is beyond the scope of this chapter, but has been reviewed previously [2, 9].

Neuropsychiatric Startle Disorders

Neuropsychiatric startle disorders are an interesting group of disorders characterized by a combination of neurologic and psychiatric symptoms, triggered by a startling stimulus. These disorders often develop later in life and include culture-specific syndromes, startle-induced tics, functional startle syndromes, and anxiety syndromes/post-traumatic stress disorder [2, 9]. The culture-specific syndromes are a particularly intriguing group with non-habituating exaggerated startle followed by variable behavioral responses including "forced obedience," echolalia, echopraxia, and/or jumping, including entities such as Latah in Southeast Asia and the Jumping Frenchmen of Maine. Much less is known about Myriachit in Siberia. As the responses do not habituate, these individuals can be teased or tormented by repeated intentional startling [10].

Hyperekplexia

Hyperekplexia, derived from two Greek words meaning "to startle excessively," is a term used to describe a group of disorders where there is an abnormal excessive startle response and episodes of stiffness [2]. It was first reported in 1958 by Kirstein and Silverskjold in a Swedish family and later by Suhren et al. in 1966 when the term "hyperekplexia" was coined [11, 12].

Etiology and Genetics

Hyperekplexia can be hereditary, sporadic, or symptomatic due to underlying brainstem or cerebral damage. In hereditary hyperekplexia, mutations occur in genes affecting glycine inhibitory neurotransmission in the brainstem and spinal cord, leading to hyperexcitability and abnormal startle response. At the moment, mutations in three genes encoding proteins involved in structure of the glycine receptor or the functioning of glycine neurotransmission have been identified in individuals with hereditary hyperekplexia. The majority of cases of hereditary hyperekplexia (61–63%) are caused by mutations in the *GLRA1* gene, which encodes the α1 subunit of the glycine receptor. Defects in the β subunit of the glycine receptor caused by mutations in the *GLRB* gene account for 12% to 14% cases. Mutations in the *SLC6A6* gene, encoding a unidirectional presynaptic glycine transporter accounts for 25% of cases for hyperekplexia. Most cases are autosomal recessive (85%), but autosomal dominant cases are also possible (15%). Diagnosis of hereditary hyperekplexia merits genetic testing for all potentially affected individuals in the family.

In some cases of hyperekplexia, no genetic cause is identified. These cases are categorized as sporadic hyperekplexia. Clinically, sporadic hyperekplexia cases tend to manifest cardinal symptoms after the first month of life in contrast to genetically-confirmed hereditary hyperekplexia where symptoms are present at birth [13]. Cases of symptomatic hyperekplexia tend to manifest later in life and are not usually accompanied by the classic generalized stiffness seen in the hereditary and sporadic entities [2]. As symptomatic hyperekplexia is due to underlying brainstem or cerebral damage, there are often other associated neurologic signs and symptoms.

Clinical Features

The core clinical features of hyperekplexia are an exaggerated non-habituating startle reflex to unexpected stimuli and stiffness. The exaggerated startle is present from birth, and in contrast to the normal startle response, leads to a generalized stiffening in the affected individual for a period after the startle. This stiffness can cause the startled person to fall "like a log" as voluntary movements are impaired during this period of stiffness, preventing their ability to break a fall with outstretched arms and increasing the risk of injury. Consciousness is preserved during the startle response and there are no subsequent tonic movements as seen with startle epilepsies. As the startle response in hyperekplexia is non-habituating even to minor stimuli, simple activities of daily life can be challenging to complete due to interruption by startle responses [2, 14].

In addition to the stiffness following a startle, neonates with hyperekplexia demonstrate generalized stiffness immediately after birth which increases with handling, producing a characteristic "stiff as a stick" position when being held. This generalized stiffness disappears in sleep. Severe attacks of stiffness can interfere with breathing and lead to apnea and cyanosis and in some extreme circumstances even sudden infant death. Fortunately, these tonic cyanotic attacks usually abate during infancy, but early diagnosis and treatment is critical in the neonatal period. Additionally, due to the increased intraabdominal pressure caused by the excessive stiffness there is increased frequency of inguinal, umbilical, hiatal hernias and congenital hip dislocations. Mild developmental delay is seen in some children with hyperekplexia, though they later catch up [2, 14].

Neonates with hyperekplexia are at increased risk for sudden death due to apnea.

Another characteristic of hyperekplexia is an exaggerated head-retraction reflex, which occurs in response to tactile stimulation of the tip of the nose, glabella, or upper lip, resulting in neck extension. In hyperekplexia, the response is exaggerated and non-habituating. Of note, the head-retraction reflex is not unique to hyperekplexia and has been reported in other disorders such as cerebral palsy [2, 14]. The generalized stiffness of hyperekplexia resolves within the first few years of life in contrast to the exaggerated startle and subsequent stiffness that persist into adulthood. Adults with hyperekplexia, however, tend to walk with a cautious, stiff-legged, mildly wide-based, but non-ataxic gait. Tone and deep tendon reflexes may be slightly increased, with flexor plantar responses [2, 14].

Treatment/Management
The mainstay of pharmacologic treatment for hyperekplexia is clonazepam, which potentiates the inhibitory neurotransmitter GABA. Clonazepam has been shown in a small double-blind placebo-controlled study to effectively decrease the magnitude of the startle response [15]. Clonazepam dosing can vary, but suggested daily doses range from 0.5 mg up to 6 mg per day [9]. Other drugs including clobazam, vigabatrin, valproate, and carbamazepine have also been used in the treatment of hyperekplexia in case reports and open studies [15–17].

The exaggerated startle and subsequent prolonged stiffness can be ameliorated during an attack by forced flexion of the head and legs towards the trunk. This technique, termed the "Vigevano maneuver," can be life-saving for neonates and infants during a tonic cyanotic attack. All families and health-care providers who provide care for children affected by hyperekplexia should be taught how to employ this maneuver [18]. Not surprisingly, significant fear of falling can be seen in adults with hyperekplexia. Although not evaluated by randomized trials, physical and cognitive therapy can be considered to help increase confidence in walking and balance and subsequently improve gait [14].

The Vigevano maneuver, grabbing the head and legs and flexing both towards the trunk, can terminate an apneic episode in a hyperekplexic infant.

Future Studies

While the Vigevano maneuver and clonazepam are effective in management of hyperekplexia, there is much interest in more targeted therapies for this disorder given the known involvement of dysfunctional glycine neurotransmission. Currently, there are several glycine receptor modulators under investigation, and these hold promise for treating hyperekplexia in the future [19]. Additionally, recent research has shown that the mutant glycine receptor in hyperekplexia disinhibits the brainstem by interacting with the GABA-A receptor and impairing its function. Thus, disruption of this interaction may be an additional potential therapeutic target for treatment [20].

Conclusion

Startle disorders are a heterogeneous group of disorders unified by an abnormal or exaggerated startle response. Hyperekplexia, a rare, usually hereditary startle disorder, characterized by exaggerated startle and stiffness when unrecognized and untreated can result in sudden death from tonic apneic cyanotic attacks. This movement disorder emergency can be managed with prompt recognition and treatment with clonazepam, and engaging the Vigevano maneuver during the attack.

References

1. Wilkins DE, Hallett M, Wess MM. Audiogenic startle reflex of man and its relationship to startle syndromes. A review Brain. 1986;109(Pt 3):561–73.
2. Bakker MJ, van Dijk JG, van den Maagdenberg AM, Tijssen MA. Startle syndromes. Lancet Neurol. 2006;5(6):513–24.
3. Brown P, Rothwell JC, Thompson PD, Britton TC, Day BL, Marsden CD. New observations on the normal auditory startle reflex in man. Brain. 1991;114(Pt 4):1891–902.
4. Jacobson E. Response to sudden unexpected stimulus. J Exp Psychol. 1926;9:19–25.
5. Brown P, Rothwell JC, Thompson PD, Britton TC, Day BL, Marsden CD. The hyperekplexias and their relationship to the normal startle reflex. Brain. 1991;114(Pt 4):1903–28.
6. Brown P, Day BL, Rothwell JC, Thompson PD, Marsden CD. The effect of posture on the normal and pathological auditory startle reflex. J Neurol Neurosurg Psychiatry. 1991;54(10):892–7.
7. Brown P. The startle syndrome. Mov Disord. 2002;17(Suppl 2):S79–82.

8. Lang PJ, Bradley MM, Cuthbert BN. Emotion, attention, and the startle reflex. Psychol Rev. 1990;97(3):377–95.

9. Dreissen YE, Tijssen MA. The startle syndromes: physiology and treatment. Epilepsia. 2012;53(Suppl 7):3–11.

10. Lanska DJ. Jumping Frenchmen, Miryachit, and Latah: culture-specific Hyperstartle-plus syndromes. Front Neurol Neurosci. 2018;42:122–31.

11. Kirstein L, Silfverskiold BP. A family with emotionally precipitated drop seizures. Acta Psychiatr Neurol Scand. 1958;33(4):471–6.

12. Suhren OBG, Tuynman A. Hyperexplexia: a hereditary startle syndrome. J Neurol Sci. 1966;3:577–605.

13. Thomas RH, Chung SK, Wood SE, Cushion TD, Drew CJ, Hammond CL, et al. Genotype-phenotype correlations in hyperekplexia: apnoeas, learning difficulties and speech delay. Brain. 2013;136(Pt 10):3085–95.

14. Balint B, Thomas R. Hereditary Hyperekplexia overview. In: Adam MP, Ardinger HH, Pagon RA, Wallace SE, LJH B, Stephens K, et al., editors. GeneReviews((R)). Seattle (WA); 1993.

15. Tijssen MA, Schoemaker HC, Edelbroek PJ, Roos RA, Cohen AF, van Dijk JG. The effects of clonazepam and vigabatrin in hyperekplexia. J Neurol Sci. 1997;149(1):63–7.

16. Mine J, Taketani T, Yoshida K, Yokochi F, Kobayashi J, Maruyama K, et al. Clinical and genetic investigation of 17 Japanese patients with hyperekplexia. Dev Med Child Neurol. 2015;57(4):372–7.

17. Stewart WA, Wood EP, Gordon KE, Camfield PR. Successful treatment of severe infantile hyperekplexia with low-dose clobazam. J Child Neurol. 2002;17(2):154–6.

18. Vigevano F, Di Capua M, Dalla Bernardina B. Startle disease: an avoidable cause of sudden infant death. Lancet. 1989;1(8631):216.

19. Lynch JW, Zhang Y, Talwar S, Estrada-Mondragon A. Glycine receptor drug discovery. Adv Pharmacol. 2017;79:225–53.

20. Zou G, Chen Q, Chen K, Zuo X, Ge Y, Hou Y, et al. Human Hyperekplexic mutations in Glycine receptors disinhibit the brainstem by hijacking GABAA receptors. iScience. 2019;19:634–46.

Pseudodystonic Emergencies

20

Jong-Min Kim and Beomseok Jeon

Patient Vignettes

Patient 1

A 6-year-old boy presented to the outpatient department for head tilt. Since the age of 2, a head tilt to the right side had been noted. When he was 4 years old, cervical spine imaging was performed, and a congenital laminar fusion on the right at the C2–3 vertebrae was found (Fig. 20.1). At age 6, a posterior in situ fusion of C2–3 vertebrae with an iliac bone graft was performed. However, his head tilt was not relieved, and the patient was referred to a neurologist. On examination, he had a head tilt to the right side with painful contraction of the neck muscles. Manual rotation of the neck to either side and attempts to straighten the neck caused severe pain. The images performed before and after the operation were reviewed. An enhancing lesion anterior to the atlas, axis, and C3 vertebra was discovered. It appeared to be an inflammatory lesion, whose exact etiology was not clear. Anti-inflammatory drugs and muscle relaxant were started. Painful contractions of the neck muscles were somewhat reduced, resulting in mild improvement in his head tilt. Still, future management remains a challenge.

Supplementary Information The online version of this chapter (https://doi.org/10.1007/978-3-030-75898-1_20) contains supplementary material, which is available to authorized users.

J.-M. Kim · B. Jeon (✉)
Department of Neurology, Seoul National University College of Medicine, Seoul, South Korea
e-mail: brain@snu.ac.kr

Fig. 20.1 Radiographic findings from patient 1. Three-dimensional reconstructed CT image demonstrates fusion of the right laminae at C2–3 vertebrae (posterolateral aspect of cervical spine)

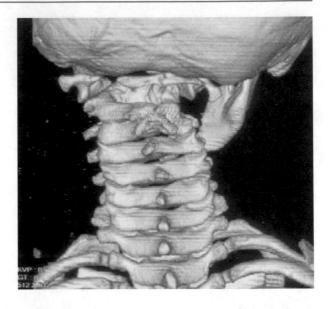

Patient 2

A 54-year-old woman came to the emergency room with severe muscle spasms of the neck and inability to speak or swallow. She had been previously healthy until progressive muscle spasms developed about a week prior to the visit. Examination revealed a retrocollic neck posture with inability to move the neck in any direction. She also had difficulty in opening her mouth due to trismus. She later recalled that she had suffered a minor scratch on her left shoulder about a week before developing her symptoms. Continuous trains of muscle firing were seen on electromyography (EMG), and she was diagnosed with localized tetanus. High doses of diazepam relieved much of the pain and spasm. She improved gradually over the next 3 months.

Concept of Pseudodystonia

Dystonia is a syndrome of sustained muscle contractions, causing abnormal postures, with twisting and repetitive movements [1]. The etiological classification divides the causes of dystonia into four major categories: primary (or idiopathic), dystonia-plus syndromes, secondary (or symptomatic), and heredodegenerative diseases in which dystonia is a prominent feature [2]. However, there are other diseases, both neurological and non-neurological, in which sustained abnormal postures may be present that mimic dystonia. Fahn proposed the term "pseudodystonia" to describe "disorders that can mimic torsion dystonia, but are not generally considered to be a true dystonia" [2]. Berlot et al. suggested a classification of pseudodystonia based on its underlying pathophysiological mechanisms [3].

Table 20.1 Pseudodystonia

1. Stiff-person syndrome
2. Isaacs' syndrome, myotonic dystrophy, congenital myotonia
3. Sandifer syndrome
4. Musculoskeletal or developmental abnormality (Satoyoshi syndrome, atlanto-axial subluxation in Down syndrome, congenital Klippel–Feil syndrome, congenital muscular torticollis, juvenile rheumatoid arthritis, congenital laminar fusion, ligament absence, laxity, damage, syringomyelia, Chiari malformation, Dupuytren's contracture, compensatory act for strabismus and diplopia)
5. Atlanto-axial rotatory subluxation, spontaneous, or associated with trauma, juvenile rheumatoid arthritis, acute arthritis of high cervical spine, inflammatory head and neck process
6. Tetanus, localized, cephalic, generalized
7. Neoplastic torticollis (posterior fossa tumor, spinal cord astrocytoma)
8. Infectious/inflammatory torticollis (infectious atlanto-axial rotatory fixation with or without subluxation (Grisel's syndrome), nonspecific pharyngitis, tonsillitis or adenoiditis, retropharyngeal or tonsillar abscess, parotitis, mastoiditis or otitis media, cervical adenitis, acute rheumatic fever, syphilitic pharyngeal ulcer, influenza, acute encephalomyelitis with rigidity)
9. Seizures manifesting as sustained twisting postures
10. Torticollis from arteriovenous fistula at craniocervical junction

Pseudodystonia includes stiff-person syndrome, Isaacs' syndrome, Sandifer's syndrome, atlanto-axial rotatory subluxation, tetanus, torticollis due to spinal cord astrocytoma, acute infectious torticollis, and other numerous conditions (Table 20.1). Musculoskeletal abnormalities of the spine (atlanto-axial subluxation in Down's syndrome, congenital Klippel–Feil syndrome, juvenile rheumatoid arthritis), ocular muscular torticollis (compensatory posturing of the head for strabismus and diplopia), syringomyelia, and Chiari malformation can induce torticollis, and are other examples of pseudodystonic conditions.

Stiff-person syndrome is characterized by progressive rigidity and muscle spasms affecting the axial and limb muscles [4–6]. Patients typically evidence marked lordosis, caused by axial rigidity. Symptoms may be confined to one limb or even present on one side of the body, mimicking limb dystonia or hemidystonia. Isaacs' syndrome is a peripheral nerve hyperexcitability syndrome that presents with cramps, fasciculations, and myokymia [7–9]. Needle EMG reveals neuromyotonic discharges, myokymic discharges, and abnormal spontaneous activity. Neuromyotonic and myokymic discharges are caused by ectopic discharges from motor axons. Isaacs' syndrome is often associated with elevated voltage-gated potassium channel-complex antibodies. Myotonia is characterized by impaired relaxation of muscles after voluntary contraction or electrical stimulation due to repetitive depolarization of the muscle membrane [10–12]. In myotonic dystrophy, myotonia improves with repeated exercise and is worsened by exposure to cold. Myotonia congenita is an inherited disorder of muscle membrane hyperexcitability caused by reduced sarcolemmal chloride conductance. Multifocal motor neuropathy was reported to present with prominent cramping resembling dystonia [13].

Children with Sandifer syndrome present with torticollis and gastro-esophageal reflux, where torticollis possibly provides relief from abdominal discomfort caused by gastro-esophageal reflux [14–17]. Satoyoshi syndrome is characterized by painful muscle spasms, alopecia, amenorrhea, malabsorption, and secondary skeletal abnormalities mimicking a skeletal dysplasia [18–21]. Muscle spasms produce abnormal posturing of the affected limbs and trunk muscles. Klippel-Feil syndrome is a congenital defect in the segmentation of the cervical spine, and the atlanto-axial displacement may resemble cervical dystonia [22–24]. Congenital muscular torticollis is characterized by ipsilateral cervical lateral flexion and contralateral cervical rotation due to unilateral shortening of the sternocleidomastoid muscle [25–27]. Uziel et al. reported a 6-year-old girl with acute torticollis as the manifestation of systemic onset juvenile rheumatoid arthritis [28]. Chiari malformations are characterized by descent of the cerebellar tonsils or vermis into the cervical spinal canal [29–32]. These malformations can be associated with hydrocephalus, spina bifida, hydromyelia, syringomyelia, curvature of the spine (kyphosis and scoliosis) and tethered cord syndrome. Dupuytren's contracture, characterized by fibrosis of the palmar and digital fascia, may lead to hand deformities in which fingers cannot be fully extended, resulting in a flexion deformity [33, 34]. Head tilt or head rotation may appear as a compensatory phenomenon preventing diplopia in patients with trochlear or abducens nerve palsy [35–39]. Bayrakci et al. reported a patient with an arteriovenous fistula at the craniocervical junction presenting with torticollis [40]. For the cause of torticollis, they suggested compression of the right accessory nerve, meningeal irritation by a bulging vascular structure, and change in blood supply of the pons and medulla affecting cranial nerve nuclei (vestibular nuclear complex).

Pseudodystonic Emergencies

Some pseudodystonic disorders may present as emergencies. Atlanto-axial rotatory subluxation, tetanus, neoplastic torticollis, and infectious/inflammatory torticollis are pseudodystonic conditions requiring urgent workup and treatment (Table 20.2).

Table 20.2 Pseudodystonic emergencies

1. Atlanto-axial rotatory subluxation, spontaneous, or associated with trauma, juvenile rheumatoid arthritis, acute arthritis of high cervical spine, inflammatory head and neck process
2. Tetanus: localized, cephalic, generalized
3. Neoplastic torticollis (posterior fossa tumor, spinal cord astrocytoma)
4. Infectious/inflammatory torticollis (infectious atlanto-axial rotatory fixation with or without subluxation (Grisel's syndrome), nonspecific pharyngitis, tonsillitis or adenoiditis, retropharyngeal or tonsillar abscess, parotitis, mastoiditis or otitis media, cervical adenitis, acute rheumatic fever, syphilitic pharyngeal ulcer, influenza, acute encephalomyelitis with rigidity)

Atlanto-axial rotatory subluxation is a serious cause of torticollis in childhood [41–45]. Children are susceptible to this condition due to the degree of freedom of the atlas and axis and the laxity of their spinal ligaments. The trauma needed to produce atlanto-axial subluxation can be trivial, and the condition may occur spontaneously without trauma. The typical manifestations of atlanto-axial rotatory subluxation are head tilt, contralateral head rotation, and mild neck flexion. The neck muscles appear loose. The spinous process of the axis may be palpable in the same direction as the head rotation. The patient may be unable to rotate the neck past midline. The consequence of missed atlanto-axial rotatory subluxation in children can be devastating. Early diagnosis can, however, produce complete recovery. Axial traction combined with rotation to the neutral position is the treatment of choice. If the diagnosis is delayed for more than a month, axial traction is not helpful and an operation for atlanto-axial fusion is necessary, with the consequence of limitation in range of motion of the neck.

Tetanus may affect a limb, the neck (localized), or the face (cephalic) or it may be generalized [46–50]. Generalized tetanus presents with pain or stiffness over the back or the neck, usually followed by trismus and autonomic disturbances. Cephalic or localized tetanus may be misdiagnosed as focal dystonia. Trismus mimics jaw dystonia. Fiorillo and Robinson reported a 10-year-old boy who developed continuous painful spasm of the foot after an injury [46]. Initially, the diagnosis was delayed. He was eventually treated with tetanus immunoglobulin and antibiotics, although foot spasms continued for 4 months. You et al. reported a 58-year-old woman who initially presented craniocervical tetanic spasms of unknown cause [47]. Two days after admission, she developed severe laryngospasm suddenly, requiring bedside emergency tracheostomy.

Spinal cord tumor may present as torticollis [51–54]. Shafrir and Kaufman reported a tragedy in an infant with congenital torticollis due to spinal cord astrocytoma [51]. Chiropractic manipulation prior to the correct diagnosis triggered a respiratory arrest and quadriplegia due to tumor necrosis. The authors suggest that all children with torticollis, even those with congenital torticollis, should have a radiological evaluation before any physical therapy is started.

The most common cause of an emergency presentation of torticollis is an infectious or inflammatory process of the head or neck [55–62]. Torticollis may follow nonspecific pharyngitis, tonsillitis or adenoiditis, parotitis, mastoiditis or otitis media, acute rheumatic fever, or influenza. A soft tissue mass in the cervical area, such as a retropharyngeal or tonsillar abscess, may irritate neck muscles resulting in postures mimicking cervical dystonia. All children presenting with acute nontraumatic torticollis should be assumed to have an inflammatory process of the head or the neck. Initial management must include cervical immobilization. Computed tomography (CT) or magnetic resonance imaging (MRI) is necessary to delineate the atlanto-axial joint, as plain radiographs are insufficient. All patients with acute or persistent torticollis must be assumed to harbor an atlanto-axial rotatory subluxation until proven otherwise.

Evaluation and Treatment of Pseudodystonic Emergencies

All patients presenting with acute torticollis should be assumed to have a traumatic or inflammatory head and neck process. Initial management should include cervical immobilization. All children with torticollis, even those with congenital torticollis, must have a neurological and radiological evaluation before any physical mobilization. CT or MRI is necessary to delineate the atlanto-axial joint, and to identify space-occupying lesions in the head and neck. All patients with persistent torticollis must be assumed to harbor an atlanto-axial rotatory subluxation until proven otherwise. By following these guidelines, and maintaining a high level of suspicion, patients presenting with pseudodystonia can be safely and effectively managed.

Acute torticollis: First, immobilize. Second, perform a neurologic examination and CT or MRI. Assume that the patient has an atlanto-axial rotatory subluxation until proven otherwise. No chiropractic manipulation should be performed until everything is clear.

The diagnosis of tetanus is clinical. It requires a history of injury or wound and at least of one of the following signs: trismus (inability to open the mouth) or risus sardonicus (sustained facial muscle spasm) or painful muscular contractions. Tetanus may occur in patients who are unable to recall a specific injury or wound. Therefore, it is crucial to first think of tetanus even if there is no history. For treatment, human tetanus immunoglobulin, also called tetanus antitoxin, should be administered by intramuscular injection or intravenously as soon as possible. To reduce toxin production, antibiotics are given; metronidazole, tetracyclines, macrolides, clindamycin, cephalosporins, and chloramphenicol are effective. Benzodiazepines can be used to control muscle spasm. Airway and autonomic dysfunction, such as blood pressure and body temperature fluctuations, should be carefully managed.

First, suspect tetanus even with no history of injury or wound. Then, administer tetanus immunoglobulin and antibiotic. Keep an eye on airway and autonomic dysfunction.

References

1. Fahn S. Concept and classification of dystonia. Adv Neurol. 1988;50:1–8.
2. Fahn S, Bressman SB, Marsden CD. Classification of dystonia. Adv Neurol. 1998;78:1–10.
3. Berlot R, Bhatia KP, Kojović M. Pseudodystonia: A new perspective on an old phenomenon. Parkinsonism Relat Disord. 2019;62:44–50.
4. Baizabal-Carvallo JF, Jankovic J. Stiff-person syndrome: insights into a complex autoimmune disorder. J Neurol Neurosurg Psychiatry. 2015;86(8):840–8.
5. Kenda J, Kojović M, Graus F, Gregorič KM. (Pseudo) hemidystonia associated with anti-glutamic acid decarboxylase antibodies--a case report. Eur J Neurol. 2015;22(12):1573–4.

6. Di Luca DG, Bette S, Singer C, Luca C. Teaching NeuroImages: Severe spasms resembling status dystonicus as an unusual presentation of stiff-person syndrome. Neurology. 2019;92(7):e748.

7. Tuite PJ, Navarette C, Bril V, Lang AE. Idiopathic generalized myokymia (Isaacs' syndrome) with hand posturing resembling dystonia. Mov Disord. 1996;11(4):448–9.

8. Ahmed A, Simmons Z. Isaacs syndrome: a review. Muscle Nerve. 2015;52(1):5–12.

9. Katirji B. Peripheral nerve hyperexcitability. Handb Clin Neurol. 2019;161:281–90.

10. Lossin C, George AL Jr. Myotonia congenita. Adv Genet. 2008;63:25–55.

11. Thornton CA. Myotonic dystrophy. Neurol Clin. 2014;32(3):705–19. viii

12. Rempe T, Subramony SH. "Status myotonicus" in Na $_v$ 1.4-M1592V channelopathy. Neuromuscul Disord. 2020;30(5):424–6.

13. Garg N, Heard RNS, Kiers L, Gerraty R, Yiannikas C. Multifocal motor neuropathy presenting as Pseudodystonia. Mov Disord Clin Pract. 2016;4(1):100–4.

14. Deskin RW. Sandifer syndrome: a cause of torticollis in infancy. Int J Pediatr Otorhinolaryngol. 1995;32(2):183–5.

15. Shahnawaz M, van der Westhuizen LR, Gledhill RF. Episodic cervical dystonia associated with gastro-oesophageal reflux. A case of adult-onset Sandifer syndrome. Clin Neurol Neurosurg. 2001;103(4):212–5.

16. Mindlina I. Diagnosis and management of Sandifer syndrome in children with intractable neurological symptoms. Eur J Pediatr. 2020;179(2):243–50.

17. Tumturk A, Kaya Ozcora G, Kacar Bayram A, Kabaklioglu M, Doganay S, Canpolat M, et al. Torticollis in children: an alert symptom not to be turned away. Childs Nerv Syst. 2015;31(9):1461–70.

18. Merello M, Garcia H, Nogues M, Leiguarda R. Masticatory muscle spasm in a non-Japanese patient with Satoyoshi syndrome successfully treated with botulinum toxin. Mov Disord. 1994;9:104–5.

19. Ehlayel MS, Lacassie Y. Satoyoshi syndrome: an unusual postnatal multisystemic disorder. Am J Med Genet. 1995;57(4):620–5.

20. Drost G, Verrips A, van Engelen BG, Stegeman DF, Zwarts MJ. Involuntary painful muscle contractions in Satoyoshi syndrome: a surface electromyographic study. Mov Disord. 2006;21(11):2015–8.

21. Bledsoe IO. Phenomenology of muscle Spasmsin Satoyoshi syndrome and treatment with botulinum toxin injections. Mov Disord Clin Pract. 2020;7(5):555–6.

22. Tracy MR, Dormans JP, Kusumi K. Klippel-Feil syndrome: clinical features and current understanding of etiology. Clin Orthop Relat Res. 2004;424:183–90.

23. Lopez-Vicchi M, Da Prat G, Gatto EM. Pseudodystonic posture secondary to Klippel-Feil syndrome and Diastematomyelia. Tremor Other Hyperkinet Mov (N Y). 2015;5:325.

24. Frikha R. Klippel-Feil syndrome: a review of the literature. Clin Dysmorphol. 2020;29(1):35–7.

25. Brougham DI, Cole WG, Dickens DR, Menelaus MB. Torticollis due to a combination of sternomastoid contracture and congenital vertebral anomalies. J Bone Joint Surg Br. 1989;71(3):404–7.

26. Nilesh K, Mukherji S. Congenital muscular torticollis. Ann Maxillofac Surg. 2013;3(2):198–200.

27. Sargent B, Kaplan SL, Coulter C, Baker C. Congenital Muscular Torticollis: Bridging the Gap Between Research and Clinical Practice. Pediatrics. 2019;144(2):e20190582.

28. Uziel Y, Rathaus V, Pomeranz A, Solan H, Wolach B. Torticollis as the sole initial presenting sign of systemic onset juvenile rheumatoid arthritis. J Rheumatol. 1998;25:166–8.

29. Kiwak KJ, Deray MJ, Shields WD. Torticollis in three children with syringomyelia and spinal cord tumor. Neurology. 1983;33(7):946–8.

30. Hill MD, Kumar R, Lozano A, Tator CH, Ashby P, Lang AE. Syringomyelic dystonia and athetosis. Mov Disord. 1999;14(4):684–8.

31. Alexiou GA, Prodromou N. Torticollis as an initial sign of Chiari I malformation. Pediatr Emerg Care. 2009;25(3):215.

32. Mancarella C, Delfini R, Landi A. Chiari Malformations. Acta Neurochir Suppl. 2019;125:89–95.

33. Townley WA, Baker R, Sheppard N, Grobbelaar AO. Dupuytren's contracture unfolded. BMJ. 2006;332(7538):397–400.
34. Mella JR, Guo L, Hung V. Dupuytren's contracture: an evidence based review. Ann Plast Surg. 2018;81(6S Suppl 1):S97–S101.
35. Varrato J, Galetta S. Fourth nerve palsy unmasked by botulinum toxin therapy for cervical torticollis. Neurology. 2000;55(6):896.
36. Straumann D, Bockisch CJ, Weber KP. Dynamic aspects of trochlear nerve palsy. Prog Brain Res. 2008;171:53–8.
37. Lau FH, Fan DS, Sun KK, Yu CB, Wong CY, Lam DS. Residual torticollis in patients after strabismus surgery for congenital superior oblique palsy. Br J Ophthalmol. 2009;93(12):1616–9.
38. Erkan Turan K, Taylan Sekeroglu H, Koc I, Kilic M, Sanac AS. The frequency and causes of abnormal head position based on an ophthalmology clinic's findings: is it overlooked? Eur J Ophthalmol. 2017;27(4):491–4.
39. Diora JR, Plager DA. Sudden-onset trochlear nerve palsy: clinical characteristics and treatment implications. J AAPOS. 2019;23(6):321.e1–321.e5.
40. Bayrakci B, Aysun S, First M. Arteriovenous fistula: a cause of torticollis. Pediatr Neurol. 1999;20(2):146–7.
41. Grogaard B, Dullerud R, Magnaes B. Acute torticollis in children due to atlanto-axial rotary fixation. Arch Orthop Trauma Surg. 1993;112:185–8.
42. Sobolewski BA, Mittiga MR, Reed JL. Atlantoaxial rotary subluxation after minor trauma. Pediatr Emerg Care. 2008;24(12):852–6.
43. Missori P, Marruzzo D, Peschillo S, Domenicucci M. Clinical remarks on acute post-traumatic atlanto-axial rotatory subluxation in pediatric-aged patients. World Neurosurg. 2014;82(5):e645–8.
44. Neal KM, Mohamed AS. Atlantoaxial rotatory subluxation in children. J Am Acad Orthop Surg. 2015;23(6):382–92.
45. Kinon MD, Nasser R, Nakhla J, Desai R, Moreno JR, Yassari R, et al. Atlantoaxial Rotatory Subluxation: A Review for the Pediatric Emergency Physician. Pediatr Emerg Care. 2016;32(10):710–6.
46. Fiorillo L, Robinson JL. Localized tetanus in a child. Ann Emerg Med. 1999;33:460–3.
47. You S, Kim MJ, Jang EH, Lim YM, Chung SJ. Teaching video NeuroImages: cephalic tetanus as a pseudodystonic emergency. Neurology. 2011;77:e77–8.
48. Adeleye AO, Azeez AL. Fatal tetanus complicating an untreated mild open head injury: a case-illustrated review of cephalic tetanus. Surg Infect. 2012;13(5):317–20.
49. Rodrigo C, Fernando D, Rajapakse S. Pharmacological management of tetanus: an evidence-based review. Crit Care. 2014;18(2):217.
50. Yen LM, Thwaites CL. Tetanus Lancet. 2019;393(10181):1657–68.
51. Shafrir Y, Kaufman BA. Quadriplegia after chiropractic manipulation in an infant with congenital torticollis caused by a spinal cord astrocytoma. J Pediatr. 1992;120:266–9.
52. Cammarota A, Gershanik OS, García S, Lera G. Cervical dystonia due to spinal cord ependymoma: involvement of cervical cord segments in the pathogenesis of dystonia. Mov Disord. 1995;10(4):500–3.
53. Kumandaş S, Per H, Gümüş H, Tucer B, Yikilmaz A, Kontaş O, et al. Torticollis secondary to posterior fossa and cervical spinal cord tumors: report of five cases and literature review. Neurosurg Rev. 2006;29(4):333–8. discussion 338
54. Fąfara-Leś A, Kwiatkowski S, Maryńczak L, Kawecki Z, Adamek D, Herman-Sucharska I, et al. Torticollis as a first sign of posterior fossa and cervical spinal cord tumors in children. Childs Nerv Syst. 2014;30(3):425–30.
55. Berry DS, Moriarty RA. Atlantoaxial subluxation related to pharyngitis: Grisel's syndrome. Clin Pediatr. 1999;38:673–5.
56. Kelly CP, Isaacman DJ. Group B streptococcal retropharyngeal cellulitis in a young infant: a case report and review of the literature. J Emerg Med. 2002;23(2):179–82.
57. Battiata AP, Pazos G. Grisel's syndrome: the two-hit hypothesis--a case report and literature review. Ear Nose Throat J. 2004;83(8):553–5.

58. Pilge H, Prodinger PM, Bürklein D, Holzapfel BM, Lauen J. Nontraumatic subluxation of the atlanto-axial joint as rare form of acquired torticollis: diagnosis and clinical features of the Grisel's syndrome. Spine (Phila Pa 1976). 2011;36(11):E747–51.
59. Ortiz GL, Pratts I, Ramos E. Grisel's syndrome: an unusual cause of torticollis. J Pediatr Rehabil Med. 2013;6(3):175–80.
60. Iaccarino C, Francesca O, Piero S, Monica R, Armando R, de Bonis P, et al. Grisel's syndrome: non-traumatic atlantoaxial rotatory subluxation-report of five cases and review of the literature. Acta Neurochir Suppl. 2019;125:279–88.
61. Ishikawa Y, Miyakoshi N, Hongo M, Kasukawa Y, Kudo D, Shimada Y. Pyogenic atlanto-axial rotational dislocation representing adult torticollis with vertebral artery occlusion: a case report and review. World Neurosurg. 2020;144:82–7.
62. Al-Driweesh T, Altheyab F, Alenezi M, Alanazy S, Aldrees T. Grisel's syndrome post otolaryngology procedures: a systematic review. Int J Pediatr Otorhinolaryngol. 2020;137:110225.

Functional Movement Disorders

21

Christopher D. Stephen, Daniel Schneider,
and Daniel T. Williams

Patient Vignette

A 73-year-old female with depression, anxiety, and post-traumatic stress disorder had the acute onset of jerking movements of all four limbs immediately after receiving propofol anesthesia for an elective colonoscopy as surveillance for her rectal cancer. After the procedure was completed, on awakening she had further sudden onset "tonic clonic" jerking on attempting to stand. A Code Stroke was called and she was admitted to the medicine service, where stroke workup was negative. Although the diagnosis was unclear, it was felt to possibly be related to a medication effect of the propofol. She was discharged to inpatient rehabilitation, and throughout her stay she had uncontrolled shaking of the arms and legs, which made walking very challenging even with a walker. She noted that as soon as she tried to bear weight the shaking would begin and she would have to sit down. This led to her being wheelchair-bound for roughly 5 months. She was treated with physical therapy and occupational therapy and considerably improved, although she still experienced episodes of shaking which could be worse variably in the arms, legs, or trunk. The severity of the shaking fluctuated during an episode, and her walking and balance were worse. Fatigue, stress, and cold temperatures tended to trigger the episodes, and lorazepam and going to bed seemed to help. She had no family history of

C. D. Stephen (✉)
Ataxia Center, Dystonia Center, Movement Disorders Unit, and Functional Neurological Disorder Research Program, Department of Neurology, Massachusetts General Hospital and Harvard Medical School, Boston, MA, USA
e-mail: cstephen@mgh.harvard.edu

D. Schneider (Deceased)
Department of Neurology, Robert Wood Johnson Medical School, New Brunswick, NJ, USA

D. T. Williams
Department of Psychiatry, Columbia University Medical Center, New York, NY, USA

© Springer Nature Switzerland AG 2022
S. J. Frucht (ed.), *Movement Disorder Emergencies*, Current Clinical Neurology,
https://doi.org/10.1007/978-3-030-75898-1_21

movement disorders or other neurological disorders. She was examined in outpatient neurology 1 year and 2 months after symptom onset. There was evidence of multi-domain cognitive deficits, involving a vague history, frontal/executive dysfunction requiring frequent prompting and motor impersistence, low-frequency anomia, and reduced verbal fluency, scoring 22/30 on the Montreal Cognitive Assessment. There was inconsistent and variable leg shaking, which changed in semiology, with unusual jerking, involving the trunk/torso, arms, and legs with inconsistent and variable body part involvement triggered by reflex testing, tone testing, and various other parts of the examination. There was a clearly distractible bilateral postural tremor. There was highly variable dysmetria, with highly inconsistent and variable tremor and stiffness, at times appearing perfectly accurate and others missing the examiner's finger by a wide margin. There was unusual slowness, with ponderous and effortful hand and leg movements and clumsiness bilaterally, in sharp contrast to clearly normal spontaneous movements. Gait was markedly abnormal and inconsistent. When walking into the visit, gait appeared normal; however when this was formally examined, she had substantial difficulty standing, owing to uncontrolled truncal jerking movements, involving the legs and trunk, which resolved when concentrating and greatly improved when jogging. Unusual flailing movements with Romberg testing, astasia abasia on tandem gait, and retropulsion on pull testing were markedly variable. There was diffuse give-way weakness in the lower extremities, with preserved underlying strength and highly variable proprioception testing.

She was felt to have a functional movement disorder (FMD) with characteristic signs and a typical history with sudden onset of symptoms, rapid escalation with significant variability (and subsequent dramatic improvement, going from wheelchair-bound to being able to walk unaided with physical therapy), in addition to provocation with examination. She reported a considerable improvement with lorazepam, also consistent. This appeared to have been precipitated by her elective colonoscopy and occurred in the setting of depression, anxiety, and PTSD. However, she did have multi-domain cognitive deficits, involving predominantly frontal/executive dysfunction with concern for an underlying neurocognitive disorder. She was referred for rehabilitation therapy focusing on functional neurological disorder (FND) techniques and to the specialist FND Clinic. With therapy, self-guided cognitive behavioral therapy, and work on her anxiety, her episodes greatly improved.

This case appropriately illustrates the complex features of mixed FMD in an older patient, who initially presented for emergent assessment and had been highly debilitated.

Introduction

The appearance of a chapter on FMD, a subset of FND, in a text concerning movement disorders emergencies may surprise some readers. Yet upon reflection it should not. Although specific data are lacking, FMDs may represent the most common movement disorder emergency encountered by neurologists, as these patients frequently present acutely, with an unclear diagnosis, often with dramatic, debilitating and uncontrolled movements, or involving painful spasms or crises.

FNDs represent a subgroup of disorders in which neurological symptoms such as gait difficulties, limb weakness, and abnormal movements are *inconsistent* over time and *incongruent* with the range of manifestations of organic neurological disorders [1]. Although no brain or other central nervous system lesions account for the symptoms of FND, these disorders lie at the interface between neurology and psychiatry [2] and constitute a core neuropsychiatric disorder [3]. FMDs account for up to 20% of movement disorder new patient visits [4–6] and psychogenic non-epileptic seizures/non-epileptic attacks (of which classification and differentiation from paroxysmal movement disorders are challenging), which represent 30–50% of all referrals to epilepsy monitoring units for evaluation [7] or emergency departments (ED) [8]. Overall, functional neurological disorders account for roughly 9% of all inpatient neurology admissions [6, 8]. Despite their common nature, FMD patients usually experience long delays in diagnosis, and even when a diagnosis is established, the divergent assessments and conflicting diagnoses can sow doubt in the patient's mind and may result in delays in appropriate treatment [9]. A psychiatric etiology is relevant in most cases, but the underlying pathophysiology is unknown. FMD and other FNDs are rarely associated with a factitious disorder or malingering, although this can be considered if compelling features suggest medical deception or feigning illness [10, 11].

O━━━◄   Functional movement disorders are inconsistent and incongruent.

Most neurologists can recall the experience of being urgently requested to consult in one's office or local emergency department (ED) on a patient who is eventually given the diagnosis of FND. Patients with FMD often present with unusual, rapidly escalating and debilitating symptoms, presenting for urgent or emergency assessment. Their frequent sudden-onset symptoms also lead to ED presentations, as the patient may fear a serious or potentially life-threatening process (such as a stroke or seizure) [12, 13]. Iatrogenic harm and misdiagnosis may also result in unnecessary procedures, including intubation (particularly in the setting of PNES), frequent prescription of controlled drugs (narcotics and benzodiazepines) for the treatment of pain [9], and also the increased propensity for debility, including falls (a common fallacy being that patients with FND do not fall). FMD may also occur in the setting of concerning medical illness, such as in the setting of COVID-19, which further complicates diagnosis [14–17].

The severity of FMD (which is frequently greater than those of their "organic" counterparts) [9] is not the only reason for a precise diagnosis. FMDs are more common in females but are not uncommon in males (with certain male phenotypes more likely such as functional gait or myoclonus [18]). They can be seen across the age range, from young children [19] to old age [20]. Indeed, in older individuals, where other neurological conditions such as stroke are far more likely, neurology consultation is frequent [13].

It is important to note that the distress experienced by patients and their families can be equivalent to or exceed that of other emergent neurological conditions. The consequences of misdiagnosis and delay of treatment are no less severe [21, 22]. Importantly, FMDs represent a rare situation in neurology – a condition with potentially effective treatments without side effects, and the possibility of a cure. Rapid recognition and institution of appropriate multidisciplinary treatment can help prevent disability and other untoward repercussions [23]. During the course of this chapter, we will explore what is known about these conditions, focusing on information to assist in the diagnosis and treatment in emergent situations.

A Note on Terminology

Before beginning, we need to take a moment to clarify definitions. Throughout this chapter, we will use the term "functional" to describe movements that are without a clear structural etiology and believed to be of psychiatric origin, and hence exist in a grey area between psychiatry and neurology. There are a number of psychiatric diagnoses that fit these criteria, but the most well-known example is the previous term "conversion disorder" (by International Classification of Disease (ICD) 9th Edition [ICD-9-CM] coding) or the newer term "functional neurological symptom disorder" (since the updated 2015 ICD-10CM coding) [24]. Both of these formulations are psychiatric diagnosis codes. Patients have neurological symptoms despite frequent psychiatric associations, and this duality has led to FMDs and FND being described as a "crisis" in neurology [4]. Dr. Mark Hallett expressed this elegantly: "Why do psychogenic movement disorders constitute a crisis? The nature of the crisis is that there are many patients, we don't understand the pathophysiology, we often don't know how to make the diagnosis, we don't know how to treat the patients, the patients don't want to hear that they have a psychiatric disorder and they go from doctor to doctor, psychiatrists don't seem interested anyway, and the prognosis is terrible. Psychogenic movement disorders can look like virtually any movement disorder, from myoclonus to bradykinesia, but the etiology is thought to be psychiatric rather than organic" [4]. Although this crisis has improved somewhat over the years, sadly the situation still exists. A defining characteristic of FND is that the symptoms are not deliberately or consciously feigned, but occur outside of the patient's awareness or subconscious. This is in contrast to malingering and factitious disorder, where the movements are voluntarily produced [10, 11]. There has historically been concern from providers that patients with FND are feigning illness; however, this is very rare and should only be considered where fraudulent and willful secondary gain is identified [10, 11].

The label functional includes diagnoses that were previously considered "psychogenic" [25], "non-organic" [26], "hysterical" [27], and "conversion" [28]. These terms are inaccurate and much less palatable to patients [29]. If patients are unhappy with a diagnostic term, they may not accept or engage with treatment, hence the "name issue" is important [29, 30]. FNDs represent disorders of brain function as opposed to structural lesions of the central nervous system (brain, spinal cord, nerve roots, and peripheral nerves). From a symptom perspective, they may encompass much of psychosomatic illness presenting with neurological symptoms. There has been increasing research on the pathophysiology of FNDs, which are brain-based disorders, in essence, disorders of attention or self-agency [31]. Thus, classifying symptoms as "organic" or "non-organic" is a distinction that is difficult to justify based on our modern understanding of neurophysiology. Despite increasing interest in this very important area, understanding of mechanism is limited, including how they arise (both involving predisposing vulnerabilities and precipitating factors) or how they are perpetuated [32].

Pathophysiology

In FMD, structural abnormalities are absent (i.e., imaging, laboratory testing, neurophysiology [electromyography (EMG), electroencephalography (EEG), and evoked potentials] are normal). When the term "conversion disorder" was used, psychodynamic explanations focused on the transformation or "conversion" of unconscious psychic phenomena into somatic complaints [33]. An abnormality residing purely in the psyche (hence the reason why the term "psychogenic") has fallen out of favor by many of the leaders in the field [31]. Recent literature has focused on the neurobiological substrates of functional motor disorders. Here, we must make a distinction between negative motor symptoms (e.g., weakness) and positive motor symptoms (e.g., tremor, dystonia, parkinsonism, dyskinesia, myoclonus, and tics) [34]. While functional seizures (PNES) are within the spectrum of motor FND, a full investigation of these phenomena is outside the scope of this chapter.

Research on the pathophysiology of FND is advancing, with developing findings indicating an abnormal neurobiological basis and altered neural networks [31, 35]. Studies of the functional neuroanatomy of FND reveal increased amygdala reactivity and connectivity to premotor regions [36, 37], increased cingulo-insular connectivity to motor/premotor regions [38, 39], impairments in self-agency perception involving the role of the right temporoparietal junction [40, 41], including a potential method of treatment using transcranial magnetic stimulation [42].

Theories to explain functional weakness have focused largely on functional imaging findings that support mechanisms limiting the generation of motor intention [43, 44] or impairing the execution of motor intentions [45, 46]. Studies have also suggested abnormal processing of sensory [47, 48] and cognitive information [49–52] in patients with these conditions. Further research into "positive" functional motor disorders, mechanisms for abnormal limbic processing [28], as well as mechanisms to explain the interruption of conscious awareness [40] has been investigated. Studies have also assessed abnormal cerebral blood flow [35], including in patients with functional gait [53]. There is also a case report of two patients with abnormal dopamine transporter (DaT) scan uptake, despite clinically definite functional parkinsonism and improvement of scans over time with improvement of their symptoms [54].

A final note should be made about studies that have included subjects with voluntary production of symptoms as a comparator group to those with presumed functional symptoms [40, 43, 46, 51]. Differences found on functional imaging provides support for differentiation of patients with consciously and unconsciously produced symptoms, and provides hope that a physiological test might be devised to help differentiate these conditions in the future.

Diagnosis

Accurate diagnosis of FMD is fundamentally important for treatment. Virtually all movement disorders seen by neurologists have a functional equivalent. Even movements very difficult to voluntarily reproduce like palatal tremor [55, 56] or eye movements mimicking opsoclonus (generally related to convergence spasm) have been documented as functional [57]. Physicians frequently fear making a diagnosis of a FMD given the concern that a misdiagnosis could irreparably damage the physician–patient relationship or even lead to legal repercussions. However, the opposite should be equally concerning. The misdiagnosis of a functional condition as "organic" can lead to significant iatrogenic harm through unnecessary treatments including medications, interventions, and surgeries [58, 59]. Even with prompt and appropriate treatment, a cure is by no means certain. Failure to consider a functional etiology may lead to a significant delay in providing disease-altering treatment.

There have been several iterations of diagnostic criteria for FMD [60]. In 1988, Fahn and Williams produced the first official criteria, although these were only for functional dystonia [61], and included the diagnostic categories: documented, clinically established, probable, and possible functional dystonia. For documented and clinically established FMD, incongruence or inconsistency of movements with classical organic dystonia were specifically highlighted to make a diagnosis [62]. Additional supportive criteria included functional neurological signs and symptoms, or "obvious psychiatric disturbance" [61]. Diagnostic criteria were revised in 1995, and documented and clinically established categories were combined as "clinically definite" FMD [63]. Clinically possible FMD involved "obvious emotional disturbance," which is least reliable in diagnosing FMD [62, 63]. Shill and Gerber proposed new diagnostic criteria for FMD, although they removed the necessity for incongruence/inconsistency, and "necessary and sufficient" core symptoms included pain, fatigue, exposure to a disease model, and potential for secondary gain; multiple somatizations and psychiatric disturbance were secondary [62]. Inconsistency and incongruence of the movement abnormalities are felt by many neurologists to be the most important factors required of an FMD diagnosis [62]. Gupta and Lang's 2009 criteria focused on clinically definite criteria and emphasized a laboratory-supported diagnosis while minimizing the importance of emotional disturbance and patient history [64]. A concern of the authors was that false positive diagnoses were sometimes related to patients presenting with an "organic" neurological disorder with associated psychiatric symptoms [62]. Typically, diagnostic certainty is graded on a scale of

Table 21.1 Diagnostic certainty for functional movement disorders

CLASS I: Clinically documented – persistently relieved by psychotherapy and/or other adjunctive therapies like suggestion or administration of placebo

CLASS II: Clinically established – physical exam and history consistent with functional movement disorder

CLASS III: Probable – inconsistent and incongruent movements but no other supporting features, consistent and congruent movements but other physical exam features supportive of functional etiology, consistent and congruent movements in a patient with multiple other known somatizations

CLASS IV: Possible – presence of psychiatric disturbance in the patient but no obvious signs or symptoms that clearly support a functional etiology

Adapted from Williams et al. [63]

possible, probable, and "clinically definite" ("documented" and "clinically established"), as shown in Table 21.1 [61, 64].

FMD may have associated historical features [9, 65]; however, diagnosis is based on specific "rule-in" neurological examination features [66] which are inconsistent with an organic movement disorder [62, 67]. Most neurologists do not have access to electrophysiological laboratory testing to confirm a functional diagnosis [68]. Accelerometers have been found to be of value, but application in the outpatient setting [34] is challenging.

The diagnosis of FMD is beset with many challenges, even for the experienced neurologist. FMD may commonly be mistaken for "organic" movement disorders including essential tremor, Parkinson's disease, and dystonia (which is, in the opinion of the author and other expert neurologists, the most diagnostically challenging of the FMDs [69]). Genetic disorders presenting with rapid symptom onset or paroxysmal symptoms can be mistakenly diagnosed as FMD, for example, paroxysmal dystonia/dyskinesia [70, 71], potentially treatable metabolic movement disorders [72], rapid-onset dystonia-parkinsonism [73], and acute drug-induced and tardive dystonias [74]. Atypical presentations of common conditions, bizarre "organic" gait disorders, or an "organic" neurological disorder occurring in the setting of significant psychiatric symptoms may be misconstrued as functional. In contrast, uncommon presentations of FMD such a parkinsonism, tics, chorea, ataxia, or abnormal eye movements, in addition to extremes of age may be falsely diagnosed as "organic" [75]. FMDs not infrequently coexist with organic movement and neurological disorders, such as Parkinson's disease presenting with sometimes dramatic and rapidly progressive functional overlay (FMD co-occurs with Parkinson's disease in 1.4–7.5%), often affecting the adjacent body part [76]; or paroxysmal FMD/functional seizures (psychogenic non-epileptic seizures) in the setting of epilepsy (20% of functional seizures also have symptomatic epilepsy) [77].

These challenges may be particularly prevalent in the emergency setting, where there is limited time available to take a thorough history, address concurrent psychiatric symptoms, comprehensively assess the patient and specifically look for functional signs (particularly if the assessor does not have the necessary expertise to elucidate these) [12]. The general recommendation is that only a specialist with expertise in distinguishing FMDs should make the diagnosis [62]. However, in the emergency setting, general neurologists or residents/trainees are the first to assess the patient [78]. Even when seeing a movement disorders specialist, diagnostic uncertainty is high, particularly in the most atypical and challenging cases [79, 80]. It is important to note that the first impression a patient with FMD has with a neurologist is crucial, as the power of an accurate FMD diagnosis exerts a dramatic impact on disease trajectory. In addition, misdiagnoses and diagnostic delays frequently lead to unnecessary investigations [9], increased healthcare costs [1], iatrogenic harm, and poor prognosis [59, 81].

The FMD diagnosis must be made by a neurologist, as a psychiatrist is not qualified to differentiate "organic" from functional movement disorders. Fortunately, recent studies reveal that when physicians make the diagnosis, they tend to be correct. Stone performed a meta-analysis of reports in the literature since 1965 and found that only about 4% of patients reported after 1970 were misdiagnosed as functional [82]. Unfortunately, there are no data evaluating the frequency of neurologists initially diagnosing a patient with an "organic" movement disorder and then revising their diagnosis to functional.

Once a neurological diagnosis of FMD has been established, the psychiatrist helps to manage the comorbid psychiatric symptoms, as part of an integrated, multidisciplinary approach [83]. A psychiatrist can also put the symptoms into a larger context, including the frequent co-occurrence of somatoform disorders such as somatization disorder and evaluate other comorbid psychiatric disorders, including anxiety (most common), mood, psychotic (rarely associated), and personality disorders [1, 2]. Emergent psychiatric symptoms such as suicidality and psychosis should be assessed during the evaluation and may be very important. The presence of these symptoms, or any indication that the patient might be a danger to self or others, requires urgent psychiatric evaluation, and psychiatric assessment and management should occur concurrently with neurological assessment and diagnosis. Need for psychotherapy, including cognitive behavioral therapy, can also be directed by psychiatry [3].

A concern among neurologists is that patients with FMD may actually be malingering or have factitious disorder [10, 11]. Ultimately the diagnosis of malingering/factious disorder is challenging, as patients with these diagnoses frequently present to the ED, signs are the same as that of FMD (although purposely feigned, as opposed to subconscious), neurologists are not well trained and patients may be in a psychological state of "self-deception" and the presence of symptoms is directly associated with secondary gain [11]. Although outside of the scope of this chapter, clues to malingering include a history of fabrication or lying in the past, marked inconsistency between patient historical reports to different providers, and patient avoidance of relevant investigations [10] as outlined in detail by Bass and Wade [84].

As appropriate diagnosis of FMD is vital in the treatment pathway, as this may avoid unnecessary harm and suffering from incorrect diagnosis. We therefore turn to specific historical and "rule in" clinical-examination-based clues to aid the neurologist in making the correct diagnosis [66, 67].

General Diagnostic Features of FMD

The FMD diagnosis is not a "diagnosis of exclusion," but instead is based on a mixture of positive and negative findings, as applies to any other medical condition. Table 21.2 lists a number of general features in the history and physical examination that might make one consider a functional diagnosis, and Table 21.3

Table 21.2   General clinical clues to functional movement disorders

Historical features
Abrupt onset of maximal symptom severity
Static, non-progressive course
Spontaneous remissions/recurrences
Inconsistent symptoms with "organic" neurological disorders
Psychiatric symptoms (caution, may also be present in "organic" disorders)
Physical precipitating event (injury [often trivial], procedure, surgery, drug side effect) or emotionally traumatizing experience
Atypical triggers
Paroxysmal movement disorder with onset above age 21
Association with somatizations and functional somatic disorders (fibromyalgia, irritable bowel syndrome, chronic fatigue, etc.)
Employed in allied health professions (extreme caution, possible imprinting)
May co-occur with "organic" neurological disorders
General examination features
Movements inconsistent with those seen in "organic" disorders
  Variable frequency, amplitude, phenomenology (direction/distribution)
  Distractibility – movement reduces/resolves with concurrent distraction maneuvers (contralateral finger tapping in time with examiner, Luria sequencing), cognitive distraction (serial sevens, other tasks requiring significant concentration) or when patient not being directly observed
  Provocation with examination or attention directed at the affected body part
  Entrainment of abnormal movement (particularly tremor but can also occur with myoclonus/jerks and also other movements)
Movements incongruous with "organic" movement disorders
  Frequent mixed/combined movement disorder (multiple semiologies), which is rare in movement disorders in general
  Paroxysmal episodes precipitated by examination, startle, or suggestibility
  Suggestibility (movements come on after applying a tuning fork, with reflex testing, or startle)
  Specific abnormal movements suggestive of FMD (fixed dystonia at onset, bizarre gait with astasia abasia, facial spasms moving from one side of the face to the other, convergence spasm)
  Delayed/excessive startle, such as after reflex testing
  Associated unusual speech disorder, such as stuttering speech, or verbal gibberish (particularly when provoked by examining speech specifically)
Other "rule in" non-movement functional neurological signs
  Give-way collapsing weakness
  Non-anatomic sensory loss (midline splitting, "tuning fork" test)
  "Tubular" visual field loss
Disability out of proportion to objective examination findings
Excessive fatigue or exhaustion

Adapted from Gupta and Lang. [64]

Table 21.3 Clinical clues to specific functional movement disorder subtypes

Tremor	*Parkinsonism*
Entrainment Reduction, pauses, or disappearance with distraction Absence of finger tremors (when they would otherwise be expected) Increase in tremor with inertial loading Clear action tremor with normal spontaneous movements, without tremor Consistent amplitude at rest, posture, or action	Tremor equally present at rest, posture, and action Lack of re-emergent tremor Distraction, concentration, and walking do not activate resting tremor Oppositional paratonia, without rigidity Unusual, ponderous bradykinesia, which may appear effortful (no decrement) No improvement in arm swing with jogging/running Normal dopamine transporter (DaT) scan
Dystonia	*Tics*
Fixed posture at onset Lower extremity onset in an adult Tonic facial movements alternating from one side to the other Other features see Fig. 21.1	No history of childhood tics Lack of rostrocaudal motor tic distribution Lack of, or unusual premonitory urge Very distractible but not suppressible Frequently associated with other FMD Rarely respond to typical tic-suppressing medications
Gait	*Weakness*
Knee buckling Uneconomical and maladaptive movements with standard gait Consistently falls always away from examiner or away from harm Zigzag gait or constant scissoring with each step Astasia abasia with tandem gait Improvement and change in the gait with dual tasking (finger snapping, cognitive distraction, etc.) Improvement walking in squatting position Inconsistent and unusual Romberg and retropulsion pull testing	Collapsing/give-way weakness Hoover's sign "Dragging" monoplegic gait Dropping plegic arm always avoids striking self Ipsilateral Sternocleidomastoid weakness Inability to move affect limb once placed into a posture Abductor sign
Myoclonus/jerks	*Paroxysmal*
Often axial jerks of the trunk, hips, and knees of the trunk, hips, and knees Precipitated by reflex testing	Episodes highly variable in semiology and duration Episodes provoked by examination

lists features of interest in specific FMD phenotypes. None of these signs or symptoms are sufficient in themselves for a diagnosis, and unfortunately there is no definitive sign that indicates functional disease. It is therefore important to gather as much information as possible from history and physical examination, both supporting functional disease and ruling out other potential causes, before making a diagnosis. Simply noting that one has never seen a patient with a certain symptom is not sufficient for a diagnosis, nor is noting a single sign (such as give-way/collapsing weakness) and basing one's entire diagnosis on that sign. An illustration of this latter concept is a study by Gould in 1986 [85]. They assessed 30 patients following an acute structural lesion to the CNS (25/30 with an acute stroke) and evaluated seven historical and physical signs typically associated with functional disease (i.e., history of hypochondriasis, secondary gain, *la belle indifference*, non-anatomic sensory loss, pain or vibration splitting the midline, changing boundaries of hypoalgesia, give-way weakness). They found that all patients had at least one of these findings; one patient had all seven, with an average of more than three signs and symptoms. Despite this fact, none of these patients were misdiagnosed as FND, as there were other associated features on history and examination leading away from an entirely functional etiology (although the above study does suggest that the patients assessed likely had some degree of functional overlay). It therefore behooves the clinician to assess the entire history, examination, and results of investigations to save making a premature FND diagnosis and to be cautious when data suggesting a functional cause are limited, particularly in the case of trainees who lack the breadth of neurological experience of rare and unusual phenomenologies [78].

⊶⊷   Function movement disorder is not a diagnosis of exclusion.

General features of an FND include a sudden onset of maximal symptom intensity, with rapid symptom progression and a subsequent static course [10]. There is also a frequent association with a physical precipitating event, such as an injury (often trivial/innocuous), surgery or procedure (injection, lumbar puncture, etc.) but also sudden emotional traumatizing experience (death of a relative or friend, abuse, loss of a job or sudden financial hardship), or a reminder of such events [86]. As a note of caution, peripheral trauma can result in a variety of "organic" movement disorders, in addition to FMDs [87–89]. Spontaneous, iatrogenic, or life-event-related remissions are also very rare in "organic" movement disorders (almost exclusively dystonias, such as cervical dystonia or blepharospasm [90]); however, a substantially fluctuating course, sometimes with periods of complete symptomatic resolution, is relatively common in FMD [65]. In addition, while the presence of a family history of movement disorders is usually supportive of "organic" movement disorders, there are very rare cases of familial clustering of FMD [91].

The most common FMDs in the largest clinical case series are tremor, followed by dystonia, myoclonus, gait disorder, parkinsonism, tics, and other less frequent forms [75]. A fundamental clinical feature of FMDs is that they are inconsistent with their corresponding "organic" movement disorder (age of onset, disease course, etc.), such as rapid-onset parkinsonism occurring in a young patient (rare in idiopathic Parkinson's disease or other forms of parkinsonism), often with multiple different movement disorders phenomenologies and without clear signs of an "organic" disorder (such as should generally be abundantly clear in disorders such as rapid-onset dystonia-parkinsonism [92]). There is also marked variability in phenomenology (for instance, tremors which start out with wrist flexion/extension and change to wrist abduction/adduction), frequency (at times low frequency then at others high frequency), amplitude (markedly varying amplitude from minimal to dramatically large), and duration (occurring continuously, then in trains or with inexplicably and variable gaps between movement disorders). There can be atypical triggers, or unusual relieving maneuvers, particularly in the case of paroxysmal FMDs [70]. There is also a co-occurrence with other functional symptoms/FMDs [93], such as an unusual speech disorder (stuttering speech or verbal gibberish [particularly when provoked by formally examining speech]), give-way weakness, non-anatomic sensory loss (such as midline splitting, or when applying a tuning fork across the contiguous frontal bone, differential sensation on either side), or "tubular" visual field loss (similar size of field loss close up or far away, defying physical laws) [94]. There can also be an association with somatizations and functional somatic disorders (fibromyalgia/chronic unexplained pain, chronic fatigue, functional gastrointestinal disorders) [95]. The abnormal movements may be suggestible, increasing with attention (such as when examining the applicable body part), or resolve with distraction/concentration (unusual with "organic" movement disorder), or when the patient does not feel that they are being observed (which can also be seen in factitious disorder) [11]. Stress and anxiety frequently increase both functional and "organic" movements. There can also be a placebo or atypical response to medication (e.g., instantaneous dramatic resolution of a paroxysmal episode with lorazepam, or inappropriate and inconsistent worsening with other medication trials). There is also the added complication of FMD in patients with "organic" motor disorders, such as Parkinson's disease [76], multiple sclerosis [96], or stroke [97]. Indeed, those with comorbid "organic" neurological disorders may be older, more likely to have psychiatric symptoms and often have a longer time to FMD diagnosis in comparison to "pure" FMDs [97].

Although history taking in an emergent setting will be necessarily truncated, patients with FMD have many complaints. A very useful framework for conducting a FND history is described by Stone and colleagues [93]. They recommend to "drain the symptoms dry," an approach which may not be possible in the ED, which allows the patient to unburden themselves quickly of all their symptoms. This gives a broad picture early on (and may prevent new symptoms appearing later) and at least the assessor should document the neurological review of systems [93]. Such a "pan-positive" review of symptoms in itself may be a "red flag" [98], although there is disagreement as to whether this can distinguish patients with FND [98, 99]. It is also important to ask about disability, as this will give an early indication as to severity of the movements [93]. As described above, it is important for the ED assessor to inquire regarding symptom onset (often sudden) and course (static vs. progressive), to ask about dissociation (patients feeling not in control of their movements or episodes where they have reduced awareness and are overwhelmed) [93]. It is also important to gauge what happened with previous doctors (if this is the first assessment), as this can help build rapport, understanding what treatments may not be acceptable [93]. Clinicians should ask about emotional symptoms and any perceived correlation with the movements with care. This will invariably require time if done appropriately; time spent early making the diagnosis clear and unequivocal (if possible) can potentially spare the patient from not accepting the diagnosis and ultimately reduce disease duration. Following a detailed history, the next step is to look specifically for "rule in" clinical examination features of FMD [6]. We discuss these in detail according to individual FMD phenotype.

Functional Tremor

Functional tremor is the most common FMD phenotype [100] representing more than 10% of tremor referrals to movement disorders clinics [101]. Functional tremor may often suddenly present after traumatic events [101]. The clinical presentation of functional tremor may be variable. Symptoms can be intermittent or continuous, and affect a single body part, multiple limbs, or even the entire body [101]. There are frequent phenomenological differences and inconsistencies with "organic" tremor. A fundamental quality of an "organic" tremor is the consistency of core phenomenology, whereas FT may change in character (rest, postural, kinetic), variability (changing frequency, amplitude, and direction of movement of the tremor) and increasing with attention, such as with examination or when the body part is examined. Unlike a parkinsonian tremor or essential tremor, the tremor is often intermittent (occurring in episodes), irregular, and inconsistent. Functional tremor may decrease with distraction or suggestion; however, this requires distraction tasks of sufficient difficulty. In some cases, even mildly distracting tasks (such as finger tapping or doing other large movements) can be sufficient; however, in more difficult to distract functional tremors, this requires a greater degree of distraction cause such as performing Luria sequencing or random sequential finger movements in time with the examiner. If there is a superimposed functional/psychogenic slowness of movement on the contralateral side, this may limit the ability of the task to produce the desired effect. Another diagnostic sign frequently present in functional tremor is entrainment, where the frequency of the tremor adopts that of the frequency of active contralateral movements. Other clues such as absence of finger, voice, or facial tremor [101], constant amplitude with changes from rest to posture to action, failure of the tremor to attenuate when the limb is weighted, and excessive exhaustion when tremor is activated during examination have also been described [63, 100, 102–104].

Physiological testing can provide valuable assistance in making the diagnosis [103, 105]. Measures of the regularity, frequency, and amplitude of the tremor as well as entrainment, distraction, weighting, or co-activation (underlying antagonistic muscle activation whenever the tremor is present) may aid in diagnosis [101]. Unfortunately, neurophysiological or kinematic assessment is only available clinically in a small number of clinical centers.

Functional Dystonia

Despite being the second most common FMD (30%) after functional tremor, this is among the most challenging FMD diagnostically [65, 69]. Frucht and colleagues have produced a comprehensive survey of functional dystonia (FD), which provides invaluable guidance to the examining practitioner [65]. One of the reasons why functional dystonia is so difficult to diagnose clinically is that the usual techniques to diagnose FMD (distractibility and entrainment) are frequently absent. In the setting of fixed dystonia, they are often completely absent [65]. In addition, if fixed posturing is sustained for long enough, patients may develop secondary contractures, which can further limit assessment and mimic "organic" dystonia [106]. To help guide diagnosis, a risk prediction algorithm designed to increase the examiner's index of suspicion of functional dystonia has been produced [9], where sudden resolution/recurrence or abrupt onset are more indicative of functional dystonia. Functional dystonia also has a poorer outcome than other functional motor disorders [60, 69], and the presence of chronic pain or chronic regional pain syndrome is particularly associated with a poor outcome [107].

Making the diagnosis of functional dystonia is difficult and ideally requires a movement disorder specialist [62, 65]. The reason for this lies in the nature of dystonia itself. Dystonia, at least primary dystonia, could be considered a "functional" disorder in the traditional sense, as it is a disease without evidence of a structural lesion on pathology or imaging, related instead to an abnormal motor program [65]. All dystonia was believed to be functional for this very reason up until the mid-twentieth century. Factors such as the *geste antagoniste* (a phenomenon where sensory stimulation on a specific area of the body can reduce or alleviate the dystonic symptoms) and the presence of a "null point" (where the symptoms seem to resolve when the affected body part is placed in a specific posture) appeared to some to support its characterization as functional [108]. However, the pendulum swung in the opposite direction and many believed that all dystonia was "organic." In the 1980s, it became clear that although most cases of dystonia are "organic," a subset could only be understood as a clear FMD [61, 109, 110].

Given this history, we should not be surprised that the diagnosis of functional dystonia can be difficult, particularly if one is not familiar with the usual phenomenology of dystonia [65]. Incongruent twisting movements occurring along multiple axes, symptoms beginning with a fixed posture (something that usually only occurs later in patients with "organic" dystonia), and symptoms beginning in the lower limbs in an adult [65] are often functional. Typical features of functional dystonia include rapid onset (sudden or over a few days), female sex, a minor precipitating event, resting dystonia at onset, no overflow dystonia, pain/hyperesthesia (may fulfill criteria for chronic regional pain syndrome type I [CRPS-I]), immediate dramatic responses to placebo, and poor response to botulinum toxin injections [65]. There are multiple functional dystonia subtypes and diagnostic features of the main subtypes are shown in Fig. 21.1.

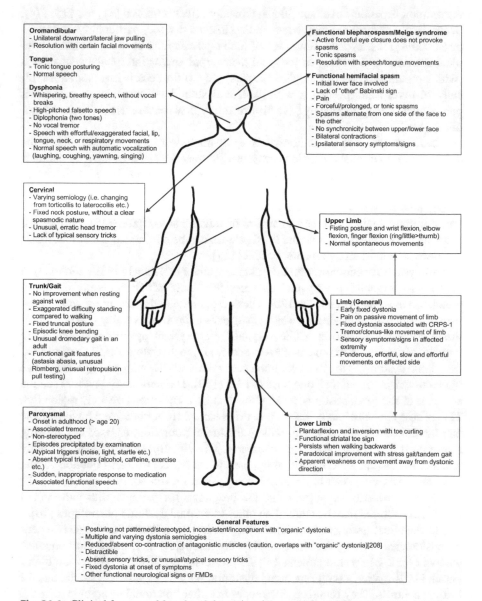

Oromandibular
- Unilateral downward/lateral jaw pulling
- Resolution with certain facial movements

Tongue
- Tonic tongue posturing
- Normal speech

Dysphonia
- Whispering, breathy speech, without vocal breaks
- High-pitched falsetto speech
- Diplophonia (two tones)
- No vocal tremor
- Speech with effortful/exaggerated facial, lip, tongue, neck, or respiratory movements
- Normal speech with automatic vocalization (laughing, coughing, yawning, singing)

Cervical
- Varying semiology (i.e. changing from torticollis to laterocollis etc.)
- Fixed neck posture, without a clear spasmodic nature
- Unusual, erratic head tremor
- Lack of typical sensory tricks

Trunk/Gait
- No improvement when resting against wall
- Exaggerated difficulty standing compared to walking
- Fixed truncal posture
- Episodic knee bending
- Unusual dromedary gait in an adult
- Functional gait features (astasia abasia, unusual Romberg, unusual retropulsion pull testing)

Paroxysmal
- Onset in adulthood (> age 20)
- Associated tremor
- Non-stereotyped
- Episodes precipitated by examination
- Atypical triggers (noise, light, startle etc.)
- Absent typical triggers (alcohol, caffeine, exercise etc.)
- Sudden, inappropriate response to medication
- Associated functional speech

Functional blepharospasm/Meige syndrome
- Active forceful eye closure does not provoke spasms
- Tonic spasms
- Resolution with speech/tongue movements

Functional hemifacial spasm
- Initial lower face involved
- Lack of "other" Babinski sign
- Pain
- Forceful/prolonged, or tonic spasms
- Spasms alternate from one side of the face to the other
- No synchronicity between upper/lower face
- Bilateral contractions
- Ipsilateral sensory symptoms/signs

Upper Limb
- Fisting posture and wrist flexion, elbow flexion, finger flexion (ring/little>thumb)
- Normal spontaneous movements

Limb (General)
- Early fixed dystonia
- Pain on passive movement of limb
- Fixed dystonia associated with CRPS-1
- Tremor/clonus-like movement of limb
- Sensory symptoms/signs in affected extremity
- Ponderous, effortful, slow and effortful movements on affected side

Lower Limb
- Plantarflexion and inversion with toe curling
- Functional striatal toe sign
- Persists when walking backwards
- Paradoxical improvement with stress gait/tandem gait
- Apparent weakness on movement away from dystonic direction

General Features
- Posturing not patterned/stereotyped, inconsistent/incongruent with "organic" dystonia
- Multiple and varying dystonia semiologies
- Reduced/absent co-contraction of antagonistic muscles (caution, overlaps with "organic" dystonia)[208]
- Distractible
- Absent sensory tricks, or unusual/atypical sensory tricks
- Fixed dystonia at onset of symptoms
- Other functional neurological signs or FMDs

Fig. 21.1 Clinical features of functional dystonia subtypes. (Adapted from Frucht et al. [65])

Functional cranial dystonia (functional facial spasm, functional blepharospasm, oromandibular/tongue) is characterized by lower facial involvement which may be asymmetric, and is often paroxysmal. Semiology may involve tonic spasms, with brief periods of normal facial muscle activity, fixed posturing, unilateral or bilateral tonic lip pulling, associated speech difficulties [65, 111] and may mimic hemifacial spasm [112]. Mobile functional dystonia frequently affects the lower limbs (but may involve any body part); however, in "organic" dystonia, adult leg dystonia is uncommon in patients over age 30 and typically affects children [11, 65, 113, 114]. Secondary foot dystonia may occur in Parkinson's disease, particularly in young-onset cases [115]. Typical semiology of limb dystonia includes foot inversion with plantar flexion and curling of toes and metacarpal and/or interphalangeal flexion (with a predilection for the ring/little fingers) [65]. If the neck is involved, this typically involves tonic posturing with ipsilateral shoulder elevation and prominent pain. Functional dystonia may have bizarre, or atypical sensory tricks (geste antagoniste) [116].

Fixed postures add an additional layer of diagnostic complication. When the diagnosis of functional dystonia is suspected, it may be useful to have the patients evaluated under anesthesia. Even if the condition might be functional, patients are still at risk for developing contractures [106]. If the clinician suspects a contracture, exam under anesthesia is critical prior to initiation of treatment, since contractures will not improve with standard treatment of functional symptoms [9]. Further, for some patients, knowledge that the fixed posture can be eliminated under anesthesia can have an important therapeutic benefit [117].

Paroxysmal functional dystonia/dyskinesia tends to occur in mid-adulthood, in contrast to "organic" paroxysmal dyskinesia/dystonia which generally occurs in childhood or adolescence [118–120]. Therefore, individuals presenting with paroxysmal dystonia/dyskinesia above age 21 suggests a functional etiology, in the appropriate context. In addition, while "organic" paroxysmal dyskinesia/dystonia are very rare, they are common in FMDs and functional dystonia [65]. Paroxysmal functional dystonia is the most common paroxysmal FMD, with paroxysmal events often comprising more than one form of FMD [70]. The semiology involves sudden episodes of abnormal postures, resembling dystonia, involving any body region [65, 121]. These episodes can be difficult to differentiate from PNES and have variable and inconsistent semiology with widely fluctuating duration, as opposed to being stereotyped in their "organic" counterparts [65, 70]. Episodes may have highly unusual and inconsistent triggers, as opposed to the typical triggers (alcohol, coffee, exercise, fever, etc.) seen in "organic" paroxysmal movement disorders [70, 121]. There are some data suggesting that the prognosis for patients with paroxysmal functional dystonia may be better than other functional dystonia phenotypes [70].

Physiological testing in functional dystonia has been limited as adjunctive neurophysiological testing does not reliably differentiate functional from "organic" dystonia [65]. Espay and colleagues [122] assessed cortical and spinal inhibitory circuits in 10 patients with functional dystonia, 8 with "organic" dystonia, and 12 healthy controls. They found no differences in either functional or organic patients, despite clear differences compared to controls. However, three small studies have shown some potential promise for physiological testing. One revealed abnormal brain plasticity in "organic" patients but not functional patients [123]. Another found more synchronous EMG changes between arm muscles and higher signal-to-noise ratios in "organic" dystonia compared to a single functional dystonia patient [124]. A third revealed an abnormal blink reflex on EMG testing in patients with "organic" blepharospasm (i.e., eyelid dystonia) vs. those with presumed functional disease [125]. Although all three of these studies were small, if replicated on a larger scale they might indicate a way for physiologic testing to assist in making the diagnosis.

Functional Gait Disorder

Functional gait disorder is another common form of FMD and frequently coexists with FMDs (functional tremor, dystonia, parkinsonism, tics), although it can be seen in isolation [126]. By their nature, functional disorders affecting gait and balance are frequently abrupt in onset, quickly and significantly disabling, frequently requiring walking aids and may result in patients being wheelchair-bound. For this reason, they are a particularly common cause for ED referral and assessment, as they result in patients being unable to walk safely, requiring rehabilitation, home services, or social support [1]. Furthermore, there is a misconception that patients with functional gait never fall or injure themselves. However, this can certainly happen (particularly in older FMD patients, for a variety of reasons) and highlights both the seriousness of this form of FMD, and that such accidents represent another reason why these patients may present to the ED.

O━━━▼   Patients with functional gait disorders can fall and injure themselves.

There are essentially two different forms of functional gait disorder: functional gait in the setting of other FMD or functional weakness, or rarer those with purely a functional gait without other functional motor symptoms [127]. Hence, the presence of other functional features makes gait difficulties more likely to be functional. A cornerstone of assessment is that the features of a functional gait are inconsistent with other common "organic" causes of gait disorder [126]. Common examples include uneconomical and maladaptive movements, significant fluctuation of impairment, excessive effort with "huffing and puffing" (low sensitivity) [128], hesitation (a phenomenon like freezing that does not improve after the first step), unusual scissoring (such as scissoring with every step inconsistent with a spastic gait), patients complaining of poor balance or falls yet displaying evidence of preserved balance control, astasia-abasia with tandem gait, improvement and change in gait with dual tasking (finger snapping or tapping the thigh, cognitive distraction tasks such as serial sevens), or paradoxical ability to dance [129].

This may also be associated with common abnormal and inconsistent examination maneuvers used to assess gait and balance. There may be a functional Romberg sign, with exaggerated sway even with feet apart and substantially worse with eyes closed, improvement with distraction, consistently falling toward or away from the examiner regardless of the examiner's position, or large amplitude swaying building up after a latency [129]. There may be similarly uneconomical and exaggerated movement with retropulsion on pull testing, sometimes in contrast to a relatively stable appearing gait. Patients may also inexplicably be able to normally push themselves on a chair normally, despite substantial gait difficulties, which are at odds with what is seen in "organic" gait disorders, where they have difficulties with the chair and when walking [130].

Common distinct phenotypes of functional gait disorder include [127]:

1. "Walking-on-ice" – narrow-based with arms held out and oscillation from side to side
2. Foot dragging gait – in the setting of unilateral functional leg weakness, where in contrast to hemiparesis (when typically, the affected leg will circumduct) the leg is frequently internally rotated and dragged behind the patient
3. Knee buckling gait – knee bending or collapsing, which may begin as soon as the patient walks or after some distance, increasing fall risk resulting in injury
4. Leg tremor – involving the standing leg, with a delay in initiating swing phase on the non-weight-bearing leg and where walking faster may stop the movement
5. Functional slowness – moving in "slow motion" with movements unusually slow and stiff, sometimes in sharp contrast to normal leg agility and toe tapping

In a large series of functional gait disorder patients, excessive slowness of movement was found to be more common in patients with a functional gait disorder, while knee buckling was the most common pure functional gait disorder, followed by astasia-abasia [131]. In another case series, dystonia was the most common FMD interfering with gait, followed by tremor and myoclonus [128]. In addition, Daum and colleagues sought to assess the sensitivity and specificity of typical signs elicited in functional gait disorders, which were very specific but often quite insensitive. Leg dragging gait and psychogenic Romberg were reliable signs, sudden knee buckling was suggestive, and other signs required interpretation with caution (robotic gait, walking on ice, flailing arms, and sudden side steps) [66, 67].

Functional gait disorder should be contrasted with a cautious gait, fear of falling, or "post-fall syndrome" [132]. In older patients who have had a severe and injurious fall or recurrent falls, fear of falling is very common and may be incapacitating, rendering people wheelchair-bound [133]. There may be an overlap, with functional gait disorder sometimes resulting from such fear of falling. Similarly, there can be substantial gait difficulties in patients with perceptual disturbances without a movement disorder, including sensory ataxia, decreased visual acuity, vestibular dysfunction, or pure oscillopsia (where patients with downbeat nystagmus may have considerable gait difficulties) [134], or pain causing an antalgic gait [135]. There are other specific examination signs seen in "organic" gait disorders in a useful review by Nonnekes and colleagues [135].

Functional Myoclonus/Jerks

Functional myoclonus or jerks are the third most common FMD [136]. The typical age of onset is middle age [137] and unusually for FMD, tends to affect men more than women [138]. Onset is generally sudden, often after minor physical trauma or psychiatric disturbance, generally with a static course [136]. Jerks can involve any part of the body, although more typically involve axial jerks, with non-rhythmic flexion jerks of the trunk, hips, or knees. Movements are inconsistent with "organic" myoclonus, where asynchronous and non-rhythmic jerks are highly variable in amplitude and frequency and more commonly present when supine [136, 139]. Functional jerks may also commonly be precipitated by reflex testing and may be quite easily distractible with cognitive tasks (reciting the months of the year backwards or serial sevens), sometimes causing sudden resolution or entrainment [136, 139]. In comparison, "organic" myoclonus often begins slowly (other than Lance-Adams posthypoxic myoclonus), has a consistent phenomenology, may be focal, segmental, axial, or generalized, may be stimulus-sensitive and may improve with clonazepam, levetiracetam, or zonisamide [136]. It can be difficult to distinguish functional myoclonus from propriospinal myoclonus (a rare disorder with flexor jerks involving the trunk, hips, and knees), which is felt to be generated at the spinal cord level from propriospinal pathways, often with abnormal spinal imaging (in secondary cases) and a characteristic appearance on electromyography (EMG) [139]. Neurophysiology can be a useful tool to differentiate these disorders but is not available in the emergency setting. EMG findings in idiopathic propriospinal myoclonus reveal a fixed muscle activation pattern, slow conduction velocity (<15 m/s), burst duration of 1000 ms, and synchronous activation of agonist and antagonist muscles [140]. These features are not present in functional jerks/myoclonus – instead, jerk-locked electroencephalography (EEG)-EMG reveals a Bereitschaftspotential preceding the jerk, in keeping with motor preparatory activity [139]. Other abnormal hyperkinetic movements including tics or chorea should also be ruled out before assigning a diagnosis of functional myoclonus [136].

Functional Parkinsonism

Functional parkinsonism is a rare FMD phenotype (1.5–7% of FMD patients) and along with functional dystonia, one of the most challenging FMDs to diagnose. In sharp contrast to typical Parkinson's disease (PD), mean age of onset is in the 40s [141]. Frequently, diagnosis is delayed, and in a case series only 25% received a diagnosis at their initial visit [142]. The presence of a negative DaT scan can be useful in the diagnosis [143] but does not discriminate other mimics of PD. Abrupt onset of maximal symptom severity is common, often involving tremor [141]. This sudden onset and frequent association with other movement disorders may lead to various investigations in search of an esoteric cause of parkinsonism, including genetic (rapid-onset dystonia-parkinsonism [92]), autoimmune, or paraneoplastic disease [144, 145].

Tremor in functional parkinsonism tends to involve the dominant hand, is unusual and inconsistent often of equal severity at rest, posture, and action (without the pause with arms outstretched of a re-emergent parkinsonian resting tremor [146]). In contrast, typical PD tremor increases with attention, distraction/concentration, and walking [141, 147]. In functional parkinsonism the distractibility may be subtle, requiring complex motor (Luria sequencing, complicated alternating finger movement, or rhythmic tapping) or cognitive tasks (serial sevens, complicated calculations) to produce brief pauses in tremor in the most persistent cases. Tremor can be variable in frequency and distribution (pronation/supination or wrist flexion/extension) and may sometimes spread to the contralateral limb if the affected limb is held in place, often without a finger tremor [101]. In addition, there is no true rigidity, instead oppositional paratonia with active resistance to passive movement and a tendency to decrease with augmentation/facilitation maneuvers (in contrast to increasing or unmasking rigidity with reinforcement in true parkinsonism) [141,

147]. When assessing for bradykinesia, labored, ponderous, effortful slowness often has a fixed reduction in amplitude which does not change, and at odds with normal velocity spontaneous movements [141, 147]. Speech can be unusual, quiet or a mute whisper with other functional features such as stuttering. Gait may be slow and stiff or shuffling but does not generally have freezing; while there is frequently decreased arm swing, this does not improve with jogging or running as seen in PD [141]. There can also be an exaggerated retropulsion on pull testing, sometimes with dramatic flailing arms and instability even with a slight pull, rolling back on the heels when performing this test (effectively turning the test into a "trust fall"). There may be astasia-abasia with tandem gait, similar to other functional gait disorders described above. If there is concurrent significant depression, there may also be true hypomimia [148]. Patients may have a pronounced placebo response to interventions, such as complete resolution after a single tablet of levodopa, or conversely no response at all to levodopa [147]. There may also be a dramatic placebo effect (or no effect) with other interventions, such as deep brain stimulation [149, 150] and transcranial magnetic stimulation [151]. Given these complexities, movement disorders experts should make the diagnosis of functional parkinsonism.

As a note of caution, FNDs may occur in 1.4–7% of PD patients [76, 147, 152]. Wissel and colleagues in a case series of 53 PD-FND described several important features of PD associated with FND (PD-FND) [76]. PD-FND was frequently associated with psychiatric symptoms including anxiety and depression, with stressful events, a higher prevalence of somatoform disorders and tended to have higher healthcare utilization [76]. Patients were predominantly female (68%), had a longer delay to PD diagnosis, and FND symptoms were abrupt in onset in 55%. FND preceded or co-occurred with PD onset in 34% and almost always involved the symptomatic side of their PD symptoms [76]. Patients had multiple functional phenotypes in 60%, gait disorder (40%), tremor (40%), functional overlay of parkinsonism (21%), dystonia (15%), speech impairment (11%), myoclonus (6%), and more frequently had dyskinesias (41.9% in PD-FND vs 17.9% in PD) [76]. Functional symptoms generally remained static (55%) and PD-FND patients had significantly higher levodopa doses than standard PD (972 ± 701 vs. 741 ± 559 mg daily) [76].

Aside from tremor analysis, the only physiological tests that have been used in this disorder are F-DOPA PET [153] and SPECT DaT scans [143, 154–156] to look for evidence of decreased activity of the dopamine system. The assumption is that functional parkinsonism should not have decreased dopamine activity, while "organic" parkinsonism should. Criticisms have arisen both from reports of some patients with presumed parkinsonism who do not have abnormal scans (i.e., symptoms without evidence of dopaminergic deficit [SWEDDs]) [157] and from a report from Schneider and colleagues of two patients with abnormal scans but with clinically documented functional parkinsonism, with scans reverting to normal with an improvement in symptoms or time [54]. PD and FND can co-exist, further leading to diagnostic uncertainty.

Functional Tics

Tic disorders are considered "unvoluntary" movements, as they are within the range of volitional control and can be suppressed and it is not unsurprising that functional tics are often very difficult to differentiate from "organic" tic disorders [136]. This is made even more difficult as these two conditions share traits and may overlap, as is present in other "organic" movement disorders [158, 159]. In addition, an exacerbation of tics typically occurs suddenly and may trigger an ED assessment, particularly in children with neuropsychiatric symptoms as seen in the controversial diagnosis of pediatric autoimmune neuropsychiatric disorder associated with streptococcal infections (PANDAS) [160]. Uncontrolled movements and vocalizations occurring suddenly in adults can also prompt emergency assessment [161, 162]. In addition to increases in other FMDs during COVID-19, there has been a notable increase in both "organic" and functional tics [16].

Patients with tic disorders invariably have a history of tics in childhood [163], generally with onset below age 10, are more common in males, typically have a family history of tics, and are rarely sudden in onset [164]. In Tourette's syndrome and other tic disorders, a rostrocaudal motor tic distribution involves the face, movements and vocalizations are commonly associated with a premonitory urge, and tics can usually be briefly suppressed. Attention deficit with hyperactivity or obsessive-compulsive disorder are common, and tics wax and wane, frequently responding to medications (antipsychotics, A2-adrenergic agonists, and botulinum toxin) [158, 164]. In sharp contrast, functional tics generally occur in females, often young adults, rarely have a family history of tics, and are frequently sudden in onset [158, 164]. The nature of the movements in functional tics are also different, as they are commonly distractible or suggestible, not suppressible, and rarely respond to typical tic-suppressing medications [164]. In addition, in functional tics, there is not a rostrocaudal gradient involving the face, but frequently involves the trunk and extremities and interferes with voluntary action ("blocking" tics) [158, 165]. Abnormal movements that are not typical of tics include wild thrashing or inconsistent, non-stereotyped patterns [166]. Other factors such as purely vocal tics or tics starting in adulthood can be suggestive, but both have been described in the literature as occurring with "organic" tics [163]. The diagnosis is therefore made by reviewing the history and physical examination for supporting signs or symptoms that might indicate functional tics. While extremely rare, echo- or coprophenomena can be seen in functional tics, there can be shared risk factors (anxiety, obsessionality, impulsivity, and precipitating life events) and treatment can also overlap, as cognitive behavioral therapy (habit-reversal therapy, exposure-response prevention) and treatment of anxiety and depression can benefit both disorders [158].

Functional Weakness

Sudden weakness is a common cause for presentation to the ED for evaluation to appropriately rule out stroke; however, there are many stroke mimics, including motor FND [167, 168]. FNDs have turned out to be one of the most common stroke mimics, accounting for up to 40% of non-stroke cases in different series [169, 170].

They are more commonly female and younger than the typical stroke cohort, may also account for repeated presentations [171] and may even be given thrombolytics, given the understandable time constraints to adequately assess these patients during these emergency situations [172]. Functional weakness should also be on the differential diagnosis of weakness with concern for spinal cord, cauda equina or nerve route etiology, particularly in scan-negative cases, or can also involve functional overlay on top of "organic" spinal weakness [173].

The diagnostic literature for functional weakness is broad, with multiple signs and symptoms being championed over the years as helpful in making the diagnosis [171, 174–176]. Functional weakness is more commonly hemiparetic than monoparetic and can also include a functional gait disorder [171]. In addition to this, Stone and colleagues [171] assessed nine "positive physical signs" in a study of 109 patients with a diagnosis of functional weakness. These included four motor signs (i.e., collapsing/give-way weakness, dragging monoplegic gait, Hoover's sign [weakness of voluntary hip extension but normal involuntary hip extension strength during contralateral hip flexion], and hand strike [a seemingly limp arm avoiding the face when dropped from a height]), four sensory symptoms (i.e., ipsilateral increased vibration sense, ipsilateral decreased vibration sensation, midline-splitting sensory loss, and ipsilateral decreased temperature sensation), and one cognitive symptom (i.e., *la belle indifférence*). The motor signs were common (collapsing weakness and Hoover's sign occurred in 70% and 56% of patients, respectively), while the sensory symptoms were less common and in comparison, *la belle indifférence* was infrequent, found in only three patients [171].

While there are many clinical maneuvers to assess functional weakness, few have been validated in formal studies, although Daum and colleagues also attempted to assess the sensitivity and specificity of "rule in" functional examination signs [66, 67]. This is important because occasionally physicians will treat a favorite sign or symptom as pathognomonic of functional disease, when in fact there is little evidence to support this type of thinking. For instance, in Gould's 1986 paper [85], one of the signs they looked for in their patients with known CNS lesions was "give-way weakness." This is the tendency to provide submaximal effort during confrontational strength testing and is often considered a sign of functional weakness. They found that 10 of the 30 patients displayed this sign, despite known structural etiology of their injuries. They found that 60 patients (56%) displayed a "Hoover's sign," but they also found that 1 of 7 controls also had the sign. Despite these early findings, Daum and colleagues conducted a systematic review assessing the reported functional signs [66] and then compared 20 FND patients with 20 controls to assess the inter-observer agreement and prevalence of the signs [67]. They described 14 validated signs, revealing low sensitivity but high specificity and overall considered give-way weakness, drift without pronation and Hoover's sign as highly reliable, the Spinal Injuries Test [177] being reliable, and hand stroke (arm drop) being insufficiently reliable and requiring interpretation with caution [67]. It is also always important to bear in mind that a patient can have both functional and "organic" illness, so one must use caution when interpreting these diagnostic signs – humility and caution are needed when interpreting the significance of any single sign.

Physiological testing has been more helpful in ruling out functional weakness than ruling it in. Imaging studies and neurophysiology tests designed to evaluate the integrity of the nervous system (such as EMG and evoked potentials) should all be negative or have findings that do not account for the patient's complaints. The use of motor-evoked potentials (MEPs) can be of potential utility, with normal MEPs in the setting of a paretic limb, if there is no definitive neurophysiological or imaging cause for a patient's weakness [34]. There has also been at least one attempt to use physiological testing to quantify the results of the clinical exam. Ziv [178] examined ways to quantify testing for the Hoover's sign as well as equivalent tests in the upper extremities.

Management of Functional Movement Disorders in the Emergency Setting

Anderson and colleagues provided a comprehensive assessment of treatment of FMD in the emergency setting [12]. First, it is important to rule out serious "organic" pathology, such as stroke or seizures [12]. If there is high diagnostic suspicion of FMD, this should be explained to the patient and if there is diagnostic uncertainty but an FND is still a consideration, this should also be discussed. Once the diagnosis has been made, the first step in the treatment is appropriately delivering the diagnosis, which is particularly important in the ED setting [12, 179, 180]. A useful framework to guide discussion of the FND diagnosis and the initial management plan is eloquently described by Stone and Carson [180, 181]. Despite the time constraints, making a functional diagnosis with high diagnostic suspicion is vitally important, as particularly in the initial stages of functional disease making an alternative diagnosis may sow doubt and may reinforce and perpetuate unhelpful illness beliefs or health fears [12]. Communication of a diagnosis should also be collaborative with the ED physicians, for consistency of messaging [12]. Given fluctuation of FMD symptoms (and particularly in paroxysmal FMD or PNES which may result in an entirely normal examination on later assessment), detailed documentation including the presence of "rule in" clinical signs can be very important to the outpatient neurology provider to assign the clinical features and history to the most likely diagnosis [12]. A useful approach to communication in the ED setting includes emphasizing that FND is real, common, brain-based, and treatable, which may include using a simplified analogy (software vs. hardware problem), that diagnosis is based on specific neurological examination findings and also underscoring the difference between FMD and other serious "organic" disorders that the patient is concerned about (and explaining why these are not the case), which (if the provider is sufficiently skilled and confident in making an FMD diagnosis) will allay the patient's fears [113, 180, 182]. Providing education materials through websites such as www.neurosymptoms.org or www.fndhope.org can also be helpful and will allow the patient to read up about FND and understand why this fits with their presentation. It may also potentially mitigate unhelpful Internet research, which may result in confusion and increasing patient fear of an undiagnosed serious "organic" neurological disorder (although FMD is also serious in its own right, given the propensity for significant disability) [65]. Ultimately, the patient's acceptance and understanding of the diagnosis is crucial to the management of FMDs and may obviate searching for alternative diagnoses and subsequent adherence to treatment. A useful guide to the initial neurological management of FND is shown in Table 21.4, highlighting an emerging standard of multidisciplinary care, involving therapeutic roles for

Table 21.4 Guidance for the initial management of motor FND

1. Assessment and (ideally) unambiguous diagnosis
Useful guide shown by Stone and Carson [180, 181]
The *most important* initial treatment is patient understanding and acceptance
Explanation that genuine disorder with potential for reversibility
Positive diagnosis based on the presence of typical signs that, in and of themselves, indicate the potential for reversibility
Avoid assumption that psychological stressors in the patient's life are causing symptoms. Symptoms themselves are often the main stressor
Insisting that there must be others may lead to frustration and an angry patient
Exploration of mechanisms, e.g., triggering of symptoms by pain, injury, or dissociation and a discussion of how symptoms manifest as "abnormal motor signals" in the nervous system
Provide written documentation to patient (such as fact sheets from www.neurosymptoms. org)
2. Commencement of the multidisciplinary management
Treat as early as possible; best results <3 months after symptom onset
Avoid invasive therapeutic procedures
Minimize medications where possible
Anti-depressants/anti-anxiety medications may be beneficial for the treatment of psychiatric symptoms
Physical aids/wheelchairs may be a barrier to recovery [181]
(Possible use of placebo treatments controversial) [191]
Start and plan treatment of comorbidities, including comorbid "organic" neurological disorders
Set up outpatient neurology follow-up
Physical therapy, occupational therapy, speech and language pathology tailored to symptoms and using FND-specific techniques and strategies (provide rehabilitation therapists with relevant consensus guidelines to guide treatment) (Nielsen et al. [184] and Nicholson et al. [189])
Psychiatric assessment as necessary (particularly if significant psychiatric symptomatology) for planning of outpatient psychiatry and psychological interventions (behavior modification, cognitive behavioral therapy, etc.) and transferred to the outpatient setting
Introduce self-guided cognitive behavioral therapy [196]
Examination under general or local anesthesia can be considered in fixed dystonia [117, 182, 184]
Electroconvulsive therapy, if clinically indicated from a psychiatric standpoint [198]
3. Complex treatments (deferred to outpatient setting)
Plan multimodal pain management techniques (including cognitive behavioral therapy)
Paroxysmal FMD – treatment as per non-epileptic attacks
Manual by Curt LaFrance "Taking Control of your Seizures: Workbook" and "Nonepileptic Seizures: Therapist Guide"
If available, in complex/difficult to diagnose cases, a specialist FND clinic can be a useful resource [201]
In select cases – planned admission for FND-specific inpatient multidisciplinary rehabilitation programs [202]

education, physical therapy (PT), occupational therapy (OT), and psychotherapy (cognitive behavioral therapy and related psychotherapy) [183]. Core medical involvement includes neurology (and outpatient follow-up arrangements should be made in house) and psychiatry (particularly for uncontrolled psychiatric symptoms, equally arranging a transition to the outpatient setting).

Treatment may be limited if the patient is only assessed in the ED and not admitted [12] but if the patient is to be admitted, there should again be clear communication with the admitting neurology, medicine, or other team and if there is diagnostic uncertainty, following a different inpatient management pathway [32]. Further inpatient observation can be useful in FMD to allow multiple assessments to observe consistency of functional examination signs and inconsistency with "organic" disease, as well as for appropriate further investigations (such as relevant magnetic resonance imaging), limiting investigations with potential for iatrogenic harm, such as lumbar punctures, where possible) [32].

In either setting, a multidisciplinary approach is required [12, 32] and the diagnostic concerns should also be clearly relayed to rehabilitation specialists, so that appropriate FND-specific treatment can be commenced. In the ED, physical therapy/physiotherapy (PT) evaluation for patients with weakness, gait, or other pertinent symptoms, and occupational therapy (OT) for those with upper extremity motor impairments may reinforce a functional diagnosis and triage patients' needs [12]. Fortunately, there are now consensus recommendations on the PT treatment of motor FND [184]. There have been clinical trial data suggesting efficacy of PT [185], as well as FND-specific inpatient rehabilitation programs [186] and for transition to the outpatient setting [187]. A protocol for a multicenter clinical trial of PT for FND is underway [188]. OT can also frequently be important in rehabilitation [23] and Nicholson and colleagues have recently published consensus guidelines [189]. In the absence of rehabilitation therapists with experience in the specific techniques used in FND, copies of these guidelines can be very important to guide inpatient and subsequent outpatient therapy, as standard approaches (such as for stroke, Parkinson's disease), can frequently be unsuccessful and in some cases, counterproductive. Depending on the patient's symptoms, patients with speech or swallowing symptoms may benefit from targeted speech and language pathology input, using additional FND-specific techniques [190].

The use of placebos in the diagnosis and treatment of FMD is controversial. Inadvertent observation of the inappropriate effects of medications (such as rapid resolution or sudden worsening after treatment, inconsistent with the known physiological effects) should be recognized [191]. Frucht and colleagues have also provided specific advice for the multidisciplinary treatment of functional dystonia [65]. In the inpatient setting, the use of general or local anesthesia after consultation with orthopedic surgery may cause complete relaxation of posturing in fixed dystonia, which may aid in diagnosis and also in the determination of the presence of contractures [117, 182, 184]. If fixed posturing is not treated, contractures may develop [106]. Although patients may be very debilitated by their symptoms, physical aids/wheelchairs may be a barrier to recovery in the outpatient setting, although unavoidable in the cases of safety concerns [181]. Requests for second opinions should be welcomed but the number of these opinions should be limited and targeted, with consultations sought from experts in rare movement disorders, as well as FND (FD paper), as otherwise this can lead to confusion on the part of the patient and contribute to the excessive healthcare utilization seen in FMD patients [1, 9]. One of the most devastating consequences of this condition is unnecessary medical and surgical procedures, and this risk can increase with the more doctors they see [9].

The multimodal treatment of pain in FMD should be started in the ED/inpatient setting but oral medications should be minimized and controlled drugs (opiates/opioids and benzodiazepines) should be avoided for numerous reasons [9]. In the case of debilitating chronic pain, outpatient treatment programs including rehabilitation and CBT may be valuable, including Mind-Body programs [192, 193]. Although oral medications should be minimized, anti-depressants and anti-anxiety medications can be useful in treating psychiatric symptoms [194, 195]. Introducing the idea of self-guided cognitive behavioral therapy (the self-guided CBT workbook, "Overcoming Functional Neurological Symptoms: A Five Area Approach," based on the UK clinical trial by Sharpe et al.) can be useful, particularly if the patient is receptive. We suggest that this can be a useful guide for patients' self-help CBT and can also be used during individual psychotherapy [196]. There are also plans for clinical trials of CBT [197]. Discharge planning should involve multidisciplinary coordination and includes outpatient neurology, psychiatry (as needed, if assessed in the ED/inpatient setting), and rehabilitation [187]. In cases of severe and decompensated psychiatric symptoms, as deemed necessary from a clinical standpoint, there are cases of spontaneous remission of FND symptoms with electroconvulsive therapy [198, 199] and improvement in somatoform disorders [200].

If available in the area, a specialist FND clinic can be a useful resource in complex or difficult to diagnose cases [201]. In select cases, a planned admission for FND-specific inpatient multidisciplinary rehabilitation programs can be of value (combining neuropsychiatry, psychology, PT, OT and, in some cases, speech therapy) and the experienced centers who offer this have published impressive results [202].

Conclusion

In summary, there is evidence that an intensive, multidimensional treatment approach is helpful, although data are limited. A treatment approach centered on neurology and psychiatry management, with PT, OT, and speech therapy as applicable as well as psychotherapy is recommended. Medication treatment is reasonable, particularly if there are significant comorbid psychiatric symptoms. The holistic treatment of pain and other tailored treatments tailored to specific FMD treatments should be considered. Unfortunately, despite treatment, the prognosis of functional motor symptoms is generally poor, with a systematic review suggesting that roughly 40% of patients remain the same or worse at follow-up [86].

References

1. Stephen CD, Fung V, Lungu CI, Espay AJ. Assessment of emergency department and inpatient use and costs in adult and pediatric functional neurological disorders. JAMA Neurol. 2021;78(1):88–101. https://doi.org/10.1001/jamaneurol.2020.3753. PMID: 33104173; PMCID: PMC7589058.
2. Perez DL, Keshavan MS, Scharf JM, Boes AD, Price BH. Bridging the great divide: what can neurology learn from psychiatry? J Neuropsychiatry Clin Neurosci. 2018;30(4):271–8.
3. Perez DL, Aybek S, Nicholson TR, Kozlowska K, Arciniegas DB, LaFrance WC Jr. Functional neurological (conversion) disorder: a core neuropsychiatric disorder. J Neuropsychiatry Clin Neurosci. 2020;32(1):1–3. https://doi.org/10.1176/appi.neuropsych.19090204. PMID: 3196424.
4. Hallett M. Psychogenic movement disorder: a crisis for neurology. Curr Neurol Neurosci Rep. 2006;6(4):269–71.
5. Factor SA, Podskalny GD, Molho ES. Psychogenic movement disorders: frequency, clinical profile, and characteristics. J Neurol Neurosurg Psychiatry. 1995;59:406–12.
6. Lempert T. Psychogenic disorders in neurology: frequency and clinical spectrum. Acta Neurol Scand. 1990;82:335–40.
7. Benbadis SR, O'Neill E, Tatum WO, Heriaud L. Outcome of prolonged video-EEG monitoring at a typical referral epilepsy center. Epilepsia. 2004;45(9):1150–3.
8. Beharry J, Palmer D, Wu T, Wilson D, Le Heron C, Mason D, et al. Functional neurological disorders presenting as emergencies to secondary care. Eur J Neurol. 2021; https://doi.org/10.1111/ene.14728. Epub ahead of print.
9. Stephen CD, Perez DL, Chibnik LB, Sharma N. Functional dystonia: a case-control study and risk prediction algorithm. Ann Clin Transl Neurol. 2021; https://doi.org/10.1002/acn3.51307. Epub ahead of print. PMID: 33724724.
10. Stone J, Carson A. Functional neurologic symptoms: assessment and management. Neurol Clin. 2011;29(1):1–18, vii.
11. Bass C, Halligan P. Factitious disorders and malingering in relation to functional neurologic disorders. Handb Clin Neurol. 2016;139:509–20.
12. Anderson JR, Nakhate V, Stephen CD, Perez DL. Functional (psychogenic) neurological disorders: assessment and acute management in the emergency department. Semin Neurol. 2019;39(1):102–14.
13. Cock HR, Edwards MJ. Functional neurological disorders: acute presentations and management. Clin Med (Lond). 2018;18(5):414–7. https://doi.org/10.7861/clinmedicine.18-5-414. PMID: 30287439; PMCID: PMC6334101.
14. Piscitelli D, Perin C, Tremolizzo L, Peroni F, Cerri CG, Cornaggia CM. Functional movement disorders in a patient with COVID-19. Neurol Sci. 2020;41(9):2343–4.
15. Valente KD, Alessi R, Baroni G, Marin R, Dos Santos B, Palmini A. The COVID-19 outbreak and PNES: the impact of a ubiquitously felt stressor. Epilepsy Behav. 2021;117:107852. https://doi.org/10.1016/j.yebeh.2021.107852. Epub ahead of print.
16. Heyman I, Liang H, Hedderly T. COVID-19 related increase in childhood tics and tic-like attacks. Arch Dis Child. 2021:archdischild-2021-321748. Epub ahead of print. PMID: 33677431.
17. Clark JR, Liotta EM, Reish NJ, Shlobin NA, Hoffman SC, Orban ZS, et al. Abnormal movements in hospitalized COVID-19 patients: a case series. J Neurol Sci. 2021;423:117377. https://doi.org/10.1016/j.jns.2021.117377. Epub ahead of print.
18. Baizabal-Carvallo JF, Jankovic J. Gender differences in functional movement disorders. Mov Disord Clin Pract. 2019;7(2):182–7. https://doi.org/10.1002/mdc3.12864. PMID: 32071937; PMCID: PMC7011817.
19. Leary PM. Conversion disorder in childhood – diagnosed too late, investigated too much? J R Soc Med. 2003;96:436–8.

20. Batla A, Stamelou M, Edwards MJ, Pareés I, Saifee TA, Fox Z, et al. Functional movement disorders are not uncommon in the elderly. Mov Disord. 2013;28(4):540–3.
21. Carson AJJ. Do medically unexplained symptoms matter? A prospective cohort study of 300 new referrals to neurology outpatient clinics. J Neurol Neurosurg Psychiatry. 2000;68:207–10.
22. Anderson KE, Gruber-Baldini AL, Vaughan CG, Reich SG, Fishman PS, Weiner WJ, et al. Impact of psychogenic movement disorders versus Parkinson's on disability, quality of life, and psychopathology. Mov Disord. 2007;22:2204–9.
23. Demartini B, Batla A, Petrochilos P, Fisher L, Edwards MJ, Joyce E. Multidisciplinary treatment for functional neurological symptoms: a prospective study. J Neurol. 2014;261(12):2370–7. https://doi.org/10.1007/s00415-014-7495-4. Epub 2014 Sep 20. PMID: 25239392; PMCID: PMC4242999.
24. Stone J, Hallett M, Carson A, Bergen D, Shakir R. Functional disorders in the neurology section of ICD-11: a landmark opportunity. Neurology. 2014;83(24):2299–301. https://doi.org/10.1212/WNL.0000000000001063. PMID: 25488992; PMCID: PMC4277679.
25. Fahn S, Olanow CW. "Psychogenic movement disorders": they are what they are. Mov Disord. 2014;29(7):853–6. https://doi.org/10.1002/mds.25899. Epub 2014 May 5. PMID: 24797587.
26. White A. The use of thiopentone in the treatment of non-organic locomotor disorders. J Psychosom Res. 1988;32:249–53.
27. Walters AS, Boudwin J, Wright D, Jones K. Three hysterical movement disorders. Psychol Rep. 1988;62:979–85.
28. Voon V. Emotional stimuli and motor conversion disorder. Brain. 2010;133:1526–36.
29. Stone J, Wojcik W, Durrance D, Carson A, Lewis S, MacKenzie L, et al. What should we say to patients with symptoms unexplained by disease? The "number needed to offend". BMJ. 2002;325(7378):1449–50. https://doi.org/10.1136/bmj.325.7378.1449. PMID: 12493661; PMCID: PMC139034.
30. LaFaver K, Hallett M. Functional or psychogenic: what's the better name? Mov Disord. 2014;29(13):1698–9. https://doi.org/10.1002/mds.26035. Epub 2014 Sep 21. PMID: 25242623; PMCID: PMC5681356.
31. Voon V, Cavanna AE, Coburn K, Sampson S, Reeve A, LaFrance WC Jr, (On behalf of the American Neuropsychiatric Association Committee for Research). Functional neuro-anatomy and neurophysiology of functional neurological disorders (conversion disorder). J Neuropsychiatry Clin Neurosci. 2016;28(3):168–90. https://doi.org/10.1176/appi.neuro-psych.14090217. Epub 2016 Feb 22. PMID: 26900733.
32. McKee K, Glass S, Adams C, Stephen CD, King F, Parlman K, et al. The inpatient assessment and management of motor functional neurological disorders: An interdisciplinary perspective. Psychosomatics. 2018;59(4):358–68.
33. Mace C. All in the mind? The history of hysterical conversion as a clinical concept. In: Halligan PW, Bass C, Marshall JC, editors. Contemporary approaches to the study of hysteria: clinical and theoretical perspectives. Oxford: Oxford University Press; 2001. p. 1–11.
34. Perez DL, Aybek S, Popkirov S, Kozlowska K, Stephen CD, Anderson J, et al; (On behalf of the American Neuropsychiatric Association Committee for Research). A review and expert opinion on the neuropsychiatric assessment of motor functional neurological disorders. J Neuropsychiatry Clin Neurosci. 2021;33(1):14–26. https://doi.org/10.1176/appi.neuro-psych.19120357. Epub 2020 Aug 11. PMID: 32778007.
35. Bègue I, Adams C, Stone J, Perez DL. Structural alterations in functional neurologi-cal disorder and related conditions: a software and hardware problem? Neuroimage Clin. 2019;22:101798. https://doi.org/10.1016/j.nicl.2019.101798. Epub 2019 Mar 28. PMID: 31146322; PMCID: PMC6484222.
36. Aybek S, Nicholson TR, Zelaya F, O'Daly OG, Craig TJ, David AS, et al. Neural correlates of recall of life events in conversion disorder. JAMA Psychiat. 2014;71(1):52–60. https://doi.org/10.1001/jamapsychiatry.2013.2842. PMID: 24258270.
37. Hassa T, Sebastian A, Liepert J, Weiller C, Schmidt R, Tüscher O. Symptom-specific amyg-dala hyperactivity modulates motor control network in conversion disorder. Neuroimage Clin.

2017;15:143–50. https://doi.org/10.1016/j.nicl.2017.04.004. PMID: 28529870; PMCID: PMC5429234.

38. Li R, Li Y, An D, Gong Q, Zhou D, Chen H. Altered regional activity and inter-regional functional connectivity in psychogenic non-epileptic seizures. Sci Rep. 2015;5:11635. https://doi.org/10.1038/srep11635. PMID: 26109123; PMCID: PMC4480007.

39. van der Kruijs SJ, Bodde NM, Vaessen MJ, Lazeron RH, Vonck K, Boon P, et al. Functional connectivity of dissociation in patients with psychogenic non-epileptic seizures. J Neurol Neurosurg Psychiatry. 2012;83(3):239–47. https://doi.org/10.1136/jnnp-2011-300776. Epub 2011 Nov 5. PMID: 22056967.

40. Voon V, Gallea C, Hattori N, Bruno M, Ekanayake V, Hallett M. The involuntary nature of conversion disorder. Neurology. 2010;74(3):223–8. https://doi.org/10.1212/WNL.0b013e3181ca00e9. PMID: 20083798; PMCID: PMC2809033.

41. Maurer CW, LaFaver K, Ameli R, Epstein SA, Hallett M, Horovitz SG. Impaired self-agency in functional movement disorders: A resting-state fMRI study. Neurology. 2016;87(6):564–70. https://doi.org/10.1212/WNL.0000000000002940. Epub 2016 Jul 6. PMID: 27385746; PMCID: PMC4977370.

42. Zito GA, Anderegg LB, Apazoglou K, Müri RM, Wiest R, Holtforth MG, Aybek S. Transcranial magnetic stimulation over the right temporoparietal junction influences the sense of agency in healthy humans. J Psychiatry Neurosci. 2020;45(4):271–8. https://doi.org/10.1503/jpn.190099.

43. Spence SA. Hysterical paralyses as disorders of action. Cogn Neuropsychiatry. 1999;4:203–26.

44. Burgmer M, Konrad C, Jansen A, Kugel H, Sommer J, Heindel W, et al. Abnormal brain activation during movement observation in patients with conversion paralysis. NeuroImage. 2006;29:1336–43.

45. Marshall JC, Halligan PW, Fink GR, Wade DT, Frackowiak RS. The functional anatomy of a hysterical paralysis. Cognition. 1997;64:B1–8.

46. Stone J, Zeman A, Simonotto E, Meyer M, Azuma R, Flett S, et al. FMRI in patients with motor conversion symptoms and controls with simulated weakness. Psychosom Med. 2007;69:961–9.

47. Tiihonen J, Kuikka J, Viinamaki H, Lehtonen J, Partanen J. Altered cerebral blood flow during hysterical paresthesia. Biol Psychiatry. 1995;37:134–5.

48. Vuilleumier P, Chicherio C, Assal F, Schwartz S, Slosman D, Landis T. Functional neuroanatomical correlates of hysterical sensorimotor loss. Brain. 2001;124:1077–90.

49. Kanaan RA, Craig TK, Wessely SC, David AS. Imaging repressed memories in motor conversion disorder. Psychosom Med. 2007;69:202–5.

50. de Lange FP, Roelofs K, Toni I. Increased self-monitoring during imagined movements in conversion paralysis. Neuropsychologia. 2007;45:2051–8.

51. Cojan Y, Waber L, Carruzzo A, Vuilleumier P. Motor inhibition in hysterical conversion paralysis. NeuroImage. 2009;47:1026–37.

52. de Lange FP, Toni I, Roelofs K. Altered connectivity between prefrontal and sensorimotor cortex in conversion paralysis. Neuropsychologia. 2010;48:1782–8.

53. Yazici KM, Kostakoglu L. Cerebral blood flow changes in patients with conversion disorder. Psychiatry Res. 1998;83:163–8.

54. Schneider D, Haberfeld E, Fahn S. Treating the patient, not the scan: two patients with psychogenic parkinsonism in spite of abnormal pet scans. Mov Disord. 2011;26:S345.

55. Williams DR. Psychogenic palatal tremor. Mov Disord. 2004;19:333–5.

56. Pirio Richardson S, Mari Z, Matsuhashi M, Hallett M. Psychogenic palatal tremor. Mov Disord. 2006;21:274–6.

57. Teodoro T, Cunha JM, Abreu LF, Yogarajah M, Edwards MJ. Abnormal eye and cranial movements triggered by examination in people with functional neurological disorder. Neuroophthalmology. 2018;43(4):240–3.

58. Fahn S, Jankovic J. Principles and practice of movement disorders. Philadelphia: Churchill Livingstone; 2007. p. 597–611.

59. Bramstedt KA, Ford PJ. Protecting human subjects in neurosurgical trials: the challenge of psychogenic dystonia. Contemp Clin Trials. 2006;27(2):161–4.
60. Schmerler DA, Espay AJ. Functional dystonia. Handb Clin Neurol. 2016;139:235–45.
61. Fahn S, Williams DT. Psychogenic dystonia. Adv Neurol. 1988;50:431–55.
62. Espay A, Lang A. Phenotype-specific diagnosis of functional (psychogenic) movement disorders. Curr Neurol Neurosci Rep. 2015;15(6):32.
63. Williams DT, Ford B, Fahn S. Phenomenology and psychopathology related to psychogenic movement disorders. Adv Neurol. 1995;65:231–57.
64. Gupta A, Lang AE. Psychogenic movement disorders. Curr Opin Neurol. 2009;22(4):430–6. https://doi.org/10.1097/WCO.0b013e32832dc169. PMID: 19542886.
65. Frucht L, Perez DL, Callahan J, MacLean J, Song PC, Sharma N, et al. Functional dystonia: differentiation from primary dystonia and multidisciplinary treatments. Front Neurol. 2021;11:605262.
66. Daum C, Hubschmid M, Aybek S. The value of 'positive' clinical signs for weakness, sensory and gait disorders in conversion disorder: a systematic and narrative review. J Neurol Neurosurg Psychiatry. 2014;85:180–90.
67. Daum C, Gheorghita F, Spatola M, Stojanova V, Medlin F, Vingerhoets F, et al. Interobserver agreement and validity of bedside 'positive signs' for functional weakness, sensory and gait disorders in conversion disorder: a pilot study. J Neurol Neurosurg Psychiatry. 2015;86(4):425–30.
68. Espay AJ, Goldenhar LM, Voon V, Schrag A, Burton N, Lang AE. Opinions and clinical practices related to diagnosing and managing patients with psychogenic movement disorders: an international survey of movement disorder society members. Mov Disord. 2009;24(9):1366–74.
69. Newby R, Alty J, Kempster P. Functional dystonia and the borderland between neurology and psychiatry: new concepts. Mov Disord. 2016;31(12):1777–84.
70. Ganos C, Aguirregomozcorta M, Batla A, Stamelou M, Schwingenschuh P, Münchau A, et al. Psychogenic paroxysmal movement disorders– clinical features and diagnostic clues. Parkinsonism Relat Disord. 2014;20(1):41–6.
71. Gardiner AR, Jaffer F, Dale RC, Labrum R, Erro R, Meyer E, et al. The clinical and genetic heterogeneity of paroxysmal dyskinesias. Brain. 2015;138(Pt 12):3567–80.
72. Jinnah HA, Albanese A, Bhatia KP, Cardoso F, Da Prat G, de Koning TJ, et al. Treatable inherited rare movement disorders. Mov Disord. 2018;33(1):21–35.
73. Sweney MT, Newcomb TM, Swoboda KJ. The expanding spectrum of neurological phenotypes in children with ATP1A3 mutations, alternating hemiplegia of childhood, rapid-onset dystonia-parkinsonism, CAPOS and beyond. Pediatr Neurol. 2015;52(1):56–64.
74. Mulroy E, Balint B, Bhatia KP. Tardive syndromes. Pract Neurol. 2020;20(5):368–76.
75. Baizabal-Carvallo JF, Fekete R. Recognizing uncommon presentations of psychogenic (functional) movement disorders. Tremor Other Hyperkinet Mov (N Y). 2015;5:279. https://doi.org/10.7916/D8VM4B13. PMID: 25667816; PMCID: PMC4303603.
76. Wissel BD, Dwivedi AK, Merola A, Chin D, Jacob C, Duker AP, et al. Functional neurological disorders in Parkinson disease. J Neurol Neurosurg Psychiatry. 2018;89(6):566–71.
77. Kutlubaev MA, Xu Y, Hackett ML, Stone J. Dual diagnosis of epilepsy and psychogenic nonepileptic seizures: systematic review and meta-analysis of frequency, correlates, and outcomes. Epilepsy Behav. 2018;89:70–8.
78. Perez DL, Hunt A, Sharma N, Flaherty A, Caplan D, Schmahmann JD. Cautionary notes on diagnosing functional neurologic disorder as a neurologist-in-training. Neurol Clin Pract. 2020;10(6):484–7.
79. Morgante F, Edwards MJ, Espay AJ, Fasano A, Mir P, Martino D. Diagnostic agreement in patients with psychogenic movement disorders. Mov Disord. 2012;27(4):548–52.
80. van der Salm SM, de Haan RJ, Cath DC, van Rootselaar AF, Tijssen MA. The eye of the beholder: inter-rater agreement among experts on psychogenic jerky movement disorders. J Neurol Neurosurg Psychiatry. 2013;84(7):742–7.

81. Shill H, Gerber P. Evaluation of clinical diagnostic criteria for psychogenic movement disorders. Mov Disord. 2006;21(8):1163–8.
82. Stone J, Smyth R, Carson A, Lewis S, Prescott R, Warlow C, et al. Systematic review of misdiagnosis of conversion symptoms and "hysteria". BMJ. 2005;331:989.
83. O'Neal MA, Baslet G. Treatment for patients with a functional neurological disorder (conversion disorder): an integrated approach. Am J Psychiatry. 2018;175(4):307–14.
84. Bass C, Wade DT. Malingering and factitious disorder. Pract Neurol. 2019;19(2):96–105.
85. Gould R, Miller BL, Goldberg MA, Benson DF. The validity of hysterical signs and symptoms. J Nerv Ment Dis. 1986;174:593–7.
86. Gelauff J, Stone J, Edwards M, Carson A. The prognosis of functional (psychogenic) motor symptoms: a systematic review. J Neurol Neurosurg Psychiatry. 2014;85(2):220–6.
87. van Rooijen DE, Geraedts EJ, Marinus J, Jankovic J, van Hilten JJ. Peripheral trauma and movement disorders: a systematic review of reported cases. J Neurol Neurosurg Psychiatry. 2011;82(8):892–8.
88. Bhatia KP, Bhatt MH, Marsden CD. The causalgia-dystonia syndrome. Brain. 1993;116(Pt 4):843–51.
89. Ganos C, Edwards MJ, Bhatia KP. Posttraumatic functional movement disorders. Handb Clin Neurol. 2016;139:499–507.
90. Mainka T, Erro R, Rothwell J, Kühn AA, Bhatia KP, Ganos C. Remission in dystonia – systematic review of the literature and meta-analysis. Parkinsonism Relat Disord. 2019;66:9–15.
91. Stamelou M, Cossu G, Edwards MJ, Murgia D, Pareés I, Melis M, et al. Familial psychogenic movement disorders. Mov Disord. 2013;28(9):1295–8.
92. Haq IU, Snively BM, Sweadner KJ, Suerken CK, Cook JF, Ozelius LJ, et al. Revising rapid-onset dystonia-parkinsonism: broadening indications for ATP1A3 testing. Mov Disord. 2019;34(10):1528–36.
93. Stone J, Carson A, Sharpe M. Functional symptoms and signs in neurology: assessment and diagnosis. J Neurol Neurosurg Psychiatry. 2005;76(Suppl 1):i2–12.
94. Bruce BB, Newman NJ. Functional visual loss. Neurol Clin. 2010;28(3):789–802.
95. Czarnecki K, Hallett M. Functional (psychogenic) movement disorders. Curr Opin Neurol. 2012;25(4):507–12.
96. Walzl D, Solomon AJ, Stone J. Functional neurological disorder and multiple sclerosis: a systematic review of misdiagnosis and clinical overlap. J Neurol. 2021; https://doi.org/10.1007/s00415-021-10436-6. Epub ahead of print. PMID: 33611631.
97. Tinazzi M, Geroin C, Erro R, Marcuzzo E, Cuoco S, Ceravolo R, et al. Functional motor disorders associated with other neurological diseases: beyond the boundaries of "organic" neurology. Eur J Neurol. 2020; https://doi.org/10.1111/ene.14674.
98. Robles L, Chiang S, Haneef Z. Review-of-systems questionnaire as a predictive tool for psychogenic nonepileptic seizures. Epilepsy Behav. 2015;45:151–4.
99. Carson AJ, Stone J, Hansen CH, Duncan R, Cavanagh J, Matthews K, et al. Somatic symptom count scores do not identify patients with symptoms unexplained by disease: a prospective cohort study of neurology outpatients. J Neurol Neurosurg Psychiatry. 2015;86(3):295–301.
100. Bhatia KP, Schneider SA. Psychogenic tremor and related disorders. J Neurol. 2007;254(5):569–74.
101. Deuschl G, Köster B, Lücking CH, Scheidt C. Diagnostic and pathophysiological aspects of psychogenic tremors. Mov Disord. 1998;13(2):294–302.
102. Kim YJ, Pakiam AS, Lang AE. Historical and clinical features of psychogenic tremor: a review of 70 cases. Can J Neurol Sci. 1999;26:190–5.
103. Piboolnurak P, Rothey N, Ahmed A, Ford B, Yu Q, Xu D, et al. Psychogenic tremor disorders identified using tree-based statistical algorithms and quantitative tremor analysis. Mov Disord. 2005;20:1543–9.
104. Kenney C, Diamond A, Mejia N, Davidson A, Hunter C, Jankovic J. Distinguishing psychogenic and essential tremor. J Neurol Sci. 2007;263:94–9.
105. Hallett M. Physiology of psychogenic movement disorders. J Clin Neurosci. 2010;17(8):959–65.

106. Ziegler JS, von Stauffenberg M, Vlaho S, Böhles H, Kieslich M. Dystonia with secondary contractures: a psychogenic movement disorder mimicking its neurological counterpart. J Child Neurol. 2008;23(11):1316–8.
107. Ibrahim NM, Martino D, van de Warrenburg BPC, Quinn NP, Bhatia KP, Brown RJ, et al. The prognosis of fixed dystonia: a follow-up study. Parkinsonism Relat Disord. 2009;15(8):592–7.
108. Ganos C, Edwards MJ, Bhatia K. The phenomenology of functional (psychogenic) dystonia. Mov Disord Clin Pract. 2014;1(1):36–44.
109. Lang AE. Psychogenic dystonia: a review of 18 cases. Can J Neurol Sci. 1995;22:136–43.
110. Munts AG. How psychogenic is dystonia? Views from past to present. Brain. 2010;133:1552–64.
111. Fasano A, Tinazzi M. Functional facial and tongue movement disorders. Handb Clin Neurol. 2016;139:353–65.
112. Tan EK, Jankovic J. Psychogenic hemifacial spasm. J Neuropsychiatry Clin Neurosci. 2001;13(3):380–4.
113. Stephen CD, Sharma N, Callahan J, Carson AJ, Perez DL. A case of functional dystonia with associated functional neurological symptoms: diagnostic and therapeutic challenges. Harv Rev Psychiatry. 2017;25(5):241–51.
114. Thomas M, Jankovic J. Psychogenic movement disorders: diagnosis and management. CNS Drugs. 2004;18(7):437–52.
115. Tolosa E, Compta Y. Dystonia in Parkinson's disease. J Neurol. 2006;253(Suppl 7):VII7–13.
116. Munhoz RP, Lang AE. Gestes antagonistes in psychogenic dystonia. Mov Disord. 2004;19(3):331–2.
117. Fahn S. Role of anesthesia in the diagnosis of treatment of psychogenic movement disorders. In: Hallett M, Fahn S, Jankovic J, Lang A, Cloninger CR, Yudofsky S, editors. Psychogenic movement disorders: neurology and neuropsychiatry. Philadelphia: Lippincott Williams & Wilkins; 2006. p. 256–61.
118. Bruno MK, Hallett M, Gwinn-Hardy K, Sorensen B, Considine E, Tucker S, et al. Clinical evaluation of idiopathic paroxysmal kinesigenic dyskinesia: new diagnostic criteria. Neurology. 2004;63(12):2280–7.
119. Bruno MK, Lee HY, Auburger GW, Friedman A, Nielsen JE, Lang AE, et al. Genotype-phenotype correlation of paroxysmal nonkinesigenic dyskinesia. Neurology. 2007;68(21):1782–9.
120. Verrotti A, D'Egidio C, Agostinelli S, Gobbi G. Glut1 deficiency: when to suspect and how to diagnose? Eur J Pediatr Neurol. 2012;16(1):3–9.
121. Thenganatt MA, Jankovic J. Psychogenic movement disorders. Neurol Clin. 2015;33(1):205–24.
122. Espay AJ, Morgante F, Purzner J, Gunraj CA, Lang AE, Chen R. Cortical and spinal abnormalities in psychogenic dystonia. Ann Neurol. 2006;59(5):825–34.
123. Quartarone A, Rizzo V, Terranova C, Morgante F, Schneider S, Ibrahim N, et al. Abnormal sensorimotor plasticity in organic but not in psychogenic dystonia. Brain. 2009;132:2871–7.
124. Kobayashi K, Lang AE, Hallett M, Lenz FA. Thalamic neuronal and EMG activity in psychogenic dystonia compared with organic dystonia. Mov Disord. 2011;26:1348–52.
125. Schwingenschuh P, Katschnig P, Edwards MJ, Teo JT, Korlipara LV, Rothwell JC, et al. The blink reflex recovery cycle differs between essential and presumed psychogenic blepharospasm. Neurology. 2011;76:610–4.
126. Nonnekes J, Růžička E, Serranová T, Reich SG, Bloem BR, Hallett M. Functional gait disorders: a sign-based approach. Neurology. 2020;94(24):1093–9.
127. Edwards M. Functional (psychogenic) gait disorder: diagnosis and management. Handb Clin Neurol. 2018;159:417–23. https://doi.org/10.1016/B978-0-444-63916-5.00027-6. PMID: 30482331.
128. Baizabal-Carvallo JF, Alonso-Juarez M, Jankovic J. Functional gait disorders, clinical phenomenology, and classification. Neurol Sci. 2020;41(4):911–5.
129. Lempert T, Brandt T, Dieterich M, Huppert D. How to identify psychogenic disorders of stance and gait: a video study in 37 patients. J Neurol. 1991;238:140–6.

130. Okun MS, Rodriguez RL, Foote KD, Fernandez HH. The "chair test" to aid in the diagnosis of psychogenic gait disorders. Neurologist. 2007;13(2):87–91.
131. Baik JS, Lang AE. Gait abnormalities in psychogenic movement disorders. Mov Disord. 2007;22(3):395–9.
132. Murphy J, Isaacs B. The post-fall syndrome: a study of 36 elderly patients. Gerontology. 1982;28:265–70.
133. Sudarsky L. Psychogenic gait disorders. Semin Neurol. 2006;26(3):351–6.
134. Schniepp R, Wuehr M, Huth S, Pradhan C, Schlick C, Brandt T, et al. The gait disorder in downbeat nystagmus syndrome. PLoS One. 2014;9(8):e105463.
135. Nonnekes J, Goselink RJM, Růžička E, Fasano A, Nutt JG, Bloem BR. Neurological disorders of gait, balance and posture: a sign-based approach. Nat Rev Neurol. 2018;14(3):183–9.
136. Dreissen YEM, Cath DC, Tijssen MAJ. Functional jerks, tics, and paroxysmal movement disorders. Handb Clin Neurol. 2016;139:247–58.
137. Yu XX, Stone J. Functional myoclonus: time to stop jerking around with negative diagnosis. Parkinsonism Relat Disord. 2018;51:1–2.
138. van der Salm SM, Erro R, Cordivari C, Edwards MJ, Koelman JH, van den Ende T, et al. Propriospinal myoclonus: clinical reappraisal and review of literature. Neurology. 2014;83(20):1862–70.
139. Erro R, Edwards MJ, Bhatia KP, Esposito M, Farmer SF, Cordivari C. Psychogenic axial myoclonus: clinical features and long-term outcome. Parkinsonism Relat Disord. 2014;20(6):596–9.
140. Chokroverty S, Walters A, Zimmerman T, Picone M. Propriospinal myoclonus: a neurophysiologic analysis. Neurology. 1992;42:1591–5.
141. Thenganatt MA, Jankovic J. Psychogenic (functional) parkinsonism. Handb Clin Neurol. 2016;139:259–62. https://doi.org/10.1016/B978-0-12-801772-2.00022-9. PMID: 27719845.
142. Frasca Polara G, Fleury V, Stone J, Barbey A, Burkhard PR, Vingerhoets F, et al. Prevalence of functional (psychogenic) parkinsonism in two Swiss movement disorders clinics and review of the literature. J Neurol Sci. 2018;387:37–45. https://doi.org/10.1016/j.jns.2018.01.022. Epub 2018 Feb 3. PMID: 29571869.
143. Benaderette S, Zanotti Fregonara P, Apartis E, Nguyen C, Trocello JM, Remy P, et al. Psychogenic parkinsonism: a combination of clinical, electrophysiological, and [(123)I]-FP-CIT SPECT scan explorations improves diagnostic accuracy. Mov Disord. 2006;21(3):310–7.
144. Kannoth S, Anandakkuttan A, Mathai A, Sasikumar AN, Nambiar V. Autoimmune atypical parkinsonism – a group of treatable parkinsonism. J Neurol Sci. 2016;362:40–6.
145. Baizabal-Carvallo JF, Jankovic J. Autoimmune and paraneoplastic movement disorders: An update. J Neurol Sci. 2018;385:175–84.
146. Jankovic J, Schwartz KS, Ondo W. Re-emergent tremor of Parkinson's disease. J Neurol Neurosurg Psychiatry. 1999;67(5):646–50.
147. Ambar Akkaoui M, Geoffroy PA, Roze E, Degos B, Garcin B. Functional motor symptoms in Parkinson's disease and functional parkinsonism: a systematic review. J Neuropsychiatry Clin Neurosci. 2020;32(1):4–13.
148. Mergl R, Mavrogiorgou P, Hegerl U, Juckel G. Kinematical analysis of emotionally induced facial expressions: a novel tool to investigate hypomimia in patients suffering from depression. J Neurol Neurosurg Psychiatry. 2005;76(1):138–40.
149. Pourfar MH, Tang CC, Mogilner AY, Dhawan V, Eidelberg D. Using imaging to identify psychogenic parkinsonism before deep brain stimulation surgery. Report of 2 cases. J Neurosurg. 2012;116(1):114–8.
150. Langevin JP, Skoch JM, Sherman SJ. Deep brain stimulation of a patient with psychogenic movement disorder. Surg Neurol Int. 2016;7(Suppl 35):S824–6.
151. Bonnet C, Mesrati F, Roze E, Hubsch C, Degos B. Motor and non-motor symptoms in functional parkinsonism responsive to transcranial magnetic stimulation: a case report. J Neurol. 2016;263(4):816–7.

152. Onofrj M, Thomas A, Tiraboschi P, Wenning G, Gambi F, Sepede G, et al. Updates on somatoform disorders (SFMD) in Parkinson's disease and dementia with Lewy bodies and discussion of phenomenology. J Neurol Sci. 2011;310(1–2):166–71.

153. Lang AE, Koller WC, Fahn S. Psychogenic parkinsonism. Arch Neurol. 1995;52:802–10.

154. Booij J, Speelman JD, Horstink MW, Wolters EC. The clinical benefit of imaging striatal dopamine transporters with [123I]FP-CIT SPET in differentiating patients with presynaptic parkinsonism from those with other forms of parkinsonism. Eur J Nucl Med. 2001;28:266–72.

155. Gaig C, Martí MJ, Tolosa E, Valldeoriola F, Paredes P, Lomeña FJ, et al. 123I-Ioflupane SPECT in the diagnosis of suspected psychogenic parkinsonism. Mov Disord. 2006;21:1994–8.

156. Felicio AC, Godeiro-Junior C, Moriyama TS, Shih MC, Hoexter MQ, Borges V, et al. Degenerative parkinsonism in patients with psychogenic parkinsonism: a dopamine transporter imaging study. Clin Neurol Neurosurg. 2010;112:282–5.

157. Morgan JC, Sethi KD. Psychogenic parkinsonism. In: Hallett M, Fahn S, Jankovic J, Lang A, Cloninger CR, Yudofsky S, editors. Psychogenic movement disorders: neurology and neuropsychiatry. Philadelphia: Lippincott Williams & Wilkins; 2006. p. 62–8.

158. Ganos C, Martino D, Espay AJ, Lang AE, Bhatia KP, Edwards MJ. Tics and functional tic-like movements: can we tell them apart? Neurology. 2019;93(17):750–8.

159. McGurrin P, Attaripour S, Vial F, Hallett M. Purposely induced tics: electrophysiology. Tremor Other Hyperkinet Mov (N Y). 2020;10. https://doi.org/10.7916/tohm.v0.744. PMID: 32195038; PMCID: PMC7070698.

160. Shimasaki C, Frye RE, Trifiletti R, Cooperstock M, Kaplan G, Melamed I, et al. Evaluation of the Cunningham Panel™ in pediatric autoimmune neuropsychiatric disorder associated with streptococcal infection (PANDAS) and pediatric acute-onset neuropsychiatric syndrome (PANS): changes in antineuronal antibody titers parallel changes in patient symptoms. J Neuroimmunol. 2020;339:577138.

161. Vale TC, Pedroso JL, Knobel M, Knobel E. Late-onset psychogenic chronic phonic-tics. Tremor Other Hyperkinet Mov (N Y). 2016;6:387. https://doi.org/10.7916/D88S4PWW. PMID: 27375961; PMCID: PMC4925920.

162. Chouksey A, Pandey S. Functional movement disorders in elderly. Tremor Other Hyperkinet Mov (N Y). 2019;9. https://doi.org/10.7916/tohm.v0.691. PMID: 31413900; PMCID: PMC6691911.

163. Chouinard S, Ford B. Adult onset tic disorders. J Neurol Neurosurg Psychiatry. 2000;68(6):738–43.

164. Baizabal-Carvallo JF, Jankovic J. The clinical features of psychogenic movement disorders resembling tics. J Neurol Neurosurg Psychiatry. 2014;85(5):573–5.

165. Demartini B, Ricciardi L, Parees I, Ganos C, Bhatia KP, Edwards MJ. A positive diagnosis of functional (psychogenic) tics. Eur J Neurol. 2015;22(3):527–e36.

166. Dooley JM, Stokes A, Gordon KE. Pseudo-tics in Tourette syndrome. J Child Neurol. 1994;9:50–1.

167. Stephen CD, Caplan LR. Transient focal neurological events. Chapter 76. In: Caplan LR, Biller J, Leary MC, Lo EH, Thomas AJ, Yenari M, Zhang JH, editors. Primer on cerebrovascular diseases. 2nd ed. San Diego: Academic Press; 2017. p. 365–71.

168. Stephen CD, Caplan LR. Stroke Mimics: transient focal neurological events. Chapter 5. In: Munshi SK, Harwood R, editors. Stroke in the older person. 1st ed. New York: Oxford University Press; 2019. p. 51–64.

169. Lioutas VA, Sonni S, Caplan LR. Diagnosis and misdiagnosis of cerebrovascular disease. Curr Treat Options Cardiovasc Med. 2013;15(3):276–87.

170. Vroomen PC, Buddingh MK, Luijckx GJ, De Keyser J. The incidence of stroke mimics among stroke department admissions in relation to age group. J Stroke Cerebrovasc Dis. 2008;17(6):418–22.

171. Stone J, Warlow C, Sharpe M. The symptom of functional weakness: a controlled study of 107 patients. Brain. 2010;133:1537–51.

172. Parry AM, Murray B, Hart Y, Bass C. Audit of resource use in patients with non-organic disorders admitted to a UK neurology unit. J Neurol Neurosurg Psychiatry. 2006;77:1200–1.

173. Hoeritzauer I, Pronin S, Carson A, Statham P, Demetriades AK, Stone J. The clinical features and outcome of scan-negative and scan-positive cases in suspected cauda equina syndrome: a retrospective study of 276 patients. J Neurol. 2018;265(12):2916–26.
174. Hoover CF. A new sign for the detection of malingering and functional paresis of the lower extremities. JAMA. 1908;LI:746–7.
175. Koehler PJ, Okun MS. Important observations prior to the description of the Hoover sign. Neurology. 2004;63:1693–7.
176. Sonoo M. Abductor sign: a reliable new sign to detect unilateral non-organic paresis of the lower limb. J Neurol Neurosurg Psychiatry. 2004;75:121–5.
177. Yugué I, Shiba K, Ueta T, Iwamoto Y. A new clinical evaluation for hysterical paralysis. Spine (Phila Pa 1976). 2004;29(17):1910–3; discussion 1913.
178. Ziv I, Djaldetti R, Zoldan Y, Avraham M, Melamed E. Diagnosis of "non-organic" limb paresis by a novel objective motor assessment: the quantitative Hoover's test. J Neurol. 1998;245:797–802.
179. Stone J. Functional neurological disorders: the neurological assessment as treatment. Pract Neurol. 2016;16(1):7–17.
180. Carson A, Lehn A, Ludwig L, Stone J. Explaining functional disorders in the neurology clinic: a photo story. Pract Neurol. 2016;16(1):56–61.
181. Stone J. The bare essentials: functional symptoms in neurology. Pract Neurol. 2009;9(3):179–89. https://doi.org/10.1136/jnnp.2009.177204. PMID: 19448064.
182. Gelauff J, Dreissen YEM, Tijssen MA, Stone J. Treatment of functional motor disorders. Curr Treat Options Neurol. 2014;16(4):286.
183. Adams C, Anderson J, Madva EN, LaFrance WC Jr, Perez DL. You've made the diagnosis of functional neurological disorder: now what? Pract Neurol. 2018;18(4):323–30. https://doi.org/10.1136/practneurol-2017-001835. Epub 2018 May 15. PMID: 29764988; PMCID: PMC6372294.
184. Nielsen G, Stone J, Matthews A, Brown M, Sparkes C, Farmer R, et al. Physiotherapy for functional motor disorders: a consensus recommendation. J Neurol Neurosurg Psychiatry. 2015;86(10):1113–9.
185. Jordbru AA, Smedstad LM, Klungsøyr O, Martinsen EW. Psychogenic gait disorder: a randomized controlled trial of physical rehabilitation with one-year follow-up. J Rehabil Med. 2014;46(2):181–7.
186. Nielsen G, Ricciardi L, Demartini B, Hunter R, Joyce E, Edwards MJ. Outcomes of a 5-day physiotherapy programme for functional (psychogenic) motor disorders. J Neurol. 2015;262(3):674–81.
187. Maggio JB, Ospina JP, Callahan J, Hunt AL, Stephen CD, Perez DL. Outpatient physical therapy for functional neurological disorder: a preliminary feasibility and naturalistic outcome study in a U.S. cohort. J Neuropsychiatry Clin Neurosci. 2020;32(1):85–9.
188. Nielsen G, Stone J, Buszewicz M, Carson A, Goldstein LH, Holt K, et al; Physio4FMD Collaborative Group. Physio4FMD: protocol for a multicentre randomised controlled trial of specialist physiotherapy for functional motor disorder. BMC Neurol. 2019;19(1):242.
189. Nicholson C, Edwards MJ, Carson AJ, Gardiner P, Golder D, Hayward K, et al. Occupational therapy consensus recommendations for functional neurological disorder. J Neurol Neurosurg Psychiatry. 2020;91(10):1037–45.
190. Barnett C, Armes J, Smith C. Speech, language and swallowing impairments in functional neurological disorder: a scoping review. Int J Lang Commun Disord. 2019;54(3):309–20.
191. Kaas BM, Humbyrd CJ, Pantelyat A. Functional movement disorders and placebo: a brief review of the placebo effect in movement disorders and ethical considerations for placebo therapy. Mov Disord Clin Pract. 2018;5(5):471–8. https://doi.org/10.1002/mdc3.12641. PMID: 30515436; PMCID: PMC6207108.
192. Harris S. Psychogenic movement disorders in children and adolescents: an update. Eur J Pediatr. 2019;178(4):581–5.
193. Khachane Y, Kozlowska K, Savage B, McClure G, Butler G, Gray N, et al. Twisted in pain: the multidisciplinary treatment approach to functional dystonia. Harv Rev Psychiatry. 2019;27(6):359–81.

194. Voon V, Lang AE. Antidepressant treatment outcomes of psychogenic movement disorders. J Clin Psychiatry. 2005;66:1529–34.
195. Gilmour GS, Nielsen G, Teodoro T, Yogarajah M, Coebergh JA, Dilley MD, et al. Management of functional neurological disorder. J Neurol. 2020;267(7):2164–72. https://doi.org/10.1007/s00415-020-09772-w. Epub 2020 Mar 19. PMID: 32193596; PMCID: PMC7320922.
196. Sharpe M, Walker J, Williams C, Stone J, Cavanagh J, Murray G, et al. Guided self-help for functional (psychogenic) symptoms: a randomized controlled efficacy trial. Neurology. 2011;77(6):564–72.
197. Richardson M, Kleinstäuber M, Wong D. Nocebo-Hypothesis Cognitive Behavioral Therapy (NH-CBT) for persons with functional neurological symptoms (motor type): design and implementation of a randomized active-controlled trial. Front Neurol. 2020;11:586359.
198. Fontana RS, Clark FA, Griffeth B. Functional neurological symptom disorder spontaneously remits after electroconvulsive therapy. J ECT. 2019;35(2):e10. https://doi.org/10.1097/YCT.0000000000000527. PMID: 30095557.
199. Chiu NM, Strain JJ. Successful electroconvulsive therapy and three-yearfollow-up in a bipolar I depressed patient with comorbid conversion disorder. Neuropsychiatry (London). 2017;7(3):212–6. https://doi.org/10.4172/Neuropsychiatry.1000200.
200. Leong K, Tham JC, Scamvougeras A, Vila-Rodriguez F. Electroconvulsive therapy treatment in patients with somatic symptom and related disorders. Neuropsychiatr Dis Treat. 2015;11:2565–72. https://doi.org/10.2147/NDT.S90969. PMID: 26504388; PMCID: PMC4605246.
201. Aybek S, Lidstone SC, Nielsen G, MacGllivray L, Bassetti CL, Lang AE, et al. What is the role of a specialist assessment clinic for FND? lessons from three national referral centers. J Neuropsychiatry Clin Neurosci. 2020;32(1):79–84.
202. Williams DT, Lafaver K, Carson A, Fahn S. Inpatient treatment for functional neurologic disorders. Handb Clin Neurol. 2016;139:631–41. https://doi.org/10.1016/B978-0-12-801772-2.00051-5. PMID: 27719878.

Tardive and Neuroleptic-Induced Emergencies

22

Patrick S. Drummond and Steven J. Frucht

Patient Vignettes

Patient 1

A 26-year-old man with severe juvenile parkinsonism was maintained on a regimen of levodopa and pergolide. He was admitted to the hospital in order to adjust his Parkinson's disease medications, and pergolide was tapered off. The neurologist was called to the bedside when he subsequently experienced an acute episode of painful turning of his neck to the right, elevation of the right arm, and dystonic posturing of the left leg. His eyes remained deviated up and to the right, although he could bring them into primary gaze with difficulty. A diagnosis of oculogyric crisis secondary to pergolide withdrawal was made, and treatment with intravenous diphenhydramine terminated the crisis.

Patient 2

A 92-year-old woman presented to a movement disorder clinic in the company of her daughter. For the last 3 years, her daughter had meticulously documented episodes, occurring every 3 days and lasting for hours, during which she would obsess

Supplementary Information The online version of this chapter (https://doi.org/10.1007/978-3-030-75898-1_22) contains supplementary material, which is available to authorized users.

P. S. Drummond (✉) · S. J. Frucht
Department of Neurology, NYU Langone Health, New York, NY, USA
e-mail: patrick.drummond@nyulangone.org

© Springer Nature Switzerland AG 2022
S. J. Frucht (ed.), *Movement Disorder Emergencies*, Current Clinical Neurology,
https://doi.org/10.1007/978-3-030-75898-1_22

about a thought or object, and subsequently experience rapid irregular breathing, posturing, and jerking of her limbs. Examination in the office revealed Hoehn and Yahr stage IV parkinsonism, with a magnetic resonance imaging consistent with vascular parkinsonism. She had been taking carbidopa/levodopa 25/100 three times daily. She was admitted to the hospital in order to observe and film an episode. During the event, she was awake, followed commands intermittently, and demonstrated respiratory dysrhythmias, myoclonic jerks, and a fixed forward gaze. A diagnosis of oculogyric crisis was made, and elimination of levodopa and introduction of 0.5 mg of benztropine mesylate three times per day terminated the events. She died 2 years later, and autopsy confirmed the diagnosis of vascular parkinsonism.

Introduction

The first antipsychotic medication chlorpromazine was discovered in 1949 during French surgeon Henri-Marie Laborit's search for a "lytic cocktail" intended to dampen autonomic activity and prevent surgical shock [1]. Laborit astutely observed the secondary affective and behavioral impact of chlorpromazine and went on to recommend its use to his psychiatry colleagues at Sainte-Anne's hospital in Paris. In 1952, Pierre Deniker and Jean Delay published the first case series describing its ameliorative effects on 38 patients with chronic psychosis [2]. The term neuroleptic, meaning "that which seizes the nerve," was coined by Delay in 1955 to describe in part the parkinsonian akinesia that accompanied rapid improvement in psychosis [3].

With more widespread use of phenothiazine-derived medications and the eventual introduction of haloperidol and other first-generation antipsychotics, neurologists went on to describe a varied array of hyperkinetic movement disorders caused by exposure to centrally acting dopamine receptor-blocking agents (DRBAs). The majority were noted to be short-lived and self-limited, occurring within days or weeks of exposure and resolving with discontinuation of the DRBA. These included acute dystonic reactions [4], acute akathisia [5], and acute orobuccolingual (OBL) dyskinesias [6]. However, nearly 10 years passed before the larger spectrum of late or delayed movement disorders were more broadly recognized, termed tardive dyskinesia by Arild Faurbye in 1964 [7]. These long-duration movement disorders were seen after chronic exposure to DRBAs and frequently exacerbated by withdrawal or discontinuation of the offending agent. These included tardive dyskinesia, tardive dystonia, and tardive akathisia, now jointly referred to under the umbrella term tardive syndromes.

With the advent of second-generation antipsychotics, there was an expectation that the prevalence of tardive syndromes would fall due to their preferential serotonin receptor activity and lower affinity for dopamine D2 receptors. While they have been shown to carry a lower annual incidence rate of tardive dyskinesia [8], they have failed to produce the dramatic reduction that was initially predicted [9]. This is hypothesized to stem from increasing off-label use of antipsychotics in common conditions like treatment-resistant depression coupled with the continued use of other DRBAs such as antinausea agents metoclopramide and prochlorperazine, and calcium channel blockers flunarizine and cinnarizine.

While most neuroleptic-induced movement disorders produce mild and some-times barely noticeable symptoms, as is the case with OBL dyskinesias, more severe and bothersome movements like dystonia and akathisia can result. Rarely, emergent and potentially life-threatening syndromes can be caused by DRBAs: neuroleptic-induced respiratory and gastrointestinal phenomena, and oculogyric crisis.

Neuroleptic-Induced Respiratory Phenomena

Acute laryngeal dystonia was quickly recognized as a potential fatal respiratory side effect of neuroleptic treatment. It was first described in a patient who developed an acute dystonic reaction with laryngospasm following treatment with intravenous prochlorperazine [10]. Although rare, it has since been reported after exposure to a number of DRBAs, occurring primarily in young men, and in rare instances leading to death [11]. Patients typically present with acute stridor without an obvious pre-cipitating infectious illness or aspiration event. Examination will often provide clues to etiology if there are other segmental manifestations of dystonia such as blepharospasm, torticollis, or opisthotonos. A history of DRBA exposure should prompt high suspicion and immediate empiric treatment, but all patients should still undergo emergent endoscopy to rule out other causes of airway obstruction. Tardive forms of laryngeal dystonia have also been described in patients undergoing chronic treatment with antipsychotics [12–15]. These can present in both an acute and sub-acute fashion, more often again in younger individuals following a recent increase in dosage or change in neuroleptic.

Other less familiar tardive respiratory phenomena have also been seen in patients on long-term neuroleptic therapy. Hunter et al. were the first to report the presence of respiratory dyskinesias in 1964 in two patients weaned off phenothiazine-derived antipsychotics after several years of treatment [16]. They described unusual distur-bances of respiratory rate, rhythm, and amplitude with episodes of acute respiratory distress in which they appeared to inspire against a closed glottis resulting in apnea and cyanosis. Respiratory dyskinesias were formally classified as an extrapyramidal side effect in 1978 following a published case series better detailing their clinical presentation and successful treatment through dopamine depletion with reserpine [17]. The same year, the first emergent case of tardive respiratory dyskinesia was reported following discontinuation of chlorpromazine, culminating in a hospitaliza-tion for acute hypoxic respiratory failure due to aspiration pneumonia, and resolv-ing only after treatment with high doses of haloperidol [18].

More widespread studies have since looked at the prevalence of respiratory symptoms in patients with tardive OBL dyskinesia, estimated to occur in 2.3% of chronic institutionalized patients [19]. Clinical descriptions include tachypnea, abdominal breathing, and audible gasping, grunting, sighing, and moaning. There has been concern that respiratory dyskinesias are an underreported phenomenon, poorly recognized by psychiatrists and sometimes dismissed as a manifestation of a patient's underlying mental illness. Breathing irregularities appear to be present even in patients with tardive dyskinesia who are asymptomatic from a pulmonary standpoint, manifesting as erratic respiratory patterns with variable rate and tidal volume analogous to movements in other areas of the body [20].

Tardive respiratory dyskinesia tends to preferentially manifest in older women with a longer duration of neuroleptic treatment, often after dose reduction or discontinuation of a DRBA [21, 22]. Patients typically present with subacute onset of dyspnea, dysphagia, and aerophagia without signs of overt hypoxemia. Like tardive dyskinesia, symptoms improve at rest, worsen with stress, anxiety, and pain, and disappear with sleep. Patients with suspected respiratory dyskinesia should be examined at rest with bare chest exposed in order to observe for irregularities in speed, rhythm, and depth of breathing. Some patients may display inappropriate use of accessory inspiratory and expiratory musculature as well. Workup should include an arterial blood gas that may reveal evidence of respiratory alkalosis and a chest x-ray to rule out subclinical aspiration. Formal pulmonary function testing is often difficult to obtain due to irregular breathing patterns and co-occurrence of OBL dyskinesias. Complications include aerophagia, aspiration pneumonia, and respiratory arrest.

Neuroleptic-Induced Gastrointestinal Phenomena

Hyperkinetic movement disorders of the gastrointestinal system have been well described in patients following neuroleptic exposure, preferentially involving the striated muscles of the oral cavity, pharynx, and upper esophagus. Initial reports of dysphagia in patients with tardive dyskinesia hypothesized that involuntary tongue protrusion from OBL dyskinesias led to impaired deglutition [23]. However, several cases of isolated dysphagia have since been reported in the absence of OBL dyskinesias, supporting a diagnosis of lingual or pharyngeal dystonia in most [24–29]. During normal swallowing, the tongue pushes the food bolus through the relaxed oropharynx down into the esophagus. Patients with lingual dystonia will have difficulty retaining and manipulating food in the oral cavity with the tongue. Upon attempting to swallow, they may be unable to pass a bolus posteriorly to the oropharynx. In severe cases of lingual dystonia, patients may even force food particles forward and out of the mouth akin to eating dystonia seen in neuroacanthocytosis [30]. Patients with pharyngeal dystonia on the other hand will masticate and manipulate food normally with the tongue but be unable to move it past the overactive muscles of the posterior pharynx, trapping the bolus in the oral cavity.

When vomiting or food regurgitation is present, it is important to consider involvement of the more distal gastrointestinal tract. Esophageal dyskinesias have been documented by Horiguchi et al. in two patients with OBL dyskinesias who developed dysphagia and food regurgitation following withdrawal of chronic haloperidol therapy [31]. Uncoordinated, dyskinetic movements of the upper esophagus were observed through contrast radiography and esophageal manometry. Neuroleptic suppression resolved symptoms in one patient whereas asphyxiation of food led to death in the other.

Forms of tardive oromandibular dystonia may indirectly impact swallowing leading to weight loss and nutritional deficiency [32]. In severe jaw-closing dystonia, patients may be unable to introduce solids into the oral cavity, whereas in severe jaw-opening dystonia, mastication may be impossible leaving only liquid nutrition as an option.

Workup in all patients with suspected neuroleptic-induced gastrointestinal phenomena should include fiberoptic endoscopic evaluation of swallowing and videofluoroscopy with modified barium swallow and manometry if no etiology is found. Occasionally, both respiratory and gastrointestinal tardive phenomena may coexist, further complicating diagnosis, and sometimes requiring placement of a gastrostomy tube to maintain nutritional support until directed treatment is effective [33].

Oculogyric Crisis

Oculogyric crisis is a rare form of acute dystonia in which the eyes are conjugately deviated in a sustained, tonic posture of upward and/or lateral gaze. It occurs in paroxysms typically lasting seconds to minutes, though may rarely extend for hours at a time [34]. Clinical severity can vary from brief, subtle deviations of the eyes as an isolated symptom to more severe, painful presentations with associated dystonic posturing of the face, jaw, neck, trunk, and limbs [35]. In the more extreme manifestation, involuntary movements are often accompanied by symptoms of autonomic dysfunction such as hypertension, tachycardia, mydriasis, and diaphoresis, as well as psychiatric symptoms of anxiety, agitation, and psychosis. Although not life-threatening, patients are conscious and aware of their symptoms, often leading to panic and marked discomfort.

Oculogyric crisis was first reported in patients with encephalitis lethargica in the 1910–1930s [36] but has since been described as a result of focal brain lesions and as a manifestation of some rare metabolic and neurodegenerative disorders [37]. Although a wide array of drugs has been reported to trigger oculogyric crisis, it is most seen in conjunction with acute dystonic reactions, occurring immediately or shortly after exposure to a DRBA. There are rare reports of tardive oculogyric crises recurring chronically, in one patient up to several months after cessation of the offending neuroleptic agent [38]. Oculogyric crisis remains a clinical diagnosis and patients presenting with eye deviation and altered awareness should be appropriately worked up and treated for the possibility of focal seizures.

Treatment

Clinical history is critical in initially raising the possibility of a neuroleptic-induced movement disorder and whenever possible it is helpful to differentiate between acute versus tardive phenomena. However, several movement disorders can often coexist in one individual and their chronicity may be difficult to parse out. It is always important to ask about duration of neuroleptic treatment, last known exposure, and any recent dose adjustments or changes in therapy. When the patient is unable to provide history and no collateral information is available, the presence of psychiatric symptoms or characteristic tardive phenomena like OBL dyskinesias should prompt high suspicion of a neuroleptic-induced movement disorder.

In the emergency setting, initial management should focus on airway, breathing, and circulation. Acute laryngeal dystonia is the most life-threatening of neuroleptic-induced movement disorders and immediate treatment with intravenous antihistamines or anticholinergics will usually abort dystonia within minutes. Diphenhydramine is the most widely available treatment in most clinical settings and 25 or 50 mg delivered intravenously is often sufficient. Benztropine is equally effective and can be given intravenously or intramuscularly at a dose of 1 or 2 mg. Acute dystonic reactions including oculogyric crisis should be managed similarly, and benzodiazepines including diazepam and clonazepam may be of additional benefit in the latter [39]. Patients should continue oral anticholinergics for at least 1 week after the acute event to avoid recurrence, and the offending agent should be discontinued [40].

Treatment of acute laryngeal dystonia required intravenous administration of diphenhydramine (available in crash carts), that can be life-saving.

Management of tardive respiratory and gastrointestinal phenomena is more nuanced and there is little guidance in the literature beyond case reports. Discontinuation of the DRBA is not always beneficial and can sometimes lead to further worsening of symptoms. Anticholinergics can exacerbate tardive dyskinesia, and benzodiazepines generally provide only symptomatic relief. While neuroleptic suppression with high potency antipsychotics like haloperidol may provide short-term benefits, symptoms may ultimately reemerge and patients are at greater risk of long-term side effects from higher doses.

Evidence and clinical experience support the strategy of dopamine depletion via use of vesicular monoamine transporter 2 (VMAT2) inhibitors like tetrabenazine [41]. Although there are no published reports of their efficacy in neuroleptic-induced respiratory and gastrointestinal phenomena, it is presumed that the newer VMAT2 inhibitors deutetrabenazine and valbenazine would provide similar benefits given their proven success in treating tardive dyskinesia [42, 43]. The risk of drug-induced parkinsonism, depression and hypotension may limit the use of VMAT2 inhibitors in some patients, though they are generally well tolerated even in older individuals. For patients who are judged to require long-term neuroleptic therapy, cross titration to the atypical antipsychotic clozapine is often the ideal alternative, particularly in refractory forms of tardive dystonia. This of course carries with it several potential side effects, most notably drug-induced agranulocytosis that requires close monitoring and frequent blood draws.

Conclusion

Tardive or neuroleptic-induced emergencies, while rare, can be life-threatening. Prompt recognition and termination by intravenous anticholinergic infusion are an emergency that all neurologists should learn to recognize.

References

1. Laborit H, Huguenard P, Alluaume R. A new vegetative stabilizer; 4560 R.P. Presse Med. 1952;60(10):206–8.
2. Delay J, Deniker P, Harl JM. Therapeutic use in psychiatry of phenothiazine of central elective action (4560 RP). Ann Med Psychol (Paris). 1952;110(2 1)·112–7.
3. Delay J, Deniker P. Neuroleptic effects of chlorpromazine in therapeutics of neuropsychiatry. J Clin Exp Psychopathol. 1955;16(2):104–12.
4. Ayd FJ. A survey of drug-induced extrapyramidal reactions. JAMA. 1961;175:1054–60.
5. Steck H. Extrapyramidal and diencephalic syndrome in the course of largactil and serpasil treatments. Ann Med Psychol (Paris). 1954;112(2 5):737–44.
6. Sigwald J, Bouttier D, Raymondeaud C, Piot C. 4 Cases of facio-bucco-linguo-masticatory dyskinesis of prolonged development following treatment with neuroleptics. Rev Neurol (Paris). 1959;100:751–5.
7. Faurbye A, Rasch PJ, Petersen PB, Brandborg G, Pakkenberg H. Neurological symptoms in pharmacotherapy of psychoses. Acta Psychiatr Scand. 1964;40(1):10–27.
8. Correll CU, Schenk EM. Tardive dyskinesia and new antipsychotics. Curr Opin Psychiatry. 2008;21(2):151.
9. Carbon M, Hsieh CH, Kane JM, Correll CU. Tardive dyskinesia prevalence in the period of second-generation antipsychotic use: a meta-analysis. J Clin Psychiatry. 2017;78(3):e264.
10. Christian CD, Paulson G. Severe motility disturbance after small doses of prochlorperazine. N Engl J Med. 1958;259(17):828–30.
11. Koek RJ, Pi EH. Acute laryngeal dystonic reactions to neuroleptics. Psychosomatics. 1989;30(4):359–64.
12. Rowley H, Lynch T, Keogh I, Russell J. Tardive dystonia of the larynx in a quadriplegic patient: an unusual cause of stridor. J Laryngol Otol. 2001;115:918–9.
13. Havaki-Kontaxaki BJ, Kontaxakis VP, Christodoulou GN. Treatment of tardive pharyngo-laryngeal dystonia with olanzapine. Schizophr Res. 2004;66(2–3):199–200.
14. Tsai CS, Lee Y, Chang YY, Lin PY. Ziprasidone-induced tardive laryngeal dystonia: a case report. Gen Hosp Psychiatry. 2008;30(3):277–9.
15. Matsuda N, Hashimoto N, Kusumi I, Ito K, Koyama T. Tardive laryngeal dystonia associated with aripiprazole monotherapy. J Clin Psychopharmacol. 2012;32(2):297–8.
16. Hunter R, Earl CJ, Thronicroft S. An apparently irreversible syndrome of abnormal movements following phenothiazine medication. Proc R Soc Med. 1964;57(8):758–62.
17. Weiner WJ, Goetz CG, Nausieda PA, Klawans HL. Respiratory dyskinesias: extrapyramidal dysfunction and dyspnea. Ann Intern Med. 1978;88(3):327–31.
18. Casey DE, Rabins P. Tardive dyskinesia as a life-threatening illness. Am J Psychiatry. 1978;135(4):486–8.
19. Yassa R, Lal S. Respiratory irregularity and tardive dyskinesia. A prevalence study. Acta Psychiatr Scand. 1986;73(5):506–10.
20. Wilcox PG, Bassett A, Jones B, Fleetham JA. Respiratory dysrhythmias in patients with tardive dyskinesia. Chest. 1994;105(1):203–7.

21. Hayashi T, Nishikawa T, Koga I, Uchida Y, Yamawaki S. Prevalence of and risk factors for respiratory dyskinesia. Clin Neuropharmacol. 1996;19(5):390–8.
22. Chiu HF, Lam LC, Chan CH, Ho CK, Shum PP. Clinical and polygraphic characteristics of patients with respiratory dyskinesia. Br J Psychiatry. 1993;162:828–30.
23. Massengill R Jr, Nashold B. A swallowing disorder denoted in tardive dyskinesia patients. Acta Otolaryngol. 1969;68(5):457–8.
24. Stones M, Kennie DC, Fulton JD. Dystonic dysphagia associated with fluspirilene. BMJ. 1990;301(6753):668–9.
25. Gregory RP, Smith PT, Rudge P. Tardive dyskinesia presenting as severe dysphagia. J Neurol Neurosurg Psychiatry. 1992;55(12):1203–4.
26. Hayashi T, Nishikawa T, Koga I, Uchida Y, Yamawaki S. Life-threatening dysphagia following prolonged neuroleptic therapy. Clin Neuropharmacol. 1997;20(1):77–81.
27. Aino I, Saigusa H, Nakamura T, Matsuoka C, Komachi T, Kokawa T. Progressive dysphagia with peculiar laryngeal movement induced by tardive dystonia. Nihon Jibiinkoka Gakkai Kaiho. 2006;109(11):785–8.
28. Duggal HS, Mendhekar DN. Risperidone-induced tardive pharyngeal dystonia presenting with persistent dysphagia: a case report. Prim Care Companion J Clin Psychiatry. 2008;10(2):161–2.
29. Agarwal PA, Ichaporia NR. Flupenthixol-induced tardive dystonia presenting as severe dysphagia. Neurol India. 2010;58(5):784–5.
30. Achiron A, Melamed E. Tardive eating dystonia. Mov Disord. 1990;5(4):331–3.
31. Horiguchi J, Shingu T, Hayashi T, Kagaya A, Yamawaki S, Horikawa Y, Kitadai Y, Inoue M, Nishikawa T. Antipsychotic-induced life-threatening 'esophageal dyskinesia'. Int Clin Psychopharmacol. 1999;14(2):123–7.
32. Gonzalez-Alegre P, Schneider RL, Hoffman H. Clinical, etiological, and therapeutic features of jaw-opening and jaw-closing oromandibular dystonias: a decade of experience at a single treatment center. Tremor Other Hyperkinet Mov (N Y). 2014;4:231.
33. Samie MR, Dannenhoffer MA, Rozek S. Life-threatening tardive dyskinesia caused by metoclopramide. Mov Disord. 1987;2(2):125–9.
34. FitzGerald PM, Jankovic J. Tardive oculogyric crises. Neurology. 1989;39(11):1434–7.
35. Slow EJ, Lang AE. Oculogyric crises: a review of phenomenology, etiology, pathogenesis, and treatment. Mov Disord. 2017;32(2):193–202.
36. Berger JR, Vilensky JA. Encephalitis lethargica (von Economo's encephalitis). Handb Clin Neurol. 2014;123:745–61.
37. Barow E, Schneider SA, Bhatia KP, Ganos C. Oculogyric crises: etiology, pathophysiology and therapeutic approaches. Parkinsonism Relat Disord. 2017;36:3–9.
38. Sachdev P. Tardive and chronically recurrent oculogyric crises. Mov Disord. 1993;8(1):93–7. https://doi.org/10.1002/mds.870080117.
39. Horiguchi J, Inami Y. Effect of clonazepam on neuroleptic-induced oculogyric crisis. Acta Psychiatr Scand. 1989;80(5):521–3.
40. Pierre JM. Extrapyramidal symptoms with atypical antipsychotics: incidence, prevention and management. Drug Saf. 2005;28(3):191–208.
41. Kruk J, Sachdev P, Singh S. Neuroleptic-induced respiratory dyskinesia. J Neuropsychiatry Clin Neurosci. 1995;7(2):223–9.
42. Anderson KE, Stamler D, Davis MD, Factor SA, Hauser RA, Isojärvi J, et al. Deutetrabenazine for treatment of involuntary movements in patients with tardive dyskinesia (AIM-TD): a double-blind, randomized, placebo-controlled, phase 3 trial. Lancet Psychiatry. 2017;4(8):595–604.
43. Hauser RA, Factor SA, Marder SR, Knesevich MA, Ramirez PM, Jimenez R, et al. KINECT 3: a phase 3 randomized, double-blind, placebo-controlled trial of valbenazine for tardive dyskinesia. Am J Psychiatry. 2017;174(5):476–84.

Abductor Paresis in Shy-Drager Disease

23

Eiji Isozaki

Abbreviations

ASV	Adaptive servo-ventilation
BIS	Bispectral index
BPAP	Bilevel positive airway pressure
CPAP	Continuous positive airway pressure
CRD	Central respiratory disturbance
CSAS	Central sleep apnea syndrome
CT	Cricothyroid muscle
DISE	Drug-induced sleep endoscopy
EPAP	Expiratory positive airway pressure
FA	Floppy arytenoid
FE	Floppy epiglottis
IPAP	Inspiratory positive airway pressure
LM	Laryngomalacia
MSA	Multiple system atrophy
NPPV	Noninvasive positive pressure ventilation
OSAS	Obstructive sleep apnea syndrome
PCA	Posterior cricoarytenoid muscle
SAS	Sleep apnea syndrome
T90	Percentage of sleep time in less than 90% oxygen saturation
TA	Thyroarytenoid muscle
UAO	Upper airway obstruction
VCAI	Vocal cord abductor impairment

Supplementary Information The online version of this chapter (https://doi.org/10.1007/978-3-030-75898-1_23) contains supplementary material, which is available to authorized users.

E. Isozaki (✉)
Department of Neurology, Tokyo Metropolitan Neurological Hospital, Fuchu, Tokyo, Japan

Patient Vignette

A 74-year-old man diagnosed with multiple system atrophy (MSA) 9 years prior
was readmitted to our hospital because of pneumonia. A fiberoptic laryngoscopy
showed no laryngeal abnormalities during both wakefulness and diazepam-induced
sleep. Aspiration was subtle. Next year, he developed nocturnal stridor. On second
fiberoptic laryngoscopy, moderately severe vocal cord abductor impairment with
abduction restriction during wakefulness and paradoxical movement during sleep
was found. On an overnight recording of percutaneous arterial blood oxygen saturation (SpO$_2$), no desaturation less than 90% was demonstrated. Arterial blood gas
analysis on room air was normal. Only 1 week after discharge, he was readmitted to
our hospital because of increasing snoring. Arterial blood gas analysis on oxygen
inhalation with 2 l/m when awake showed pH = 7.39, pCO$_2$ = 51 Torr, and
pO$_2$ = 88 Torr. On physical findings, his suprasternal notch became hollow during
every inspiration. A third fiberoptic laryngoscopy during wakefulness demonstrated
severe vocal cord abductor impairment with slit-like aperture of the glottis, requiring emergency intratracheal intubation. After tracheostomy was performed, he
could speak with a speech valve. Arterial blood gas analysis on room air became
almost normal: pH = 7.46, pCO$_2$ = 45 Torr, pO$_2$ = 82 Torr. No oxygen desaturation
less than 90% of SpO$_2$ was demonstrated on an overnight recording.

Introduction

Descriptions of vocal cord dysfunction in MSA date back to the late 1960s [1, 2]. In
1979, Williams et al. [3] compiled clinical data on vocal cord paralysis from 12
patients with Shy-Drager syndrome. Pathological studies on the laryngeal muscles
showed neurogenic atrophy of the sole vocal cord abductor, the posterior cricoarytenoid muscle (PCA) [4, 5]. However, presence [4, 6, 7] or absence [5, 8] of involvement of the nucleus ambiguus remains controversial. Vocal cord abductor impairment
(VCAI) developing inspiratory stridor has drawn a lot of attention because of its
close relationship with nocturnal sudden death [9–11]. Stridor was credited as one
of the "additional features of possible MSA" in the "Second consensus statement on
the diagnosis of multiple system atrophy" from 2008 [12]. In 2019, the international
consensus statement, "stridor in multiple system atrophy" was raised [13]. In this
statement, 34 studies with evidence levels of class II to class IV from 1979 to 2016
were summarized, together with the experts' opinions.

Though VCAI develops frequently in MSA, its pathogenesis and prognosis still
remain unclear, and treatment plans do not always reach consensus. This chapter
describes an overview according to the following five subheadings: (1) clinical
aspects of VCAI, (2) pathogenesis of VCAI, (3) laryngeal abnormalities other than
VCAI, (4) treatments, (5) combination with upper airway obstruction (UAO) and
central respiratory disturbance (CRD). We use the term "VCAI" instead of "vocal
cord abductor paralysis" because vocal cord dysfunction is caused by both abductor
paralysis and adductors hyperactivity. The term "noninvasive positive pressure

ventilation" (NPPV) refers to both continuous positive airway pressure (CPAP) and bilevel positive airway pressure (BPAP), forming a counterpart with TPPV (tracheostomized positive pressure ventilation). The term "supraglottic collapse" is used as a concept including both floppy epiglottis (FE) and floppy arytenoid (FA).

Clinical Aspects of VCAI

Symptoms and Diagnosis of VCAI

The core symptom of VCAI is nocturnal stridor, often perceived by the patient's bedpartner or caregivers because of its peculiar breathing sound. While snoring observed in obstructive sleep apnea syndrome (OSAS) is equally loud as inspiratory stridor in MSA, there are fundamental differences as stridor derives from the larynx and snoring mainly from the pharynx. These differences should be distinguished in several ways (Table 23.1). Kavey et al. [14] sounded an alarm that stridor could be mistaken for snoring, and serious laryngeal dysfunction could be overlooked. Inspiratory stridor in MSA is characterized by a loud, high-pitched, harsh sound [13]. At first, stridor develops only during sleep, and later occurs during wakefulness, particularly as the patient takes a breath in conversation. Diurnal stridor may be mistaken for steroid-unresponsive asthma attacks when a clinical history of nocturnal stridor is missing. VCAI can appear at any time in the course of MSA, even as an initial [15] or an isolated [16] symptom. One of the objective findings on inspection is a retractive breathing showing inspiratory hollowing of the suprasternal notch or supraclavicular fossa (Fig. 23.1). This finding indicates the presence of severe stenosis of upper or lower respiratory tract, not specific to VCAI. On auscultation, inspiratory stridor is louder in the neck than on the chest, unlike asthma. Nocturnal stridor has been called "metallic," "croup-like [14]," "donkey-braying [5]," "dog howling," or "fur seal roaring" in quality, reflecting its high-pitched tone.

A definite diagnosis of VCAI is made by drug-induced sleep endoscopy (DISE). Using this method, we classified the severity of VCAI into four stages from stage 0 (normal) to stage 3 (severe VCAI), according to the position of the vocal cords on inspiration (Table 23.2). VCAI is characterized by abduction restriction with paradoxical movement of vocal cords showing inspiratory adduction and expiratory abduction,

Table 23.1 Difference between vocal cord abductor impairment and obstructive sleep apnea

Vocal cord abductor impairment		Obstructive sleep apnea
1. Stridor or snoring		
Sound source	Larynx (vocal cord)	Pharynx (soft palate, etc.)
Fundamental frequency	Higher (200–500 Hz)	Lower (100–300 Hz)
Body position change	Almost noneffective	Usually effective
Nasal airway tube	Noneffective	Usually effective
Daytime inspiratory stridor	Existent	Nonexistent
2. Sleep apnea	Existent, but often tachypneic	Always present
3. Relationship with REM sleep	Poorer	Closer

REM rapid eye movement

During expiration   During inspiration

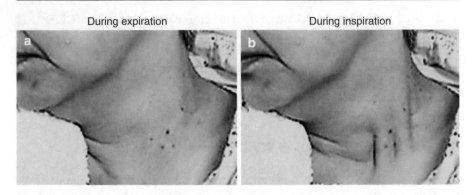

Fig. 23.1 Retractive breathing in MSA patient with vocal cord abductor impairment. Suprasternal notch and supraclavicular fossa become hollow associated with stridor during inspiration (**b**) compared to expiration (**a**) as shown in the text

Table 23.2 Stage classification of vocal cord abductor impairment on a fiberoptic laryngoscopy

Stage	Awake	Asleep	Posterior glottis findings during sleep
0 (normal)	Normal	Unchanged	
1 (mild)	Normal	Paradoxical	1a: triangular without stridor 1b: narrower with stridor
2 (moderately)	Abduction restriction	Paradoxical	2a: triangular without stridor 2b: narrower with stridor
3 (severe)	Midline fixation	Midline fixation	

and is often induced or exacerbated by sleep. The vocal glottis consists of two parts: the anterior glottis mainly involving voicing and the posterior glottis in breathing. Since patency of the posterior glottis mainly determines the severity of VCAI, we further divided stages 1 and 2 into two types according to the shape and the presence or absence of stridor: type a for triangular shape with some airway space, and type b for a slit-like shape with inspiratory stridor (Fig. 23.2) [17]. Thereby, type b (stages 1b and 2b) is more serious than type a (stages 1a and 2a). In some cases, stage 1b is more serious than stage 2a. Looking back on our patient in the clinical vignette, first fiberoptic laryngoscopy showed moderately severe VCAI (stage 2) and an overnight recording of SpO_2 was normal. Unfortunately, posterior glottis at first examination could not be observed fully, resulting in an unknown stage (2a or 2b). In retrospect, a repeat DISE and overnight recording of SpO_2 would have been useful. Another noteworthy point is the influence of sleep depth on both SpO_2 and laryngoscopic findings. If sleep depth under DISE is insufficient (shallow sleep), VCAI can be "masked." This is true in analyzing an overnight recording of SpO_2. Eastwood et al. [18] reported that increasing sleep depth by propofol anesthesia was associated with increased collapsibility of the upper airway. Sigl and Chamoun [19] introduced bispectral index (BIS), which translated a patient's electroencephalogram (EEG) signals into scaled numbers from 0 (EEG silent) to 100 (fully awake) to reflect consciousness levels and sedation depth. On the basis of these backgrounds, Lo et al. [20] proposed an objective and reproducible sedation method for DISE using propofol pump infusion to maintain optimal BIS level between 65 and 75. This method seems to be useful in evaluating the severity of UAO more objectively and semiquantitatively.

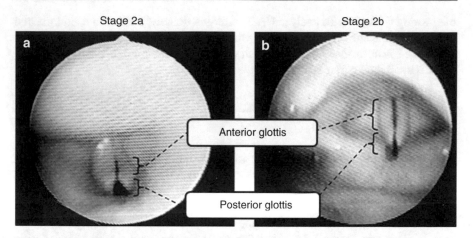

Fig. 23.2 Laryngoscopic photographs of vocal cord abductor impairment on stages 2a and 2b. Posterior glottis is still patent, indicating type a (**a**), while almost closed with a slit-like aperture, indicating type b (**b**). Anterior glottis is closed

Acoustic Analysis of Stridor

Studies on the acoustic analysis of stridor sound are few. Comparing the vibration frequency between snoring and nocturnal stridor, the latter shows 233 ± 45 Hz [21] or 260-330 Hz [22], higher than the former, agreeing with the auditory impression of a high-pitched shrill sound. Tanaka et al. [23] reported a patient in whom characteristic nocturnal stridor was useful for the early diagnosis of MSA. Koo et al. [24] divided stridor into two types using Multi-Dimensional Voice Program: rhythmic and semi-rhythmic types. Prognosis of the patients with the former was poorer than that with the latter, though there were no significant differences between types in all of the seven acoustic parameters such as fundamental frequency. With progression of VCAI, the vocal glottis comes to be much narrower, approaching the position during vocalization. Looking at this situation from another angle, inspiratory stridor can be regarded as "inspiratory vocalization," resulting in an increase of quality with some limpidity associated with a decrease of noise components [25]. This may lead to the results from Koo et al. [24] showing that the rhythmic type with poorer prognosis exhibited more regular frequency and amplitude. In contrast, many reports on the acoustic analysis of snoring in OSAS have been made. For example, a median peak frequency [26] or pitch and formant [27] differed according to the obstruction sites. Lee et al. [28] reported that the frequency spectrum of stridor was distributed only within the low-frequency band (40–300 Hz) in the mild group with sole obstruction, while widely within the low, mid, and high frequency bands in the severe group with multiple obstructions. They concluded that high maximal intensity of low-frequency snoring sounds ($\geq$60 dB) was useful as a specific surrogate of multi-level obstructions, while low mean intensity of mid-frequency snoring sounds (<45 dB) as a good predictor of a surgical response [28]. Meanwhile, there was also an opinion that acoustic analysis was relatively accurate but not a strong method for diagnosing OSA [29]. To analyze UAO multidirectionally, DISE is a useful method to find the "hidden" obstructive sites when awake. Recently, Arigliani et al. [30] introduced an all-in-one machine, which was capable of simultaneously visualizing various decisional parameters on a single monitor.

Pathogenesis of VCAI

The mechanism of VCAI is easier to understand using our see-saw model (Fig. 23.3). There are at least five factors causing VCAI: factor 1 for neurogenic atrophy of the sole abductor, PCA; factor 2 for delay of the glottic opening at the beginning of inspiration; factor 3 for isolated contraction of the tensor (cricothyroid muscle, CT); factor 4 for dystonic activity of the adductor (thyroarytenoid muscle, TA); and factor 5 for airway-protection reflex of the adductor(s) during inspiration [31, 32]. Detailed explanations for each factor follow. Factor 1: neurogenic atrophy of PCA drawn as decreased volume in Fig. 23.3 has been reported both pathologically [4, 5] and electromyographically [33, 34]. In our pathological study on the intrinsic laryngeal muscles (vocal cords abductor, adductor, and tensor muscles) taken from 41 autopsied cases of various neurodegenerative disorders, eight of the nine cases of MSA showed neurogenic atrophy limited only to PCA. Such a selectivity was not observed in any of other disorders including Parkinson's disease (10 cases), progressive supranuclear palsy (four cases), amyotrophic lateral sclerosis (10 cases), and Machado-Joseph disease (four cases) [35]. In the latter two disorders, neurogenic changes were extended to all of the three muscles. As described before, it remains controversial whether there exists a neuronal loss of the nucleus ambiguus innervating intrinsic laryngeal muscles or not. This controversy can be explained partly by the difference of mixing ratio (dominancy) of paralytic component with weakness of the abductor and nonparalytic component with dystonia of the adductors. Factor 2: the basic function of PCA is to dilate the vocal glottis just prior to the initial phase of inspiration evoked by diaphragm contraction in order to prevent upper airway collapse [36]. In MSA, contraction onset of PCA is delayed resulting in the laryngeal collapse [25]. Such a delayed activity was reported also in the patients with OSAS [37]. Therefore, applying positive pressure to the stenotic site (vocal glottis) is a rational approach to prevent laryngeal collapse, i.e., CPAP. Factor 3: CT is a glottic tensor stretching the vocal cords anteromedially. It could potentially result in more medial positioning of the vocal cords in bilateral vocal cord abductor paralysis [38, 39]. That is to say, the function of CT depends on the activity of PCA: as an abductor under intact PCA, while as an adductor under damaged PCA [40]. Thereby, CT functions as an adductor in MSA with VCAI. Factor 4: several laryngeal electromyographical studies showed continuous or inspiratory phasic activity of TA [32, 34, 41–43]. Furthermore, Merlo et al. [44] reported the usefulness of botulinum toxin injection to TA with subjective improvement and reduced tonic electromyographical activity. From these reports, laryngeal dystonia was thought to be involved partly in

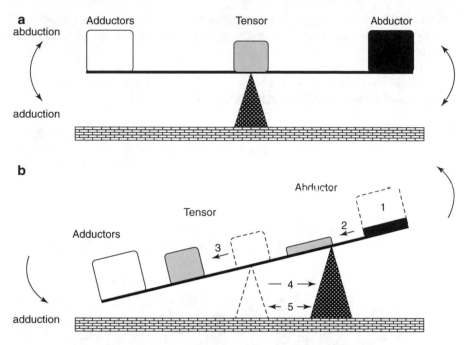

Fig. 23.3 Seesaw model of vocal cord abductor impairment. (**a**) Seesaw is well-balanced between abduction and adduction during quiet breathing. (**b**) Seesaw inclines toward the adduction during inspiration caused by activation of five factors: (1) neurogenic atrophy of the abductor, (2) delay of the glottic opening, (3) isolated contraction of the tensor, (4) dystonia of the adductor, and (5) airway-protection reflex

developing VCAI. Such a dystonic action is shown by arrow 4 in Fig. 23.3 as a shift of the fulcrum toward adduction. Factor 5: it was reported that inspiratory activity of TA disappeared after tracheostomy [31], CPAP [32], or BPAP [43]. For this reason, Shiba et al. [31] pointed out the difference in the working mechanism of CPAP between pharyngeal obstruction in OSAS and VCAI in MSA. In the former, pharyngeal obstruction is relieved by conventional air-splint effect, while in the latter VCAI showing paradoxical vocal cord movement caused by reflexive positive inspiratory activation of adductors, which can be augmented by forced inspiratory efforts under dyspneic situation [31, 32]. Bidirectional arrow 5 in Fig. 23.3 indicates functional disturbance.

In assimilating this see-saw model, there are two important points to note. First, these five factors do not always function independently, namely, factors 2 and 3 are secondary to factor 1. Factor 5 may be involved partly in factor 4. Second, mixing the ratio of paralytic and nonparalytic components changes with disease progression. It indicates that VCAI can change quantitatively and qualitatively among individual patient and even in a single patient. Therefore, some resourceful countermeasures are required when a newly appearing obstructive situation occurs. Todisco et al. [41] reported that MSA-P patients predominantly showed a paradoxical burst-like inspiratory activation of TA (dystonia pattern), while MSA-C mainly had additional neurogenic findings of vocal cord muscles (dystonia-plus pattern).

Laryngeal Abnormalities Other than VCAI

Supraglottic collapse refers to the condition where laryngeal inlet becomes plugged by the epiglottis, arytenoid regions, or both during inspiration. The epiglottis falls down to the posterior pharyngeal wall, and arytenoid regions are sucked inward to various degrees (Fig. 23.4). The former was named FE or epiglottis collapse, and the latter FA or arytenoid collapse. Prolapsing sites in Fig. 23.4c, d are almost confined to bilateral cuneiform tubercles of a small segment of aryepiglottic folds (Fig. 23.5). This segment includes the cuneiform cartilage inside, which is anatomically isolated from arytenoid cartilage. Therefore, it may be unsuitable to call such

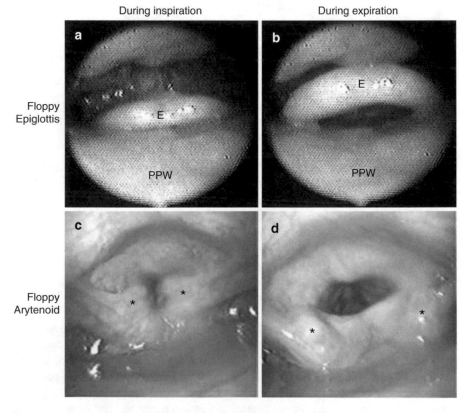

Fig. 23.4 Laryngoscopic photographs of supraglottic collapse. Floppy epiglottis: epiglottis (E) falls down to the posterior pharyngeal wall (PPW) during inspiration (**a**), with some airway patency during expiration (**b**). Floppy arytenoid: cuneiform tubercles (✲) are sucked inward during inspiration (**c**), with some airway patency during expiration (**d**)

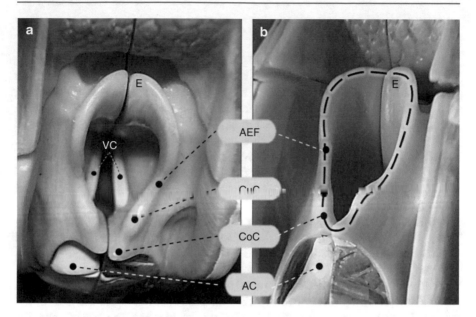

Fig. 23.5 Anatomy of the larynx (SOMSO models). Laryngeal inlet indicated by a broken circle in (**b**) is an oblique and oval-shaped plane separating larynx from pharynx. It consists of upper half of epiglottis and succeeding aryepiglottic folds (AEF) containing cuneiform cartilage (CuC) and corniculate cartilage (CoC). CuC is apart from CoC belonging to arytenoid cartilage (AC). Vocal cord (VC) is seen in the back of laryngeal inlet (**a**)

a phenomenon floppy "arytenoid." This point was described later from the point of view of classification for laryngomalacia (LM). Supraglottic collapse was observed in various disorders or conditions. In patients with MSA, we described this as "sleep-induced laryngomalacia" due to fiberscopic similarities to LM [45]. Similar reports on FE or FA in MSA have been made mainly from Japan [46–48].

FE has been expressed as other terms such as lax, flaccid, or prolapsing epiglottis, reflecting the epiglottic "limber" movements on laryngoscopy. However, floppiness was not confirmed physiologically. Frequencies of FE and FA were reported to be 25% and 15% in MSA patients, respectively [46], or 28% and 28% in MSA patients presenting with VCAI, respectively [25]. Thus, FE and FA were not as frequent as VCAI but not rare. Thanks to the introduction of DISE, supraglottic structures, particularly epiglottis, have attracted attention as clinically significant obstructive sites in OSAS. As another laryngeal abnormalities, Ward et al. [49] described "quivering" or "tremulous" movement of arytenoid regions, and subsequently similar reports have been made [50–52]. This phenomenon was considered a marker of the severity of glottic stenosis [51] or a clinical marker to delineate MSA (91.2%) from Parkinson's disease (no patients) [50, 52]. In addition, they reported that the frequency of the irregular arytenoid cartilage movement had no correlation with disease duration, patients' age, or MSA phenotypes [52]. The mechanism of this abnormal arytenoid movement remains unknown.

Supraglottic Collapse and LM

We [25] reported that supraglottic collapse observed in MSA corresponded to any of three types in the classification of LM by Olney et al. [53]. Laryngomalacia showing inspiratory inward collapse of supraglottic structures in infants was originally described in 1942. Similar phenomenon had been already known as congenital laryngeal stridor since the late 1800s. From around 1980s on, the concept of LM has been gradually extended to older children or adults, and accordingly, they have been called various names: acquired LM [54, 55], acquired idiopathic LM [56], late-onset LM [57], or adult-onset LM [58, 59]. Etiologies of LM with onset from children to adults were considerably heterogeneous and many classifications have been made [53, 54, 57–60]. These were roughly divided into two groups based on etiology and laryngoscopic findings. Richter et al. [57] classified LM into three categories: feeding-disordered LM, sleep-disordered LM, and exercise-induced LM. Meanwhile, Ferri et al. [58] divided LM into five groups: neurologic, exercise-induced, postoperative, idiopathic, and age-related LM. They mentioned that patients with neurologic etiology required tracheostomy more often than those with other etiologies [58]. These two reports indicated that etiologies for LM varied widely. Laryngoscopic classification by Olney et al. [53] has been used frequently, particularly in relationship with surgery: type 1 for prolapse of mucosa overlying arytenoid cartilages, type 2 for foreshortened aryepiglottic folds, and type 3 for posterior displacement of epiglottis. Supraglottic prolapse confined to cuneiform tubercle as shown in Fig. 23.4 was almost the same as type 1 LM in Holinger and Konior's classification [60]. They divided LM into 6 types: type 1 for inward collapse of the aryepiglottic folds, primarily cuneiform cartilages, type 2 for a long, tubular epiglottis causing obstruction, type 3 for anterior, medial collapse of the arytenoid cartilages, type 4 for posterior inspiratory displacement of the epiglottis, type 5 for short aryepiglottic folds, and type 6 for an overlay acute angle of the epiglottis. While true function of the cuneiform and the corniculate cartilages are unknown, they were thought to stiffen the aryepiglottic fold to prevent aspiration during swallowing.

The laryngeal inlet is anatomically an oblique and oval-shaped plane separating the larynx from pharynx (see Fig. 23.5). It consists of the upper half of the epiglottis and succeeding aryepiglottic folds containing cuneiform and corniculate cartilages. It appeared that such an oval-shaped laryngeal inlet is easy to be plugged with the teardrop-shaped epiglottis to avoid aspiration and to accept enough air flow by expanding an inlet area. Therefore, it can be assumed that epiglottic deformities, abnormal positions, and abnormal movements may interrupt breathing as well as swallowing functions to varying degrees.

Supraglottic Collapse and OSAS

The main UAO site in OSAS was the upper pharynx including soft palate and lateral pharyngeal walls, less often the epiglottis [61]. However, introduction of DISE clarified multilevel obstructions including the epiglottis [62–65]. Frequency of FE (epiglottis collapse) in OSAS ranged widely from 12% [66] to 42% [67]. Even in patients with upper airway resistance syndrome, which is positioned as a pre-stage of OSAS, frequency of FE was 39% [68]. CPAP did not work well or even could exacerbate epiglottis collapse in some patients with OSAS [69–71]. On the other hand, reports on FA in OSAS were limited. Only Lo et al. [20] reported that the frequency of FA (46.7%) was higher than that of FE (23.3%) in the OSAS patients and snorers who underwent DISE.

Frequency of multiplicity of UAO in OSAS was reported to be high in various degrees; 45% [72], 72% [69], 84% [63], or 96% [73]. The reasons for such a large variation might be a difference of sleep depth induced by sedative, a difference of interrater reliability on the evaluation of supraglottic collapse [74], and length of the observation time with DISE [64]. Hybášková et al. [73] examined the multiplicity of UAO in OSAS patients, resulting in 31.4% in two collapsing locations, 47.1% in three, and 17.6% in all levels (palatal, oropharyngeal, tongue base, and epiglottis).

Golz et al. [75] mentioned that common pathophysiological mechanisms might be involved between LM and OSAS because of the similarity of laryngoscopic findings and equally favorable operation effects in both diseases. Dion et al. [76] reported that abnormal corniculate and cuneiform cartilage motion developed supraglottic collapse mimicking LM induced by forceful inspiration in adult patients with noisy breathing and dyspnea with exertion. In addition, the following three findings may also support the abovementioned hypothesis by Golz et al. First, supraglottic structures were unresponsive or even hazardous to CPAP treatment [66, 72, 77–79]. Second, supraglottic collapse was often associated with other obstructive sites. Third, epiglottis showed similar deformities in LM and OSAS. The former two findings were described before, and here epiglottic deformities were described. Omega-shape is a well-known finding in LM, and was found also in MSA [25, 48]. However, there is an opinion that it was not always pathognomonic [60]. It was reported that the epiglottis can develop some deformities other than omega-shape [80]. In the patients with OSAS, two different types of epiglottis were reported: a flat type [81] and a type with an increase in the concavity of the posterior surface [82, 83]. The etiology was speculated to be degeneration of suspensory apparatus of epiglottis in the former [81], while an increased laryngeal pressure created by collapsing airway in the latter [82]. Gazayerli et al. [83] reported that epiglottis deformity was enhanced with increase of body mass index and improved after weight loss. Thus, epiglottis deformity can be either a cause or a result for UAO.

Obstructive sleep apnea syndrome is a heterogeneous disorder and has recently been reported to have various subtypes such as rapid eye movement-related OSAS [84], sleep-stage-independent OSAS [85], and positional OSAS [86]. In some OSAS patients, UAO was relieved by jaw thrust, head turning maneuver [61, 87, 88], or lateral position changes of the head [70]. Thereby, Vonk et al. [87] mentioned the usefulness of the positional therapy in the patients with OSAS presenting with epiglottis collapse. Victores et al. [89] already pointed out that hypopharyngeal (tongue base and epiglottis) collapse was the primary site that improved with change in position (positional OSAS). At present, however, there have been almost no reports on evaluating the effect of jaw thrust or head turning on UAO, particularly supraglottic collapse in MSA patients.

Treatments

Respiratory disturbance in MSA is caused by both UAO characterized by multiplicity in space and time and CRD with various combinations. Of therapeutic importance is how we manage such intermingled and changeable situations.

Treatment for VCAI

Tracheostomy has been exclusively performed for VCAI in patients with MSA [3, 17, 90]. After introduction of CPAP, however, many reports have shown the effectiveness of CPAP for VCAI [91–95] because of the simplicity and less invasiveness. Figure 23.6 shows an air-splint effect by CPAP in an MSA patient with VCAI of stage 2a. In this patient, glottic space became slightly wider in the posterior and a part of the anterior glottis. However, some MSA patients do not respond to CPAP. Silver and Levine [93] alerted that CPAP was not effective in preventing death, and that CPAP did not appear to have an impact on outcome of stridor. Iranzo [96] reported that patients might still benefit from tracheostomy if daytime stridor appeared or CPAP was not tolerated or failed to abolish nocturnal stridor. Moreover, Chitose et al. [97] reported an MSA patient presenting with severe VCAI with limited effect from CPAP, resulting in successful laser arytenoidectomy. Our previous study using an artificial vocal cord model showed that CPAP was effective for the

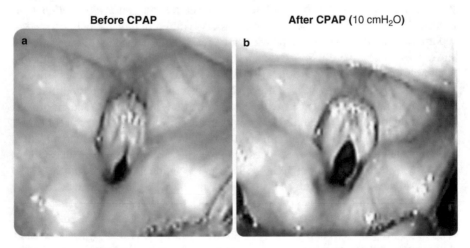

Fig. 23.6 Effect of CPAP on vocal cord abductor impairment with stage 2a. Posterior glottis showing some space (**a**) dilates after CPAP with 10 cm H_2O (**b**)

model simulating mild to moderately severe VCAI, but ineffective for severe VCAI with midline position of vocal cords [98]. Even if severe VCAI could be relieved by high positive pressure, it might be not available practically because of the intolerance or risk of lung injury.

There are several hurdles to clear in the managements on NPPV therapy: when an airway-keeping device including tracheostomy or NPPV should be introduced, what kind of device is preferable, and how re-evaluation after first treatment (for example, CPAP) is performed. It is not yet clear when an airway-keeping device should be introduced. The ideal time for therapeutic intervention is not too early and not too late. To approach an optimal point, several viewpoints should be taken into consideration, which were dominancy (mixing ratio) of paralytic and nonparalytic components, severity of dysphagia, degrees of coexistent CRD, and general condition of the patient. Kimura et al. [99] reported that the aggravation of dysphasia was an important index in judging the indication for tracheostomy in MSA patients with VCAI. We thought that stage 2b was optimal in performing tracheostomy [17, 25]. Stage 2b was a moderately severe VCAI where posterior glottis in addition to anterior glottis became narrow enough to induce vocal cord vibration during inspiration, namely inspiratory stridor (see Fig. 23.2b). In addition, following two situations may be also helpful to decide the time for introducing an airway-keeping device. One was an appearance of diurnal stridor and the other was an increase of the index T90 showing the severity of nocturnal hypoxemia. Since diurnal stridor has been known to develop in the advanced stage of VCAI, it has been thought to become an indicator to apply tracheostomy or NPPV [93, 96]. T90 means the percentage of sleep time spent at less than 90% of SpO_2 and has been frequently used as one of the parameters for the severity of OSAS. From our previous study, T90 seemed to be one of the useful parameters to perform tracheostomy when it reached nearly 20% in MSA patients with VCAI [25].

It remains unresolved whether or not CPAP is effective for VCAI despite the dominance of paralytic and nonparalytic components. Treatments for VCAI except for tracheostomy and CPAP included microscopic laryngosurgeries and botulinum toxin injection to vocal cord adductors. Many microsurgeries have been performed in the various disorders with VCAI. However, there were only four patients limited to MSA until now [97, 100–102]. Arytenoidectomy was effective in all four patients, with varying rationales for surgery: insufficient effect of previous CPAP [97], patient's refusal of CPAP and tracheostomy [101], patient's request for performing arytenoidectomy and posterior cordotomy together [102], and an alternative option after unsuccessful laterofixation [100]. Among them, Mahmud et al. [102] emphasized the advantage of their surgical procedure avoiding transient postoperative tracheostomy for laryngeal edema. At present, laryngomicrosurgery in MSA should be viewed as investigational.

With regard to treatment with botulinum toxin injections, only one MSA patient has been reported [44], although this treatment is widely performed in the patients with laryngeal dystonia including adductor breathing dystonia [103]. Botulinum toxin injection seems to be effective if VCAI is caused predominantly by nonparalytic (dystonic) components, defined by laryngeal electromyography. As with botulinum toxin injection treatment, it is not clear whether CPAP is also effective for both types of VCAI.

Treatment for FE and FA

Though FE and FA are not uncommon in MSA, there are only a few reports on treatments. According to Shimohata et al. [104], no obvious improvements were observed in three patients with severe FE, while in nine of patients with mild FE, two caused severe FE and the remaining seven improved by CPAP. Sakuta et al. [48] reported a patient with MSA under auto-CPAP for OSAS who developed dyspnea because of newly appearing VCAI and FA, resulting in an improvement with tracheostomy. This report is instructive in that the second therapeutic intervention with tracheostomy was required in the follow-up to CPAP treatment. Dedhia et al. [77] mentioned that primary epiglottis obstruction occurred in 15% of patients with OSAS who were unable to tolerate CPAP, and that head and neck cancer and MSA were two entities with high rates of obstructive sleep apnea due in part to laryngeal abnormalities. Moreover, Andersen et al. [105] reported that an OSAS patient initiated by lax epiglottis had a feeling "of being suffocated" immediately after application of CPAP, and that CPAP was a contraindication in the setting of a lax epiglottis. Collapsibility of the tongue base and epiglottis were reported to be significantly resistant to CPAP, which was overcome by increasing to 15 cmH$_2$O [71].

Figure 23.7 shows a treatment strategy for a representative MSA patient, who was assumed to develop VCAI at first, then FE or FA, and finally CRD. CPAP is preferable when VCAI is mild (stage 1) to moderately severe (stage 2a), while tracheostomy should be considered in later stages (stage 2b or more) [25]. Careful attention should be paid when inspiratory stridor becomes audible again despite CPAP. In such a situation, two background factors were considered: progression of VCAI as described above, and presence of newly appearing supraglottic collapse (FE and FA). FE and FA are often unresponsive to CPAP [71], resulting in tracheostomy. However, some MSA patients with supraglottic collapse (FE) are known to respond to CPAP [104]. Unfortunately, it is difficult to predict the difference between a CPAP responder and a CPAP non-responder. When CRD is added to mild to moderately severe VCAI, BPAP or ASV is applied. When tracheostomy was already performed because of the preceding severe VCAI or supraglottic collapse, TPPV is required if applicable. ASV has been recommended for complex SAS that is one of the OSAS types, and is strongly connected to CPAP failure.

Considering the difficulty in predicting new situations, it may be unavoidable to introduce CPAP as a back-up, rather than conventional CPAP as an initial therapeutic intervention. Direct visualization of obstructive sites and their response to positive pressure, that is, DISE with CPAP/BPAP, is useful in choosing an airway-keeping device. Civelek et al. [106] compared conventional CPAP titration and

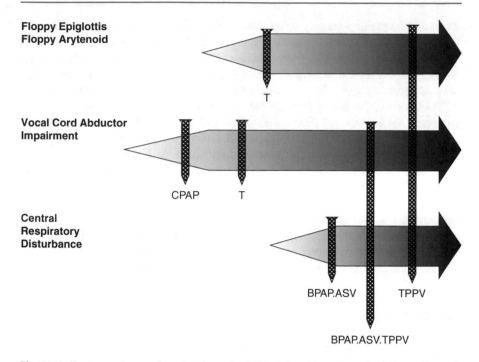

Fig. 23.7 Treatment strategy for a representative MSA patient. Treatments are performed according to both sites, severity, and multiplicity of upper airway obstruction and central respiratory disturbance with various combinations. BPAP and CPAP, bilevel and continuous positive airway pressure, respectively, T tracheostomy, ASV adaptive servo-ventilation, TPPV tracheostomized positive pressure ventilation

DISE-assisted CPAP titration, with no significant differences between them. An important point on the respiratory management is that careful follow-up with timely and indispensable examinations after initial treatment with CPAP or tracheostomy is critically important.

CPAP Failure

The term "CPAP failure" has been used in respiratory management for OSAS patients or neonates with severe respiratory failure. According to Braganza et al. [107], it is a situation with persistent obstructive sleep apnea, hypoxemia ($SpO_2 < 85\%$) or hypercapnia despite maximal CPAP. Such a CPAP non-responder group occupied about 9% [108] or 13% [109] of OSAS patients. It is empirically known that some MSA patients also did not respond to CPAP. Several factors may predict CPAP failure in OSAS: T90 value more than 43.5% [110], high body mass index [110], awake SpO_2 less than 94% [107], and PaO_2 less than 68 mmHg [107]. Dieleman et al. [62], who examined 30 patients with OSAS with CPAP failure by DISE, reported that 27% of them had FE requiring some additional therapy. Multilevel obstructions have been identified in OSAS patients, resulting in the need for multi-dimensional surgery on soft tissue, skeletal, and bariatric operations [111]. Various less invasive and elaborate surgical operations have been performed, with favorable outcomes [70, 80]. Treatments for CPAP failure other than surgical procedures include mandibular advancement and electrical stimulation of the peripheral nerve innervating upper airway muscles such as the genioglossus muscle [112].

Studies on CPAP failure in MSA have just begun. There were some differences and some similarities in CPAP failure between MSA and OSAS. Common points were multiplicity of UAO and complex SAS. However, combination of multiplicity was different between them. The most common site of collapse in the upper airway (soft palate, oropharyngeal region, tongue base, and epiglottis) was the soft palate (98%) and the most common combination of multilevel collapse was that of palatal + oropharyngeal + tongue base (33.3%), followed by that of palatal + oropharyngeal region (23.5%) in 51 patients with OSAS who underwent DISE [73]. In contrast, there have been no reports with analysis for combination of multilevel obstruction in MSA. However, the larynx (vocal cord and supraglottic structures) is clinically the most significant obstructive site in this disorder.

Combination with UAO and CRD

Respiratory disturbance in MSA is caused mainly by two mechanisms of UAO and CRD. Clinical symptoms develop as a result from mutual interactions between them. This is an important point, as optimal treatment reflects variable mixing of paralytic and nonparalytic components. There are several reports of MSA patients who developed sudden death despite tracheostomy or NPPV [10, 93]. Causes for sudden death were thought to be CRD including CSAS, central respiratory dysrhythmia, complex SAS, and impaired chemosensitivity to hypoxemia [113]. Several reports have looked for lesions for CRD, including the nucleus ambiguus [4–6], pre-Bötzinger complex, medullary serotonergic neurons [114], medullary raphe, and parabrachial nuclear complex [115].

Involvement of CRD in MSA has been suggested since the 1980s [5, 14]. In 2000, Silber and Levine [93] recommended consideration of tracheostomy for MSA patients with stridor, but also assessment for central hypoventilation and appropriate management due to deaths after tracheostomy. Iranzo et al. [116] reported that the severity of motor impairment at the initiation of treatment appeared to be the most significant limiting factor for CPAP long-term acceptance. On the other hand, a concept of complex SAS was advocated by Morgenthaler et al. in 2006 [117] they proposed inclusion and exclusion criteria, revised in 2014 [118]. Respiratory disturbances suggestive of a strong connection between UAO and CRD have been reported. Suzuki et al. [119], reported the first case of MSA presenting with complex sleep-disordered breathing (complex SAS), and called attention to the recognition of "central apnea in disguise" – disappearance of stridor was not the sole goal of MSA therapy. Hamada et al. [120] reported MSA patients with multiple sleep-related disorder symptoms such as stridor, apnea, and hypoventilation, who failed CPAP treatment because of the development of hypercapnia but responded well to advanced adaptive servo-ventilation (ASV). Advanced ASV is one of the NPPV instruments, functioning by changing both expiratory positive airway pressure (EPAP) and pressure support automatically [121]: as an auto-CPAP machine when in sufficient ventilation and as a pressure support machine in hypoventilation [120]. This instrument was originally developed for patients with cardiac failure associated with Cheyne-Stokes respiration. Since then, application of ASV has been gradually extended to patients with sleep-disordered breathing from various diseases including neuromuscular disorders requiring ventilatory support. However, there are only a few reports of patients with MSA who underwent ASV.

A significant problem is how the obstructive sites causing VCAI, FE, or FA respond to EPAP and pressure support. Our previous study using an artificial vocal cord model showed that there exists a threshold in setting-up the optimal EPAP to release the paradoxical vocal cords movement. Therefore, when respiratory mode is required to change from CPAP to BPAP because of additional CRD, EPAP should be set in excess of individual patient-specific thresholds before setting pressure support [98]. Rekik et al. [122] proposed a tailored management of stridor in MSA: fixed CPAP when stridor was isolated, auto-adjusting CPAP when it was combined with obstructive sleep apnea, and ASV when combined with central sleep apnea.

As has been described thus far, MSA shows widely extended respiratory disturbances in the UAO diversity, CRD diversity, and functional diversity straddling over UAO and CRD. In addition, CPAP can be a double-edged sword for UAO, particularly FE. Thereby, logical therapeutic strategies with less invasive and sophisticated devices for entangled respiratory disturbances in MSA are needed.

Conclusion

Respiratory disturbances in MSA derive from both upper airway obstruction and involvement of central respiratory centers. Vocal cord abductor impairment is caused by five factors based on paralytic and nonparalytic components. Upper airway obstruction accompanied by dynamic changes with progression results in the quantitative and qualitatively diverse findings among individual patient and even in a single patient. There is a clear need for prediction and comprehensive treatments of respiratory disturbance in MSA.

References

1. Bannister R, Ardill L, Fentem P. Defective autonomic control of blood vessels in idiopathic orthostatic hypotension. Brain. 1967;90:725–46.
2. Martin JB, Travis RH, van den Noort S. Centrally mediated orthostatic hypotension. Arch Neurol. 1968;19:163–73.

3. Williams A, Hanson D, Calne DB. Vocal cord paralysis in the Shy-Drager syndrome. J Neurol Neurosurg Psychiatry. 1979;42:151–3.
4. Isozaki E, Matsubara S, Hayashida T, Oda M, Hirai S. Morphometric study of nucleus ambiguus in multiple system atrophy presenting with vocal cord abductor paralysis. Clin Neuropathol. 2000;19:213–20.
5. Bannister R, Gibson W, Michaels L, Oppenheimer DR. Laryngeal abductor paralysis in multiple system atrophy. A report on three necropsied cases, with observations on the laryngeal muscles and the nuclei ambigui. Brain. 1981;104:351–68.
6. Lapresle J, Annabi A. Olivopontocerebellar atrophy with velopharyngolaryngeal paralysis: a contribution to the somatotopy of the nucleus ambiguous. J Neuropathol Exp Neurol. 1979;38:401–6.
7. Ikeda K, Iwasaki Y, Kuwajima A, Iguchi H, Sunohara N, Nonaka I, et al. Preservation of branchimotor neurons of the nucleus ambiguus in multiple system atrophy. Neurology. 2003;61:722–3.
8. Benarroch EE, Schmeichel AM, Parisi JE. Preservation of branchimotor neurons of the nucleus ambiguus in multiple system atrophy. Neurology. 2003;60:115–7.
9. Munschauer FE, Loh L, Bannister R, Newsom-Davis J. Abnormal respiration and sudden death during sleep in multiple system atrophy with autonomic failure. Neurology. 1990;40:677–9.
10. Shimohata T, Ozawa T, Nakayama H, Tomita M, Shinoda H, Nishizawa M. Frequency of nocturnal sudden death in patients with multiple system atrophy. J Neurol. 2008;255:1483–5.
11. Isozaki E, Miyamoto K, Osanai R, Hayashida T, Tanabe H. Clinical studies of 23 patients with multiple system atrophy presenting with vocal cord paralysis. Rinsho Shinkeigaku. 1991;31:249–54. Japanese.
12. Gilman S, Wenning GK, Low PA, Brooks DJ, Mathias CJ, Trojanowski JQ, et al. Second consensus statement on the diagnosis of multiple system atrophy. Neurology. 2008;71:670–6.
13. Cortelli P, Buonaura GC, Benarroch EE, Giannini G, Iranzo A, Low PA, et al. Stridor in multiple system atrophy: consensus statement on diagnosis, prognosis, and treatment. Neurology. 2019;93:630–9.
14. Kavey NB, Whyte J, Blitzer A, Gidro-Frank S. Sleep-related laryngeal obstruction presenting as snoring or sleep apnea. Laryngoscope. 1989;99:851–4.
15. Wu YR, Chen CM, Ro LS, Chen ST, Tang LM. Vocal cord paralysis as an initial sign of multiple system atrophy in the central nervous system. J Formos Med Assoc. 1996;95:804–6.
16. Hughes RG, Gibbin KP, Lowe J. Vocal fold abductor paralysis as a solitary and fatal manifestation of multiple system atrophy. J Laryngol Otol. 1998;112:177–8.
17. Isozaki E, Hayashi M, Hayashida T, Tanabe H, Hirai S. Vocal cord abductor paralysis in multiple system atrophy--paradoxical movement of vocal cords during sleep. Rinsho Shinkeigaku. 1996;36:529–33. Japanese.
18. Eastwood PR, Platt PR, Shepherd K, Maddison K, Hillman DR. Collapsibility of the upper airway at different concentrations of propofol anesthesia. Anesthesiology. 2005;103:470–7.
19. Sigl JC, Chamoun NG. An introduction to bispectral analysis for the electroencephalogram. J Clin Monit. 1994;10:392–404.
20. Lo YL, Ni YL, Wang TY, Lin TY, Li HY, White DP, et al. Bispectral index in evaluating effects of sedation depth on drug-induced sleep endoscopy. J Clin Sleep Med. 2015;11:1011–20.
21. Isozaki E. Clinicopathological, electromyological, and phoniatric studies on bilateral vocal cord paralysis in multiple system atrohy. Kita Kanto Igaku. 1991;41:389–409. Japanese.
22. Kakitsuba N, Sadaoka T, Kanai R, Fujiwara Y, Takahashi H. Peculiar snoring in patients with multiple system atrophy: its sound source, acoustic characteristics, and diagnostic significance. Ann Otol Rhinol Laryngol. 1997;106:380–4.
23. Tanaka H, Nishio H, Sasanabe R, Shiomi T. A case of multiple systemic atrophy (MSA) analyzed by acoustic sound for nocturnal inspiratory stridor. Nihon Kokyuki Gakkai Zasshi. 2007;45:604–8. Japanese.

24. Koo DL, Lee JY, Joo EY, Hong SB, Nam H. Acoustic characteristics of stridor in multiple system atrophy. PLoS One. 2016;11:e0153935. https://doi.org/10.1371/journal.pone.0153935. eCollection 2016.
25. Isozaki E. Upper airway obstruction in multiple system atrophy. Adv Neurol Sci. 2006;50:409–19. Japanese.
26. Agrawal S, Stone P, McGuinness K, Morris J, Camilleri AE. Sound frequency analysis and the site of snoring in natural and induced sleep. Clin Otolaryngol Allied Sci. 2002;27:162–6.
27. Won TB, Kim SY, Lee WH, Han DH, Kim DY, Kim JW, et al. Acoustic characteristics of snoring according to obstruction site determined by sleep videofluoroscopy. Acta Otolaryngol. 2012;132(Suppl 1):S13–20.
28. Lee LA, Lo YL, Yu JF, Lee GS, Ni YL, Chen NH, et al. Snoring sounds predict obstruction sites and surgical response in patients with obstructive sleep apnea hypopnea syndrome. Sci Rep. 2016;6:30629. https://doi.org/10.1038/srep30629.
29. Jin II, Lee LA, Song L, Li Y, Peng J, Zhong N, et al. Acoustic analysis of snoring in the diagnosis of obstructive sleep apnea syndrome: a call for more rigorous studies. J Clin Sleep Med. 2015;11:765–71.
30. Arigliani M, Toraldo DM, Montevecchi F, Conte L, Galasso L, Rosa FD, et al. A new technological advancement of the drug-induced sleep endoscopy (DISE) procedure: the "all in one glance" strategy. Int J Environ Res Public Health. 2020;17:4261.
31. Shiba K, Isono S, Nakazawa K. Paradoxical vocal cord motion: a review focused on multiple system atrophy. Auris Nasus Larynx. 2007;34:443–52.
32. Isono S, Shiba K, Yamaguchi M, Tanaka A, Hattori T, Konno A, et al. Pathogenesis of laryngeal narrowing in patients with multiple system atrophy. J Physiol. 2001;536(Pt 1):237–49.
33. Guindi GM, Higenbottam TW, Payne JK. A new method for laryngeal electromyography. Clin Otolaryngol Allied Sci. 1981;6:271–8.
34. Alfonsi E, Terzaghi M, Cosentino G, Tassorelli C, Manni R, Pozzi N, et al. Specific patterns of laryngeal electromyography during wakefulness are associated to sleep disordered breathing and nocturnal stridor in multiple system atrophy. Parkinsonism Relat Disord. 2016;31:104–9.
35. Isozaki E, Hayashi M, Hayashida T, Oda M, Hirai S. Myopathology of the intrinsic laryngeal muscles in neurodegenerative diseases, with reference to the mechanism of vocal cord paralysis. Rinsho Shinkeigaku. 1998;38:711–8. Japanese.
36. Eichenwald EC, Howell RG, Kosch PC, Ungarelli RA, Lindsey J, Stark R. Developmental changes in sequential activation of laryngeal abductor muscle and diaphragm in infants. J Appl Physiol. 1992;73:1425–31.
37. Hudgel DW. Differential activation of respiratory muscles during wakefulness and sleep. Prog Clin Biol Res. 1990;345:233–9.
38. Sahin M, Aydogdu I, Akyildiz S, Erdinc M, Ozturk K, Ogut F. Electromyography-guided botulinum toxin injection into the cricothyroid muscles in bilateral vocal fold abductor paralysis. Clin Exp Otorhinolaryngol. 2017;10:193–202.
39. Benninger MS, Hanick A, Hicks DM. Cricothyroid muscle botulinum toxin injection to improve airway for bilateral recurrent laryngeal nerve paralysis. A case series. J Voice. 2016;30:96–9.
40. Crumley RL. Laryngeal synkinesis: its significance to the laryngologist. Ann Otol Rhinol Laryngol. 1989;98:87–92.
41. Todisco M, Alfonsi E, Isaias IU, Zangaglia R, Minafra B, Cosentino G, et al. Vocal cord electromyographic correlates of stridor in multiple system atrophy phenotypes. Parkinsonism Relat Disord. 2020;70:31–5.
42. Isozaki E, Osanai R, Horiguchi S, Hayashida T, Hirose K, Tanabe H. Laryngeal electromyography with separated surface electrodes in patients with multiple system atrophy presenting with vocal cord paralysis. J Neurol. 1994;241:551–6.

43. Nonaka M, Imai T, Shintani T, Kawamata M, Chiba S, Matsumoto H. Non-invasive positive pressure ventilation for laryngeal contraction disorder during sleep in multiple system atrophy. J Neurol Sci. 2006;247:53–8.
44. Merlo IM, Occhini A, Pacchetti C, Alfonsi E. Not paralysis, but dystonia causes stridor in multiple system atrophy. Neurology. 2002;58:649–52.
45. Tobisawa S, Isozaki E, Naito R, Hayashi H. Sleep-induced laryngomalacia in multiple system atrophy [abstract]. Rinsho Shinkeigaku. 2005;45:1166. [Japanese].
46. Shimohata T, Shinoda H, Nakayama H, Ozawa T, Terajima K, Yoshizawa H, et al. Daytime hypoxemia, sleep-disordered breathing, and laryngopharyngeal findings in multiple system atrophy. Arch Neurol. 2007;64:856–61.
47. Shimohata T, Nakayama H, Aizawa N, Nishizawa M. Discontinuation of continuous positive airway pressure treatment in multiple system atrophy. Sleep Med. 2014;15:1147–9.
48. Sakuta H, Miyamoto M, Suzuki K, Miyamoto T, Nakajima I, Nakamura T, et al. Obese woman presenting as vocal cord abductor paralysis and floppy arytenoid associated with early signs of multiple system atrophy. Rinsho Shinkeigaku. 2012;52:421–4. Japanese.
49. Ward PH, Hanson DG, Berci G. Observations on central neurologic etiology for laryngeal dysfunction. Ann Otol Rhinol Laryngol. 1981;90:430–41.
50. Warnecke T, Vogel A, Ahring S, Gruber D, Heinze H-J, Dziewas R, et al. The shaking palsy of the larynx-potential biomarker for multiple system atrophy: a pilot study and literature review. Front Neurol. 2019;10:241.
51. Ozawa T, Shinoda H, Tomita M, Shimohata T, Nakayama H, Nishizawa M. Tremulous arytenoid movements predict severity of glottic stenosis in multiple system atrophy. Mov Disord. 2010;25:1418–23.
52. Gandor F, Vogel A, Claus I, Ahring S, Gruber D, Heinze HJ, et al. Laryngeal movement disorders in multiple system atrophy: a diagnostic biomarker? Mov Disord. 2020; https://doi.org/10.1002/mds.28220. Online ahead of print.
53. Olney DR, Greinwald JH Jr, Smith RJ, Bauman NM. Laryngomalacia and its treatment. Laryngoscope. 1999;109:1770–5.
54. Woo P. Acquired laryngomalacia: epiglottis prolapse as a cause of airway obstruction. Ann Otol Rhinol Laryngol. 1992;101:314–20.
55. Chetty KG, Kadifa F, Berry RB, Mahutte CK. Acquired laryngomalacia as a cause of obstructive sleep apnea. Chest. 1994;106:1898–9.
56. Siou GS, Jeannon JP, Stafford FW. Acquired idiopathic laryngomalacia treated by laser aryepiglottoplasty. J Laryngol Otol. 2002;116:733–5.
57. Richter GT, Rutter MJ, deAlarcon A, Orvidas LJ, Thompson DM. Late-onset laryngomalacia: a variant of disease. Arch Otolaryngol Head Neck Surg. 2008;134:75–80.
58. Ferri GM, Prakash Y, Levi JR, Tracy LF. Differential diagnosis and management of adult-onset laryngomalacia. Am J Otolaryngol. 2020;41:102469.
59. Hey SY, Oozeer NB, Robertson S, MacKenzie K. Adult-onset laryngomalacia: case reports and review of management. Eur Arch Otorhinolaryngol. 2014;271:3127–32.
60. Holinger LD, Konior RJ. Surgical management of severe laryngomalacia. Laryngoscope. 1989;99:136–42.
61. Hohenhorst W, Ravesloot MJL, Kezirian EJ, de Vries N. Drug-induced sleep endoscopy in adults with sleep-disordered breathing: techniques and the VOTE classification system. Oper Tech Otolaryngol. 2012;23:11–8.
62. Dieleman E, Veugen CCAFM, Hardeman JA, Copper MP. Drug-induced sleep endoscopy while administering CPAP therapy in patients with CPAP failure. Sleep Breath. 2020. https://doi.org/10.1007/s11325-020-02098-x. Online ahead of print.
63. Koo SK, Choi JW, Myun NS, Lee HJ, Kim YJ, Kim YJ. Analysis of obstruction site in obstructive sleep apnea syndrome patients by drug induced sleep endoscopy. Am J Otolaryngol. 2013;34:626–30.
64. Heo SJ, Park CM, Kim JS. Time-dependent changes in the obstruction pattern during drug-induced sleep endoscopy. Am J Otolaryngol. 2014;35:42–7.

65. Amos JM, Durr ML, Nardone HC, Baldassari CM, Duggins A. Systematic review of drug-induced sleep endoscopy scoring systems. Otolaryngol Head Neck Surg. 2018;158:240–8.
66. Roustan V, Barbieri M, Incandela F, Missale F, Camera H, Braido F, et al. Transoral glossoepiglottopexy in the treatment of adult obstructive sleep apnoea: a surgical approach. Acta Otorhinolaryngol Ital. 2018;38:38–44.
67. Xu HJ, Jia RF, Yu H, Gao Z, Huang WN, Peng H, et al. Investigation of the source of snoring sound by drug-induced sleep nasendoscopy. ORL J Otorhinolaryngol Relat Spec. 2015;77:359–65.
68. Spinowitz S, Kim M, Park SY. Patterns of upper airway obstruction on drug-induced sleep endoscopy in patients with sleep-disordered breathing with AHI <5. OTO Open. 2017;1:2473974X17721483. https://doi.org/10.1177/2473974X17721483. eCollection Jul-Sep 2017.
69. Bachar G, Feinmesser R, Shpitzer T, Yaniv E, Nageris B, Eidelman L. Laryngeal and hypopharyngeal obstruction in sleep disordered breathing patients, evaluated by sleep endoscopy. Eur Arch Otorhinolaryngol. 2008;265:1397–402.
70. Torre C, Camacho M, Liu SYC, Huon LK, Capasso R. Epiglottis collapse in adult obstructive sleep apnea: a systematic review. Laryngoscope. 2016;126:515–23.
71. Torre C, Liu SY, Kushid CA, Nekhendzy V, Huon LK, Capass R. Impact of continuous positive airway pressure in patients with obstructive sleep apnea during drug-induced sleep endoscopy. Clin Otolaryngol. 2017;42:1218–23.
72. Salamanca F, Costantini F, Bianchi A, Amaina T, Colombo E, Zibordi F. Identification of obstructive sites and patterns in obstructive sleep apnoea syndrome by sleep endoscopy in 614 patients. Acta Otorhinolaryngol Ital. 2013;33:261–6.
73. Hybášková J, Jor O, Novák V, Zeleník K, Matouše P, Komínek P. Drug-induced sleep endoscopy changes the treatment concept in patients with obstructive sleep Apnoea. Biomed Res Int. 2016;2016:6583216. https://doi.org/10.1155/2016/6583216. Epub 2016 Dec 14.
74. Koo SK, Lee SH, Koh TK, Kim YJ, Moon JS, Lee HB, et al. Inter-rater reliability between experienced and inexperienced otolaryngologists using Koo's drug-induced sleep endoscopy classification system. Eur Arch Otorhinolaryngol. 2019;276:1525–31.
75. Golz A, Goldenberg D, Westerman ST, Catalfumo FJ, Netzer A, Westerman LM, et al. Laser partial epiglottidectomy as a treatment for obstructive sleep apnea and laryngomalacia. Ann Otol Rhinol Laryngol. 2000;109:1140–5.
76. Dion GR, Eller RL, Thomas RF. Diagnosing aerodynamic supraglottic collapse with rest and exercise flexible laryngoscopy. J Voice. 2012;26:779–84.
77. Dedhia RC, Rosen CA, Soose RJ. What is the role of the larynx in adult obstructive sleep apnea? Laryngoscope. 2014;124:1029–34.
78. Verse T, Pirsig W. Age-related changes in the epiglottis causing failure of nasal continuous positive airway pressure therapy. J Laryngol Otol. 1999;113:1022–5.
79. Jeong SH, Sung CM, Lim SC, Yang HC. Partial epiglottectomy improves residual apnea-hypopnea index in patients with epiglottis collapse. J Clin Sleep Med. 2020; https://doi.org/10.5664/jcsm.8640. Online ahead of print.
80. Kanemaru S, Kojima H, Fukushima H, Tamaki H, Tamura Y, Yamashita M, et al. A case of floppy epiglottis in adult: a simple surgical remedy. Auris Nasus Larynx. 2007;34:409–11.
81. Delakorda M, Ovsenik N. Epiglottis shape as a predictor of obstruction level in patients with sleep apnea. Sleep Breath. 2019;23:311–7.
82. Gazayerli M, Bleibel W, Elhorr A, Maxwell D, Seifeldin R. A correlation between the shape of the epiglottis and obstructive sleep apnea. Surg Endosc. 2006;20:836–7.
83. Gazayerli M, Bleibel W, Elhorr A, Elakkary E. The shape of the epiglottis reflects improvement in upper airway obstruction after weight loss. Obes Surg. 2006;16:945–7.
84. Su CS, Liu KT, Panjapornpon K, Andrews N, Schaefer NF. Functional outcomes in patients with REM-related obstructive sleep apnea treated with positive airway pressure therapy. J Clin Sleep Med. 2012;8:243–7.
85. Gupta R, Lahan V, Sindhwani G. Sleep-stage-independent obstructive sleep apnea: an unidentified group? Neurol Sci. 2013;34:1543–50.

86. Uzer F, Toptas AB, Okur U, Bozkurt S, Dogrul E, Turhan M, et al. Comparison of positional and rapid eye movement-dependent sleep apnea syndromes. Ann Thorac Med. 2018;13:42–7.
87. Vonk PE, Venema JAMU, Hoekema A, Ravesloot MJL, van de Velde-Muusers JA, de Vries N. Jaw thrust versus the use of a boil-and-bite mandibular advancement device as a screening tool during drug-induced sleep endoscopy. J Clin Sleep Med. 2020;16:1021–7.
88. Park D, Kim JS, Heo SJ. The effect of the modified jaw-thrust maneuver on the depth of sedation during drug-induced sleep endoscopy. J Clin Sleep Med. 2019;15:1503–8.
89. Victores AJ, Hamblin J, Gilbert J, Switzer C, Takashima M. Usefulness of sleep endoscopy in predicting positional obstructive sleep apnea. Otolaryngol Head Neck Surg. 2014;150:487–93.
90. Jin K, Okabe S, Chida K, Abe N, Kimpara T, Ohnuma A, et al. Tracheostomy can fatally exacerbate sleep-disordered breathing in multiple system atrophy. Neurology. 2007;68:1618–21.
91. Ghorayeb I, Yekhlef F, Bioulac B, Tison F. Continuous positive airway pressure for sleep-related breathing disorders in multiple system atrophy: long-term acceptance. Sleep Med. 2005;6:359–62.
92. Iranzo A, Santamaria J, Tolosa E. Continuous positive air pressure eliminates nocturnal stridor in multiple system atrophy. Lancet. 2000;356:1329–30.
93. Silber MH, Levine S. Stridor and death in multiple system atrophy. Mov Disord. 2000;15:699–704.
94. Kuźniar TJ, Morgenthaler TI, Prakash UBS, Pallanch JF, Silber MH, Peikert MT. Effects of continuous positive airway pressure on stridor in multiple system atrophy-sleep laryngoscopy. Case Rep J Clin Sleep Med. 2009;5:65–7.
95. Heo SJ, Kim JS, Lee BJ, Park D. Isolated stridor without any other sleeping breathing disorder diagnosed using drug-induced sleep endoscopy in a patient with multiple system atrophy: A case report. Medicine (Baltimore). 2020;99:e19745. https://doi.org/10.1097/MD.0000000000019745.
96. Iranzo A. Management of sleep-disordered breathing in multiple system atrophy. Sleep Med. 2005;6:297–300.
97. Chitose S, Kikuchi A, Ikezono K, Umeno H, Nakashima T. Effect of laser arytenoidectomy on respiratory stridor caused by multiple system atrophy. J Clin Sleep Med. 2012;8:713–5.
98. Isozaki E, Tobisawa S, Nishizawa M, Nakayama H, Fukui K, Takanishi A. Experimental vocal cord abduction impairment with an artificial vocal cord. Rinsho Shinkeigaku. 2009;49:407–13. Japanese.
99. Kimura Y, Sugiura M, Ohmae Y, Kato T, Kishimoto S. When should tracheotomy be performed in bilateral vocal cord paralysis involving multiple system atrophy? Nihon Jibiinkoka Gakkai Kaiho. 2007;110:7–12. Japanese.
100. Umeno H, Ueda Y, Mori K, Chijiwa K, Nakashima T, Kotby NM. Management of impaired vocal fold movement during sleep in a patient with Shy-Drager syndrome. Am J Otolaryngol. 2000;21(5):344–8.
101. Stomeo F, Rispoli V, Sensi M, Pastore A, Malagutti N, Pelucchi S. Subtotal arytenoidectomy for the treatment of laryngeal stridor in multiple system atrophy: phonatory and swallowing results. Braz J Otorhinolaryngol. 2016;82:116–20.
102. Mahmud A, Strens LHA, Tedla M. Laser arytenoidectomy and posterior cordotomy in a patient with bilateral vocal cord paralysis due to multiple system atrophy. BMJ Case Rep. 2015;2015:bcr2014206156. https://doi.org/10.1136/bcr-2014-206156.
103. Blitzer A, Brin MF, Simonyan K, Ozelius LJ, Frucht SJ. Phenomenology, genetics, and CNS network abnormalities in laryngeal dystonia: a 30-year experience. Laryngoscope. 2018;128(Suppl 1):S1–9.
104. Shimohata T, Tomita M, Nakayama H, Aizawa N, Ozawa T, Nishizawa M. Floppy epiglottis as a contraindication of CPAP in patients with multiple system atrophy. Neurology. 2011;76:1841–2.
105. Andersen AP, Alving J, Lildholdt T, Wulff CH. Obstructive sleep apnea initiated by a lax epiglottis. A contraindication for continuous positive airway pressure. Chest. 1987;91:621–3.

106. Civelek S, Emre IE, Dizdar D, Cuhadaroglu C, Eksioglu BK, Eraslan AK, et al. Comparison of conventional continuous positive airway pressure to continuous positive airway pressure titration performed with sleep endoscopy. Laryngoscope. 2012;122:691–5.

107. Braganza MV, Hanly PJ, Fraser KL, Tsai WH, Pendharkar SR. Predicting CPAP failure in patients with suspected sleep hypoventilation identified on ambulatory testing. J Clin Sleep Med. 2020; https://doi.org/10.5664/jcsm.8616. Online ahead of print.

108. Schäfer H, Ewig S, Hasper E, Lüderitz B. Failure of CPAP therapy in obstructive sleep apnoea syndrome: predictive factors and treatment with bilevel-positive airway pressure. Respir Med. 1998;92:208–15.

109. Slouka D, Honnerova M, Hrabe V, Matas A. The prediction of treatment failure of the continuous positive airways pressure. Bratisl Lek Listy. 2014;115:704–7.

110. Slouka D, Honnerova M, Hosek P, Matas A, Slama K, Landsmanova J, et al. Risk factors for failure of continuous positive airway pressure treatment in patients with ostructive sleep apnoea. Biomed Pap Med Fac Univ Palacky Olomouc Czech Repub. 2018;162:134–8.

111. Li HY, Lee LA, Tsa MS, Chen NH, Chuang LP, Fang TJ, et al. How to manage continuous positive airway pressure (CPAP) failure -hybrid surgery and integrated treatment. Auris Nasus Larynx. 2020;47:335–42.

112. Keymel S, Kelm M, Randerath WJ. Non-CPAP therapies in obstructive sleep apnoea: an overview. Pneumologie. 2013;67:50–7. German.

113. Tsuda T, Onodera H, Okabe S, Kikuchi Y, Itoyama Y. Impaired chemosensitivity to hypoxia is a marker of multiple system atrophy. Ann Neurol. 2002;52:367–71.

114. Tada M, Kakita A, Toyoshima Y, Onodera O, Ozawa T, Morita T, Nishizawa M, et al. Depletion of medullary serotonergic neurons in patients with multiple system atrophy who succumbed to sudden death. Brain. 2009;132:1810–9.

115. Benarroch EE. Multiple system atrophy: a disorder targeting the brainstem control of survival. Clin Auton Res. 2019;29:549–51.

116. Iranzo A, Santamaria J, Tolosa E, Vilaseca I, Valldeoriola F, Martí MJ, et al. Long-term effect of CPAP in the treatment of nocturnal stridor in multiple system atrophy. Neurology. 2004;63:930–2.

117. Morgenthaler TI, Kagramanov V, Hanak V, Decker PA. Complex sleep apnea syndrome: is it a unique clinical syndrome? Sleep. 2006;29:1203–9.

118. Morgenthaler TI, Kuzniar TJ, Wolfe LF, Willes L, McLain WC 3rd, Goldberg R. The complex sleep apnea resolution study: a prospective randomized controlled trial of continuous positive airway pressure versus adaptive servoventilation therapy. Sleep. 2014;37:927–34.

119. Suzuki M, Saigusa H, Shibasaki K, Kodera K. Multiple system atrophy manifesting as complex sleep-disordered breathing. Auris Nasus Larynx. 2010;37:110–3.

120. Hamada S, Takahashi R, Mishima M, Chin K. Use of a new generation of adaptive servo ventilation for sleep-disordered breathing in patients with multiple system atrophy. BMJ Case Rep. 2015;2015:bcr2014206372. https://doi.org/10.1136/bcr-2014-206372.

121. Javaheri S, Goetting MG, Khayat R, Wylie PE, Goodwin JL, Parthasarathy S. The performance of two automatic servo-ventilation devices in the treatment of central sleep apnea. Sleep. 2011;34:1693–8.

122. Rekik S, Martin F, Dodet P, Redolfi S, Semenescu SL, Corvol JC. Stridor combined with other sleep breathing disorders in multiple system atrophy: a tailored treatment? Sleep Med. 2018;42:53–60.

Dopa-Responsive Dystonia and Related Disorders

Yoshiaki Furukawa, Mark Guttman, Yuji Tomizawa, and Stephen J. Kish

Patient Vignettes

Patient 1

A 6-year-old girl with gait disturbance was introduced by an orthopedist in 1990, before the discovery of causative genes in dopa-responsive dystonia (DRD). Although early motor development was normal, she had Trendelenburg's symptoms due to a congenital dislocation of the left hip (acetabular dysplasia). In addition, she developed flexion-inversion of the left foot at age 3, which became aggravated toward the evening and was alleviated in the morning after sleep. Her postural dystonia spread to other limbs within 3 years but was more pronounced in the legs. Neurologic examination also revealed symmetric hyperreflexia without extensor plantar responses, and rigid hypertonicity in the legs. Investigations, including copper metabolism and brain MRI, were normal. Therapeutic trials with levodopa and tetrahydrobiopterin (BH4; the cofactor for tyrosine hydroxylase [TH]) were considered, and a lumbar puncture was performed to measure CSF pterins. She

Supplementary Information The online version of this chapter (https://doi.org/10.1007/978-3-030-75898-1_24) contains supplementary material, which is available to authorized users.

Y. Furukawa (✉) · Y. Tomizawa
Department of Neurology, Juntendo Tokyo Koto Geriatric Medical Center, Tokyo, Japan

Department of Neurology, Faculty of Medicine, Juntendo University, Tokyo, Japan
e-mail: furukawa@juntendo.gmc.ac.jp

M. Guttman
Centre for Movement Disorders, Toronto, ON, Canada

S. J. Kish
Human Brain Laboratory, Centre for Addiction and Mental Health, University of Toronto, Toronto, ON, Canada

© Springer Nature Switzerland AG 2022
S. J. Frucht (ed.), *Movement Disorder Emergencies*, Current Clinical Neurology,
https://doi.org/10.1007/978-3-030-75898-1_24

remarkably responded to low doses of levodopa but not to acute BH4 administration. After increasing the dosage of levodopa (20 mg/kg/day, without a decarboxylase inhibitor [DCI]) and undergoing an operation (acetabuloplasty) for the complicated condition, she became completely normal and was diagnosed as DRD. The diagnosis was supported by CSF data (decreased total biopterin and neopterin) and was confirmed later by genetic analysis [1, 2].

Patient 2

A 45-year-old woman states that her long-standing foot dystonia has deteriorated over the last year. She also describes that she has developed a tremor involving her right arm in the last few months. She manifested her dystonic posturing (in-turning) at age 7, and the initial treatment strategy has been beneficial, until recently, with trihexyphenidyl. She noticed that her foot dystonia was worse in the late afternoon and evening. She discloses a family history of overt dystonia in her brother, father, and paternal grandfather. Her two daughters (identical twins) have occasionally manifested mild dystonic posture of the foot after extreme exercise. On examination she showed dystonia of the feet, with the right being worse. She had increased tone in her right leg and arm. Rapid alternating movements were slow in the right foot and hand and in the left foot to a lesser extent. She had a mild postural tremor of her right hand. Her walking revealed dystonic posturing of the right foot. Investigations included normal brain CT and copper metabolism studies. She was successfully switched from trihexyphenidyl to levodopa with a DCI and has had no dystonia or parkinsonism on examination. The clinical diagnosis of DRD was confirmed by genetic analysis [3].

Introduction

DRD is a clinical syndrome characterized by childhood-onset dystonia and a dramatic and sustained response to low doses of levodopa [4–7]. This clinical syndrome typically presents with gait disturbance due to foot dystonia, later development of some parkinsonian features, and diurnal fluctuation of symptoms (worsening of symptoms toward the evening and their alleviation in the morning after sleep) (Table 24.1). In general, the sustained levodopa responsiveness without motor adverse effects of chronic levodopa therapy (motor response fluctuations and dopa-induced dyskinesias) distinguishes DRD from early-onset parkinsonism/early-onset Parkinson's disease (EOPD) with dystonia [2, 8, 9]. Because patients with DRD respond so well to treatment with levodopa, and because failure to recognize this disorder causes unacceptable morbidity, we choose to classify DRD as a movement disorder emergency.

There are three known causative loci for DRD (locus heterogeneity): (1) the *GCH1* gene on chromosome 14q22.1-q22.2, which encodes GTP cyclohydrolase 1

Table 24.1 Clinical features of classic dopa-responsive dystonia (DRD)

1. Onset generally in childhood following normal early motor development
2. Onset of dystonia in a limb, typically foot dystonia resulting in gait disturbance
3. Later development of some parkinsonian features; tremor is mainly postural
4. Presence of brisk deep-tendon reflexes in the legs, ankle clonus, and/or the striatal toe[a] in many patients
5. Characteristic diurnal fluctuation of symptoms (aggravation of symptoms toward the evening and their alleviation in the morning after sleep); the magnitude of diurnal fluctuation is variable and usually attenuates with age and disease progression
6. Gradual progression to generalized dystonia, typically more pronounced dystonia in the legs throughout the disease course
7. A dramatic and sustained response (complete or near-complete responsiveness of symptoms) to low doses of levodopa
8. Maximum benefit is generally achieved by less than 300–400 mg/day[b] of levodopa with a decarboxylase inhibitor
9. Typically, absence of motor adverse effects of chronic levodopa therapy (motor response fluctuations and dopa-induced dyskinesias) under optimal doses of levodopa
10. Female predominance of clinically affected individuals in autosomal dominant GTPCH1-deficient DRD (the major form of DRD)

GTPCH1 GTP cyclohydrolase 1
[a]Dystonic extension of the big toe, which may be misinterpreted as a Babinski response (see "Clinical Observations" in the text)
[b]See "Treatment" in the text

(GTPCH1), the rate-limiting enzyme in the biosynthetic pathway for BH4; (2) the *TH* gene on 11p15.5, coding for the enzyme TH that catalyzes the rate-limiting step in catecholamine biosynthesis; and (3) the *SPR* gene on 2p14-p12, encoding sepiapterin reductase (SR), which is involved in the last step (a two-step reduction) in cofactor BH4 biosynthesis (Fig. 24.1) [9–15]. Many patients with DRD have demonstrated dominantly inherited *GCH1* mutations (GTPCH1-deficient DRD [DYT5a; DYT-GCH1]; the major form of DRD), whereas a relatively small number of DRD patients have shown recessively inherited *TH* mutations (TH-deficient DRD [DYT5b; DYT-TH]; the mild form of TH deficiency) or *SPR* mutations (SR-deficient DRD [DYT-SPR]; the very mild form of SR deficiency) [9, 11, 12, 15–20]. Because no mutations in either *GCH1*, *TH*, or *SPR* have been identified in some patients with DRD, a therapeutic trial with low-dose levodopa is still important practical approach to the diagnosis of this treatable disorder. Since clinical suspicion is a key to the diagnosis, physicians should know not only the classic phenotype of GTPCH1-, TH-, and SR-deficient DRD but also the broad phenotypic spectrum in GTPCH1, TH, and SR deficiencies.

Any pediatric patient diagnosed with dystonia without clear etiology should receive an observed trial of levodopa to rule out DRD.

This chapter summarizes clinical characteristics in DRD and related disorders and recent advances in the genetics and biochemistry of these disorders.

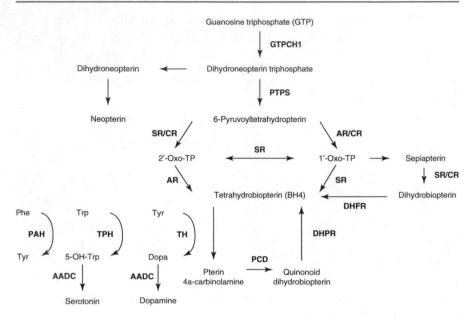

Fig. 24.1 Biosynthesis and regeneration of tetrahydrobiopterin (BH4) and BH4-dependent hydroxylation of aromatic amino acids. AADC aromatic amino acid decarboxylase, AR aldose reductase, CR carbonyl reductase, DHFR dihydrofolate reductase, DHPR dihydropteridine reductase, GTPCH1 GTP cyclohydrolase 1, PAH phenylalanine hydroxylase, PCD pterin-4a-carbinolamine dehydratase, Phe phenylalanine, PTPS 6-pyruvoyltetrahydropterin synthase, SR sepiapterin reductase, TH tyrosine hydroxylase, TPH tryptophan hydroxylase, Trp tryptophan, Tyr tyrosine, 1'-oxo-TP 2'-hydroxy-1'-oxopropyltetrahydrobiopterin, 2'-oxo-TP 1'-hydroxy-2'-oxopropyltetrahydrobiopterin, 5-OH-Trp 5-hydroxytryptophan

Clinical Observations

Classic DRD

In 1971, Segawa et al. [21] and Castaigne et al. [22] independently reported clinical characteristics of one family each with DRD, which they called at that time "hereditary progressive basal ganglia disease with marked fluctuation" and "progressive extrapyramidal disorder," respectively. Advances in the genetics and biochemistry of DRD have demonstrated that the former had autosomal dominant GTPCH1 deficiency and the latter had autosomal recessive TH deficiency [11, 23, 24]. In both families, a dramatic and sustained response to low doses of levodopa without motor side effects during chronic levodopa treatment had been confirmed [5, 21–26].

In patients with classic DRD, there is no abnormality in the perinatal and postnatal period (see Table 24.1). Early motor development (e.g., sitting and crawling) is generally normal. The average age of onset of typical DRD is approximately 6 years [5, 6]. Initial symptoms in most patients with childhood-onset DRD are gait difficulty due to dystonia in the leg, typically flexion-inversion of the foot (talipes equinovarus). Because of this dystonic posturing, patients often wear the outer side of their shoes down easily. A relatively small number of patients have onset with arm or neck dystonia, tremor (mainly postural), or slowness of movements. In childhood-onset patients, gradual progression to generalized dystonia occurs, but dystonia is typically more pronounced in the lower limbs throughout the disease course. There is a tendency to fall, and standing position with equinovarus posturing of the feet can induce increased lumbar lordosis, flexion of the hip joints, and hyperextension of the knee joints. A variable degree of rigidity and slowness of movements are recognized in the affected limbs. Rapid fatiguing of effort with repetitive motor tasks (e.g., foot tapping) is often observed. On neurologic examination, in addition to dystonic and parkinsonian elements, some clinical findings suggestive of pyramidal signs in the lower extremities (brisk deep-tendon reflexes, ankle clonus, spasticity, and/or [intermittent] extensor plantar responses) are detected in many patients. Normal efferent corticospinal activity using magnetoelectrical stimulation of motor cortex has suggested a nonpyramidal basis for these findings [27]. Dystonic extension of the big toe in DRD (the striatal toe [28]), which occurs spontaneously or is induced by plantar stimulation, may be misinterpreted as an extensor plantar response. Typical diurnal fluctuation of symptoms (aggravation of symptoms toward the evening and alleviation of symptoms in the morning after sleep) occurs in approximately 80% of patients. The magnitude of diurnal fluctuation generally attenuates with age and disease progression.

⚷ Diurnal fluctuation is characteristic of DRD. The degree of fluctuation is variable, with some patients being normal in the morning and others being only less severely affected in the morning compared to later in the day. Some cases only show exercise-induced exacerbation or manifestation of dystonia, or complain of prominent stiffness and fatigue after exercise.

A predominance of clinically affected females is observed in autosomal dominant DRD. The female-to-male ratio has been reported to be 1.3:1–8.3:1 [5, 6, 24, 29–32]. Estimates suggest that DRD is recognized worldwide and the prevalence in both England and Japan is 0.5 per million and that 5–10% of dystonia patients in childhood or adolescence have DRD [4, 28]. Recently, however, Dobričić et al. [32] have reported that the prevalence of GTPCH1-deficient DRD in Serbia was 2.96 per million; there was no evidence for a common founder, but haplotype analysis indicated that some of the patients had common ancestors. Generally, the severity of gait disturbance and dystonia in adolescent-onset cases is milder than that in childhood-onset cases. Patients with adolescent-onset DRD seldom develop severe generalized dystonia. However, dystonia in female patients can be markedly exacerbated after taking oral contraceptives [29, 33, 34]. Teenage-onset patients with slow progression may become more symptomatic in mid-adulthood due to development of overt parkinsonian features [35]. In general, there are no intellectual, cerebellar, sensory, or autonomic disturbances in classic DRD patients.

Phenotypic Heterogeneity

The following wide range of symptoms and signs has been reported in DRD families, especially in those associated with dominantly inherited *GCH1* mutations.

Adult-Onset Parkinsonism

There are two types of adult-onset parkinsonism, "benign" parkinsonism and "neurodegenerative" parkinsonism, in GTPCH1-deficient DRD pedigrees [36]. An earlier linkage study demonstrated "benign" adult-onset parkinsonism (showing slow progression and no motor adverse effects of levodopa) as a phenotypic expression of autosomal dominant DRD [10]. Patients with this phenotype manifest no dystonic symptoms prior to the onset of their parkinsonism, including resting tremor, in mid- or late adulthood [10, 37, 38]. Cases with "benign" parkinsonism due to heterozygous *GCH1* mutations markedly respond to low doses of levodopa and remain functionally normal for a long period of time without developing motor response fluctuations, freezing episodes, or dopa-induced dyskinesias under optimal doses of levodopa [29, 39–44]. An age-related decline of striatal biopterin during adulthood could contribute to this parkinsonian phenotype [16, 45]. Positron emission tomography (PET) and single-photon emission computed tomography (SPECT) investigations using presynaptic dopaminergic markers demonstrated normal results in "benign" parkinsonism [38, 46–51]. In some GTPCH1-deficient DRD pedigrees, patients with "neurodegenerative" parkinsonism or dystonia-parkinsonism associated with *GCH1* pathogenic variants have been found, and in contrast to observations in "benign" parkinsonism, these patients demonstrated abnormal ^{18}F-fluorodopa PET or dopamine transporter (DAT) SPECT imaging [49, 50, 52–57]. Investigations on *GCH1*, including genome-wide association studies, have highlighted this gene as a low-risk susceptibility locus for Parkinson's disease (PD) [57–61].

Follow-Up of the Patient in the Second Vignette The proband (patient 2) in the second vignette [3] later developed motor adverse effects of chronic levodopa therapy, severe wearing off, and dopa-induced dyskinesias, which necessitated bilateral globus pallidus internus deep brain stimulation treatment. Although we have not performed DAT imaging on her, this patient could have "neurodegenerative" dystonia-parkinsonism associated with a *GCH1* mutation.

DRD Simulating Cerebral Palsy or Spastic Paraplegia

There were DRD patients who were initially misdiagnosed as having cerebral palsy (the spastic diplegic form) or spastic paraplegia (the familial or apparently sporadic form) because of hyperreflexia, clonus, spasticity, and/or extensor plantar responses in the legs [40, 43, 62–66]. As mentioned, a nonpyramidal basis for these findings in DRD has been suggested [27]. An extensor plantar response observed in DRD often disappears after starting levodopa administration, suggesting that the previous finding may be a dystonic phenomenon (the striatal toe) rather than a Babinski response. Mutations in *GCH1*, *TH*, and *SPR* have been identified in patients with DRD simulating cerebral palsy (including other forms) or spastic paraplegia [19, 20, 40, 43, 64–69]. Thus, although the differential diagnosis of cerebral palsy and of spastic paraplegia should include DRD, this appears to be still underappreciated.

Various Types of Focal Dystonia

The clinical phenotype of DRD associated with heterozygous mutations in *GCH1* has been extended to include various types of focal dystonia (e.g., adult-onset guitarist's cramp) and spontaneous remission of dystonia and/or parkinsonism (sometimes with a relapse in the later course of illness) [29, 39, 40, 70–73]. However, in our experience, pure writer's cramp and isolated scoliosis were not always associated with *GCH1* mutations found in the probands with the classic phenotype [16, 43, 74].

Other Involuntary Movements

In rare instances, exaggerated startle responses, involuntary jerky movements, or cerebellar signs were observed in GTPCH-deficient DRD [75–77]. Leuzzi et al. [76] reported a GTPCH1-deficient DRD patient who showed delayed attainment of early motor milestones and myoclonus-dystonia responding to levodopa; myoclonus-dystonia as a phenotype of GTPCH1-deficient DRD was recognized only in this case [13, 31, 78].

Non-motor Symptoms

In GTPCH1-deficient DRD, conflicting results have been reported on non-motor symptoms. Psychiatric and behavioral symptoms (depressive disorders, panic attacks, obsessive-compulsive disorder, etc.), sleep disorders, migraine, and/or restless legs syndrome were found in some families with *GCH1*-associated DRD [24, 29, 75, 79, 80]. Antelmi et al. [81] analyzed published data on non-motor symptoms in patients with "GTPCH1-deficient DRD" and stated that overt non-motor symptoms would suggest a diagnosis of "DRD plus" diseases (other neurotransmitter disorders that may sometimes mimic DRD) rather than of GTPCH1-deficient DRD. Tadic et al. [82] described that 6 of their 23 cases with GTPCH1-deficient DRD reported 1 or more non-motor symptoms including depression, anxiety, or migraine. However, a more recent investigation by the same researchers (a case-control study using levodopa-treated cases) did not confirm an increased frequency of non-motor symptoms [83]. Recently, Timmers et al. [84] have found a higher lifetime prevalence of psychiatric disorders and daytime sleepiness in adults but not in children with GTPCH1-deficient DRD.

Molecular Genetics

GTPCH1-Deficient DRD

The enzyme GTPCH1 is encoded by a single copy gene, *GCH1*, which is composed of six exons spanning approximately 30 kilobases [85]. This enzyme catalyzes the rate-limiting step in the biosynthetic pathway for BH4 (see Fig. 24.1). BH4 is the natural cofactor not only for TH but also for phenylalanine hydroxylase (PAH) and tryptophan hydroxylase (TPH), and most patients with autosomal recessive GTPCH1 deficiency (usually homozygotes) have BH4-dependent hyperphenylalaninemia (HPA) and severe neurologic dysfunction [85–88]. In contrast to these patients, GTPCH1-deficient DRD patients (usually heterozygotes) never develop HPA. There is another phenotype of GTPCH1 deficiency, dystonia with motor delay, associated with compound heterozygosity or rarely homozygosity for *GCH1* mutations [29, 33, 42, 89–94]. In patients with these GTPCH1 deficiencies (i.e., GTPCH1-deficient DRD [mild], dystonia with motor delay [moderate], and GTPCH1-deficient HPA [severe]), more than 250 *GCH1* mutations have been reported [9]. Penetrance in patients with GTPCH1-deficient DRD was reported to be higher in females than in males (87% vs. 38% [30]), indicating gender-related incomplete penetrance; similar rates have been confirmed in this autosomal dominant disorder (87% vs. 35% [24]). No clear correlations between specific clinical features and types of *GCH1* mutations have been established in GTPCH1-deficient DRD.

In reports on DRD, in which sequence analysis of *GCH1* was conducted in a relatively large number of families, mutations in the coding region (including the splice sites) of this gene were found in approximately 60% of pedigrees with DRD [95]; the *GCH1* mutation detection rate by this sequence analysis ranged from 20% [96] to 80% [16, 24, 97]. For *GCH1* "coding region mutation-negative" DRD families, possible explanations (as suggested previously [7, 16, 95]) are the following: (1) a large genomic deletion in *GCH1* [3, 14, 32, 44, 66, 72, 97–102] or an intragenic duplication [75] or inversion of *GCH1*; (2) a mutation in noncoding regulatory regions of *GCH1* [40, 66, 70, 90, 103–105]; (3) a recessively inherited mutation in *TH* or *SPR* (see below); and (4) a mutation in, as yet undetermined, regulatory genes having an influence on *GCH1* expression or other genes, the products of which interact with GTPCH1 and can modify the enzyme function. Since our first report of a large heterozygous *GCH1* deletion in the four-generation DRD family (shown in "Patient Vignettes") [3], a variety of methods, including multiplex ligation-dependent probe amplification, have been used to detect a *GCH1* exon deletion/duplication; mutation detection rate by gene-targeted deletion/duplication analysis ranged from 0% [106, 107] to 38% [44]. A large genomic deletion in *GCH1* is an important subtype, and deletion/duplication analysis should be conducted in all of the patients with *GCH1* coding region mutation-negative DRD; in fact, after conducting additional *GCH1* analysis, Furukawa [95], Hagenah et al. [97], and Clot et al. [66] found *GCH1* mutations in 80–90% of their DRD pedigrees. When Wider et al. [14] restudied a Swiss family with DRD, which Grötzsch et al. [108] had mapped to locus named DYT14 on chromosome 14q13 (outside the *GCH1* gene on 14q22.1-q22.2 [11]), a heterozygous deletion of exons 3–6 of *GCH1* was identified.

🔑 Approximately 13% of genetically confirmed probands with GTPCH1-deficient DRD had *GCH1* variants (exon or whole-gene deletions/duplications) detected by deletion/duplication analysis [9]; thus, if sequence analysis (including whole-exome sequencing) is not diagnostic, gene-targeted deletion/duplication analysis (e.g., multiplex ligation-dependent probe amplification) or comprehensive genomic deletion/duplication analysis (e.g., exome array) should be conducted.

TH-Deficient DRD

Human *TH* consists of 14 exons spanning approximately 8.5 kilobases [19, 95]. The enzyme TH, a BH4-dependent monooxygenase, catalyzes the rate-limiting step in catecholamine biosynthesis (see Fig. 24.1). TH deficiency is associated with a wide phenotypic spectrum. Based on the severity of symptoms and signs as well as responsiveness to levodopa therapy, the clinical phenotypes can be classified into TH-deficient DRD (mild form), TH-deficient infantile parkinsonism with motor delay (severe form), and TH-deficient progressive infantile encephalopathy (very severe form) [19]. More than 20 patients with genetically confirmed TH-deficient DRD have been reported [12, 17, 22, 23, 26, 64, 106, 109–120]. In these patients, early psychomotor development is normal, and onset of symptoms is usually between ages 12 months and 12 years. Intellect is generally not impaired in patients with TH-deficient DRD; of note, Schiller et al. [109] have reported a TH-deficient DRD case with mild cognitive impairment due to infantile rhesus incompatibility. In rare instances, sustained upward ocular deviations (oculogyric crises) are observed. Typical diurnal fluctuation of symptoms has been reported in approximately one third of patients with TH-deficient DRD (a much lower incidence than recognized in GTPCH1-deficient DRD). In contrast to GTPCH1-deficient DRD [24, 30, 39], female predominance is not a clinical characteristic in TH-deficient DRD [19, 95]. A dramatic and sustained response to low doses of levodopa without any motor adverse effects for more than 30 years has been confirmed in TH-deficient DRD patients [23, 109, 121], including two affected brothers originally reported by Castaigne et al. [22]. In a family with TH-deficient DRD, the mutated recombinant enzyme showed approximately 15% of specific activity compared with the wild type in a coupled in vitro transcription-translation assay system [12, 112].

There have been some reports of adult-onset DRD patients associated with *TH* mutations [122, 123]. Bally et al. [123] have described a "heterozygote" for a *TH* pathogenic variant (c.296del [p.Leu99Argfs*15]) who developed DRD at age

38 years. Interestingly, the same *TH* deletion was previously found in a boy with DRD (compound heterozygote) and in his father with exercise-induced stiffness responding to levodopa (heterozygote) [64]. It has been suggested that a subtle phenotypic effect in heterozygotes for autosomal recessive disorders may be more common than is generally considered [64, 124].

SR-Deficient DRD

The very mild form of autosomal recessive SR deficiency is a rare cause of DRD [9, 18, 20]. The human dimeric enzyme SR is encoded by *SPR* which consists of three exons [87]. Arrabal et al. [18] reported one family with a strikingly mild phenotype (without motor and cognitive delay) of SR deficiency associated with compound heterozygosity for *SPR* pathogenic variants; one was a missense mutation, and the other was a partially penetrant splicing mutation. Even in this pedigree with SR-deficient DRD, an affected family member showed decreased levels of the neurotransmitter metabolites homovanillic acid (HVA) and 5-hydroxyindoleacetic acid (5-HIAA) in CSF. Levodopa and 5-hydroxytryptophan were administered for the affected individual, but 5-hydroxytryptophan was not tolerated. Other cases with recessively inherited SR deficiency usually develop more severe symptoms [67, 125–130].

Recently, Shalash et al. [131] have reported a rare heterozygous *SPR* mutation as a cause of autosomal dominant SR-deficient DRD with incomplete penetrance and a common heterozygous variant in the dihydrofolate reductase gene (*DHFR*) as a potential modifier, affecting the penetrance of the pathogenic *SPR* variant; the presence of another case with DRD due to dominantly inherited SR deficiency was suggested previously [132].

Genetically Related Disorders

Severe GTPCH1 Deficiency (GTPCH1-Deficient HPA)

Patients with autosomal recessive GTPCH1 deficiency generally develop BH4-dependent HPA in the first 6 months of life [85–88, 95]. There was no detectable GTPCH1 activity in liver biopsy specimens in cases with GTPCH1-deficient HPA. This disorder presents with severe dysfunction, including convulsions, mental retardation, swallowing difficulties, developmental motor delay, truncal hypotonia, limb hypertonia, involuntary movements, and autonomic symptoms. In the first report of recessively inherited GTPCH1 deficiency by Niederwieser et al. [86], hyperreflexia with an extensor plantar response was also described. In contrast to dominantly inherited GTPCH1-deficient DRD patients, administration of levodopa, 5-hydroxytryptophan, and BH4 is necessary for recessively inherited GTPCH1-deficient HPA patients [7, 86, 87].

Moderate GTPCH1 Deficiency (Dystonia with Motor Delay)

A phenotype of GTPCH1 deficiency (dystonia with motor delay), which is clinically and biochemically intermediate between GTPCH1-deficient DRD (mild) and GTPCH1-deficient HPA (severe), has been found in compound heterozygotes and rarely homozygotes for *GCH1* mutations [29, 33, 42, 89–94]. This phenotype is characterized by developmental motor delay, limb dystonia (with truncal hypotonia) that progresses to generalized dystonia, and no overt HPA in infancy. Such cases could be misdiagnosed initially as having cerebral palsy. In three compound heterozygotes [33, 42, 90], their mothers and maternal grandmothers (all heterozygotes) developed DRD symptoms, suggesting that intrafamilial phenotypic heterogeneity in some GTPCH1-deficient DRD pedigrees may be explained by an additional *GCH1* mutation [7, 95]. Kong et al. [133] have reported a boy with a heterozygous *GCH1* missense mutation, who was floppy in his early infancy and had developmental motor delay, in a GTPCH1-deficient DRD family. This boy might have an additional large deletion/duplication in *GCH1* on the other allele. It is worth noting that one compound heterozygote responded remarkably to low doses of levodopa and made further improvement in motor function when BH4 was chronically added to maintenance levodopa treatment [33, 134].

Contiguous Gene Deletion Syndrome Relating to GTPCH1 Deficiency

Lohmann et al. [135] identified chromosome rearrangements, which included a large deletion encompassing *GCH1* and adjacent genes, in a pedigree with seemingly non-Mendelian inheritance of DRD associated with digital and eye abnormalities; the proband in this family was previously reported to have a heterozygous deletion of all six exons of *GCH1* [97].

Other BH4-Related Enzyme Deficiencies Including Severe SR Deficiency

Patients with autosomal recessive BH4-related enzyme deficiencies (so called BH4 deficiencies [87]), including recessively inherited severe GTPCH1 deficiency (see above), develop BH4-dependent HPA in the first 6 months of life; an exception is autosomal recessive SR deficiency (in which BH4 is synthesized through the salvage pathway in peripheral tissues where dihydrofolate reductase activity is preserved [87, 125, 126, 128, 136, 137]). These patients typically present with severe neurologic dysfunction (e.g., psychomotor retardation, convulsions, microcephaly, swallowing difficulties, hypersomnia, cognitive impairment, truncal hypotonia, limb hypertonia, paroxysmal stiffening, involuntary movements, oculogyric crises); diurnal fluctuation of symptoms and/or dystonia "partially" responding to levodopa can be seen in some cases [7, 67, 95, 125–130, 138, 139]. For patients with the severe form of autosomal recessive SR deficiency, oral administration of both levodopa and 5-hydroxytryptophan is necessary because of very low levels of HVA and 5-HIAA in CSF [67, 128]. BH4 treatment and neurotransmitter replacement therapy (levodopa and 5-hydroxytryptophan) are indispensable for patients with other autosomal recessive BH4-related enzyme deficiencies [7, 87].

Very Severe TH Deficiency (TH-Deficient Progressive Infantile Encephalopathy)

More than 20 patients with molecularly confirmed TH-deficient progressive infantile encephalopathy have been reported [115, 117, 120, 140–153]. The onset is before age 3–6 months. Fetal distress is recognized in most; patients may demonstrate feeding difficulties, hypotonia, and/or growth retardation affecting head circumference, height, and/or weight from birth. Determining the age of onset is sometimes difficult because of complicated perinatal events. Patients have marked delay in motor development, truncal hypotonia, severe hypokinesia, limb hypertonia, hyperreflexia with extensor plantar responses, oculogyric crises, bilateral ptosis, intellectual disability, and paroxysmal periods of lethargy (with increased sweating and drooling) alternating with irritability (lethargy-irritability crises [115]). In general, dystonia is not a prominent clinical feature; however, in the most severely affected infants, dystonic crises (every 4–5 days) have been reported [115, 147]. Other involuntary movements can be observed in some. Although autonomic disturbances occur, especially in the periods of lethargy-irritability crises, the clinical characteristics of impaired production of peripheral catecholamines (e.g., abnormalities in the maintenance of blood pressure) are not present [115, 140]. Usually, typical diurnal fluctuation of symptoms is not recognized. Patients are extremely sensitive to levodopa therapy; thus, treatment with levodopa is often limited by intolerable dyskinesias. Some cases develop severe dyskinesias even at doses of 0.2–1.5 mg/kg/day levodopa (with a DCI); no or only minimum improvement can be detected in these cases [140, 142, 147].

Severe TH Deficiency (TH-Deficient Infantile Parkinsonism with Motor Delay)

More than 50 patients with genetically confirmed TH-deficient infantile parkinsonism with motor delay have been reported [66, 110, 115–117, 120, 148, 150, 154–171]. In general, the pregnancies of affected individuals are uncomplicated. Perinatal and early postnatal periods are usually normal. Onset in most patients is between ages 3 and 12 months. In this severe form, motor milestones are overtly delayed in infancy. All patients demonstrate truncal hypotonia as well as parkinsonian symptoms and signs. Although dystonia is recognized in most, it tends to be less prominent. Brisk deep-tendon reflexes, spasticity, and/or extensor plantar responses are frequently detected. Oculogyric crises are often observed. Ptosis and other features of mild autonomic dysfunction can be recognized. Intellectual disability is found in many of the affected individuals. Typical diurnal fluctuation of symptoms is not observed in most patients. Of note, diurnal variation of axial hypotonia but not of limb dystonia has been described in one case [66, 163]. Patients demonstrate a marked response to levodopa. However, in contrast to TH-deficient DRD, the responsiveness is generally not complete, and/or it takes several months or even years for the full effects of treatment to become established. Some cases are hypersensitive to levodopa and are prone to intolerable dyskinesias; because of this hypersensitivity, such cases should be treated with very low initial doses of levodopa [66, 117, 163]. Because null variants of *TH* are lethal as shown in *TH* (−/−) knockout mice [172], patients associated with mutations of this gene appear to have some residual TH activity. In fact, in a patient with TH-deficient infantile parkinsonism with motor delay, the mutated TH revealed 0.3–16% of wild-type enzyme activity in three complementary expression systems [154].

Atypical Forms of Severe TH Deficiency

TH-Deficient Myoclonus-Dystonia
Stamelou et al. [173] reported three sibs with severe TH deficiency who presented with truncal hypotonia, developmental motor delay, generalized dystonia, and prominent myoclonic jerks in infancy. The proband had a normal birth but was floppy. After beginning levodopa treatment at age 13 years, all of her symptoms, including cognitive dysfunction, markedly improved. She could walk some steps with help but had generalized dystonia, choreoathetoid movements, slowing in finger-tapping, and myoclonic jerks even 5 years after starting levodopa therapy.

TH Deficiency with Exacerbation by Viral Infections
Diepold et al. [174] reported one patient with developmental psychomotor delay, truncal hypotonia, parkinsonism, and dystonic posturing of the hands. These symptoms were induced and/or exacerbated by viral infections. Although he demonstrated a remarkable response to levodopa, this case still had truncal hypotonia and developmental delay 6 months after starting levodopa treatment.

TH Deficiency with a Biphasic Clinical Course
Giovanniello et al. [175] described one case with TH deficiency showing a biphasic course. Psychomotor development was normal in early infancy. In the second year of life, he demonstrated toe-walking, frequent falls, and developmental language delay. At age 11 years, he developed involuntary movements over the course of a few months. When examined at age 13 years, he had generalized choreoathetosis, myoclonic jerks, dysarthria, gaze paresis, oculogyric crises, and borderline IQ. He showed hypersensitivity to levodopa and could be treated only with very low doses.

Laboratory Investigations

Routine blood counts and chemistries, plasma and urine amino acids, and serum copper and ceruloplasmin are normal in patients with DRD.

CSF Analysis

Before the discovery of *GCH1* mutations, a functional abnormality of brain GTPCH1 was suggested by decreased levels of CSF total biopterin and neopterin in autosomal dominant DRD [1, 8, 176–178]. Total biopterin (BP) includes BH4, quinonoid dihydrobiopterin, and 7,8-dihydrobiopterin, and total neopterin (NP) consists of degradation products (dihydroneopterin and neopterin) of dihydroneopterin triphosphate, which is synthesized from GTP by GTPCH1 [179] (see Fig. 24.1). Most of brain BP exists as BH4 and more than 70% of CSF NP exists as the dihydro form [179]. Generally, NP is considered to reflect GTPCH1 activity, and there have been no negative reports on the results of CSF NP measurement (low NP concentrations) in all GTPCH1-deficient disorders [1, 2, 33, 65, 79, 180–184], except for one report showing a borderline value in an atypical case with dominantly inherited GTPCH1 deficiency [76]. Decreased NP levels in CSF are not observed in other types of BH4 deficiency [16, 18, 125, 128]. Measurements of both BP and NP in CSF are useful for the differential diagnoses of the following diseases responsive to levodopa [2, 7, 8, 35]: GTPCH1-deficient disorders (low BP and NP), TH-deficient disorders (normal BP and NP), and PD or EOPD (low BP associated with normal NP), including autosomal recessive parkin type of EOPD caused by *PRKN* mutations. Precise determination of CSF levels of neurotransmitter metabolites (before starting levodopa therapy) is diagnostic of TH-deficient disorders (low HVA and 3-methoxy-4-hydroxyphenylethyleneglycol associated with normal 5-HIAA) [7, 19, 115, 117, 154, 155, 158]. Detection of sepiapterin in CSF is useful for the diagnosis of SR-deficient disorders (in which brain sepiapterin in the salvage pathway accumulates owing to very low dihydrofolate reductase activity in the brain) [87, 125, 126, 128, 136, 137].

Activity Assay

Ichinose et al. [11] reported that GTPCH1 activity levels in phytohemagglutinin (PHA)-stimulated mononuclear blood cells were decreased in DRD patients having *GCH1* mutations. Using cultured lymphoblasts, however, Bezin et al. [185] have suggested that the PHA induction alone misrepresents the actual status of GTPCH1 activity. Activity of GTPCH1 in PHA-stimulated mononuclear blood cells was lower in normal females than in normal males in one report [11]. Nevertheless, there was no difference of this activity between females and males in another report from the same group [186]. Unfortunately, non-stimulated GTPCH1 activity in mononuclear blood cells is too low to be measured. Measurement of GTPCH1 activity in cytokine-stimulated fibroblasts was reported to be useful for the diagnosis [80, 181]. In coexpression studies, it has been demonstrated that GTPCH1 with dominantly inherited *GCH1* mutations but not recessively inherited ones inactivated the wild-type enzyme, suggesting a critical role of this dominant negative effect in autosomal dominant GTPCH1-deficient DRD [187–189]. However, Suzuki et al. [190] has suggested that such a dominant negative effect is unlikely to explain low enzyme activity in PHA-stimulated mononuclear blood cells from GTPCH1-deficient DRD patients (<20% of controls [11]) and that a reduction of the amount of GTPCH1 protein found in these cells may contribute to the mechanism of dominant inheritance. The enzyme TH is mainly expressed in the brain and the adrenal medulla, and direct measurement of its activity is not a diagnostic option. Reduced levels of SR activity in fibroblasts have been reported in patients with SR-deficient disorders [18, 128].

Phenylalanine Loading Test

Patients with DRD never develop HPA. However, a subclinical defect in phenylalanine metabolism (due to partial BH4 deficiency in the liver) can be detected in GTPCH1-deficient and SR-deficient DRD patients by the phenylalanine loading test, analyzing plasma phenylalanine-to-tyrosine ratios for 6 or 4 h following an oral phenylalanine load (100 mg/kg) [18, 191–193]. The reason for the difference in susceptibility to a BH4-deficient condition between TH and PAH could relate to different Km (Michaelis constant) values of the hydroxylases for BH4 [95].

Neuroimaging

Brain CT and MRI are normal in patients with DRD. PET and SPECT investigations using presynaptic dopaminergic markers have shown normal or near-normal results in the striatum of DRD and "benign" parkinsonism due to *GCH1* mutations (see *GCH1*-associated "benign" parkinsonism and "neurodegenerative" parkinsonism in "Phenotypic Heterogeneity") [38, 46–52, 182, 194–196]. These PET and SPECT findings are consistent with normal striatal levels of aromatic amino acid decarboxylase (AADC), DAT, and vesicular monoamine transporter in autopsied patients with GTPCH1-deficient DRD, indicating that striatal dopamine nerve terminals are preserved in this disorder [35, 41]. Examinations of PET and SPECT using presynaptic dopaminergic markers revealed no abnormalities even in more severely affected cases with autosomal recessive SR deficiency [128, 197]. Using [^{11}C]-raclopride PET, elevated D2 receptor binding has been found in the striatum of patients with DRD [47, 196, 198]. This increased receptor binding could be due to receptor upregulation and/or diminished competition for the tracer as a consequence of low synaptic dopamine concentration. An approach using network analysis of [^{18}F]-fluorodeoxyglucose PET images was not sufficiently sensitive for diagnosis of GTPCH1-deficient DRD [31, 199].

Neuropathology

Neuropathologic investigations showed a normal population of cells with reduced melanin and no evidence of Lewy body formation in the substantia nigra of four symptomatic cases with typical GTPCH1-deficient DRD and one asymptomatic case with a *GCH1* mutation (in a family with classic DRD linked to the *GCH1* locus [10]) [14, 35, 41, 108, 200, 201]. No degenerative changes in the substantia nigra were observed even in a 90-year-old GTPCH1-deficient DRD patient having a disease duration of 82 years [201]. Recently, Schreglmann et al. [121] have found a pallor of neuromelanin containing neurons without decreased cell density in the substantia nigra of one patient with TH-deficient DRD; clinical and genetic characteristics of this patient were reported previously by Schiller et al. [109]. There have been no reports of neuropathologic findings in SR-deficient DRD.

Neurochemistry

Neurochemical data from two of the four symptomatic cases with GTPCH1-deficient DRD and the *GCH1*-associated asymptomatic case are available [35, 41, 200, 202]. In the putamen, BP and NP concentrations were substantially lower in the two patients (mean: −84% and −62%) than in age-matched normal controls. Striatal subregional dopamine data pointed to an involvement of the caudal portion of the putamen as the striatal subregion that was most affected by dopamine loss in both patients (−88%) [35, 200]. Dopamine content in this striatal subdivision was normal in an autopsied individual with *DYT1* dystonia [203]. It is known that the caudal putamen is most affected by loss of dopamine in patients with PD [204–207]. In the asymptomatic *GCH1* mutation carrier, decreases in BP and NP levels in the putamen (−82% and −57%) paralleled those in the two symptomatic cases [41]. However, in this asymptomatic case, dopamine content in the caudal subdivision of the putamen was not as severely reduced (−44%) as in the symptomatic cases. Consistent with other postmortem data suggesting that greater than 60–80% of striatal dopamine loss is necessary for overt motor symptoms to occur [205], the maximal 44% dopamine reduction in the striatum of the asymptomatic *GCH1* mutation carrier was not sufficient to produce any symptoms of GTPCH1-deficient DRD.

In contrast to patients with PD [208, 209], striatal levels of AADC, DAT, and vesicular monoamine transporter were normal in the two symptomatic cases with GTPCH1-deficient DRD, indicating that dopaminergic terminals in the striatum are preserved in this disorder [35]. However, TH protein levels were markedly decreased in the putamen of both symptomatic cases (>−97%). These biochemical findings have suggested that striatal dopamine reduction in GTPCH1-deficient DRD is caused not only by decreased TH activity due to low cofactor content but also by actual loss of TH protein without nerve terminal loss. The human brain data are compatible with TH protein loss but preserved AADC in brains of BH4-deficient mice [210–213]. In contrast to the symptomatic cases, TH protein content in the putamen was only moderately reduced in the asymptomatic case (−52%) [41].

Striatal TH protein reduction in GTPCH1-deficient DRD may be caused by a diminished regulatory effect of BH4 on the steady-state level (stability/expression) of TH molecules [35]. Because TH protein concentrations in the substantia nigra, where striatal TH molecules are synthesized, were normal in both symptomatic cases, BH4 could control stability rather than expression of this enzyme [16, 35]. This is supported by a report showing loss of TH protein but not of *TH* mRNA in brains of BH4-deficient mice [211–213]. The neurochemical findings in the asymptomatic *GCH1* mutation carrier suggest that the extent of striatal TH protein loss may be critical in determining the symptomatic state of GTPCH1-deficient DRD [41]. As BH4 is also the cofactor for TPH, it has been assumed that partial BH4 deficiency in GTPCH1-deficient DRD results in lowering of brain serotonin. However, all serotonin markers (serotonin, TPH, and serotonin transporter [206, 214]) have been found to be normal in the striatum of GTPCH1-deficient DRD [202].

In a 16-week-old miscarried human fetus having compound heterozygous *TH* mutations, protein levels of dopaminergic markers, including TH, in the mesencephalon and pons were reported to be lower than those in "one" control subject [151]; a sister of this fetus had the same mutations in *TH* and developed TH-deficient progressive infantile encephalopathy [146]. In contrast, almost normal content of mutant TH protein in the substantia nigra and distinct loss of this enzyme in the striatum were recognized in encephalopathy *TH* knockin mice [215]. Moreover, in DRD *TH* knockin mice [216, 217], normal number of TH-positive neurons in the substantia nigra and severely reduced TH immunostaining, associated with normal DAT staining, in the striatum were observed. There have been no reports of neurochemical data in patients with classic TH-deficient DRD and SR deficiency.

Diagnosis

The diagnoses of GTPCH1-deficient DRD, TH-deficient DRD, and SR-deficient DRD can be established by identification of *GCH1*, *TH*, and *SPR* mutations, respectively, by gene-targeted testing or comprehensive genomic testing (e.g., exome sequencing); approximately 87% of genetically proven probands with GTPCH1-deficient DRD had *GCH1* mutations detected by sequence analysis, and the remaining 13% had *GCH1* mutations identified by deletion/duplication analysis (e.g., multiplex ligation-dependent probe amplification) [9]. Unfortunately, however, not all patients with DRD have demonstrated pathogenic variants of *GCH1*, *TH*, or *SPR*. Biochemical testing (see "Laboratory Investigations") should be conducted in these mutation-negative cases, and a therapeutic trial with low doses of levodopa based on clinical suspicion is still crucial to the diagnosis of DRD.

Once *GCH1*, *TH*, and *SPR* mutations have been identified in probands, prenatal diagnoses for pregnancy are possible, and some results of prenatal testing have been reported [146, 153, 169]. Using next-generation sequencing, Nedelea et al. [153] found a heterozygous *GCH1* variant (reported previously [65, 76]) and also a homozygous *TH* variant (not described in the literature) in a proband (the first child) with progressive infantile encephalopathy. In this family, the prenatal testing revealed that a fetus (the second child) was a heterozygote for the *TH* variant; the second child was delivered at term, and early postnatal evolution was normal. Based on the available information, both *GCH1* and *TH* variants identified in the proband were classified as "variants of unknown clinical significance," and deletion/duplication analysis of these genes revealed no additional mutations. Thus, interpretation of genetic results is sometimes difficult, and a multidisciplinary approach in the context of new diagnostic techniques is recommended [31, 153].

The major differential diagnoses of DRD include EOPD, *DYT1* dystonia, cerebral palsy, and spastic paraplegia. Patients with EOPD responding markedly to levodopa, especially those with onset below age 20 years, often develop gait disturbance due to foot dystonia as the initial symptom [2, 8, 9]. Furthermore, these EOPD patients can demonstrate mild to moderate diurnal fluctuation (sleep benefit) prior to levodopa administration. Thus, the clinical differentiation between EOPD patients with dystonia and DRD patients in the early course of disorder is sometimes difficult. In general, the most reliable clinical distinction between EOPD (particularly autosomal recessive parkin type of EOPD due to *PRKN* mutations) and DRD is the occurrence of motor adverse effects of chronic levodopa therapy (wearing-off and on-off phenomena and dopa-induced dyskinesias) in EOPD. Under optimal doses, typically, patients with DRD on long-term levodopa treatment do not develop these complications. A dramatic and sustained response to low doses of levodopa in DRD distinguishes this disorder from all other forms of dystonia, including *DYT1* dystonia, and from cerebral palsy as well as spastic paraplegia.

Because of characteristic diurnal fluctuation of symptoms, childhood- or adolescent-onset DRD is occasionally misdiagnosed as psychological reaction or hysteria, especially in the early course of illness.

Treatment

There is general agreement that patients with childhood-onset dystonic symptoms of unknown etiology should be treated with low doses of levodopa [5–7, 31, 218–220] (whereas Maas et al. argue against such an empiric trial of levodopa [221]). Initial use of a dose of 25 mg levodopa with a DCI (levodopa/DCI) two to three times daily and gradual increase to higher doses have been recommended [218] (Table 24.2). Although DRD patients may develop dyskinesias (mainly choreic movements) at the initiation of levodopa treatment, such dyskinesias subside following dose reduction and do not reappear with later slow-dose increments [5–7]: note that these transient dyskinesias are different from those with motor response fluctuations observed in PD and EOPD patients during chronic levodopa therapy. It has been reported that amantadine suppressed severe dopa-induced choreic dyskinesias, which developed at initiation of levodopa treatment, in two compound heterozygotes for *GCH1* mutations having dystonia and motor delay [89]. Because some children with DRD showed remarkable responsiveness to smaller doses and a

Table 24.2 Treatment for classic dopa-responsive dystonia (DRD)

Symptom	Treatment	Dose of levodopa with a decarboxylase inhibitor (DCI)/directions
Dystonia/parkinsonism	Levodopa	Initial suggested dose of levodopa with a DCI (levodopa/DCI)
		1. DRD children: 25 mg, 2–3 times daily (Nygaard et al. [218])
		2. DRD children: 25 mg, once a day (Furukawa et al. [223, 224])
		DRD adults: 50 mg, 1–2 times daily
		3. DRD children <6 years: 1–10 mg/kg daily, administered in multiple doses
		(Wijemanne and Jankovic [31])
		DRD children ≥6 years and adults: 50 mg, 1–3 times daily
		Gradual titration to higher doses of levodopa/DCI is recommended
		Motor benefit can be recognized immediately or within a few days of starting therapy
		Full benefit occurs within several days to a few months after beginning treatment
Transient dyskinesias[a] at levodopa initiation	Reduction of levodopa dose	Dyskinesias associated with levodopa initiation subside following dose reduction
		Such transient dyskinesias do not reappear with later slow increments in dose

[a]Note that these dyskinesias are different from those observed in Parkinson's disease during chronic levodopa treatment

child manifesting dystonia and motor delay developed very severe dyskinesias (which lasted 4 days) after receiving a single 50 mg dose of levodopa/DCI [33, 222], we have suggested starting a therapeutic trial using a dose of 25 mg levodopa/DCI, once a day, for dystonia children without developmental motor delay and of 12.5 mg levodopa/DCI, once a day, or even less for those with overt motor delay in infancy [223, 224]. In fact, the child manifesting dystonia and motor delay was successfully treated with an initial dosage of 8 mg/day of levodopa/DCI [33]. Recently, Wijemanne and Jankovic [31] have suggested an initial dose of 1–10 mg/kg levodopa/DCI daily, administered in multiple doses, for children aged below 6 years and of 50 mg levodopa/DCI one to three times daily for children aged above 6 years. For adult patients, an initial dose of 50 mg levodopa/DCI, once or twice a day [223, 224], or the same dose, once to three times a day [31], has been recommended. In DRD patients, motor benefit can be recognized immediately or within a few days, and full benefit occurs within several days to a few months after beginning levodopa administration. Maximum benefit (complete or near-complete responsiveness of symptoms) is generally achieved by less than 300 mg/day of levodopa/DCI (see Table 24.1) or by less than 20–30 mg/kg/day of levodopa without a DCI [5, 6, 218]. According to Nygaard and Duvoisin [225], no dose of levodopa/DCI greater than 400 mg/day was necessary for DRD patients. Some genetically confirmed patients with GTPCH1-deficient DRD needed 400 mg/day or more of levodopa/DCI [29, 43,

222]. A continued stable response to levodopa therapy and no complications for more than 30 years have been confirmed in patients with GTPCH1-deficient DRD and TH-deficient DRD [5, 21–26, 29, 109, 121, 201]. Even DRD cases untreated for more than 40 years showed a remarkable response at initiation of levodopa treatment [5, 6, 14, 108]. In 20 pregnancies reported in 12 patients with GTPCH1-deficient DRD, levodopa therapy was continued without adverse effects in most, and no fetal abnormalities were recognized [29]. Exacerbation of symptoms after taking oral contraceptives was found in some female cases with GTPCH1-deficient DRD [29, 33, 34].

Physicians should avoid discontinuing levodopa therapy and using anti-dopaminergic agents (including some antipsychotic medications) in patients with DRD.

Although DRD patients can respond to anticholinergics and dopamine agonists, the efficacy of levodopa is usually superior to that of these other drugs [5, 29, 218]. The limited clinical literature demonstrates that acute BH4 treatment may be much less effective than levodopa therapy for patients with GTPCH1-deficient DRD, including the apparently sporadic patient shown in the first vignette [2, 176, 226]. In this genetically proven patient, BH4 (40 mg/kg/day) was orally administered for 5 consecutive days [2]. Although the dosage of BH4 should be sufficient to enter the brain [227–229], no functional benefit was found from this acute oral BH4 administration. Even after intravenous infusion of BH4 in GTPCH1-deficient DRD patients, HVA concentrations in CSF were unchanged despite marked elevation of BP levels in CSF [226]. The low efficacy of such acute administration of BH4 (adequate to cross the blood-brain barrier) may be explained by striatal TH protein loss in GTPCH1-deficient DRD, which would be expected to limit any acute stimulatory effect of the cofactor BH4 on dopamine biosynthesis [35]. In contrast, the remarkable efficacy of levodopa (which bypasses TH in the biosynthetic pathway of dopamine) can be explained by the normal protein levels of AADC, for which levodopa is a substrate [35]. Assuming that BH4 does, in fact, influence the steady-state level of TH protein in the human brain, it could be expected that repeated administration of BH4, if sufficiently prolonged, might upregulate TH protein content in the nigrostriatal dopaminergic terminals in GTPCH1-deficient DRD.

Conclusion

Since the discovery of *GCH1*, *TH*, and *SPR* mutations responsible for DRD, our understanding of this disorder has greatly increased. However, the underlying mechanisms of phenotypic heterogeneity (e.g., two types of adult-onset parkinsonism in GTPCH1-deficient DRD [36]) in DRD pedigrees are still unknown; there may be additional genetic and/or environmental factors that can modulate the outcome of pathogenic variants in the causative genes for DRD. As clinical suspicion is a key to the diagnosis of this treatable disorder, physicians should know the broad phenotypic spectrum in GTPCH1-, TH-, and SR-deficient DRD families. Moreover, because (1) administration of levodopa and "5-hydroxytryptophan" is necessary for severe autosomal recessive SR deficiency, (2) administration of levodopa, 5-hydroxytryptophan, and "BH4" is indispensable for other severe autosomal recessive BH4-related enzyme deficiencies (including GTPCH1-deficient HPA), and (3) very low-dose levodopa must be used initially for infantile-onset cases with severe or very severe autosomal recessive TH deficiency having overt delay in motor development (TH-deficient infantile parkinsonism with motor delay or TH-deficient progressive infantile encephalopathy), physicians should also know symptoms and signs of the genetically related disorders. No pathogenic variants have been found by molecular genetic testing in some patients with DRD. Therefore, a therapeutic trial of levodopa at low dose is still an important practical approach to the diagnosis of DRD.

References

1. Furukawa Y, Nishi K, Kondo T, Mizuno Y, Narabayashi H. CSF biopterin levels and clinical features of patients with juvenile parkinsonism. Adv Neurol. 1993;60:562–7.
2. Furukawa Y, Shimadzu M, Rajput AH, Shimuzu Y, Tagawa T, Mori H, et al. GTP-cyclohydrolase I gene mutations in hereditary progressive and dopa-responsive dystonia. Ann Neurol. 1996;39:609–17. https://doi.org/10.1002/ana.410390510.
3. Furukawa Y, Guttman M, Sparagana SP, Trugman JM, Hyland K, Wyatt P, et al. Dopa-responsive dystonia due to a large deletion in the GTP cyclohydrolase I gene. Ann Neurol. 2000;47:517–20. https://doi.org/10.1002/1531-8249(200004)47:43.0.CO;2-B
4. Nygaard TG. Dopa-responsive dystonia. Delineation of the clinical syndrome and clues to pathogenesis. Adv Neurol. 1993;60:577–85.
5. Segawa M, Nomura Y. Hereditary progressive dystonia with marked diurnal fluctuation. In: Segawa M, editor. Hereditary progressive dystonia with marked diurnal fluctuation. New York: Parthenon Publishing; 1993. p. 3–19.
6. Nygaard T, Snow B, Fahn S, Calne D. Dopa-responsive dystonia: clinical characteristics and definition. In: Segawa M, editor. Hereditary progressive dystonia with marked diurnal fluctuation. New York: Parthenon Publishing; 1993. p. 21–35.
7. Furukawa Y, Kish SJ. Dopa-responsive dystonia: recent advances and remaining issues to be addressed. Mov Disord. 1999;14:709–15. https://doi.org/10.1002/1531-8257(199909)14:53.0.CO;2-T.
8. Furukawa Y, Mizuno Y, Narabayashi H. Early-onset parkinsonism with dystonia. Clinical and biochemical differences from hereditary progressive dystonia or DOPA-responsive dystonia. Adv Neurol. 1996;69:327–37.
9. Furukawa Y. GTP cyclohydrolase 1-deficient Dopa-responsive dystonia – GeneReviews® – NCBI bookshelf n.d. https://www.ncbi.nlm.nih.gov/books/NBK1508/ (accessed 1 Apr, 2020).
10. Nygaard TG, Wilhelmsen KC, Risch NJ, Brown DL, Trugman JM, Gilliam TC, et al. Linkage mapping of dopa-responsive dystonia (DRD) to chromosome 14q. Nat Genet. 1993;5:386–91. https://doi.org/10.1038/ng1293-386.
11. Ichinose H, Ohye T, Takahashi EI, Seki N, Aki HT, Segawa M, et al. Hereditary progressive dystonia with marked diurnal fluctuation caused by mutations in the GTP cyclohydrolase I gene. Nat Genet. 1994;8:236–42. https://doi.org/10.1038/ng1194-236.
12. Lüdecke B, Dworniczak B, Bartholomé K. A point mutation in the tyrosine hydroxylase gene associated with Segawa's syndrome. Hum Genet. 1995;95:123–5. https://doi.org/10.1007/BF00225091.

13. Furukawa Y, Rajput AH. Inherited myoclonus-dystonia: how many causative genes and clinical phenotypes? Neurology. 2002;59:1130–1. https://doi.org/10.1212/WNL.59.8.1130.

14. Wider C, Melquist S, Hauf M, Solida A, Cobb SA, Kachergus JM, et al. Study of a Swiss dopa-responsive dystonia family with a deletion in GCH1: redefining DYT14 as DYT5. Neurology. 2008;70:1377–83. https://doi.org/10.1212/01.wnl.0000275527.35752.c5.

15. Larsh T, Friedman N, Fernandez H. Child neurology: genetically determined dystonias with childhood onset. Neurology. 2020;94(20):892–5. https://doi.org/10.1212/WNL.0000000000009040.

16. Furukawa Y. Genetics and biochemistry of dopa-responsive dystonia: significance of striatal tyrosine hydroxylase protein loss. Adv Neurol. 2003;91:401–10.

17. Furukawa Y, Kish SJ, Fahn S. Dopa-responsive dystonia due to mild tyrosine hydroxylase deficiency. Ann Neurol. 2004;55:147–8. https://doi.org/10.1002/ana.10820.

18. Arrabal L, Teresa L, Sánchez-Alcudia R, Castro M, Medrano C, Gutiérrez-Solana L, et al. Genotype-phenotype correlations in sepiapterin reductase deficiency. A splicing defect accounts for a new phenotypic variant. Neurogenetics. 2011;12:183–91. https://doi.org/10.1007/s10048-011-0279-4.

19. Furukawa Y, Kish S. Tyrosine hydroxylase deficiency – GeneReviews® – NCBI bookshelf n.d. https://www.ncbi.nlm.nih.gov/books/NBK1437/ (accessed 1 Apr, 2020).

20. Nakagama Y, Hamanaka K, Mimaki M, Shintaku H, Miyatake S, Matsumoto N, et al. Leaky splicing variant in sepiapterin reductase deficiency: are milder cases escaping diagnosis? Neurol Genet. 2019;5(2) https://doi.org/10.1212/NXG.0000000000000319.

21. Segawa M, Ohmi K, Itoh S, Aoyama M, Hayakawa H. Childhood basal ganglia disease with remarkable response to L-dopa, hereditary basal ganglia disease with marked diurnal fluctuation. Shinryo (Tokyo). 1971;24:667–72.

22. Castaigne P, Rondot P, Ribadeau-Dumas JL, Saïd G. Affection extrapyramidale évoluant chez deux jeunes frères; effects remarquables du traitement par la L-Dopa. Rev Neurol. 1971;124:162–6.

23. Swaans RJM, Rondot P, Renier WO, Heuvel LPWJ, Steenbergen-Spangers GCH, Wevers RA. Four novel mutations in the Tyrosine Hydroxylase gene in patients with infantile parkinsonism. Ann Hum Genet. 2000;64:25–31. https://doi.org/10.1046/j.1469-1809.2000.6410025.x.

24. Segawa M, Nomura Y, Nishiyama N. Autosomal dominant guanosine triphosphate cyclohydrolase I deficiency (Segawa disease). Ann Neurol. 2003;54(Suppl 6):S32–45. https://doi.org/10.1002/ana.10630.

25. Segawa M, Hosaka A, Miyagawa F, Nomura Y, Imai H. Hereditary progressive dystonia with marked diurnal fluctuation. Adv Neurol. 1976;14:215–33.

26. Rondot P, Ziegler M. Dystonia--L-dopa responsive or juvenile parkinsonism? J Neural Transm Suppl. 1983;19:273–81.

27. Muller K, Homberg V, Lenard HG. Motor control in childhood onset dopa-responsive dystonia (Segawa syndrome). Neuropediatrics. 1989;20:185–91. https://doi.org/10.1055/s-2008-1071289.

28. Nygaard TG, Marsden CD, Duvoisin RC. Dopa-responsive dystonia. Adv Neurol. 1988;50:377–84.

29. Trender-Gerhard I, Sweeney MG, Schwingenschuh P, Mir P, Edwards MJ, Gerhard A, et al. Autosomal-dominant GTPCH1-deficient DRD: clinical characteristics and long-term outcome of 34 patients. J Neurol Neurosurg Psychiatry. 2009;80:839–45. https://doi.org/10.1136/jnnp.2008.155861.

30. Furukawa Y, Lang AE, Trugman JM, Bird TD, Hunter A, Sadeh M, et al. Gender-related penetrance and de novo GTP-cyclohydrolase I gene mutations in dopa-responsive dystonia. Neurology. 1998;50:1015–20. https://doi.org/10.1212/WNL.50.4.1015.

31. Wijemanne S, Jankovic J. Dopa-responsive dystonia--clinical and genetic heterogeneity. Nat Rev Neurol. 2015;11:414–24. https://doi.org/10.1038/nrneurol.2015.86.

32. Dobričić V, Tomić A, Branković V, Kresojević N, Janković M, Westenberger A, et al. GCH1 mutations are common in Serbian patients with dystonia-parkinsonism: challenging

previously reported prevalence rates of DOPA-responsive dystonia. Parkinsonism Relat Disord. 2017;45:81–4. https://doi.org/10.1016/j.parkreldis.2017.09.017.

33. Furukawa Y, Kish SJ, Bebin EM, Jacobson RD, Fryburg JS, Wilson WG, et al. Dystonia with motor delay in compound heterozygotes for GTP-cyclohydrolase I gene mutations. Ann Neurol. 1998;44:10–6. https://doi.org/10.1002/ana.410440107.

34. Postuma RB, Furukawa Y, Rogaeva E, St. George-Hyslop PH, Farrer MJ, Lang AE. Dopa-responsive dystonia presenting with prominent isolated bilateral resting leg tremor: evidence for a role of parkin? Mov Disord. 2003;18:1070–2. https://doi.org/10.1002/mds.10478.

35. Furukawa Y, Nygaard TG, Gütlich M, Rajput AH, Pifl C, DiStefano L, et al. Striatal biopterin and tyrosine hydroxylase protein reduction in dopa- responsive dystonia. Neurology. 1999;53:1032–41. https://doi.org/10.1212/wnl.53.5.1032.

36. Furukawa Y, Kish SJ. Parkinsonism in GTP cyclohydrolase 1-deficient DOPA-responsive dystonia. Brain. 2015;138:e351. https://doi.org/10.1093/brain/awu325.

37. Nygaard TG, Trugman JM, de Yebenes JG, Fahn S. Dopa-responsive dystonia: the spectrum of clinical manifestations in a large North American family. Neurology. 1990;40:66–9. https://doi.org/10.1212/wnl.40.1.66.

38. Nygaard TG, Takahashi H, Heiman GA, Snow BJ, Fahn S, Calne DB. Long-term treatment response and fluorodopa positron emission tomographic scanning of parkinsonism in a family with dopa-responsive dystonia. Ann Neurol. 1992;32:603–8. https://doi.org/10.1002/ana.410320502.

39. Steinberger D, Weber Y, Korinthenberg R, Deuschl G, Benecke R, Martinius J, et al. High penetrance and pronounced variation in expressivity of GCH1 mutations in five families with dopa-responsive dystonia. Ann Neurol. 1998;43:634–9. https://doi.org/10.1002/ana.410430512.

40. Tassin J, Dürr A, Bonnet AM, Gil R, Vidailhet M, Lücking CB, et al. Levodopa-responsive dystonia. GTP cyclohydrolase I or parkin mutations? Brain. 2000;123:1112–21. https://doi.org/10.1093/brain/123.6.1112.

41. Furukawa Y, Kapatos G, Haycock JW, Worsley J, Wong H, Kish SJ, et al. Brain biopterin and tyrosine hydroxylase in asymptomatic dopa-responsive dystonia. Ann Neurol. 2002;51:637–41. https://doi.org/10.1002/ana.10175.

42. Furukawa Y, Guttman M, Wong H, Farrell SA, Furtado S, Kish SJ. Serum prolactin in symptomatic and asymptomatic dopa-responsive dystonia due to a GCH1 mutation. Neurology. 2003;61:269–70. https://doi.org/10.1212/01.WNL.0000073983.82532.49.

43. Grimes DA, Barclay CL, Duff J, Furukawa Y, Lang AE. Phenocopies in a large GCH1 mutation positive family with dopa responsive dystonia: confusing the picture? J Neurol Neurosurg Psychiatry. 2002;72:801–4. https://doi.org/10.1136/jnnp.72.6.801.

44. Wu-Chou Y-H, Yeh T-H, Wang C-Y, Lin J-J, Huang C-C, Chang H-C, et al. High frequency of multiexonic deletion of the GCH1 gene in a Taiwanese cohort of dopa-response dystonia. Am J Med Genet Part B Neuropsychiatr Genet. 2010; https://doi.org/10.1002/ajmg.b.31058.

45. Furukawa Y, Kish SJ. Influence of development and aging on brain biopterin: implications for dopa-responsive dystonia onset. Neurology. 1998;51:632–4. https://doi.org/10.1212/WNL.51.2.632.

46. O'Sullivan JD, Costa DC, Gacinovic S, Lees AJ. SPECT imaging of the dopamine transporter in juvenile-onset dystonia. Neurology. 2001;56:266–7. https://doi.org/10.1212/WNL.56.2.266.

47. de La Fuente-Fernández R, Furtado S, Guttman M, Furukawa Y, Lee CS, Calne DB, et al. VMAT2 binding is elevated in dopa-responsive dystonia: visualizing empty vesicles by PET. Synapse (New York, NY). 2003;49:20–8. https://doi.org/10.1002/syn.10199.

48. Kang J-H, Kang S-Y, Kang H-K, Koh Y-S, Im J-H, Lee MC. A novel missense mutation of the GTP cyclohydrolase I gene in a Korean family with hereditary progressive dystonia/dopa-responsive dystonia. Brain and Development. 2004;26:287–91. https://doi.org/10.1016/S0387-7604(03)00167-0.

49. Lewthwaite AJ, Lambert TD, Rolfe EB, Olgiati S, Quadri M, Simons EJ, et al. Novel GCH1 variant in Dopa-responsive dystonia and Parkinson's disease. Parkinsonism Relat Disord. 2015;21:394–7. https://doi.org/10.1016/j.parkreldis.2015.01.004.

50. Terbeek J, Hermans S, van Laere K, Vandenberghe W. Parkinson's disease in GTP cyclohydrolase 1 mutation carriers. Brain. 2015;138:e350. https://doi.org/10.1093/brain/awu324.

51. Ahn TB, Chung SJ, Koh SB, Park HY, Cho JW, Lee JH, et al. Residual signs of dopa-responsive dystonia with GCH1 mutation following levodopa treatment are uncommon in Korean patients. Parkinsonism Relat Disord. 2019;65:248–51. https://doi.org/10.1016/j.parkreldis.2019.06.005.

52. Lin JJ, Lu CS, Tsai CH. Variability of presynaptic nigrostriatal dopaminergic function and clinical heterogeneity in a dopa-responsive dystonia family with GCH-1 gene mutation. J Neurol. 2018;265:478–85. https://doi.org/10.1007/s00415-017-8723-5.

53. Kikuchi A, Takeda A, Fujihara K, Kimpara T, Shiga Y, Tanji H, et al. Arg(184)His mutant GTP cyclohydrolase I, causing recessive hyperphenylalaninemia, is responsible for dopa-responsive dystonia with parkinsonism: a case report. Mov Disord. 2004;19:590–3. https://doi.org/10.1002/mds.10712.

54. Hjermind LE, Johannsen LG, Blau N, Wevers RA, Lucking C-B, Hertz JM, et al. Dopa-responsive dystonia and early-onset Parkinson's disease in a patient with GTP cyclohydrolase I deficiency? Mov Disord. 2006;21:679–82. https://doi.org/10.1002/mds.20773.

55. Eggers C, Volk AE, Kahraman D, Fink GR, Leube B, Schmidt M, et al. Are Dopa-responsive dystonia and Parkinson's disease related disorders? A case report. Parkinsonism Relat Disord. 2012;18:666–8. https://doi.org/10.1016/j.parkreldis.2011.10.003.

56. Ceravolo R, Nicoletti V, Garavaglia B, Reale C, Kiferle L, Bonuccelli U. Expanding the clinical phenotype of DYT5 mutations: is multiple system atrophy a possible one? Neurology. 2013;81:301–2. https://doi.org/10.1212/WNL.0b013e31829bfd7c.

57. Mencacci NE, Isaias IU, Reich MM, Ganos C, Plagnol V, Polke JM, et al. Parkinson's disease in GTP cyclohydrolase 1 mutation carriers. Brain. 2014;137:2480–92. https://doi.org/10.1093/brain/awu179.

58. Nalls MA, Pankratz N, Lill CM, Do CB, Hernandez DG, Saad M, et al. Large-scale meta-analysis of genome-wide association data identifies six new risk loci for Parkinson's disease. Nat Genet. 2014;46:989–93. https://doi.org/10.1038/ng.3043.

59. Guella I, Sherman HE, Appel-Cresswell S, Rajput A, Rajput AH, Farrer MJ. Parkinsonism in GTP cyclohydrolase 1 mutation carriers. Brain. 2015;138:e349. https://doi.org/10.1093/brain/awu341.

60. Chang D, Nalls MA, Hallgrímsdóttir IB, Hunkapiller J, van der Brug M, Cai F, et al. A meta-analysis of genome-wide association studies identifies 17 new Parkinson's disease risk loci. Nat Genet. 2017;49:1511–6. https://doi.org/10.1038/ng.3955.

61. Blauwendraat C, Heilbron K, Vallerga CL, Bandres-Ciga S, von Coelln R, Pihlstrøm L, et al. Parkinson's disease age at onset genome-wide association study: defining heritability, genetic loci, and α-synuclein mechanisms. Mov Disord. 2019;34:866–75. https://doi.org/10.1002/mds.27659.

62. Fink JK, Filling-Katz MR, Barton NW, Macrae PR, Hallett M, Cohen WE. Treatable dystonia presenting as spastic cerebral palsy. Pediatrics. 1988;82:137–8.

63. Nygaard TG, Waran SP, Levine RA, Naini AB, Chutorian AM. Dopa-responsive dystonia simulating cerebral palsy. Pediatr Neurol. 1994;11:236–40. https://doi.org/10.1016/0887-8994(94)90109-0.

64. Furukawa Y, Graf WD, Wong H, Shimadzu M, Kish SJ. Dopa-responsive dystonia simulating spastic paraplegia due to tyrosine hydroxylase (TH) gene mutations. Neurology. 2001;56:260–3. https://doi.org/10.1212/WNL.56.2.260.

65. Bandmann O, Nygaard TG, Surtees R, Marsden CD, Wood NW, Harding AE. Dopa-responsive dystonia in British patients: new mutations of the GTP-cyclohydrolase I gene and evidence for genetic heterogeneity. Hum Mol Genet. 1996;5:403–6. https://doi.org/10.1093/hmg/5.3.403.

66. Clot F, Grabli D, Cazeneuve C, Roze E, Castelnau P, Chabrol B, et al. Exhaustive analysis of BH4 and dopamine biosynthesis genes in patients with Dopa-responsive dystonia. Brain. 2009;132:1753–63. https://doi.org/10.1093/brain/awp084.

67. Friedman JR. What is not in the name? Dopa-responsive dystonia may respond to more than L-Dopa. Pediatr Neurol. 2016;59:76–80. https://doi.org/10.1016/j.pediatrneurol.2015.12.016.

68. Fan Z, Greenwood R, Felix ACG, Shiloh-Malawsky Y, Tennison M, Roche M, et al. GCH1 heterozygous mutation identified by whole-exome sequencing as a treatable condition in a patient presenting with progressive spastic paraplegia. J Neurol. 2014;261:622–4. https://doi.org/10.1007/s00415-014-7265-3.

69. Wassenberg T, Schouten MI, Helmich RC, Willemsen MAAP, Kamsteeg EJ, van de Warrenburg BPC. Autosomal dominant GCH1 mutations causing spastic paraplegia at disease onset. Parkinsonism Relat Disord. 2020;74:12–5. https://doi.org/10.1016/j.parkreldis.2020.03.019.

70. Bandmann O, Valente EM, Holmans P, Surtees RA, Walters JH, Wevers RA, et al. Dopa responsive dystonia: a clinical and molecular genetic study. Ann Neurol. 1998;44:649–56. https://doi.org/10.1002/ana.410440411.

71. Steinberger D, Topka H, Fischer D, Müller U. GCH1 mutation in a patient with adult-onset oromandibular dystonia. Neurology. 1999;52:877–9. https://doi.org/10.1212/wnl.52.4.877.

72. Klein C, Hedrich K, Kabakçi K, Mohrmann K, Wiegers K, Landt O, et al. Exon deletions in the GCHI gene in two of four Turkish families with dopa-responsive dystonia. Neurology. 2002;59:1783–6. https://doi.org/10.1212/01.WNL.0000035629.04791.3F.

73. Krim E, Aupy J, Clot F, Bonnan M, Burbaud P, Guehl D. Mutation in the GCH1 gene with dopa-responsive dystonia and phenotypic variability. Neurol Genet. 2018;4 https://doi.org/10.1212/NXG.0000000000000231.

74. Furukawa Y, Kish SJ, Lang AE. Scoliosis in a dopa-responsive dystonia family with a mutation of the GTP cyclohydrolase I gene. Neurology. 2000;54:2187. https://doi.org/10.1212/WNL.54.11.2187.

75. Ling H, Polke JM, Sweeney MG, Haworth A, Sandford CA, Heales SJR, et al. An intragenic duplication in guanosine triphosphate cyclohydrolase-1 gene in a dopa-responsive dystonia family. Mov Disorder. 2011;26:905–9. https://doi.org/10.1002/mds.23593.

76. Leuzzi V, Carducci C, Carducci C, Cardona F, Artiola C, Antonozzi I. Autosomal dominant GTP-CH deficiency presenting as a dopa-responsive myoclonus-dystonia syndrome. Neurology. 2002;59:1241–3. https://doi.org/10.1212/WNL.59.8.1241.

77. Chaila EC, McCabe DJH, Delanty N, Costello DJ, Murphy RP. Broadening the phenotype of childhood-onset dopa-responsive dystonia. Arch Neurol. 2006;63:1185–8. https://doi.org/10.1001/archneur.63.8.1185.

78. Luciano MS, Ozelius L, Sims K, Raymond D, Liu L, Saunders-Pullman R. Responsiveness to levodopa in epsilon-sarcoglycan deletions. Mov Disord. 2009;24:425–8. https://doi.org/10.1002/mds.22375.

79. Hahn H, Trant MR, Brownstein MJ, Harper RA, Milstien S, Butler IJ. Neurologic and psychiatric manifestations in a family with a mutation in exon 2 of the guanosine triphosphate-cyclohydrolase gene. Arch Neurol. 2001;58:749–55. https://doi.org/10.1001/archneur.58.5.749.

80. van Hove JLK, Steyaert J, Matthijs G, Legius E, Theys P, Wevers R, et al. Expanded motor and psychiatric phenotype in autosomal dominant Segawa syndrome due to GTP cyclohydrolase deficiency. J Neurol Neurosurg Psychiatry. 2006;77:18–23. https://doi.org/10.1136/jnnp.2004.051664.

81. Antelmi E, Stamelou M, Liguori R, Bhatia KP. Nonmotor symptoms in Dopa-responsive dystonia. Mov Disord Clin Pract. 2015;2:347–56. https://doi.org/10.1002/mdc3.12211.

82. Tadic V, Kasten M, Brüggemann N, Stiller S, Hagenah J, Klein C. Dopa-responsive dystonia revisited: diagnostic delay, residual signs, and nonmotor signs. Arch Neurol. 2012;69:1558–62. https://doi.org/10.1001/archneurol.2012.574.

83. Brüggemann N, Stiller S, Tadic V, Kasten M, Münchau A, Graf J, et al. Non-motor phenotype of dopa-responsive dystonia and quality of life assessment. Parkinsonism Relat Disord. 2014;20:428–31. https://doi.org/10.1016/j.parkreldis.2013.12.014.

84. Timmers ER, Kuiper A, Smit M, Bartels AL, Kamphuis DJ, Wolf NI, et al. Non-motor symptoms and quality of life in dopa-responsive dystonia patients. Parkinsonism Relat Disord. 2017;45:57–62. https://doi.org/10.1016/j.parkreldis.2017.10.005.

85. Ichinose H, Ohye T, Matsuda Y, Hori TA, Blau N, Burlina A, et al. Characterization of mouse and human GTP cyclohydrolase I genes. Mutations in patients with GTP cyclohydrolase I deficiency. J Biol Chem. 1995;270:10062–71. https://doi.org/10.1074/jbc.270.17.10062.

86. Niederwieser A, Blau N, Wang M, Joller P, Atarés M, Cardesa-Garcia J. GTP cyclohydrolase I deficiency, a new enzyme defect causing hyperphenylalaninemia with neopterin, biopterin, dopamine, and serotonin deficiencies and muscular hypotonia. Eur J Pediatr. 1984;141:208–14. https://doi.org/10.1007/BF00572762.

87. Blau N, Thöny B, Cotton RGH, Hyland K. Disorders of tetrahydrobiopterin and related biogenic amines. In: Scriver C, Beaudet A, Sly W, Valle D, Childs B, Vogelstein B, editors. The metabolic and molecular bases of inherited disease, vol. 2. 8th ed. New York: McGraw-Hill; 2001. p. 1725–76.

88. Opladen T, Hoffmann GF, Blau N. An international survey of patients with tetrahydrobiopterin deficiencies presenting with hyperphenylalaninaemia. J Inherit Metab Dis. 2012;35:963–73. https://doi.org/10.1007/s10545-012-9506-x.

89. Furukawa Y, Filiano JJ, Kish SJ. Amantadine for levodopa-induced choreic dyskinesia in compound heterozygotes for GCH1 mutations. Mov Disord. 2004;19:1256–8. https://doi.org/10.1002/mds.20194.

90. Bodzioch M, Lapicka-Bodzioch K, Rudzinska M, Pietrzyk JJ, Bik-Multanowski M, Szczudlik A. Severe dystonic encephalopathy without hyperphenylalaninemia associated with an 18-bp deletion within the proximal GCH1 promoter. Mov Disord. 2011;26:337–40. https://doi.org/10.1002/mds.23364.

91. Nardocci N, Zorzi G, Blau N, Fernandez Alvarez E, Sesta M, Angelini L, et al. Neonatal dopa-responsive extrapyramidal syndrome in twins with recessive GTPCH deficiency. Neurology. 2003;60:335–7. https://doi.org/10.1212/01.WNL.0000044049.99690.AD.

92. Horvath GA, Stockler-Ipsiroglu SG, Salvarinova-Zivkovic R, Lillquist YP, Connolly M, Hyland K, et al. Autosomal recessive GTP cyclohydrolase I deficiency without hyperphenylalaninemia: evidence of a phenotypic continuum between dominant and recessive forms. Mol Genet Metab. 2008;94:127–31. https://doi.org/10.1016/j.ymgme.2008.01.003.

93. Opladen T, Hoffmann G, Hörster F, Hinz A-B, Neidhardt K, Klein C, et al. Clinical and biochemical characterization of patients with early infantile onset of autosomal recessive GTP cyclohydrolase I deficiency without hyperphenylalaninemia. Mov Disord. 2011;26:157–61. https://doi.org/10.1002/mds.23329.

94. Flotats-Bastardas M, Hebert E, Raspall-Chaure M, Munell F, Macaya A, Lohmann K. Novel GCH1 compound heterozygosity mutation in infancy-onset generalized dystonia. Neuropediatrics. 2018;49:296–7. https://doi.org/10.1055/s-0038-1626709.

95. Furukawa Y. Update on dopa-responsive dystonia: locus heterogeneity and biochemical features. Adv Neurol. 2004;94:127–38.

96. Skrygan M, Bartholomé B, Bonafé L, Blau N, Bartholomé K. A splice mutation in the GTP cyclohydrolase I gene causes dopa-responsive dystonia by exon skipping. J Inherit Metab Dis. 2001;24:345–51. https://doi.org/10.1023/A:1010544316387.

97. Hagenah J, Saunders-Pullman R, Hedrich K, Kabakci K, Habermann K, Wiegers K, et al. High mutation rate in dopa-responsive dystonia: detection with comprehensive GCHI screening. Neurology. 2005;64:908–11. https://doi.org/10.1212/01.WNL.0000152839.50258.A2.

98. Steinberger D, Trübenbach J, Zirn B, Leube B, Wildhardt G, Müller U. Utility of MLPA in deletion analysis of GCH1 in dopa-responsive dystonia. Neurogenetics. 2007;8:51–5. https://doi.org/10.1007/s10048-006-0069-6.

99. Zirn B, Steinberger D, Troidl C, Brockmann K, von der Hagen M, Feiner C, et al. Frequency of GCH1 deletions in Dopa-responsive dystonia. J Neurol Neurosurg Psychiatry. 2008;79:183–6. https://doi.org/10.1136/jnnp.2007.128413.

100. Liu X, Zhang S-S, Fang D-F, Ma M-Y, Guo X-Y, Yang Y, et al. GCH1 mutation and clinical study of Chinese patients with dopa-responsive dystonia. Mov Disord. 2010;25:447–51.
https://doi.org/10.1002/mds.22976.

101. Shi WT, Cai CY, Li MS, Ling C, Li WD. Han Chinese patients with dopa-responsive
dystonia exhibit a low frequency of exonic deletion in the GCH1 gene. Genet Mol Res.
2015;14:11185–90. https://doi.org/10.4238/2015.September.22.12.

102. Wang W, Xin B, Wang H. Dopa-responsive dystonia: a male patient inherited a novel GCH1
deletion from an asymptomatic mother. J Mov Disord. 2020; https://doi.org/10.14802/
jmd.19069.

103. Theuns J, Crosiers D, Debaene L, Nuytemans K, Meeus B, Sleegers K, et al. Guanosine
triphosphate cyclohydrolase 1 promoter deletion causes DOPA-responsive dystonia. Mov
Disord. 2012;27:1451–6. https://doi.org/10.1002/mds.25147.

104. Sharma N, Armata IA, Multhaupt-Buell TJ, Ozelius LJ, Xin W, Sims KR. Mutation in J
upstream region of GCHI gene causes familial dopa-responsive dystonia. Mov Disord.
2011;26:2140 1. https://doi.org/10.1002/mds.23786.

105. Jones L, Goode L, Davila E, Brown A, McCarthy DM, Sharma N, et al. Translational
effects and coding potential of an upstream open reading frame associated with DOPA
Responsive Dystonia. Biochim Biophys Acta Mol basis Dis. 1863;2017:1171–82. https://doi.
org/10.1016/j.bbadis.2017.03.024.

106. Yan Y-P, Zhang B, Mao Y-F, Guo Z-Y, Tian J, Zhao G-H, et al. A novel tyrosine hydroxylase variant in a group of Chinese patients with dopa-responsive dystonia. Int J Neurosci.
2017;127:694–700. https://doi.org/10.1080/00207454.2016.1236381.

107. Yoshino H, Nishioka K, Li Y, Oji Y, Oyama G, Hatano T, et al. GCH1 mutations in dopa-
responsive dystonia and Parkinson's disease. J Neurol. 2018;265:1860–70. https://doi.
org/10.1007/s00415-018-8930-8.

108. Grötzsch H, Pizzolato G-P, Ghika J, Schorderet D, Vingerhoets FJ, Landis T, et al.
Neuropathology of a case of dopa-responsive dystonia associated with a new genetic locus,
DYT14. Neurology. 2002;58:1839–42. https://doi.org/10.1212/wnl.58.12.1839.

109. Schiller A, Wevers RA, Steenbergen GCH, Blau N, Jung HH. Long-term course of L-dopa-
responsive dystonia caused by tyrosine hydroxylase deficiency. Neurology. 2004;63:1524–6.
https://doi.org/10.1212/01.WNL.0000142083.47927.0A.

110. Verbeek MM, Steenbergen-Spanjers GCH, Willemsen MAAP, Hol FA, Smeitink J, Seeger
J, et al. Mutations in the cyclic adenosine monophosphate response element of the tyrosine
hydroxylase gene. Ann Neurol. 2007;62:422–6. https://doi.org/10.1002/ana.21199.

111. Bartholomé K, Lüdecke B. Mutations in the tyrosine hydroxylase gene cause various forms
of L-dopa-responsive dystonia. Adv Pharmacol (San Diego, Calif). 1998;42:48–9. https://doi.
org/10.1016/s1054-3589(08)60692-4.

112. Knappskog PM, Flatmark T, Mallet J, Lüdecke B, Bartholomé K. Recessively inherited
L-DOPA-responsive dystonia caused by a point mutation (Q381K) in the tyrosine hydroxylase gene. Hum Mol Genet. 1995;4:1209–12. https://doi.org/10.1093/hmg/4.7.1209.

113. Rondot P, Aicardi J, Goutières F, Ziegler M. Dopa-sensitive dystonia. Rev Neurol.
1992;148:680–6.

114. Wu Z-Y, Lin Y, Chen W-J, Zhao G-X, Xie H, Murong S-X, et al. Molecular analyses of
GCH-1, TH and parkin genes in Chinese dopa-responsive dystonia families. Clin Genet.
2008;74:513–21. https://doi.org/10.1111/j.1399-0004.2008.01039.x.

115. Willemsen MA, Verbeek MM, Kamsteeg EJ, de Rijk-Van Andel JF, Aeby A, Blau N, et al.
Tyrosine hydroxylase deficiency: a treatable disorder of brain catecholamine biosynthesis.
Brain. 2010;133:1810–22. https://doi.org/10.1093/brain/awq087.

116. Haugarvoll K, Bindoff LA. A novel compound heterozygous tyrosine hydroxylase mutation (p.R441P) with complex phenotype. J Parkinsons Dis. 2011;1:119–22. https://doi.
org/10.3233/JPD-2011-11006.

117. Yeung WL, Wong VCN, Chan KY, Hui J, Fung CW, Yau E, et al. Expanding phenotype and
clinical analysis of tyrosine hydroxylase deficiency. J Child Neurol. 2011;26:179–87. https://
doi.org/10.1177/0883073810377014.

118. Sun ZF, Zhang YH, Guo JF, Sun QY, Mei JP, Zhou HL, et al. Genetic diagnosis of two dopa-responsive dystonia families by exome sequencing. PLoS One. 2014;9:e106388. https://doi.org/10.1371/journal.pone.0106388.

119. Couto CM, Vargas AP, dos Santos CF, de Assis Cunha OL, Braga LW. A Severe L-Dopa responsive dystonia with slow and continuous improvement in a patient with a novel mutation in the tyrosine hydroxylase gene. Mov Disord Clin Pract. 2019;6:486–7. https://doi.org/10.1002/mdc3.12769.

120. Chen Y, Bao X, Wen Y, Wang J, Zhang Q, Yan J. Clinical and genetic heterogeneity in a cohort of Chinese children with dopa-responsive dystonia. Front Pediatr. 2020;8:83. https://doi.org/10.3389/fped.2020.00083.

121. Schreglmann S, Jaunmuktane Z, Jung H, Strand C, Holton J, Bhatia K. Neuropathology of dopa-responsive dystonia due to Tyrosine hydroxylase deficiency. Mov Disord. 2018;33:Abstract #771. https://doi.org/10.1002/mds.116.

122. Katus LE, Frucht SJ. An unusual presentation of tyrosine hydroxylase deficiency. J Clin Mov Disord. 2017;4 https://doi.org/10.1186/s40734-017-0065-z.

123. Bally JF, Breen DP, Schaake S, Trinh J, Rakovic A, Klein C, et al. Mild dopa-responsive dystonia in heterozygous tyrosine hydroxylase mutation carrier: evidence of symptomatic enzyme deficiency? Parkinsonism Relat Disord. 2020;71:44–5. https://doi.org/10.1016/j.parkreldis.2020.01.017.

124. Furukawa Y, Tomizawa Y. Comment on "Mild dopa-responsive dystonia in heterozygous tyrosine hydroxylase mutation carrier: evidence of symptomatic enzyme deficiency?".Parkinsonism Relat Disord. 2020;74:81–82. https://doi.org/10.1016/j.parkreldis.2020.03.027.

125. Bonafé L, Thöny B, Penzien JM, Czarnecki B, Blau N. Mutations in the sepiapterin reductase gene cause a novel tetrahydrobiopterin-dependent monoamine-neurotransmitter deficiency without hyperphenylalaninemia. Am J Hum Genet. 2001;69:269–77. https://doi.org/10.1086/321970.

126. Neville BGR, Parascandalo R, Farrugia R, Felice A. Sepiapterin reductase deficiency: a congenital dopa-responsive motor and cognitive disorder. Brain. 2005;128:2291–6. https://doi.org/10.1093/brain/awh603.

127. Dill P, Wagner M, Somerville A, Thöny B, Blau N, Weber P. Child neurology: paroxysmal stiffening, upward gaze, and hypotonia: hallmarks of sepiapterin reductase deficiency. Neurology. 2012;78:e29–32. https://doi.org/10.1212/WNL.0b013e3182452849.

128. Friedman J, Roze E, Abdenur JE, Chang R, Gasperini S, Saletti V, et al. Sepiapterin reductase deficiency: a treatable mimic of cerebral palsy. Ann Neurol. 2012;71:520–30. https://doi.org/10.1002/ana.22685.

129. Abeling NG, Duran M, Bakker HD, Stroomer L, Thöny B, Blau N, et al. Sepiapterin reductase deficiency an autosomal recessive DOPA-responsive dystonia. Mol Genet Metab. 2006;89:116–20. https://doi.org/10.1016/j.ymgme.2006.03.010.

130. Koht J, Rengmark A, Opladen T, Bjørnarå KA, Selberg T, Tallaksen CME, et al. Clinical and genetic studies in a family with a novel mutation in the sepiapterin reductase gene. Acta Neurol Scand Suppl. 2014;129:7–12. https://doi.org/10.1111/ane.12230.

131. Shalash AS, Rösler TW, Müller SH, Salama M, Deuschl G, Müller U, et al. c.207C>G mutation in sepiapterin reductase causes autosomal dominant dopa-responsive dystonia. Neurol Genet. 2017;3:e197. https://doi.org/10.1212/nxg.0000000000000197.

132. Steinberger D, Blau N, Goriuonov D, Bitsch J, Zuker M, Hummel S, et al. Heterozygous mutation in 5′-untranslated region of sepiapterin reductase gene (SPR) in a patient with dopa-responsive dystonia. Neurogenetics. 2004;5:187–90. https://doi.org/10.1007/s10048-004-0182-3.

133. Kong CK, Ko CH, Tong SF, Lam CW. Atypical presentation of dopa-responsive dystonia: generalized hypotonia and proximal weakness. Neurology. 2001;57:1121–4. https://doi.org/10.1212/WNL.57.6.1121.

134. Trugman JM, Hyland K, Furukawa Y. A curable cause of dystonia. In: Reich S, editor. Movement disorders: 100 instructive cases. London: Informa Healthcare; 2008. p. 93–7.

135. Lohmann K, Redin C, Tönnies H, Bressman SB, Subero JIM, Wiegers K, et al. Complex and dynamic chromosomal rearrangements in a family with seemingly non-mendelian inheritance of Dopa-responsive dystonia. JAMA Neurol. 2017;74:806–12. https://doi.org/10.1001/jamaneurol.2017.0666.

136. Blau N, Bonafé L, Thöny B. Tetrahydrobiopterin deficiencies without hyperphenylalaninemia: diagnosis and genetics of DOPA-responsive dystonia and sepiapterin reductase deficiency. Mol Genet Metab. 2001;74:172–85. https://doi.org/10.1006/mgme.2001.3213.

137. Zorzi G, Redweik U, Trippe H, Penzien JM, Thöny B, Blau N. Detection of sepiapterin in CSF of patients with sepiapterin reductase deficiency. Mol Genet Metab. 2002;75:174–7. https://doi.org/10.1006/mgme.2001.3273.

138. Roze E, Vidailhet M, Blau N, Moller LB, Doummar D, de Villemeur TB, et al. Long-term follow-up and adult outcome of 6-pyruvoyl-tetrahydropterin synthase deficiency. Mov Disord. 2006;21:263–6. https://doi.org/10.1002/mds.20699.

139. Hanihara T, Inoue K, Kawanishi C, Sugiyama N, Miyakawa T, Onishi H, et al. 6-Pyruvoyl-tetrahydropterin synthase deficiency with generalized dystonia and diurnal fluctuation of symptoms: a clinical and molecular study. Mov Disord. 1997;12:408–11. https://doi.org/10.1002/mds.870120321.

140. Hoffmann GF, Assmann B, Bräutigam C, Dionisi-Vici C, Häussler M, de Klerk JBC, et al. Tyrosine hydroxylase deficiency causes progressive encephalopathy and dopa-nonresponsive dystonia. Ann Neurol. 2003;54(Suppl 6):S56–65. https://doi.org/10.1002/ana.10632.

141. Bräutigam C, Steenbergen-Spanjers GC, Hoffmann GF, Dionisi-Vici C, van den Heuvel LP, Smeitink JA, et al. Biochemical and molecular genetic characteristics of the severe form of tyrosine hydroxylase deficiency. Clin Chem. 1999;45:2073–8.

142. de Lonlay P, Nassogne MC, van Gennip AH, van Cruchten AC, Billette De Villemeur T, Cretz M, et al. Tyrosine hydroxylase deficiency unresponsive to L-dopa treatment with unusual clinical and biochemical presentation. J Inherit Metab Dis. 2000;23:819–25. https://doi.org/10.1023/A:1026760602577.

143. Dionisi-Vici C, Hoffmann GF, Leuzzi V, Hoffken H, Bräutigam C, Rizzo C, et al. Tyrosine hydroxylase deficiency with severe clinical course: clinical and biochemical investigations and optimization of therapy. J Pediatr. 2000;136:560–2. https://doi.org/10.1016/S0022-3476(00)90027-1.

144. Janssen RJ, Wevers RA, Häussler M, Luyten JA, Steenbergen-Spanjers GC, Hoffmann GF, et al. A branch site mutation leading to aberrant splicing of the human tyrosine hydroxylase gene in a child with a severe extrapyramidal movement disorder. Ann Hum Genet. 2000;64:375–82. https://doi.org/10.1046/j.1469-1809.2000.6450375.x.

145. Häussler M, Hoffmann GF, Wevers RA. L-dopa and selegiline for tyrosine hydroxylase deficiency. J Pediatr. 2001;138:451–2. https://doi.org/10.1067/mpd.2001.110776.

146. Møller LB, Romstad A, Paulsen M, Hougaard P, Ormazabal A, Pineda M, et al. Pre- and postnatal diagnosis of tyrosine hydroxylase deficiency. Prenat Diagn. 2005;25:671–5. https://doi.org/10.1002/pd.1193.

147. Zafeiriou DI, Willemsen MA, Verbeek MM, Vargiami E, Ververi A, Wevers R. Tyrosine hydroxylase deficiency with severe clinical course. Mol Genet Metab. 2009;97:18–20. https://doi.org/10.1016/j.ymgme.2009.02.001.

148. Chi C-S, Lee H-F, Tsai C-R. Tyrosine hydroxylase deficiency in Taiwanese infants. Pediatr Neurol. 2012;46:77–82. https://doi.org/10.1016/j.pediatrneurol.2011.11.012.

149. Szentiványi K, Hansíková H, Krijt J, Vinšová K, Tesařová M, Rozsypalová E, et al. Novel mutations in the tyrosine hydroxylase gene in the first Czech patient with tyrosine hydroxylase deficiency. Prague Med Rep. 2012;113:136–46. https://doi.org/10.14712/23362936.2015.28.

150. Pons R, Syrengelas D, Youroukos S, Orfanou I, Dinopoulos A, Cormand B, et al. Levodopa-induced dyskinesias in tyrosine hydroxylase deficiency. Mov Disord. 2013;28:1058–63. https://doi.org/10.1002/mds.25382.

151. Tristán-Noguero A, Díez H, Jou C, Pineda M, Ormazábal A, Sánchez A, et al. Study of a fetal brain affected by a severe form of tyrosine hydroxylase deficiency, a rare cause of early parkinsonism. Metab Brain Dis. 2016;31:705–9. https://doi.org/10.1007/s11011-015-9780-z.

152. Leuzzi V, Mastrangelo M, Giannini MT, Carbonetti R, Hoffmann GF. Neuromotor and cognitive outcomes of early treatment in tyrosine hydroxylase deficiency type B. Neurology. 2017;88:501–2. https://doi.org/10.1212/WNL.0000000000003539.

153. Nedelea F, Veduta A, Duta S, Vayna AM, Panaitescu A, Peltecu G, et al. Prenatal genetic testing for dopa-responsive dystonia – clinical judgment in the context of next generation sequencing. J Med Life. 2018;11:343–5. https://doi.org/10.25122/jml-2018-0076.

154. Lüdecke B, Knappskog PM, Clayton PT, Surtees RA, Clelland JD, Heales SJ, et al. Recessively inherited L-DOPA-responsive parkinsonism in infancy caused by a point mutation (L205P) in the tyrosine hydroxylase gene. Hum Mol Genet. 1996;5:1023–8. https://doi.org/10.1093/hmg/5.7.1023.

155. Bräutigam C, Wevers RA, Jansen RJT, Smeitink JAM, de Rijk-van Andel JF, Gabreëls FJM, et al. Biochemical hallmarks of tyrosine hydroxylase deficiency. Clin Chem. 1998;44:1897–904.

156. Surtees R, Clayton P. Infantile parkinsonism-dystonia: tyrosine hydroxylase deficiency. Mov Disord. 1998;13:350. https://doi.org/10.1002/mds.870130226.

157. van den Heuvel LPWJ, Luiten B, Smeitink JAM, de Rijk-van Andel JF, Hyland K, Steenbergen-Spanjers GCH, et al. A common point mutation in the tyrosine hydroxylase gene in autosomal recessive L-DOPA-responsive dystonia in the Dutch population. Hum Genet. 1998;102:644–6. https://doi.org/10.1007/s004390050756.

158. Wevers RA, de Rijk-van Andel JF, Bräutigam C, Geurtz B, van den Heuvel LPWJ, Steenbergen-Spanjers GCH, et al. A review of biochemical and molecular genetic aspects of tyrosine hydroxylase deficiency including a novel mutation (291delC). J Inherit Metab Dis. 1999;22:364–73. https://doi.org/10.1023/A:1005539803576.

159. de Rijk-Van Andel JF, Gabreëls FJM, Geurtz B, Steenbergen-Spanjers GCH, van den Heuvel LPWJ, Smeitink JAM, et al. L-dopa-responsive infantile hypokinetic rigid parkinsonism due to tyrosine hydroxylase deficiency. Neurology. 2000;55:1926–8. https://doi.org/10.1212/WNL.55.12.1926.

160. Grattan-Smith PJ, Wevers RA, Steenbergen-Spanjers GC, Fung VSC, Earl J, Wilcken B. Tyrosine hydroxylase deficiency: clinical manifestations of catecholamine insufficiency in infancy. Mov Disord. 2002;17:354–9. https://doi.org/10.1002/mds.10095.

161. Yeung WL, Lam CW, Hui J, Tong SF, Wu SP. Galactorrhea-a strong clinical clue towards the diagnosis of neurotransmitter disease. Brain and Development. 2006;28:389–91. https://doi.org/10.1016/j.braindev.2005.10.012.

162. Ribasés M, Serrano M, Fernández-Alvarez E, Pahisa S, Ormazabal A, García-Cazorla A, et al. A homozygous tyrosine hydroxylase gene promoter mutation in a patient with dopa-responsive encephalopathy: clinical, biochemical and genetic analysis. Mol Genet Metab. 2007;92:274–7. https://doi.org/10.1016/j.ymgme.2007.07.004.

163. Doummar D, Clot F, Vidailhet M, Afenjar A, Durr A, Brice A, et al. Infantile hypokinetic-hypotonic syndrome due to two novel mutations of the tyrosine hydroxylase gene. Mov Disord. 2009;24:943–5. https://doi.org/10.1002/mds.22455.

164. Pons R, Serrano M, Ormazabal A, Toma C, Garcia-Cazorla A, Area E, et al. Tyrosine hydroxylase deficiency in three Greek patients with a common ancestral mutation. Mov Disord. 2010;25:1086–90. https://doi.org/10.1002/mds.23002.

165. Najmabadi H, Hu H, Garshasbi M, Zemojtel T, Abedini SS, Chen W, et al. Deep sequencing reveals 50 novel genes for recessive cognitive disorders. Nature. 2011;478:57–63. https://doi.org/10.1038/nature10423.

166. Ormazabal A, Serrano M, Garcia-Cazorla A, Campistol J, Artuch R, Castro de Castro P, et al. Deletion in the tyrosine hydroxylase gene in a patient with a mild phenotype. Mov Disord. 2011;26:1558–60. https://doi.org/10.1002/mds.23564.

167. Giovanniello T, Claps D, Carducci C, Carducci C, Blau N, Vigevano F, et al. A new tyrosine hydroxylase genotype associated with early-onset severe encephalopathy. J Child Neurol. 2012;27:523–5. https://doi.org/10.1177/0883073811420717.

168. Ortez C, Duarte ST, Ormazábal A, Serrano M, Pérez A, Pons R, et al. Cerebrospinal fluid synaptic proteins as useful biomarkers in tyrosine hydroxylase deficiency. Mol Genet Metab. 2015;114:34–40. https://doi.org/10.1016/j.ymgme.2014.10.014.

169. Zhang W, Zhou Z, Li X, Huang Y, Li T, Lin Y, et al. Dopa-responsive dystonia in Chinese patients: including a novel heterozygous mutation in the GCH1 gene with an intermediate phenotype and one case of prenatal diagnosis. Neurosci Lett. 2017;644:48–54. https://doi.org/10.1016/j.neulet.2017.01.019.

170. Feng B, Sun G, Kong Q, Li Q. Compound heterozygous mutations in the TH gene in a Chinese family with autosomal-recessive dopa-responsive dystonia A case report. Medicine (United States). 2018;97. https://doi.org/10.1097/MD.0000000000012870.

171. Kuwabara K, Kawarai T, Ishida Y, Miyamoto R, Oki R, Orlacchio A, et al. A novel compound heterozygous TH mutation in a Japanese case of dopa-responsive dystonia with mild clinical course. Parkinsonism Relat Disord. 2018;46:87–9. https://doi.org/10.1016/j.parkreldis.2017.10.019.

172. Zhou QY, Quaife CJ, Palmiter RD. Targeted disruption of the tyrosine hydroxylase gene reveals that catecholamines are required for mouse fetal development. Nature. 1995;374:640–3. https://doi.org/10.1038/374640a0.

173. Stamelou M, Mencacci NE, Cordivari C, Batla A, Wood NW, Houlden H, et al. Myoclonus-dystonia syndrome due to tyrosine hydroxylase deficiency. Neurology. 2012;79:435–41. https://doi.org/10.1212/WNL.0b013e318261714a.

174. Diepold K, Schütz B, Rostasy K, Wilken B, Hougaard P, Güttler F, et al. Levodopa-responsive infantile parkinsonism due to a novel mutation in the tyrosine hydroxylase gene and exacerbation by viral infections. Mov Disord. 2005;20:764–7. https://doi.org/10.1002/mds.20416.

175. Giovanniello T, Leuzzi V, Carducci C, Carducci C, di Sabato ML, Artiola C, et al. Tyrosine hydroxylase deficiency presenting with a biphasic clinical course. Neuropediatrics. 2007;38:213–5. https://doi.org/10.1055/s-2007-991151.

176. LeWitt PA, Miller LP, Levine RA, Lovenberg W, Newman RP, Papavasiliou A, et al. Tetrahydrobiopterin in dystonia: identification of abnormal metabolism and therapeutic trials. Neurology. 1986;36:760–4. https://doi.org/10.1212/wnl.36.6.760.

177. Fink JK, Barton N, Cohen W, Lovenberg W, Burns RS, Hallett M. Dystonia with marked diurnal variation associated with biopterin deficiency. Neurology. 1988;38:707–11. https://doi.org/10.1212/wnl.38.5.707.

178. Furukawa Y, Mizuno Y, Nishi K, Narabayashi H. A clue to the pathogenesis of dopa-responsive dystonia. Ann Neurol. 1995;37:139–40. https://doi.org/10.1002/ana.410370131.

179. Furukawa Y, Shimadzu M, Hornykiewicz O, Kish SJ. Molecular and biochemical aspects of hereditary progressive and dopa-responsive dystonia. Adv Neurol. 1998;78:267–82.

180. Blau N, Ichinose H, Nagatsu T, Heizmann CW, Zacchello F, Burlina AB. A missense mutation in a patient with guanosine triphosphate cyclohydrolase I deficiency missed in the newborn screening program. J Pediatr. 1995;126:401–5. https://doi.org/10.1016/S0022-3476(95)70458-2.

181. Bonafé L, Thöny B, Leimbacher W, Kierat L, Blau N. Diagnosis of dopa-responsive dystonia and other tetrahydrobiopterin disorders by the study of biopterin metabolism in fibroblasts. Clin Chem. 2001;47:477–85.

182. Jeon BS, Jeong JM, Park SS, Kim JM, Chang YS, Song HC, et al. Dopamine transporter density measured by [123I]β-CIT single-photon emission computed tomography is normal in dopa-responsive dystonia. Ann Neurol. 1998;43:792–800. https://doi.org/10.1002/ana.410430614.

183. Hirano M, Imaiso Y, Ueno S. Differential splicing of the GTP cyclohydrolase I RNA in dopa-responsive dystonia. Biochem Biophys Res Commun. 1997;234:316–9. https://doi.org/10.1006/bbrc.1997.6632.

184. Ihara M, Kohara N, Urano F, Ichinose H, Takao S, Nishida T, et al. Neuroleptic malignant syndrome with prolonged catatonia in a dopa-responsive dystonia patient. Neurology. 2002;59:1102–4. https://doi.org/10.1212/WNL.59.7.1102.

185. Bezin L, Nygaard TG, Neville JD, Shen H, Levine RA. Reduced lymphoblast neopterin detects GTP cyclohydrolase dysfunction in dopa-responsive dystonia. Neurology. 1998;50:1021–7. https://doi.org/10.1212/WNL.50.4.1021.

186. Hibiya M, Ichinose H, Ozaki N, Fujita K, Nishimoto T, Yoshikawa T, et al. Normal values and age-dependent changes in GTP cyclohydrolase I activity in stimulated mononuclear blood cells measured by high-performance liquid chromatography. J Chromatogr B Biomed Sci Appl. 2000;740:35–42. https://doi.org/10.1016/S0378-4347(99)00572 1.

187. Hirano M, Yanagihara T, Ueno S. Dominant negative effect of GTP cyclohydrolase I mutations in dopa-responsive hereditary progressive dystonia. Ann Neurol. 1998;44:365–71. https://doi.org/10.1002/ana.410440312.

188. Hirano M, Ueno S. Mutant GTP cyclohydrolase I in autosomal dominant dystonia and recessive hyperphenylalaninemia. Neurology. 1999;52:182–4. https://doi.org/10.1212/wnl.52.1.182.

189. Hwu WL, Chiou YW, Lai SY, Lee YM. Dopa-responsive dystonia is induced by a dominant-negative mechanism. Ann Neurol. 2000;48:609–13. https://doi.org/10.1002/1531-8249(200010)48:43.0.CO;2-H.

190. Suzuki T, Ohye T, Inagaki H, Nagatsu T, Ichinose H. Characterization of wild-type and mutants of recombinant human GTP cyclohydrolase I: relationship to etiology of dopa-responsive dystonia. J Neurochem. 1999;73:2510–6. https://doi.org/10.1046/j.1471-4159.1999.0732510.x.

191. Hyland K, Fryburg JS, Wilson WG, Bebin EM, Arnold LA, Gunasekera RS, et al. Oral phenylalanine loading in dopa-responsive dystonia: a possible diagnostic test. Neurology. 1997;48:1290–7. https://doi.org/10.1212/WNL.48.5.1290.

192. Bandmann O, Goertz M, Zschocke J, Deuschl G, Jost W, Hefter H, et al. The phenylalanine loading test in the differential diagnosis of dystonia. Neurology. 2003;60:700–2. https://doi.org/10.1212/01.WNL.0000048205.18445.98.

193. Saunders-Pullman R, Blau N, Hyland K, Zschocke J, Nygaard T, Raymond D, et al. Phenylalanine loading as a diagnostic test for DRD: interpreting the utility of the test. Mol Genet Metab. 2004;83:207–12. https://doi.org/10.1016/j.ymgme.2004.07.010.

194. Snow BJ, Nygaard TG, Takahashi H, Calne DB. Positron emission tomographic studies of dopa-responsive dystonia and early-onset idiopathic parkinsonism. Ann Neurol. 1993;34:733–8. https://doi.org/10.1002/ana.410340518.

195. Turjanski N, Bhatia K, Burn DJ, Sawle GV, Marsden CD, Brooks DJ. Comparison of striatal 18F-dopa uptake in adult-onset dystonia-parkinsonism, Parkinson's disease, and dopa-responsive dystonia. Neurology. 1993;43:1563–8. https://doi.org/10.1212/wnl.43.8.1563.

196. Kishore A, Nygaard TG, de La Fuente-Fernandez R, Naini AB, Schulzer M, Mak E, et al. Striatal D2 receptors in symptomatic and asymptomatic carriers of dopa- responsive dystonia measured with [11C]-raclopride and positron-emission tomography. Neurology. 1998;50:1028–32. https://doi.org/10.1212/WNL.50.4.1028.

197. Lee W-T, Weng W-C, Peng S-F, Tzen K-Y. Neuroimaging findings in children with paediatric neurotransmitter diseases. J Inherit Metab Dis. 2009;32:361–70. https://doi.org/10.1007/s10545-009-1106-z.

198. Künig G, Leenders KL, Antonini A, Vontobel P, Weindl A, Meinck HM. D2 receptor binding in dopa-responsive dystonia. Ann Neurol. 1998;44:758–62. https://doi.org/10.1002/ana.410440509.

199. Asanuma K, Ma Y, Huang C, Carbon-Correll M, Edwards C, Raymond D, et al. The metabolic pathology of dopa-responsive dystonia. Ann Neurol. 2005;57:596–600. https://doi.org/10.1002/ana.20442.

200. Rajput AH, Gibb WR, Zhong XH, Shannak KS, Kish S, Chang LG, et al. Dopa-responsive dystonia: pathological and biochemical observations in a case. Ann Neurol. 1994;35:396–402. https://doi.org/10.1002/ana.410350405.

201. Segawa M, Nomura Y, Hayashi M. Dopa-responsive dystonia is caused by particular impairment of nigrostriatal dopamine neurons different from those involved in Parkinson disease:

evidence observed in studies on Segawa disease. Neuropediatrics. 2013;44:61–6. https://doi.org/10.1055/s-0033-1337337.

202. Furukawa Y, Rajput AH, Tong J, Tomizawa Y, Hornykiewicz O, Kish SJ. A marked contrast between serotonergic and dopaminergic changes in dopa-responsive dystonia. Neurology. 2016;87:1060–1. https://doi.org/10.1212/WNL.0000000000003065.

203. Furukawa Y, Hornykiewicz O, Fahn S, Kish SJ. Striatal dopamine in early-onset primary torsion dystonia with the DYT1 mutation. Neurology. 2000;54:1193–5. https://doi.org/10.1212/WNL.54.5.1193.

204. Kish SJ, Shannak K, Hornykiewicz O. Uneven pattern of dopamine loss in the striatum of patients with idiopathic Parkinson's disease. Pathophysiologic and clinical implications. N Engl J Med. 1988;318:876–80. https://doi.org/10.1056/NEJM198804073181402.

205. Hornykiewicz O. Biochemical aspects of Parkinson's disease. Neurology. 1998;51 https://doi.org/10.1212/wnl.51.2_suppl_2.s2.

206. Kish SJ, Tong J, Hornykiewicz O, Rajput A, Chang L-J, Guttman M, et al. Preferential loss of serotonin markers in caudate versus putamen in Parkinson's disease. Brain. 2008;131:120–31. https://doi.org/10.1093/brain/awm239.

207. Tong J, Furukawa Y, Sherwin A, Hornykiewicz O, Kish SJ. Heterogeneous intrastriatal pattern of proteins regulating axon growth in normal adult human brain. Neurobiol Dis. 2011;41:458–68. https://doi.org/10.1016/j.nbd.2010.10.017.

208. Zhong XH, Haycock JW, Shannak K, Robitaille Y, Fratkin J, Koeppen AH, et al. Striatal dihydroxyphenylalanine decarboxylase and tyrosine hydroxylase protein in idiopathic Parkinson's disease and dominantly inherited olivopontocerebellar atrophy. Mov Disord. 1995;10:10–7. https://doi.org/10.1002/mds.870100104.

209. Wilson JM, Levey AI, Rajput A, Ang L, Guttman M, Shannak K, et al. Differential changes in neurochemical markers of striatal dopamine nerve terminals in idiopathic Parkinson's disease. Neurology. 1996;47:718–26. https://doi.org/10.1212/WNL.47.3.718.

210. Hyland K, Gunasekera RS, Engle T, Arnold LA. Tetrahydrobiopterin and biogenic amine metabolism in the hph-1 mouse. J Neurochem. 1996;67:752–9. https://doi.org/10.1046/j.1471-4159.1996.67020752.x.

211. Sumi-Ichinose C, Urano F, Kuroda R, Ohye T, Kojima M, Tazawa M, et al. Catecholamines and serotonin are differently regulated by tetrahydrobiopterin. A study from 6-pyruvoyltetrahydropterin synthase knockout mice. J Biol Chem. 2001;276:41150–60. https://doi.org/10.1074/jbc.M102237200.

212. Sumi-Ichinose C, Urano F, Shimomura A, Sato T, Ikemoto K, Shiraishi H, et al. Genetically rescued tetrahydrobiopterin-depleted mice survive with hyperphenylalaninemia and region-specific monoaminergic abnormalities. J Neurochem. 2005;95:703–14. https://doi.org/10.1111/j.1471-4159.2005.03402.x.

213. Sato K, Sumi-Ichinose C, Kaji R, Ikemoto K, Nomura T, Nagatsu I, et al. Differential involvement of striosome and matrix dopamine systems in a transgenic model of dopa-responsive dystonia. Proc Natl Acad Sci U S A. 2008;105:12551–6. https://doi.org/10.1073/pnas.0806065105.

214. Kish SJ, Furukawa Y, Chang LJ, Tong J, Ginovart N, Wilson A, et al. Regional distribution of serotonin transporter protein in postmortem human brain: is the cerebellum a SERT-free brain region? Nucl Med Biol. 2005;32:123–8. https://doi.org/10.1016/j.nucmedbio.2004.10.001.

215. Korner G, Noain D, Ying M, Hole M, Flydal MI, Scherer T, et al. Brain catecholamine depletion and motor impairment in a Th knock-in mouse with type B tyrosine hydroxylase deficiency. Brain. 2015;138:2948–63. https://doi.org/10.1093/brain/awv224.

216. Rose SJ, Yu XY, Heinzer AK, Harrast P, Fan X, Raike RS, et al. A new knock-in mouse model of l-DOPA-responsive dystonia. Brain. 2015;138:2987–3002. https://doi.org/10.1093/brain/awv212.

217. Rose SJ, Harrast P, Donsante C, Fan X, Joers V, Tansey MG, et al. Parkinsonism without dopamine neuron degeneration in aged l-dopa-responsive dystonia knockin mice. Mov Disord. 2017;32:1694–700. https://doi.org/10.1002/mds.27169.

218. Nygaard TG, Marsden CD, Fahn S. Dopa-responsive dystonia: long-term treatment response and prognosis. Neurology. 1991;41:174–81. https://doi.org/10.1212/wnl.41.2_part_1.174.
219. Koy A, Lin JP, Sanger TD, Marks WA, Mink JW, Timmermann L. Advances in management of movement disorders in children. Lancet Neurol. 2016;15:719–35. https://doi.org/10.1016/S1474-4422(16)00132-0.
220. Trau SP, Gallentine WB, Mikati MA. Child neurology: a young child with an undiagnosed case of dystonia responsive to l-dopa. Neurology. 2020;94:326–8. https://doi.org/10.1212/wnl.0000000000008963.
221. Maas RPPWM, Wassenberg T, Lin JP, van de Warrenburg BPC, Willemsen MAAP. L-Dopa in dystonia: a modern perspective. Neurology. 2017;88:1865–71. https://doi.org/10.1212/WNL.0000000000003897.
222. Steinberger D, Korinthenberg R, Topka H, Berghäuser M, Wedde R, Müller U. Dopa-responsive dystonia: mutation analysis of GCH1 and analysis of therapeutic doses of L-dopa. German Dystonia Study Group. Neurology. 2000;55:1735–7. https://doi.org/10.1212/wnl.55.11.1735.
223. Furukawa Y, Guttman M, Kish S. Dopa-responsive dystonia. In: Frucht SJ, Fahn S, editors. Movement disorder emergencies: diagnosis and treatment. 1st ed. Totowa: Humana Press; 2005. p. 209–29. https://doi.org/10.1385/1-59259-902-8:209.
224. Furukawa Y, Guttman M, Nakamura S, Kish SJ. Dopa-responsive dystonia. In: Frucht SJ, editor. Movement disorder emergencies: diagnosis and treatment. 2nd ed. Totowa: Humana Press; 2013. p. 319–40. https://doi.org/10.1007/978-1-60761-835-5_24.
225. Nygaard T, Duvoisin R. Hereditary progressive dystonia/dopa-responsive dystonia. In: Joseph A, Young R, editors. Movement disorders in neurology and neuropsychiatry. 2nd ed. Malden: Blackwell Science; 1999. p. 531–7.
226. Fink JK, Ravin P, Argoff CE, Levine RA, Brady RO, Hallett M, et al. Tetrahydrobiopterin administration in biopterin-deficient progressive dystonia with diurnal variation. Neurology. 1989;39:1393–5. https://doi.org/10.1212/wnl.39.10.1393.
227. Kapatos G, Kaufman S. Peripherally administered reduced pterins do enter the brain. Science. 1981;212:955–6. https://doi.org/10.1126/science.7233193.
228. Kaufman S, Kapatos G, McInnes RR, Schulman JD, Rizzo WB. Use of tetrahydropterins in the treatment of hyperphenylalaninemia due to defective synthesis of tetrahydrobiopterin: evidence that peripherally administered tetrahydropterins enter the brain. Pediatrics. 1982;70:376–80.
229. Kondo T, Miwa H, Furukawa Y, Mizuno Y, Narabayashi H. Tetrahydrobiopterin therapy for juvenile parkinsonism. In: Segawa M, editor. Hereditary progressive dystonia with marked diurnal fluctuation. New York: Parthenon Publishing; 1993. p. 133–40.

Wilson's Disease

25

Peter Hedera

Patient Vignettes

Patient 1

A 26-year-old man presented to a neurologist with a 6-month history of mild arm tremor. He noticed that over the past year, his memory was not as good as it used to be and sometimes he had difficulty focusing mentally on tasks. His family history was notable for two relatives on his mother's side with mild tremor. Laboratory studies were normal as were routine biochemistry panels. The neurologist sitting across the desk discussed the diagnosis of tremor, unknowingly in the midst of an emergency—not an emergency room emergency but a diagnostic emergency. If the appropriate differential diagnosis had been considered, a workup would have led to the diagnosis of Wilson's disease, with institution of appropriate treatment. Instead, the neurologist falsely reassured the patient that he had essential tremor and that it would likely not be more than an inconvenience. Over time though his tremor worsened, and a second opinion was sought at an academic movement disorder center. Again, the diagnosis was delayed, until the patient finally developed worsening tremor, dysarthria, facial dystonia, and incoordination. By the time Kayser-Fleischer rings were seen by an experienced examiner and Wilson's disease was diagnosed, neurologic damage was permanent despite effective anticopper therapy.

Supplementary Information The online version of this chapter (https://doi.org/10.1007/978-3-030-75898-1_25) contains supplementary material, which is available to authorized users.

P. Hedera (✉)
Department of Neurology, University of Louisville Medical Center, Louisville, KY, USA
e-mail: peter.hedera@louisville.edu

© Springer Nature Switzerland AG 2022
S. J. Frucht (ed.), *Movement Disorder Emergencies*, Current Clinical Neurology,
https://doi.org/10.1007/978-3-030-75898-1_25

Patient 2

A diagnosis of Wilson's disease was quickly secured in a 23-year-old woman who presented with mild dysarthria and arm tremor. An appropriate workup was performed, and the neurologist described the steps that needed to be taken in order to achieve copper balance. Unbeknownst to either of them, the patient faced an emergency—a hidden therapeutic emergency. The neurologist, unfamiliar with the ability of penicillamine to cause permanent neurologic worsening, reassured the patient about her outcome. Unfortunately, within 2 weeks of beginning penicillamine, her neurologic signs acutely worsened, and she accelerated into a precipitous neurologic decline. She became anarthric with severe generalized dystonia and became functionally completely dependent. Despite attempts to reverse the situation, her condition was permanent. An independent life was destroyed by overly aggressive penicillamine treatment.

Introduction

Wilson's disease (WD) is an autosomal recessive metabolic disorder affecting approximately 1 in 30,000 individuals [1–3]. It is caused by loss of function mutations in the transmembrane ATPase copper transporter encoded by the *ATP7B* gene [4, 5]. Impaired copper transport and excretion due to defects in the hepatic excretory pathway lead to insufficient copper binding to cuproenzymes and reduced elimination of excessive copper into the bile [6, 7]. This ultimately results in chronic copper accumulation in the liver and subsequently in the brain, as well as other organs such as kidneys or cornea. Copper is an essential micronutrient and under physiologic homeostasis is mostly bound to metallothioneins in hepatocytes or ceruloplasmin in plasma. Bound copper is biologically inactive, and only free copper (known as non-ceruloplasmin bound [NCC]) is potentially toxic [6, 7]. Excessive free copper can trigger cytotoxic effects in affected organs, leading to variable clinical phenotypes with predominantly hepatic, neurologic, or psychiatric symptoms.

In contrast to many inherited metabolic conditions, WD is highly treatable with effective therapies reversing clinical manifestations or substantially improving outcomes [8–10]. Untreated, copper overload results in catastrophic neurologic symptoms and eventual death in the vast majority of patients with WD [6, 7]. Delays in initiation of decoppering therapies are associated with worse clinical outcomes and long-term residual neurologic disability [11, 12]. Early recognition of WD is critical for timely initiation of copper removal; for this reason, *the timely diagnosis of WD is a true movement disorder emergency* (patient 1). This is especially challenging as the clinical manifestations are protean, mimicking other movement disorders such as idiopathic Parkinson's disease, essential tremor, or primary dystonia [13].

The first step in WD treatment is to remove excessive copper that is associated with increased plasma NCC levels [1]. This should induce a negative copper balance with a rapid control of NCC levels, the copper fraction likely responsible for organ toxicity [14, 15]. Currently available options are chelating agents that nonspecifically chelate copper and promote urinary copper excretion. Relatively rapid onset of action favors chelating agents in the acute phase of decoppering treatment when patients are symptomatic [1–3]. However, rapid mobilization of copper from the liver can cause additional elevations in NCC in blood, resulting in further progression of the disease with subsequent neurologic deterioration [11, 16, 17]. Even if appropriate therapy is initiated in a timely manner, this paradoxical worsening is perhaps the most feared complication of chelation therapy. This phenomenon needs to be recognized very early, and the therapy needs to be adjusted to prevent irreversible neurologic deficits. This is also an emergency when treating WD patients: *lack of recognition and prompt management of neurologic deterioration is the second WD emergency* (patient 2). Most patients experiencing paradoxical neurological worsening manifest deterioration in their gait, balance, tremor, speech, and swallowing (due to oropharyngeal dystonia). Worsening of dystonia after chelation treatment may even result in generalized dystonia that is refractory to medical management, i.e., status dystonicus or dystonic storm [18, 19].

Paradoxical worsening with decoppering treatment is a dreaded complication of WD treatment. The choice of the decoppering agent and titration with careful monitoring of copper excretion require experience and guidance from an expert.

First WD Emergency: Timely Diagnosis

Clinical Presentation

Certain clinical phenotypes are suggestive of WD and should prompt further laboratory testing. The diagnosis of WD requires a high degree of clinical suspicion—it bears repeating that the clinician will never diagnose WD if they do not think of it [13]. The historical name for WD, hepatolenticular degeneration, reflects the fact that hepatic and neurologic symptoms are the two major clinical phenotypes in symptomatic patients. WD with hepatic manifestations can be seen in about 40% of all patients, while initial neurologic symptoms and signs are present in approximately 40–50%; primary psychiatric presentations can be seen in about 10% of patients [12, 20–22]. Other systemic manifestations of WD are rare and difficult to recognize without other signs of hepatic or neurologic problems [1, 2]. Aminoaciduria, nephrolithiasis, arthropathy, premature osteoporosis, and cardiomyopathy have been reported as unusual presenting symptoms of WD. Ophthalmologic features are also common, typically asymptomatic, but very useful in supporting the diagnosis. The most important are Kayser-Fleischer (KF) rings caused by asymptomatic copper deposition in Descemet's corneal membrane [23, 24]. Sunflower cataracts, caused by copper deposits in the lens, are another asymptomatic ophthalmologic presentation of WD.

Almost all WD patients with neurologic symptoms and signs have KF rings. KF rings can be visualized at the bedside even in patients with brown irises by illuminating the iris with a light positioned at the side of the eye. KF rings are classically thicker superiorly and inferiorly. They are golden brown to green in color, with a fluffy appearance that blends into the natural color of the iris.

Copper deposits in the cornea and the lens disappear with chelation, but the severity of KF rings does not correlate with clinical deficits. Clinical suspicion for WD should be highest in patients who develop hepatic or neurologic symptoms in adolescence to early adulthood [13, 20–22, 24]. However, the age of first symptoms varies widely from the first decade to the fourth and fifth decades of life. Neurologic symptoms tend to develop approximately one decade later than hepatic presentations, but there is a considerable overlap between these two major phenotypes. Atypical, late-onset WD even in the seventh and eighth decades of life has been described [25–27].

Like other clinical presentations of WD, hepatic symptoms range from asymptomatic liver disease to life-threatening hepatic failure [1, 6, 7]. Asymptomatic patients typically have only biochemical abnormalities with elevation of liver enzymes and histologic findings of steatosis on liver biopsy. Liver involvement in WD may also mimic acute viral hepatitis or autoimmune hepatitis. However, most patients with hepatic symptoms exhibit signs of chronic liver disease with cirrhosis and splenomegaly due to portal hypertension. The hepatic phenotype of WD is frequently associated with Coombs-negative hemolytic anemia that can lead to acute renal failure in extreme cases. Transient episodes of jaundice due to hemolysis may be the initial presentation in patients who do not have any other signs of liver disease. Patients with predominantly neurologic symptoms have frequent mild liver disease, but they tend to have more compensated cholestatic hepatopathy. Liver transaminase enzymes alanine transaminase (ALT) and aspartate transaminase (AST) may be normal [1]. Thus, a normal AST and ALT in patients with suspicious neurologic symptoms does not exclude WD, and further evaluation is warranted.

Presenting neurologic symptoms can be pleotropic and present a significant diagnostic challenge; *WD is the great imitator in movement disorders* [13]. Even though neurologic presentations are very heterogeneous, WD neurologic phenotype can be grouped into dystonic, tremor-dominant or pseudosclerotic, parkinsonian, and hyperkinetic (choreic) subtypes [20–22]. A dysarthric form has been also suggested as another clinical category. However, dysarthria is the most constant neurologic sign in WD, present in 90% of patients. Initial neurologic symptoms are typically subtle and nonspecific. Motor symptoms may include lack of coordination, handwriting change, dysarthria, and drooling [28]. The clinical course is progressive in untreated patients, and they typically develop more noticeable neurologic abnormalities with dystonia, tremor, and parkinsonian syndromes [29]. The most common initial problems are tremor and ataxia, seen in about 40–60% of patients, followed by dysarthria (40–58%), dystonia (15–42%), gait abnormalities (38%), parkinsonism (11–60%), and choreoathetosis (15%) [28, 30–32]. Patients may also present with new-onset seizures as the first sign of WD in about 5% of cases [29]. However, new onset of generalized tonic-clonic seizures may also indicate the evolution of paradoxical worsening during initiation of chelation therapy, discussed in detail in the following sections. Discrete or unclassified signs were observed in 11.3% of patients, further illustrating the clinical heterogeneity [32].

Behavioral and cognitive changes are commonly associated with neurologic problems and may be detected early in the course of the disease. The pattern of cognitive decline is similar to other basal ganglia disorders [33, 34]. Apathy, reduced attention, bradyphrenia, frontal lobe dysfunction with impaired social judgment, and impulse control behaviors are now commonly recognized, and they represent a significant morbidity for WD patients. Decline in school or job performance may herald cognitive changes. Tremor in WD is highly variable with rest, postural, and action tremor observed [28, 30–32]. Wing-beating tremor is a prototypical WD tremor, proximally generated, appearing when the patient holds semi-flexed outstretched arms in the "wingbeat" posture. Its amplitude increases the longer the patient holds the position, and some patients exhibit a severe flapping tremor as if they are launching into flight. Other patients exhibit a typical postural and action tremor that may easily be misdiagnosed as essential tremor. Dystonia varies from focal to generalized dystonia [28, 30–32]. Advanced WD may produce severe generalized dystonia with secondary contractures and inability to walk. Segmental or focal dystonia affecting the craniofacial region is especially common, causing severe dysphonia, dysarthria, or even a complete loss of speech with dysphagia or inability to swallow. Many WD patients exhibit an exaggerated smile, known as risus sardonicus. Dystonia associated with WD is a prototypical secondary dystonia [13]. Parkinsonism typically manifests as masked facies with hypophonic soft voice, micrographia, and shuffling or freezing gait. Hypokinetic-rigid syndromes tend to be symmetrical, but unilateral tremor can be present leading the examiner to a misdiagnosis of Parkinson's disease.

Dysarthria is typically of a mixed type with prominent dystonic and hypokinetic features [28, 30–32]. Patients with the pseudosclerotic (tremor) subtype may also exhibit signs of cerebellar dysarthria. However, there is a considerable overlap among these groups, and patients with severe WD often display mixed phenotypes. Hyperkinetic movements are more common in younger individuals who developed WD in the second decade. Ataxia is another frequently mentioned sign, but true cerebellar ataxia is rare, and incoordination and balance problems are more commonly caused by extrapyramidal signs and severe wing-beating tremor [32]. Primary psychiatric manifestations have been reported in 10% of newly diagnosed patients without detectable neurologic or hepatic manifestations [35, 36]. Later in the course of the disease, these patients may develop additional neurologic problems, but these initial neurologic signs can be subtle and easily overlooked. Psychiatric symptoms are nonspecific ranging from depression to acute psychotic episodes, leading to common misdiagnoses of bipolar disorder or schizophrenia. Overall, this is a particularly difficult type of WD to diagnose. The analysis of patients initially seen by a psychiatrist showed that the average delay of diagnosis was more than 2 years.

Diagnosis of WD

The definite diagnosis of WD is established by biochemical tests confirming signs of copper overload, including increased urinary copper excretion and elevated values of free copper (NCC) in blood [1, 2]. Even though the diagnosis remains laboratory based, the availability of genetic testing may further increase clinical certainty, especially in patients with biliary obstruction or with borderline biochemical features as can be seen in heterozygous patients [37–39].

Screening tests are recommended as the first step in confirming the diagnosis of WD [1]. Levels of ceruloplasmin plasma, the main copper-binding plasma protein containing more than 90% of total plasma copper, are most frequently used [40]. Loss of function of the *ATP7B* gene impairs copper loading to ceruloplasmin, resulting in low plasma levels. A serum ceruloplasmin level less than 20 mg/dL (200 mg/L or 2.83 µmol/L) is consistent with the diagnosis of WD, but overall the positive predictive value is very low at 5.9% [2]. Even low ceruloplasmin levels cannot confirm the diagnosis, and additional confirmatory tests are needed. Abnormally low ceruloplasmin levels less than 5 mg/dl strongly suggest WD, but it can be also associated with conditions with very low copper plasma values, especially with copper deficiency and aceruloplasminemia [41, 42]. The latter is a rare autosomal recessive condition caused by mutations in the ceruloplasmin gene. Neurologic clinical presentations of aceruloplasminemia may mimic WD but the pathogenesis is caused by iron overload. Another possible cause of low ceruloplasmin is Menkes disease, an X-linked disorder of copper transport from enterocytes to blood and through the blood-brain barrier caused by mutations in the *ATP7A* gene [43]. Heterozygotes carrying one mutated allele of *ATP7B* gene may also have borderline low values requiring further testing. Similarly, low normal ceruloplasmin value does not exclude a diagnosis of WD. Ceruloplasmin is an acute phase reactant causing higher levels, leading to false negative results. Another important cause of higher ceruloplasmin in WD is exposure to estrogens, most commonly from birth control pills [44].

Ophthalmologic evaluation, looking for Kayser-Fleischer rings, is commonly used as a screening test. KF rings may be visible as a golden-brownish pigmentation around the limbus. Some patients may not have a fully formed circle, and increased pigmentation can be seen around 6 and 12 o'clock positions. Definitive detection of Kayser-Fleischer rings should be established by slit lamp examination. They are rarely absent in patients with neurologic presentations. The presence of KF rings can only support the diagnosis of WD, because rarely they may be present in patients with chronic cholestatic liver disease.

Every patient with suspected WD needs to have a 24-h urine copper measurement and this test alone is diagnostic in most patients [1, 2]. Obstructive hepatopathy can cause diagnostic uncertainty, but this is not common for patients with neurologic signs. It is important to completely collect 24-h urine starting after the first morning voiding on the day of the collection day and complete it the next day after the first voiding. Another technical requirement is a copper-free collection vessel. Total creatinine excretion in the 24-h urine collection is typically measured to support proper urine collection. A 24-h copper value more than 100 μg/24 h (1.6 μmol/24 h) is conventionally considered diagnostic of WD, especially for patients with neurologic or psychiatric phenotypic presentations [1, 2]. Normal values for 24-h excretion are typically below 40 or 50 μg (0.64 or 0.8 μmol)/24 h. Intermediate values between 40/50 and 100 μg/24 h may be seen in heterozygous (carrier) individuals and require further investigation. Affected symptomatic children with WD may also have 24-H urine copper values below the conventional cutoff, and lowering this value in pediatric patients has been suggested [45]. D-Penicillamine challenge has been used in patients with borderline 24-h urine copper values, but this test has been validated only in children with hepatic presentations. Administration of 500 mg of D-penicillamine before urine collection and repeated once 12 h into the collection promotes cupriuria, and values of more than 1600 μg copper/24 h (25 μmol/24 h) are considered diagnostic [46]. Overall, this test is used less commonly with the availability of genetic testing for *ATP7B* mutations.

Serum NCC (non-ceruloplasmin-bound copper) or free copper assay has been proposed as a diagnostic test for WD. It is elevated above 25 μg/dL (3.94 μmol/L) in most untreated patients [1]. Normal values are 10–15 μg/dL (1.6–2.4 μmol/L), and free copper below 5 μg/dL (0.8 4 μmol/L) indicates copper deficiency. Limited availability of this test reduces its clinical utility. The free copper fraction can be also calculated from total plasma copper and ceruloplasmin values. Six copper atoms are bound to one molecule of ceruloplasmin, resulting in approximately 3.15 μg of copper weight per 1 milligram of ceruloplasmin. Thus, free copper can be estimated as a difference between the total copper and ceruloplasmin value multiplied by three. However, this needs to be interpreted with caution, especially when the levels of ceruloplasmin are low [1]. Total copper value alone is not very helpful in the diagnosis of WD because it is very variable. Liver biopsy measuring liver copper content has been considered a gold standard for the confirmation of the diagnosis and may be still required in patients with predominantly hepatic presentation. However, the diagnosis of neurological or psychiatric WD can be confirmed using 24-H urine copper excretion assay. Hepatic copper content more than 250 μg/g dry weight (4.0 μmol/g of tissue) is considered diagnostic for WD [1].

Cloning of the causative gene for WD and the rapid progress in high-throughput sequencing methods increased the importance of genetic testing in the diagnostic process. Identification of both disease-causing mutations confirms the diagnosis. Mutations in the *ATP7B* gene can be found in any of the 21 coding exons and intronic flanking sequences, resulting in a considerable allelic heterogeneity [37, 38]. Many deleterious mutations are private and limited to single families, and most patients are compound heterozygotes. Certain ethnic groups harbor more common mutations, and genetic screening can be prioritized to analyze common mutations first. Targeted mutation analysis for specific mutations, such as multiplex amplification refractory mutation system PCR, can be employed in populations with prevalent common mutations. Otherwise, every exon and adjoining intronic areas need to be sequenced. Genetic testing should be limited to confirmation of diagnosis, family screening, and unclear cases with a high degree of suspicion for WD. Both mutations need to be known if this test is used for familial screening.

Overall rate of detection of mutations in patients with biochemically confirmed disease is approaching 98%, but intronic mutations or mutations in the promoter regions still may be undetected. Whole genome sequencing can be utilized in these cases. However, biochemical laboratory methods detecting copper overload may be sufficient to confirm the diagnosis in these patients.

Most patients manifesting neurologic problems have abnormal magnetic resonance imaging (MRI) findings, and this can help to increase the suspicion for WD [47–49]. However, these MRI changes are nonspecific and WD needs to be confirmed by other laboratory methods. Similarly, a normal MRI of the brain does not rule out WD. The most common finding is hyperintensity on T2-weighted and FLAIR images involving the putamen, striatum, and globus pallidus (Fig. 25.1). Hyperintense signal in the midbrain around the red nucleus and substantia nigra may give the appearance of the "sign of the giant panda" that is most commonly seen in WD patients (Fig. 25.2). MRI structural changes only loosely correlate with neurologic deficits. Nonetheless, MRI monitoring can be very useful to detect clinical deterioration after chelation therapy (see Fig. 25.2) or for clinical improvement if patients respond favorably to decoppering therapies [49].

⚷ A normal MRI does not exclude WD.

A scoring system utilizing clinical and laboratory features, including the presence of Kayser-Fleischer rings, neurologic or neuroimaging features, hemolytic anemia, elevated liver function, elevated 24-h urine copper values, reduced ceruloplasmin, and mutation analysis has been developed [2]. The total score is generated by adding values from 0 (normal examination or absent laboratory abnormalities), 2 points (abnormal clinical signs or abnormal laboratory tests present) to 4 points if

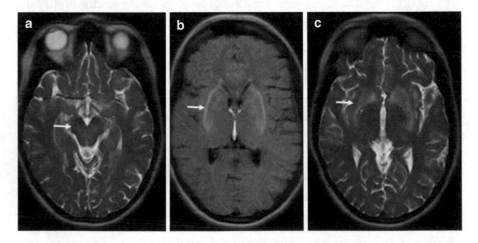

Fig. 25.1 MRI of the brain at the time of diagnosis. The patient was 20-year-old woman who was diagnosed 14 months after exhibiting first symptoms. Faint T2 hyperintensity was observed in upper brainstem (panel **a**). Increased T2 signal in basal ganglia (panels **b** and **c**) is suggestive of WD

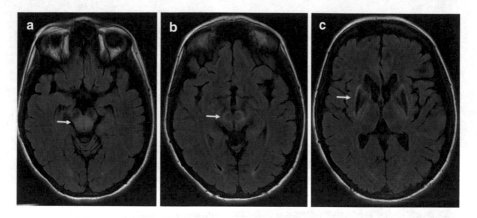

Fig. 25.2 MRI of the brain 8 months after chelation therapy was initiated. She was started on D-penicillamine at an outside institution, and within 1 month she developed severe dystonia with mutism and severe Parkinsonism. This was irreversible and her neurologic deficits were fixed. Flair imaging showed worsening of hyperintensity in the midbrain (panel **a**) with the appearance suggestive of face of the giant panda (panel **b**). Severe cystic changes were detected in basal ganglia (panel **c**)

both mutations are detected. Overall score of 4 or more points is highly suggestive for WD, and a score between 2 and 3 points is classified as probable WD where more diagnostic tests are needed [2].

Second WD Emergency: Timely Treatment

The natural history of untreated symptomatic WD is eventual death caused by liver failure or complications from disabling neurologic deficits [1, 2, 29]. Currently published therapeutic guidelines recommend life-long therapy for all patients, regardless of clinical symptoms or severity of their symptoms. Patients diagnosed and treated early may lead essentially normal lives. WD is curable by orthotopic liver transplant, but this approach is mostly reserved for fulminant liver failure, and its role as a rescue therapy for neurologic problems remains controversial [1]. Therapy should be initiated immediately after the diagnosis is confirmed, and a high degree of clinical suspicion for the diagnosis is essential. Average time from symptom onset to correct diagnosis and treatment is still around 1 year [29, 50]. This delay affects the overall success of therapy. Patients presenting with neurologic symptoms had best outcomes when the interval between first symptoms and initiation of therapy was less than 1 month. Only 20% had very favorable outcome with no abnormalities or mild residual symptoms when the diagnosis and treatment was delayed by about half a year [11, 51]. The development of neurologic symptoms is the result of elevated NCC from chronic copper accumulation. Thus, the goals of therapy are to reverse copper overload and establish a negative copper balance during which NCC values are reduced to normal levels. The tight control of NCC is critical because it is likely the main cause of copper neurotoxicity and can be a trigger of further paradoxical worsening after the therapy is started [14, 15]. Therapy for WD can be divided into an acute chelating phase followed by a chronic maintenance phase after the patients achieve improvement of their copper balance.

WD is treated with chelating agents or zinc salts. Chelators nonspecifically bind copper and promote urinary copper excretion. D-penicillamine and trientine are the two currently available chelating agents [1–3, 10, 52] [another agent, tetrathiomolybdate, has been studied but not yet approved]. Both have rapid onset of action and are used in the acute phase of decoppering therapy. They can also be used for long-term maintenance therapy. Zinc works by a different mechanism of action, as it blocks the absorption of copper from the gastrointestinal tract by triggering increased expression of metallothioneins in the enterocytes [53, 54]. Metallothioneins are cysteine-rich proteins that bind various metal ions, including copper. The dietary copper bound to metallothionein is sequestered within the intestinal cells and prevented from absorption into the blood. Negative copper balance is achieved because copper is removed through the stool after the enterocytes are shed in the intestinal lumen as a part of normal cellular turnover. This is a cumulative effect that can take up to 3 months; thus, the main role of zinc is in the maintenance phase of therapy [53]. The transition to maintenance phase of therapy is based on clinical improvement and laboratory copper values. The typical interval occurs after 2–6 months of chelating therapy, but additional clinical and laboratory improvement can be observed up to 3 months after the initiation of chelation therapy with an ongoing improvement of neurologic symptoms.

D-Penicillamine remains the most frequently prescribed chelator in the treatment of WD around the world, and its major effect is the promotion of the urinary excretion of copper [8, 55, 56]. The starting dose for patients with neurologic symptoms should be 250–500 mg/day with a careful increase by 250 mg every 5–7 days to monitor patients for possible worsening and side effects. The usual maximum dose in neurologic patients is 1500 mg/day. It is dosed three or four times per day either 1 h before meals or 2 h after meals because food reduces its absorption by almost half. Iron supplements and antacids also significantly reduce its absorption. D-Penicillamine has a strong cupreuremic effect and 24-H urine copper assay is used to monitor the therapeutic response [1, 2]. The aim of chelation therapy is to normalize NCC, but this test is not generally available. Calculated NCC based on total plasma copper and ceruloplasmin levels may be imprecise if plasma ceruloplasmin values are low. The dose is adjusted based on 24-H urine copper assay, and excretion of copper may exceed 1000 μg (16 μmol) per day at the initiation of therapy. D-Penicillamine can be also used for long-term maintenance therapy, and this dose is lower than during acute chelation. This dosing is usually 750–1000 mg/day administered in two divided doses with expected daily urine excretion between 200 μg and 500 μg (3–8 μmol). Urine copper levels below 200 μg (3 μmol)/24 h suggest overtreatment with iatrogenic copper deficiency or noncompliance with treatment [8, 9].

Frequent adverse effects are a major disadvantage of penicillamine, and up to one third of patients will eventually stop this therapy. This creates a high risk of noncompliance with a possibility of further worsening of neurologic symptoms. Acute sensitivity reactions include fever, lymphadenopathy, cutaneous eruptions, proteinuria, and signs of bone marrow suppression with neutropenia or thrombocytopenia [1]. Slower rate of dose titration or brief treatment with steroids has been suggested to mitigate these problems, but if alternative medications such as trientine are available, a change of chelating agent may be more suitable. Chronic adverse effects include nephrotoxicity with proteinuria, a lupus-like reaction with hematuria, proteinuria, positive antinuclear antibody, progeric changes in the skin, pemphigoid lesions, lichen planus, aphthous stomatitis, myasthenia gravis-like syndrome, and polymyositis. It also interferes with wound healing, and the therapy needs to be interrupted if surgery is planned D-Penicillamine also has an antipyridoxine effect, and supplementation of pyridoxine (vitamin B6) or monitoring of pyridoxine levels has been recommended [57].

Trientine is approved by the FDA as second-line therapy for patients who did not tolerate D-penicillamine. It is a chelator with a high affinity for copper, and like penicillamine the bound copper is removed through urinary excretion. Trientine has a lower cupreuremic effect than D-penicillamine, and daily copper excretion in the range of 200–500 µg (3–8 µmoles) is commonly observed in WD patients on trientine [1, 58]. The target dose of trietine during initial therapy is 750–1500 mg/day divided in two or three doses, and it also should be taken before food. Similar to D-penicillamine therapy, trientine should be started gradually in patients with neurologic symptoms, with 250 mg increments every 5–7 days. The typical maintenance dose is 750 or 1000 mg per day, and the dose is adjusted based on 24-copper urine values. Daily urinary copper excretion below 200 µg may indicate either nonadherence to therapy or induction of copper deficiency from overtreatment. Trientine tends to be well tolerated and no significant acute or chronic side effects have been observed. Bone marrow suppression with thrombocytopenia and leukopenia is rare, and it should prompt an evaluation for evolving iatrogenic copper deficiency from overtreatment.

Zinc acetate is approved by the FDA for treatment of WD but other zinc salts, available over the counter, can be used as well [53, 59]. Zinc should be taken on an empty stomach and gastric irritation with nausea is the most common side effect. The severity of gastric intolerance may be influenced by the type of salt, and zinc gluconate can be used to ameliorate gastrointestinal side effects. The typical dose of zinc acetate or zinc gluconate is 50 mg three times per day [54]. The disease control on this therapy is also monitored by 24-h copper urine assay, but given the different mechanism of action, the target copper urine values differ from monitoring parameters of chelation therapies. Zinc does not promote urinary copper excretion, and an effective treatment reduces the overall copper urinary excretion, reflecting the reduction of copper overload. Daily urinary copper excretion of less than 75 µg indicates an adequate control on zinc therapy. The most common use of zinc is for maintenance therapy after chelators have reduced NCC and induced a negative copper balance. When a patient is crossed over from a chelator to zinc, these two therapies need to overlap for a period of 2–3 months to maximize the effects on metallothionein. This is an especially suitable option for patients with neurologic phenotypes, and some patients with hepatic symptoms only may experience worsening of their disease control on zinc monotherapy.

Third WD Emergency: Paradoxical Treatment-Induced Worsening

The goals of therapy for patients with neurologic presentations are to stop the progression of neurologic disability, followed by gradual improvement of neurologic symptoms. However, treatment with currently available chelating agents is associated with a relatively high risk of deterioration of neurologic symptoms, also known as medication-induced paradoxical worsening [16, 17]. The risk for worsening on chelation therapy is higher for patients with a delayed diagnosis, but some patients deteriorate even if therapy is started in a timely fashion. The main hypothesis explaining this phenomenon is an upsurge of free NCC, caused by copper dissociation from unstable complexes with chelators, triggering a cytotoxic effect in neuronal tissue with subsequent neurologic deterioration. Correlation between the stability of NCC control without additional elevations of NCC values and favorable neurologic outcomes has been reported, but NCC assay is not readily available as a routine clinical test to monitor elevation of NCC after treatment initiation [15]. Paradoxical worsening typically occurs within the first 6 months of therapy as this is the most crucial period of chelation therapy.

The first reports of medication-induced worsening suggested that D-penicillamine has the highest risk, and as many as 20–35% of treated patients with neurologic presentations have experienced further deterioration that is often irreversible [16]. Paradoxical neurologic worsening has been also observed in patients treated with trientine, with reported incidence of 10–15% [58]. This would potentially favor trientine as first-line chelation therapy for patients with neurologic symptoms, based on previous reports of much higher risk in patients treated with D-penicillamine. The severity of presenting neurologic symptoms and the extent of structural changes detected by magnetic resonance imaging with early signal changes in the basal ganglia, thalamus, and brainstem are risk factors for paradoxical worsening (see Figs. 25.1 and 25.2). Recommended management of paradoxical neurologic worsening is to reduce the dose of the chelating agent. Additional steps include switching to a different chelating agent, especially if paradoxical worsening was induced by D-penicillamine; these patients should be switched to trientine at a lower dose. A temporary interruption of chelation can be also considered if no other treatment options are available.

More recent retrospective studies suggested that D-penicillamine, trientine, and zinc salts have very comparable incidences of paradoxical worsening, and one study found the least frequent deterioration in patients treated with D-penicillamine with the reported risk of 2% of neurologic decline, much lower than previous observations [11, 60]. The lack of head-to-head comparison between these two chelators and the retrospective nature of most of the studies make it difficult to determine whether there is a superior chelator. Thus, until more conclusive clinical data is available, the selection of first-line chelation therapy for patients with neurologic phenotypes of WD needs to be based on additional factors, including personal experience and availability.

Zinc is considered a second-line therapy after laboratory signs of copper overload have been normalized by chelators. However, zinc has been used in patients with neurologic symptoms who are at risk for paradoxical worsening or who developed this problem on typical chelators [60]. The justification of zinc as first-line therapy in these patients is to lower the risk of paradoxical worsening [61, 62]. The effects of zinc on metallothionein expression are cumulative and there is a delay of several months until zinc is fully effective. That is why some consider first-line therapy with zinc too slow to effectively control neurologic phenotypes of WD. Neurologic worsening has been also observed in patients with neurologic symptoms who were treated with zinc but is more likely caused by undertreatment [60]. Moreover, in initial treatment the doses of zinc need to be higher than for maintenance therapy and this is often poorly tolerated.

Liver transplantation corrects the genetic defect of WD and can be considered a curative procedure, even though it requires life-long immunosuppressive therapy in transplanted patients [1]. The indications for liver transplantation in hepatic forms of WD are generally well established [63]. WD patients who develop acute liver failure are candidates for transplantation because of very high mortality, and liver transplantation is a lifesaving procedure for these patients. Liver transplantation with a wild type of *ATP7B* gene promptly restores copper homeostasis with normalization of extrahepatic copper metabolism, including in the central nervous system. That is why this approach has been also advocated as a rescue therapy for neurologic patients who experienced progressive deterioration of their condition on chelation therapy [64–66]. However, the role of liver transplantation as a treatment for patients with severe neurologic deficits remains controversial. Improvement or even complete resolution after liver transplantation has been reported in some patients with severe and progressive neurologic deficits who did not respond to conventional chelation therapies. These positive outcomes are not universal, and no improvements or further progression has been also observed. The most comprehensive retrospective analysis of 18 patients with WD who underwent liver transplantation because of progressive neurologic deficits showed that four died and a major improvement was seen in eight patients [67]. The rest of the patients had less robust improvement or stabilization of their neurologic function. Thus, at present there are no consensus regarding the role of liver transplant to reverse neurologic deficits and no formal criteria of best candidates for liver transplantation for neurologic phenotypes [68].

Patients who experienced neurologic deterioration while on chelation or zinc typically show progression of orofacial dystonia, progressive dysphagia, and dysarthria. This is associated with a high risk of aspiration, and very close monitoring of swallowing is mandatory in the initial phase of WD treatment [69]. Some patients may require percutaneous endoscopic gastrostomy feeding to maintain adequate nutrition and reduce the risk of aspiration. An additional life-threating emergency is status dystonicus, reported in a handful of patients after D-penicillamine [18, 19]. This is a potentially life-threatening complication of worsening WD, presenting as an acute and severe generalized dystonia associated with rhabdomyolysis, hyperpyrexia, acute renal failure, and respiratory insufficiency. Treatment options include adjustment or change of chelating agents, as outlined above. Pharmacological therapies include benzodiazepines, baclofen, VMAT2 (vesicular monoamine transporter 2) inhibitors, or a trial with levodopa. Bilateral globus pallidus pars interna (GPi) deep brain stimulation (DBS) can benefit patients in status dystonicus that is refractory to adjustments of decoppering therapies or other pharmacological measures [70]. Outcome of medication-induced status dystonicus in WD varies from mild recovery to a fatal outcome. Similar to other examples of paradoxical worsening, status dystonicus developed within the first 2 months of chelating therapies, further emphasizing that the early stages of acute chelation therapies are most critical.

Conclusion

WD is the prototypical movement disorder challenge—a challenge to diagnose, a challenge to treat, and a challenge to monitor and maintain. However, if the clinician maintains a high index of suspicion for the condition and initiates and monitors chelation carefully, most patients can be effectively managed and live normal and productive lives.

References

1. Roberts EA, Schilsky ML. American Association for Study of Liver Diseases (AASLD). Diagnosis and treatment of Wilson's disease: an update. Hepatology. 2008;47:2089–111.
2. Ferenci P, Caca K, Loudianos G, Mieli-Vergani G, Tanner S, Sternlieb I, et al. Diagnosis and phenotypic classification of Wilson disease. Liver Int. 2003;23(3):139–42.
3. Hedera P. Update on the clinical management of Wilson's disease. Appl Clin Genet. 2017;10:9–19.
4. Bull PC, Thomas GR, Rommens JM, Forbes JR, Cox DW. The Wilson disease gene is a putative copper transporting P-type ATPase similar to the Menkes gene. Nat Genet. 1993;5(4):327–37.
5. Tanzi RE, Petrukhin K, Chernov I, Pellequer JL, Wasco W, Ross B, et al. The Wilson disease gene is a copper transporting ATPase with homology to the Menkes disease gene. Nat Genet. 1993;5(4):344–50.
6. Członkowska A, Litwin T, Dusek P, Ferenci P, Lutsenko S, Medici V, et al. Wilson disease. Nat Rev Dis Primers. 2018;4(1):21.
7. Bandmann O, Weiss KH, Kaler SG. Wilson's disease and other neurological copper disorders. Lancet Neurol. 2015;14:103–13.
8. Walshe JM, Yealland M. Chelation treatment of neurological Wilson's disease. Q J Med. 1993;86:197–204.
9. Appenzeller-Herzog C, Mathes T, Heeres MLS. Comparative effectiveness of common therapies for Wilson disease: a systematic review and meta-analysis of controlled studies. Liver Int. 2019;39:2136–52.

10. Hedera P. Clinical management of Wilson disease. Ann Transl Med. 2019;7(Suppl):S66.
11. Weiss KH, Thurik F, Gotthardt DN, Schäfer M, Teufel U, Wiegand F, EUROWILSON Consortium, et al. Efficacy and safety of oral chelators in treatment of patients with Wilson disease. Clin Gastroenterol Hepatol. 2013;11(8):1028–35, e1–2.
12. Merle U, Schaefer M, Ferenci P, Stremmel W. Clinical presentation, diagnosis and long-term outcome of Wilson's disease: a cohort study. Gut. 2007;56:115–20.
13. Hedera P. Wilson's disease: a master of disguise. Parkinsonism Relat Disorder. 2019;59:140–5.
14. Brewer GJ, Askari F, Dick RB, Sitterly J, Fink JK, Carlson M, et al. Treatment of Wilson's disease with tetrathiomolybdate: V. control of free copper by tetrathiomolybdate and a comparison with trientine. Transl Res. 2009;154(2):70–7.
15. Weiss KH, Askari FK, Czlonkowska A, Ferenci P, Bronstein JM, Bega D, et al. Bis-choline tetrathiomolybdate in patients with Wilson's disease: an open-label, multicentre, phase 2 study. Lancet Gastroenterol Hepatol. 2017;2(12):869–76.
16. Brewer GJ, Terry CA, Aisen AM, Hill GM. Worsening of neurologia syndrome in patients with Wilson's disease with initial penicillamine therapy. Arch Neurol. 1987;44:490–3.
17. Litwin T, Dziezyc K, Karlinski M, Chabik G, Czepiel W, Czlonkowska A. Early neurological worsening in patients with Wilson's disease. J Neurol Sci. 2015;355:162–16.
18. Svetel M, Sternić N, Pejović S, Kostić VS. Penicillamine induced lethal status dystonicus in a patient with Wilson's disease. Mov Disord. 2001;13:568–9.
19. Teive HA, Munhoz RP, Souza MM, Antoniuk SA, Santos ML, Teixeira MJ, et al. Status Dystonicus: study of five cases. Arq Neuropsiquiatr. 2005;63(1):26–9.
20. Pellecchia MT, Criscuolo C, Longo K, Campanella G, Filla A, Barone P. Clinical presentation and treatment of Wilson's disease: a single-centre experience. Eur Neurol. 2003;50:48–52.
21. Walshe JM. Wilson's disease. The presenting symptoms. Arch Dis Child. 1962;37:253–6.
22. Saito T. Presenting symptoms and natural history of Wilson disease. Eur J Pediatr. 1987;146:261–5.
23. Negahban K, Chern K. Cataracts associated with systemic disorders and syndromes. Curr Opin Ophthalmol. 2002;13:419–22.
24. Gow PJ, Smallwood RA, Angus PW, Smith AI, Wall AJ, Sewell RB. Diagnosis of Wilson's disease: an experience over three decades. Gut. 2000;46:415–9.
25. Ferenci P, Członkowska A, Merle U, Ferenc S, Gromadzka G, Yurdaydin C, et al. Late-onset Wilson's disease. Gastroenterology. 2007;132(4):1294–8.
26. Ala A, Borjigin J, Rochwarger A, Schilsky M. Wilson disease in septuagenarian siblings: raising the bar for diagnosis. Hepatology. 2005;41:668–70.
27. Członkowska A, Rodo M, Gromazdzka G. Late onset Wilson's disease: therapeutic implications. Mov Disord. 2008;23:896–89.
28. Oder W, Grimm G, Kollegger H, Ferenci P, Schneider B, Deecke L. Neurological and neuropsychiatric spectrum of Wilson's disease: a prospective study of 45 cases. J Neurol. 1991;238:281–7.
29. Walshe JM, Yealland M. Wilson's disease: the problem of delayed diagnosis. J Neurol Neurosurg Psychiatry. 1992;55:692–6.
30. Machado A, Chien HF, Deguti MM, Cançado E, Azevedo RS, Scaff M, et al. Neurological manifestations in Wilson's disease: report of 119 cases. Mov Disord. 2006;21(12):2192–6.
31. Burke JF, Dayalu P, Nan B, Askari F, Brewer GJ, Lorinz MT. Prognostic significance of neurologic examination in Wilson disease. Parkinsonism Relat Disord. 2011;17:551–6.
32. Członkowska A, Litwin T, Dzieżyc K, Karliński M, Bring J, Bjartmar C. Characteristics of a newly diagnosed Polish cohort of patients with neurologic manifestations of Wilson disease evaluated with the Unified Wilson's Disease Rating Scale. BMC Neurol. 2018;18:34.
33. Iwański S, Seniów J, Leśniak M, Litwin T, Członkowska A. Diverse attention deficits in patients with neurologically symptomatic and asymptomatic Wilson's disease. Neuropsychology. 2015;29:25–30.
34. Wenisch E, De Tassigny A, Trocello JM, Beretti J, Girardot-Tinant N, Woimant F. Cognitive profile in Wilson's disease: a case series of 31 patients. Rev Neurol (Paris). 2013;169:944–9.

35. Shanmugiah A, Sinha S, Taly AB, Prashanth LK, Tomar M, Arunodaya GR, et al. Psychiatric manifestations in Wilson's disease: a cross-sectional analysis. J Neuropsychiatry Clin Neurosci. 2008;20(1):81–5.
36. Svetel M, Potrebić A, Pekmezović T, Tomić A, Kresojević N, Jesić R, et al. Neuropsychiatric aspects of treated Wilson's disease. Parkinsonism Relat Disord. 2009;15(10):772–5.
37. Coffey AJ, Durkie M, Hague S, McLay K, Emmerson J, Lo C, et al. A genetic study of Wilson's disease in the United Kingdom. Brain. 2013;136(Pt 5):1476–87.
38. Thomas GR, Forbes JR, Roberts EA, Walshe JM, Cox DW. The Wilson disease gene: spectrum of mutations and their consequences. Nat Genet. 1995;9:210–7.
39. Ferenci P. Phenotype-genotype correlations in patients with Wilson's disease. Ann N Y Acad Sci. 2014;1315:1–5.
40. Cauza E, Maier-Dobersberger T, Polli C, Kaserer K, Kramer L, Ferenci P. Screening for Wilson's disease in patients with liver diseases by serum ceruloplasmin. J Hepatol. 1997;27:358–62.
41. Xu X, Pin S, Gathinji M, Fuchs R, Harris ZL. Aceruloplasminemia: an inherited neurodegenerative disease with impairment of iron homeostasis. Ann N Y Acad Sci. 2004;1012:299–305.
42. Hedera P, Peltier A, Fink JK, Wilcock S, London Z, Brewer GJ. Myelopolyneuropathy and pancytopenia due to copper deficiency and high zinc levels of unknown origin II. The denture cream is a primary source of excessive zinc. Neurotoxicology. 2009;30:996–9.
43. Menkes JH. Menkes disease and Wilson disease: two sided of the same copper coin. Part I: Menkes disease. Eur J Paediatr Neurol. 1999;3:147–58.
44. Arredondo M, Núñez H, López G, Pizarro F, Ayala M, Araya M. Influence of estrogens on copper indicators: in vivo and in vitro studies. Biol Trace Elem Res. 2010;134:252–64.
45. Manolaki N, Nikolopoulou G, Daikos GL, Panagiotakaki E, Tzetis M, Roma E, et al. Wilson disease in children: analysis of 57 cases. J Pediatr Gastroenterol Nutr. 2009;48(1):72–7.
46. Schilsky ML. Non-invasive testing for Wilson disease: revisiting the D-penicillamine challenge test. J Hepatol. 2007;47:172–3.
47. Hermann W. Morphological and functional imaging in neurological and non-neurological Wilson's patients. Ann N Y Acad Sci. 2014;131:24–9.
48. Sinha S, Taly AB, Ravishankar S, Prashanth LK, Venugopal KS, Arunodaya GR, et al. Wilson's disease: cranial MRI observations and clinical correlation. Neuroradiology. 2006;48(9):613–21.
49. Südmeyer M, Saleh A, Wojtecki L, Cohnen M, Gross J, Ploner M, et al. Wilson's disease tremor is associated with magnetic resonance imaging lesions in basal ganglia structures. Mov Disord. 2006;21(12):2134–9.
50. Prashanth LK, Taly AB, Sinha S, Arunodaya GR, Swamy HS. Wilson's disease: diagnostic errors and clinical implications. J Neurol Neurosurg Psychiatry. 2004;5:907–9.
51. Hölscher S, Leinweber B, Hefter H, Reuner U, Günther P, Weiss KH, et al. Evaluation of the symptomatic treatment of residual neurological symptoms in Wilson disease. Eur Neurol. 2010;64(2):83–7.
52. Brewer GJ, Fink JK, Hedera P. Diagnosis and treatment of Wilson disease. Semin Neurol. 1999;19:261–70.
53. Brewer GJ, Hill GM, Prasad AS, Cossack ZT, Rabbani P. Oral zinc therapy for Wilson's disease. Ann Intern Med. 1983;99:314–9.
54. Brewer GJ, Yuzbasiyan-Gurkan V, Johnson V, Dick RD, Wang Y. Treatment of Wilson's disease with zinc XII: dose regimen requirements. Am J Med Sci. 1993;305:199–202.
55. Walshe JM. Penicillamine, a new oral therapy for Wilson's disease. Am J Med. 1956;21:487–95.
56. Litin RB, Goldstein NP, Randall RV, Power MH, Diessner GR. Effect of D,L-penicillamine on the urinary excretion of copper and calcium in hepatolenticular degeneration (Wilson's disease). Neurology. 1960;10:123–6.
57. Jaffe IA, Altman K, Merryman P. The antipyridoxine effect of penicillamine in Man. J Clin Invest. 1964;43:1869–73.
58. Brewer GJ, Askari F, Lorincz MT, Carlson M, Schilsky M, Kluin KJ, et al. Treatment of Wilson disease with ammonium tetrathiomolybdate: IV. Comparison of tetrathiomolybdate

and trientine in a double-blind study of treatment of the neurologic presentation of Wilson disease. Arch Neurol. 2006;63(4):521–7.

59. Hoogenraad TU, Van Hattum J, Van den Hamer CJ. Management of Wilson's disease with zinc sulphate. Experience in a series of 27 patients. J Neurol Sci. 1987;77:137–46.

60. Czlonkowska A, Litwin T, Karliński M, Dziezyc MK, Chabik G, Czerska M. D-penicillamine versus zinc sulfate as first-line therapy for Wilson's disease. Eur J Neurol. 2014;21:599–606.

61. Hoogenraad TU. Paradigm shift in treatment of Wilson's disease: zinc therapy now treatment of choice. Brain and Development. 2006;28:141–6.

62. Avan A, de Bie RMA, Hoogenraad TU. Wilson's disease should be treated with zinc rather than Trientine or Penicillamine. Neuropediatrics. 2017;48:394–5.

63. Petrasek J, Jirsa M, Sperl J, Kozak L, Taimr P, Spicak J, et al. Revised King's College score for liver transplantation in adult patients with Wilson's disease. Liver Transpl. 2007;13(1):55–61.

64. Stracciari A, Tempestini A, Borghi A, Guarino M. Effect of liver transplantation on neurological manifestations in Wilson disease. Arch Neurol. 2000;57:384–6.

65. Laurencin C, Brunet AS, Dumortier J, Lion-Francois L, Thobois S, Mabrut JY, et al. Liver transplantation in Wilson's disease with neurological impairment: evaluation in 4 patients. Eur Neurol. 2017;77(1–2):5–15.

66. Guillaud O, Dumortier J, Sobesky R, Debray D, Wolf P, Vanlemmens C, et al. Long term results of liver transplantation for Wilson's disease: experience in France. J Hepatol. 2014;60(3):579–89.

67. Poujois A, Sobesky R, Meissner WG, Brunet AS, Broussolle E, Laurencin C, et al. Liver transplantation as a rescue therapy for severe neurologic forms of Wilson disease. Neurology. 2020;94(21):e2189–202.

68. Bandmann O, Weiss KH, Hedera P. Liver transplant for neurologic Wilson disease: hope or fallacy? Neurology. 2020;94:907–8.

69. da Silva-Júnior FP, Carrasco AE, da Silva Mendes AM, et al. Swallowing dysfunction in Wilson's disease: a scintigraphic study. Neurogastroenterol Motil. 2008;20:285–90.

70. Hedera P. Treatment of Wilson's disease motor complications with deep brain stimulation. Ann N Y Acad Sci. 2014;131:16–23.

Wilson Disease Presenting as Opsoclonus-Myoclonus Syndrome

26

Philippe A. Salles, Valentina Besa-Lehmann,
Carolina Pelayo-Varela, Prudencio Lozano-Iraguen,
Hubert H. Fernandez, and Andrés De la Cerda

Patient Vignette

A 31-year-old previously healthy man presented with an insidious 3-month history of anxiety and agoraphobia. In the last 4 weeks, he also developed upper limb action tremor and balance difficulties. This precipitous neurological decline prompted admission to the emergency unit. On examination he was very apathetic and almost mute. Smooth pursuit and saccadic ocular movements were intact, but he had bouts of ocular flutter. Mini-myoclonus in both hands and negative myoclonus in all four limbs interfered with smooth movements. He was slightly dysarthric, had mild dysmetria, intention tremor, dysdiadochokinesia, and difficulties with tandem gait. Strength, reflexes, and sensation were intact. A thorough assessment which included blood and cerebrospinal fluid tests revealed abnormal liver function, whereas other

Supplementary Information The online version of this chapter (https://doi.org/10.1007/978-3-030-75898-1_26) contains supplementary material, which is available to authorized users.

P. A. Salles
Department of Neuroscience, Clínica Dávila, Santiago, Chile

CETRAM, Santiago, Chile

Center for Neurological Restoration, Neurological Institute, Cleveland Clinic, Cleveland, OH, USA

V. Besa-Lehmann · A. De la Cerda
Department of Neuroscience, Clínica Dávila, Santiago, Chile

CETRAM, Santiago, Chile

C. Pelayo-Varela · P. Lozano-Iraguen
Department of Neuroscience, Clínica Dávila, Santiago, Chile

H. H. Fernandez (✉)
Center for Neurological Restoration, Neurological Institute, Cleveland Clinic, Cleveland, OH, USA
e-mail: fernanh@ccf.org

© Springer Nature Switzerland AG 2022
S. J. Frucht (ed.), *Movement Disorder Emergencies*, Current Clinical Neurology,
https://doi.org/10.1007/978-3-030-75898-1_26

metabolic, inflammatory, and infectious tests were all within normal limits. Signs of chronic liver disease were seen in the abdominal CT (see Fig. 26.3g), and brain MRI showed poorly delineated T2 hyperintensity in the brainstem, ascending to diencephalic structures (see Fig. 26.3a–f). Serum ceruloplasmin level was borderline (19.3 mg/dL; normal value >20 mg/dl) but no Kayser-Fleischer rings were found. His family history was remarkable for a sister who was admitted to a psychiatric unit with a history of delusions and later experienced dystonia, tremor, and seizures. Her MRI also showed nonspecific T2 hyperintensities in the brainstem and thalamus. Although an extensive workup was done, she died without a diagnosis. With this information, a genetic disease was suspected in our patient and additional investigations were obtained. Finally, an increase in the 24-hour urinary copper (1145 µg; normal value 10–30 µg) and genetic testing showing a homozygous mutation (c.3207C > A) in the *ATP7B* gene confirmed the diagnosis of Wilson disease.

Introduction

Wilson disease (WD) is a rare genetic disorder due to an inborn error of copper metabolism that typically manifests with hepatic cirrhosis and basal ganglia abnormalities [1]. The disease owes its name to the original report by the British neurologist Kinnier Wilson published in *Brain* in 1912 [2]. Wilson was the first to carry out a complete description of its clinical signs, along with descriptive photographs and histopathological reports of four patients who developed hepatic cirrhosis and extrapyramidal signs. He called the disorder "progressive lenticular degeneration" and also suspected a hereditary nature of the disease [2]. However, it is possible to find descriptions of this entity before 1912. Friedrich, in his book *A Clinical Treatise on Diseases of the Liver*, described a patient whose presentation sounded typical of WD [3]. In 1761, Morgagni catalogued several case reports of patients with liver disease and neurological signs dating back to the time of Galen [3].

WD is caused by mutations in *ATP7B* gene which encodes a transmembrane copper-transporting ATPase, leading to impaired copper homeostasis and copper overload in the liver, brain, and other organs. The clinical course of WD can vary in type and severity of symptoms, but progressive liver disease is a common feature. Patients can also present with neurologic and psychiatric symptoms [1, 4]. WD is diagnosed using staged algorithms that integrate clinical information, biochemical measures of copper metabolism, histopathological findings, and genetic testing for *ATP7B* mutations [5].

Wilson disease should be considered, if not screened, in any patient presenting with an unexplained psychiatric, neurological, and ophthalmological abnormalities (including atypical manifestations such as mutism, myoclonus, opsoclonus, or ocular flutter).

The prevalence of WD varies widely worldwide from 5 to 142 per million based on studies in different populations [6–8]. Recently, in a study done in the UK, the entire *ATP7B* coding region and adjacent splice sites were sequenced in 1000 apparently healthy neonatal controls. They found a high rate of *ATP7B* heterozygote mutation carriers (1 in 40), predicting a 1 in 7000 prevalence [8]. The prevalence of WD may be substantially higher in east Asian populations, where the prevalence is between 1:1500 [9] and 1: 3000 [10]. Some populations have a greater incidence and prevalence of WD than might be expected, possibly due to a founder effect. Some of these isolates were reported in the Greek islands of Crete [11], Sardinia [12], and Kalymnos [13], and the island of Gran Canaria [14], while the highest prevalence of genetically confirmed WD is 885 per million from the region of Rucăr in Romania [15].

WD is one of only a few treatable genetic movement disorders, making its prompt recognition and diagnosis an emergency for the patient and the clinician [1, 16]. In 1948, dimercaprol was introduced as the first possible effective treatment in WD; prior to this, all patients universally died shortly after diagnosis [17]. Due to its low prevalence and broad clinical spectrum, the diagnosis of WD is often missed even by experts [18]. This is a critical challenge, as delays in diagnosis and treatment weigh heavily on prognosis and outcome [16, 17].

Pathophysiology

Copper is an essential trace metal, required as a structural component or cofactor for many enzymatic physiological processes including angiogenesis and neuromodulation. Nonetheless when present in excess, free copper may induce oxidative stress and cellular damage [19]. Total copper balance is maintained by regulation of the rate of uptake in the small intestine from diet and its biliary excretion [20]. Usually, dietary copper is absorbed in the stomach and duodenum and transported via the portal vein to the liver where it is taken up into the hepatocyte via copper transporter 1 (CTR1). In the cytoplasm, copper is bound to the scavengers glutathione and metallothionein. Antioxidant protein 1 (ATOX1), a chaperone, delivers copper to the ATP7B, a specific transporting ATPase located in the trans-Golgi network. At low copper concentrations, ATP7B participates in the mechanism for incorporating copper into apo-ceruloplasmin to generate holo-ceruloplasmin, but at high copper concentrations, it works loading copper into vesicles for its biliary excretion [21, 22] (Fig. 26.1).

The underlying pathophysiological mechanism of WD relies on a defect in the ATP7B protein. This protein is highly expressed in hepatocytes and, at lower levels, in the kidney, placenta, brain, lung, and even heart [19, 21]. This deficiency is determined by more than 700 known associated mutations of the *ATP7B* gene [4, 23], which is located on the short arm of chromosome 13 and contains 20 introns and 21 exons [4]. Mutations are frequently missense or nonsense variants, which can affect any of the 21 exons in the gene [23]. Diverse *ATP7B* variants are expressed in different functional transporter properties [24]. Disease penetrance may be 100% but with diverse phenotype [23].

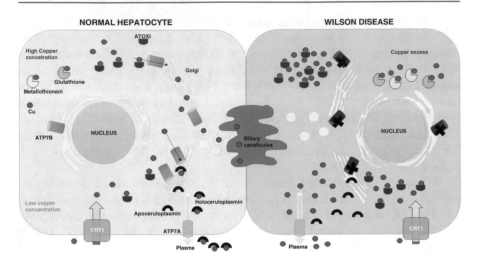

Fig. 26.1 Molecular mechanism underlying Wilson disease. Abbreviations: Cu copper, ATOX1 antioxidant protein 1, CRT1 copper transporter 1. (Modified from [22])

Reduced or dysfunctional ATP7B results in diminished serum ceruloplasmin levels, with concentrations of free serum copper usually increased, although total serum copper levels may be decreased compared with healthy controls. The overload of toxic copper in hepatic and other tissues is the major source of WD pathological tissue changes and clinical symptoms in *ATP7B* homozygous or compound heterozygous carriers [4]. Liver copper concentration is typically increased early in the disease course. It is initially distributed diffusely in the cytoplasm of hepatocytes bound to metallothionein. As copper accumulates in lysosomes, it becomes detectable by different stains such as Timm, rhodanine, and orcein. Chronic hepatocyte injury leads to hepatitis and the net accumulation in the extracellular matrix to fibrosis within the liver [4]. Determination of liver copper concentration has diagnostic implications.

Signs and Symptoms

WD may present with a variety of clinical manifestations depending on the organ affected with pathologic accumulation of copper. Therefore hepatic, neurologic, psychiatric, and ophthalmological manifestations will be the main findings. Other clinical features are hematologic disorders, osteoarthritis, tubular renal dysfunction, and cardiomyopathy, among others [25] (Table 26.1).

Symptoms usually present between the ages of 5 and 35 years. As a general rule, hepatic compromise predominates in younger patients (especially in the first decade), and neuropsychiatric symptoms in older patients (in the third decade) [26]. Most patients have a combination of features.

Table 26.1   Spectrum of manifestations in Wilson disease [1, 4]

Organ Affected	Possible Manifestations
Liver Presentation	Asymptomatic elevation of transaminases
	Asymptomatic hepatomegaly
	Steatosis
	Nonalcoholic steatohepatitis (NASH)
	Acute hepatitis
	Fulminant hepatitis
	Chronic active hepatitis
	Compensated cirrhosis
	Decompensated cirrhosis
Neurologic presentation	Isolated tremor
	Dystonic syndrome
	Parkinsonian syndrome
	Ataxic syndrome
	Combined movement disorders
	Speech disturbances
	Gait and balance disturbances
Psychiatric presentation	Cognitive impairment
	Dementia
	Personality changes
	Mood disorders
	Psychosis
Ocular presentation	Kayser-Fleischer rings
	Sunflower cataract
	Ocular movement disorders
Hematologic Presentation	Hemolytic anemia
	Thrombocytopenia
Renal presentation	Aminoaciduria
	Hypercalciuria
	Hyperphosphaturia
	Nephrolithiasis and nephrocalcinosis
	Tubular dysfunction
Cardiological presentation	Cardiomyopathy
	Cardiac arrhythmia
Endocrine presentation	Parathyroid insufficiency
	Disorders of growth
	Glucose intolerance
	Menstrual irregularity
	Delayed puberty
	Gynecomastia
Cutaneous presentation	Hyperpigmentation of lower limbs
	Azure lunulae of the nails
	Anetoderma
	Xerosis
	Acanthosis nigricans
	Subcutaneous lipomas
	Dermatomyositis
Musculoskeletal presentation	Osteoarthritis
	Chondrocalcinosis
	Osteoporosis
	Rhabdomyolysis

Hepatic manifestations are the first clinical signs in 40–50% of cases [26]. Although these disorders vary immensely [26], most patients develop a slowly progressive hepatic failure with cirrhosis and portal hypertension. Even so, acute hepatitis, hemolytic anemia, and acute fulminant hepatic failure have been described [16, 26]. Isolated mild elevations in liver tests occur in about 20% of asymptomatic *ATP7B* homozygous carriers identified by family genetic screening. Mild hepatomegaly or even unrecognized advanced liver disease may be associated [26]. Approximately 5% of WD cases present with acute liver failure, typically in the second or third decade of life. Remarkably, these patients have an accompanying nonimmune hemolytic anemia, with ratios of alkaline phosphatase to bilirubin 2.2. All of these patients have an underlying fibrosis or cirrhosis undetected until their critical presentation. Unless a timely liver transplant is performed, the evolution leads to invariable progression to death [23].

In 16–68% of patients, the liver disease does not reveal itself, and the diagnosis of WD can be made from neurologic symptoms later in life [2, 5]. In untreated cases, neurologic symptoms accumulate, leading to severe disability and eventually death [16, 27]. In some patients neurologic impairment progresses slowly over years, while in others symptoms present rapidly [5]. Among neurologic symptoms, the most distinct features are dystonia, parkinsonism, chorea, ataxia, tremor, and dysarthria [16, 27]. In a review by Lorincz of patients with neurologic WD, the most frequent manifestations were dysarthria (85–97%), dystonia (11–65%), tremor (22–55%), parkinsonism (19–62%), choreoathetosis (6–16%), and ataxia (in around 30%) [28]. Dysarthria in WD is frequently mixed with spastic, ataxic, hypokinetic, and dystonic components [28]. Dystonia may be generalized, multifocal, segmental, or focal, including vocal cord dystonia, writer's cramp, and foot dystonia. A characteristic sign in WD is the focal dystonic exaggerated smile, known as the risus sardonicus [29].

Early in neurologic WD, tremor can mimic essential tremor, with arms more frequently involved than head and legs. Asymmetry and absence of voice tremor may help in the differential. A position and task-dependent tremor may also be present [29, 30]. Though it is not the most frequent type, a "wing-beating" tremor is prototypical of WD. It is characterized by a low-frequency, high-amplitude, posture-induced proximal arm tremor, elicited by sustained abduction of the arms, with flexed elbows and palms facing downward [31]. Bradykinesia, asymmetric rigidity, tremor, and imbalance are the most common parkinsonian features [28]. Chorea is rarely present in isolation in WD and is more common in younger patients under the age of 16 [32]. Cerebellar signs, for example, overshoot of the eyes and limbs, ataxic gait or dysarthria can be found [28]. Although hepatic and neurological manifestations are the first clinical signs in most patients, psychiatric features may precede them in 15–20% of cases [6, 33]. It is common to observe behavioral and personality changes, anxiety, depression, mania and hypomanic syndrome, cognitive deficits, sleep problems, and sexual dysfunction [27, 33]. Personality disorders are common with a lifetime prevalence up to 70%, including features such as irritability or aggressiveness [34].

The ocular manifestations of WD include KF rings and sunflower cataract [35]. The former, described as golden brown, green, or yellow coloration seen at the periphery of the cornea, results from copper deposition in Descemet's membrane.

Although in some cases, they may be visible to the naked eye, a slit lamp examination is usually required. They are almost always bilateral, appearing early in the upper pole of the cornea, then inferiorly, and later circumferential [35, 36]. KF rings are a pathognomonic feature of WD. They are detected in only 20–30% of pre-symptomatic patients, 40–50% of patients with hepatic compromise, and in almost all neuropsychiatric cases [36]. They are rarely observed in other conditions, like obstructive liver diseases, monoclonal gammopathies, multiple myeloma, arci senilis, and pulmonary carcinoma [37]. Sunflower cataract, a very rare finding in WD, consists of a thin, centralized opacification surrounded by secondary opacifications arranged in a ray-like structure. It is located directly under the anterior eye capsule, and interestingly, its presence appears to have a limited effect on visual acuity [38]. Both ophthalmological signs are reversible after treatment.

Ocular motility abnormalities such as accommodation defects [39], distractibility of gaze fixation [40], abnormal anti-saccades, altered smooth pursuit movements [41], and abnormalities of vertical gaze and optokinetic nystagmus [42] have been described. Ocular flutter consists of high-frequency saccadic oscillations confined to one plane, usually horizontal, with no intersaccadic interval, usually resulting from a lesion in the pons and/or cerebellum [1]. Opsoclonus falls along the same spectrum; they share similar etiologies, topographic lesion localization, and it is possible for ocular flutter to progress to opsoclonus and vice versa [43]. Therefore, the patient described in the initial vignette presented with an opsoclonus-myoclonus syndrome. Interestingly, this presentation has not been previously reported in the literature. Yet, Samuel Alexander Kinnier Wilson described in the first case of his series "...her eyes "dance" slightly before her gaze comes to rest on a given object. On testing her, however, there is no nystagmus in any direction..." [2]. Opsoclonus-myoclonus syndrome, in addition to the ocular movements and myoclonic jerks, is usually associated with cerebellar ataxia, postural tremor, dysarthria, mutism, aphasia, encephalopathy, and behavioral disturbances. As seen in our case, it typically has a subacute and progressive presentation [44–46].

Clinical scales like the "Unified Wilson Disease Rating Scale" (UWDRS) [47] or the "Global Assessment Scale" (GAS) for WD [48] are useful to establish symptom severity during the diagnostic and follow-up phases. However, scales may underestimate symptoms like myoclonus, ocular movement disorders, or other less frequent manifestations. Likewise, the minimal UWDRS is an adequate nine-item prescreening tool for the evaluation of the neurological status in WD patients with mild to moderate neurologic symptoms [49].

Assessment

As the clinical spectrum is broad, the initial assessment depends on the clinical picture. As an example, the above case featuring a subacute onset of apathy-mutism and opsoclonus-myoclonus syndrome includes a large differential diagnosis [44, 45] of paraneoplastic, autoimmune, para-infectious, toxic, metabolic, and structural etiologies. An appropriate workup should include general metabolic and infectious blood tests, a paraneoplastic antibody panel, occult neoplasm screening, a lumbar puncture, and a brain MRI. Within the clinical assessment, looking for KF rings is a key step when WD is in the differential. They are present in 90–95% of patients with neurologic symptoms and in over half of those without neurologic symptoms [50]. However, Youn et al. found in his case series that 26.7% (12/45) of the patients with WD and neurologic symptoms had no KF rings. He also noted that these patients had a higher ceruloplasmin and serum copper level while liver cirrhosis and typical signal changes in brain MRI were less common [51]. Similar observations have been made by other authors with KF rings reported in 72 [52] to 77.8% [53] of patients manifesting neuropsychiatric symptoms. Other authors have related the presence of KF ring to the genetic status of the patients [54]. As mentioned before, KF rings are almost always bilateral, and the upper pole of the cornea is first affected. The inferior corneal quadrants are involved later by the circumferential spread [50], so it is essential to carry out a thorough examination of the entire corneal circumference, using the slit lamp by an experienced ophthalmologist. For this reason, we suspect that some reports of negative KF rings cases are due to technical issues. Considering the discussion above, the absence of KF rings should not rule out the disease. It is also important to emphasize that KF rings are not pathognomonic of WD. Other causes are listed in Table 26.3.

A brain MRI, which is usually requested at the initial assessment, is often a tremendously helpful tool. Most typical findings are listed in Table 26.2. The sign of the double panda, characteristic of this condition [55], and other classical findings on MR are shown in Figs. 26.2 and 26.3.

As there is no specific laboratory test for WD, a combination of tests reflecting disturbed copper metabolism is needed. The detection of serum ceruloplasmin levels is the most commonly used worldwide, with serum concentrations under 0.2 g/L

Table 26.2 Brain MRI characteristics according to a prospective study involving 100 patients with Wilson disease. Adapted from [56]

Brain MRI changes distribution in patients with Wilson disease	
Atrophy distribution	%
Cerebral	70
Brainstem	66
Cerebellar	52
Signal intensity changes distribution	%
Putamen	72
Caudate	61
Globus pallidus	40
Thalamus	58
Midbrain	49
Face of giant panda	12
Pons	20
Internal capsule	15
Medulla	12
Cerebellum	10
Cerebral white matter	25
Cortical lesions	9

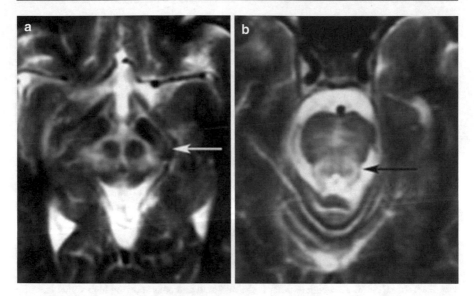

Fig. 26.2 The "double panda sign" in Wilson disease. (**a**) The midbrain "panda sign" on T2-weighted MRI has been described as preservation of normal signal intensity in the red nuclei and lateral portion of the pars reticulata of the substantia nigra, high signal in the tegmentum, and hypointensity of the superior colliculus. (**b**) The "face of the miniature panda" is seen within the pontine tegmentum. It is delineated by the relative hypointensity of the medial longitudinal fasciculi and central tegmental tracts ("eyes of the panda") in contrast with the hyperintensity of the aqueduct opening into the fourth ventricle ("nose and mouth of the panda") bounded inferiorly by the superior medullary velum. The superior cerebellar peduncles form the panda's "cheeks." The presence of "the face of the panda" on the midbrain and the "face of the miniature panda" at pons in the same patient has been called "the double panda sign." (Reprinted with permission from Jacobs et al. [55])

being suggestive for WD [5, 58, 59]. Nevertheless, about half of patients with active liver disease have levels within the low normal range, and 5–15% have levels slightly lower than normal [58, 59]. In fact, it has been shown that subnormal ceruloplasmin levels have a positive predictive value of only 6% when used as the sole screening test for WD [59]. Since ceruloplasmin is an acute-phase reactant, it may be increased in the setting of various inflammatory processes and medications, including hepatitis and steroid administration (Table 26.3). Measurement of 24-hour urinary copper excretion is often requested after finding an abnormal ceruloplasmin level, as it reflects the amount of non-ceruloplasmin-bound copper in the circulation [5]. An excretion greater than >1.6 μmol (100 mcg) supports the diagnosis, albeit it may be lower or even normal in some patients, especially in children [58, 59].

Liver biopsy is the gold standard to corroborate hepatic copper accumulation. Due to sampling errors however, estimations from a sole biopsy sample may be misrepresentative because of the heterogeneous distribution of copper within the liver, especially in the later stages of WD. Accuracy of measurement is improved with adequate specimen size (at least 1 cm of biopsy core length). A hepatic copper

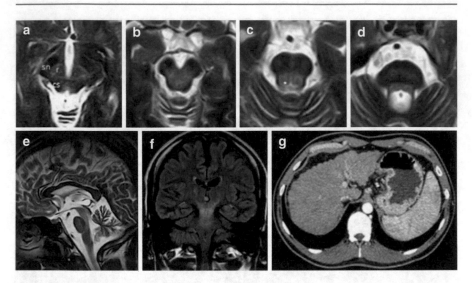

Fig. 26.3 (**a–d**) Axial T2-weighted MRI of the midbrain and pons showing high signal intensity in the tegmentum. Relative preservation of signal intensity in the red nucleus, substantia nigra, and superior colliculus is similar to the "face of the giant panda" sign description [57] (**a**). Pontine tegmentum hyperintensity with relative preservation of signal in the longitudinal medial lemniscus is similar to the "face of the miniature panda" sign description [55] (**d**). (**e**) Sagittal T2-weighted MRI showing cerebellar atrophy. (**f**) Abnormal signal increased in FLAIR in both mesencephalon and pons and mild diffuse cerebral atrophy. (**g**) The liver shows alteration in its morphology and architecture with markedly nodular edges; mild splenomegaly is also observed. Abbreviations: r red nucleus, sn substantia nigra, sc superior colliculus, * longitudinal medial fasciculus

weight >4 μmol (>250 μg) per gram of dried liver tissue is considered the best biochemical evidence for WD [59]. Histochemical techniques with copper stains are also used and are usually more accessible. The limitation of rhodamine stain is that it has a sensitivity of less than 10% as it detects only lysosomal copper deposition [60]. For this reason, hepatic copper overload cannot be excluded by histochemical evaluation alone, and the method of choice for the diagnosis of WD should be the measurement of hepatic parenchymal copper concentration. Other liver disorders, particularly those involving cholestasis, may have increased copper concentrations as well [61] (see Table 26.3).

Molecular analysis looking for pathogenic variants in the copper-transporting gene, *ATP7B*, should be considered in patients with a provisional diagnosis of WD. While the extensive coding region and the fact that more than 700 mutations have been described are major drawbacks, genetic analysis allows confirmation of the disease. Autosomal recessive diseases are not usually present in consecutive generations, but may occur in populations with high carrier *ATP7B* pathogenic variants. Not surprisingly, the presence of WD in two or more successive generations within the same family, reflecting a "pseudo-dominant" inheritance, has been reported. Therefore, the diagnosis of WD should not be ruled out merely due to a puzzling family history suggestive of an autosomal-dominant inheritance pattern.

Table 26.3 Causes of false negative and false positive results of different biomarkers used for Wilson disease diagnosis [5, 27]

Test	False negative	False positive
Serum ceruloplasmin	Normal levels Marked hepatic inflammation Overestimation by immunologic assay Steroids therapy Pregnancy, estrogen therapy	Low levels in Autoimmune hepatitis Protein loss Aceruloplasminemia Heterozygotes
24-hour urinary copper	Normal Incorrect collection Children without liver disease	Increased Hepatocellular necrosis Cholestasis Contamination
Serum "free" copper	Normal if ceruloplasmin overestimated by immunologic assay	
Hepatic copper	Due to regional variation In patients with active liver disease In patients with regenerative nodules	Cholestatic syndromes
Kayser-Fleischer rings by slit lamp examination	Absent In almost 50% of patients with hepatic presentation In 20–30% of pre-symptomatic patients In most asymptomatic siblings	Primary biliary cirrhosis Chronic cholestasis with serum bilirubin >20 mg/dL Monoclonal gammopathies Multiple myeloma Arcus senilis

Recent studies have also identified WD due to atypical forms of inheritance, such as uniparental disomy [62].

Diagnosis

Early diagnosis and treatment of WD may prevent serious long-term disability and life-threatening complications. The diagnosis can be challenging since there is no consistent gold standard test for its confirmation. Hence, no single diagnostic test can exclude or confirm this disease with 100% certainty. A combination of clinical and laboratory tests is often required instead. Ferenci et al. published the consensus on WD diagnosis established at the 8th International Meeting on WD and Menkes disease in Leipzig, Germany (2001) [63]. Those criteria were re-evaluated by Nicastro et al. on 2010, confirming that WD scoring systems provide good diagnostic accuracy, with a positive and negative predictive value of 93% and 91.6% respectively, in children [64]. Finally, in 2012 the European Association for the Study of the Liver (EASL) published the clinical practice guidelines for the diagnosis of WD, determining a diagnostic algorithm based on the Leipzig Score [5] (Table 26.4 and Fig. 26.4).

Table 26.4 EASL Wilson disease score based on the Leipzig criteria [5, 64]

Feature	Result	Score	Sensitivity and specificity
Kayser-Fleischer rings	Present	2	May be absent in up to 50% of patients with Wilson disease affecting the liver
	Absent	0	
Typical neuropsychiatric symptoms (or typical brain MRI)	Severe	2	
	Mild	1	
	Absent	0	
Coombs-negative hemolytic anemia	Present	1	Could be the presenting symptom in up to ~12%
	Absent	0	
Serum ceruloplasmin	<10 mg/dL = 2	2	Sens. 65–78.9% Spec. 96.6–100%
	10–20 mg/dL = 1	1	Sens. 77.1–99% Spec. 55.9–82.8%
	Normal (>20 mg/dl) = 0	0	
Urinary copper (in the absence of acute hepatitis)	>2x ULN	2	0.64 μmol/24 hours Sens. 78.9% Spec. 87.9%
	Normal but >5 ULN 1 day after challenge with 2 × 0.5 g D-penicillamine (Not recommended in adults)	2	1.6 μmol/24 hours Sens. 50–80% Spec. 75.6–98.3%
	1–2x ULN	1	The D-penicillamine test had only a sensitivity of 12.5%
	Normal	0	
Liver biopsy copper quantitative measurement	>5x ULN (> 4 μmol/g)	2	4 μmol/g Sens. 65.7–94.4% Spec. 52.2–98.6%
	Up to 5x ULN	1	
	(0.8–4 μmol/g) Normal (<0.8 μmol/g)	0	
Rhodanine (+) hepatocytes	Present	1	Reveal focal copper stores in <10% of patients
	Absent	0	
Mutation analysis	Homozygous pathologic mutation	4	
	Heterozygous pathologic mutation	1	
	No pathologic mutation	0	

Assessment of the Wilson disease diagnosis score
4 or more: diagnosis of Wilson disease established
3: diagnosis of Wilson disease possible; do more investigation
2 or less: diagnosis of Wilson disease unlikely

According to the EASL guidelines, the combination of typical clinical symptoms plus KF rings and a serum ceruloplasmin level less than 0.1 g/L are sufficient to establish a diagnosis [5].

The absence of low serum ceruloplasmin or Kayser-Fleisher rings does not definitively exclude the diagnosis of neurological Wilson disease.

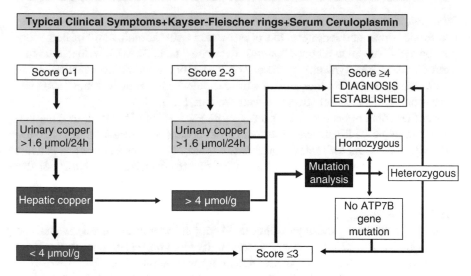

Fig. 26.4 Algorithm for Wilson disease diagnosis. (Adapted from [5])

Treatment

The aim of treatment is to remove the accumulated copper and prevent further copper gain. This is mediated by drugs that chelate copper and those that prevent gastrointestinal copper absorption [4]. Among patients with WD diagnosis, symptomatic and asymptomatic patients should be treated for life. Only patients heterozygous for *ATP7B* mutations do not require treatment as the WD diagnosis is not established. Symptomatic patients should receive an initial intensive therapy, with the aim of stabilizing liver disease and reversing or slowing down neurologic symptoms. It usually takes 1 or 2 years before maintenance treatment is introduced. In asymptomatic patients, a maintenance therapy is recommended [66].

The first drug used was a copper chelator, dimercaprol. It showed remarkable clinical improvement, but its long-term use resulted in considerable adverse events, drug tolerance, and waning clinical benefits [66]. Around the world, D-penicillamine (D-penicillamine, β,β-dimethylcysteine, β-thiovaline) is often the first-line treatment in symptomatic patients during the initial intensive phase of treatment and later as maintenance therapy, as it can be safely used for long term, even during pregnancy. It is also recommended in pre-symptomatic patients. It is a thiol with a sulfhydryl group that binds copper and facilitates its excretion into urine. This drug was introduced in 1955 by John Walshe and it marked a substantial improvement in patient's prognosis and survival [66, 67]. It should be started in a very slow ascending scheme to avoid the paradoxical neurologic deterioration observed in patients who start treatment with a high/full dose [67]. The strategy for de-coppering is to "start low and go slow" whichever is the chosen drug. Penicillamine mobilizes tissue copper stores and long-term use is associated with normalization of body copper balance. As tissue copper stores decrease, penicillamine-induced copper excretion decreases, typically by the end of 1 year [66]. Food reduces penicillamine absorption by over 50%; therefore, the drug should be given on an empty stomach. Early-onset and late-onset adverse effects are listed in Table 26.5.

Another copper-chelating agent that can be used as an alternative to penicillamine is trientine. This substance has four amino groups that form a stable ring complex with copper and facilitates cupriuresis. It is mainly used as an option in patients in whom penicillamine had to be discontinued due to adverse events, but it can also be prescribed as first-line therapy for symptomatic, asymptomatic, and pregnant patients [23, 66]. Its mechanism of action, dosing, and adverse effects are summarized in Table 26.5.

Among drugs that prevent gastrointestinal copper absorption are zinc acetate and tetrathiomolybdate. Zinc salts are absorbed by enterocytes, where they act by increasing the production of metallothionein up to 25-fold within 2 to 3 weeks of initiation of therapy. Metallothioneins are cysteine-rich proteins that bind various metal ions having a stronger affinity for copper than for zinc. The copper bound to metallothionein is sequestered within the enterocytes and prevented from absorption into the blood. The metal is subsequently lost in feces when the enterocytes are shed in the intestinal lumen during normal cellular turnover [66]. Zinc is recommended as maintenance therapy in symptomatic patients once symptoms have regressed following treatment with oral copper chelators. It has also been given as first-line therapy in asymptomatic patients.

Tetrathiomolybdate is not yet approved for WD, but this drug has been proven to block dietary copper absorption almost completely when given orally, by forming complexes with copper and proteins in the gut lumen that are not absorbed by intestinal cells and are eliminated in the feces. It requires multiple doses during day and is recommended for use for a few months only. Drug-induced neurological worsening has been reported but is possibly less common than that reported with trientine or penicillamine. Both ammonium TTM and the more recently developed choline TTM are promising therapies for WD that are in phase 2 and phase 3 multinational clinical trials. They are not as yet commercially distributed [66]. A summary of drug mechanisms of action, doses, and adverse effects is presented in Table 2.5.

It is recommended to perform monitoring at least twice a year, to determine adequacy of treatment with respect to clinical improvement and biochemical changes, to assess medication adherence, and to detect any treatment-induced adverse events. For patients on chelation therapy, elevated values for urine copper may suggest nonadherence to treatment, and hepatic deterioration may follow. Low values for urine copper excretion for patients on chelation treatment may also indicate overtreatment, and this finding is accompanied by very low values for estimates of non-ceruloplasmin-bound copper [4]. A low-copper diet can be advised but it doesn't prevent copper gain [66]. Patients with WD should generally avoid foods

Table 26.5 Drugs used in the treatment of Wilson disease [4, 25, 66, 67, 68]

Drug	Mechanism of action	Dose	Adverse effects (AE)
D-penicillamine	Chelation and urinary excretion of copper	Initial dose: ≤125 mg/day Maximum dose: 2500 mg at day divided in 3 doses Increments: 125 mg/day every 3–4 days Maintenance dose: usually up to 1000 mg/day Given on an empty stomach (Children: 20 mg/kg/body weight) Supplement with 20–25 mg of pyridoxine/day	*Early oversensitivity AE (<3 weeks):* Fever, cutaneous erosions, lymphadenopathy, neutropenia and thrombocytopenia and proteinuria *Late AE:* Nephrotoxicity, dermatologic symptoms, lupus-like syndrome, serous retinitis, myasthenia-like syndromes, polymyositis, aplastic anemia, IgA deficiency, and loss of taste Patients should be monitored regularly during treatment *Paradoxical neurological deterioration
Trientine	Chelation and urinary excretion of copper	Initial dose: 0.75–1.5 g/day in three divided doses Maximum dose: 2.4 g/day Maintenance dose: 0.5–1 g/day (Children 20 mg/kg/day)	Sideroblastic anemia (due to chelation of iron). Lupus-like reactions, hemorrhagic gastritis, loss of taste, and rashes Autoimmune disorders same as D-penicillamine but occur less frequently *Paradoxical neurological deterioration
Zinc acetate	Blockage of copper absorption by inducing metallothionein synthesis in enterocytes (adequate induction needs 3 weeks)	150 mg/day of elcmental zinc in three divided doses (In children <50 kg in body weight, the recommended dose is 75 mg)	Dyspeptic symptoms in 10% of patients Gastric ulcers, especially with zinc sulfate *Less frequent paradoxic neurological worsening than chelators
Tetrathiomolybdate	Blockage of copper absorption by forming complexes with copper and proteins in the gut lumen that are not absorbed by the intestinal cells and are eliminated in the feces	Ongoing trials	Reversible bone marrow depression, rise in aminotransferases, acute hepatitis, markedly elevated triglycerides and cholesterol levels, and seizures

with very high concentrations of copper (shellfish, nuts, chocolate, mushrooms, and organ meats) at least in the first year of treatment [4].

The main indication for liver transplantation is acute liver failure and advanced end-stage liver disease nonresponsive to medical therapy. As WD is primarily a liver disease characterized by copper defects in hepatocytes, liver transplantation can be considered a cure of the gene defect and can restore copper homeostasis [4, 25].

Symptomatic therapy of neurologic impairments depends mainly on predominant signs, such as dystonia, parkinsonism, or tremor and is based on experiences from treatment in other diseases [4].

Conclusion

Wilson disease may present with a wide spectrum of clinical manifestations. It must always be kept in mind as a differential diagnosis for any movement disorder, especially in young patients (typically under the age of 50) with concomitant hepatic compromise, even when the neurological manifestation is atypical. Establishing the diagnosis of Wilson disease is not always straightforward. Following a step-by-step diagnostic algorithm can provide clarity in challenging cases. Since Wilson disease is one of the few treatable movement disorders, early diagnosis and treatment are determinants in prognosis, preventing serious long-term disability and life-threatening complications.

References

1. Fahn S, Jankovic J, Hallett M. Principles and practice of movement disorders [Internet]. Elsevier; 2011. Available from: https://www.elsevier.com/books/principles-and-practice-of-movement-disorders/9781437723694
2. Wilson SAK. Progressive lenticular degeneration: a familial nervous disease associated with cirrhosis of the liver. Brain [Internet]. 1912;34:295–507. Available from: https://academic.oup.com/brain/article-lookup/doi/10.1093/brain/34.4.295
3. Walshe JM. History of Wilson's disease: 1912 to 2000. Mov Disord [Internet]. 2006;21:142–7. Available from: http://doi.wiley.com/10.1002/mds.20694.
4. Członkowska A, Litwin T, Dusek P, Ferenci P, Lutsenko S, Medici V, et al. Wilson disease. Nat Rev Dis Prim. 2018;4:1–20.
5. Ferenci P, Czlonkowska A, Stremmel W, Houwen R, Rosenberg W, Schilsky M, et al. EASL clinical practice guidelines: Wilson's disease. J Hepatol [Internet]. European Association for the Study of the Liver; 2012;56:671–85. Available from: https://doi.org/10.1016/j.jhep.2011.11.007
6. Lo C, Bandmann O. Epidemiology and introduction to the clinical presentation of Wilson disease. Handb Clin Neurol. 2017;142:7.
7. Sternlieb I, Scheinberg IH. Prevention of Wilson's disease in asymptomatic patients. N Engl J Med [Internet]. 1968;278:352–9. Available from: http://www.nejm.org/doi/abs/10.1056/NEJM196802152780702.
8. Coffey AJ, Durkie M, Hague S, McLay K, Emmerson J, Lo C, et al. A genetic study of Wilson's disease in the United Kingdom. Brain. 2013;136:1476–87.

9. Ohura T, Abukawa D, Shiraishi H, Yamaguchi A, Arashima S, Hiyamuta S, et al. Pilot study of screening for Wilson disease using dried blood spots obtained from children seen at outpatient clinics. J Inherit Metab Dis. 1999;22:74–80.

10. Hahn SH, Lee SY, Jang YJ, Kim SN, Shin HC, Park SY, et al. Pilot study of mass screening for Wilson's disease in Korea. Mol Genet Metab. 2002;76:133–6.

11. Dedoussis GVZ, Genschel J, Sialvera T-E, Bochow B, Manolaki N, Manios Y, et al. Wilson disease: high prevalence in a mountainous area of Crete. Ann Hum Genet [Internet]. 2005;69:268–74. Available from: http://doi.wiley.com/10.1046/j.1529-8817.2005.00171.x.

12. Loudianos G, Dessi V, Lovicu M, Angius A, Figus A, Lilliu F, et al. Molecular character-ization of Wilson disease in the Sardinian population? Evidence of a founder effect. Hum Mutat [Internet]. 1999;14:294–303. Available from: http://doi.wiley.com/10.1002/%28SICI% 291098-1004%28199910%2914%3A4%3C294%3A%3AAID-HUMU4%3E3.0.CO%3B2-9.

13. Antonietta Z, Olympia M, Lepori MB, Valentina D, Stefania D, Simona I, et al. High inci-dence and allelic homogeneity of Wilson disease in 2 isolated populations: a prerequisite for efficient disease prevention programs. J Pediatr Gastroenterol Nutr [Internet]. 2008;47:334–8. Available from: http://journals.lww.com/00005176-200809000-00012

14. García-Villarreal L, Daniels S, Shaw SH, Cotton D, Galvin M, Geskes J, et al. High preva-lence of the very rare Wilson disease gene mutation Leu708Pro in the Island of Gran Canaria (Canary Islands, Spain): a genetic and clinical study. Hepatology [Internet]. 2000;32:1329–36. Available from: http://doi.wiley.com/10.1053/jhep.2000.20152.

15. Cocoş R, Şendroiu A, Schipor S, Bohîlţea LC, Şendroiu I, Raicu F. Genotype-phenotype corre-lations in a mountain population community with high prevalence of Wilson's disease: genetic and clinical homogeneity. Dermaut B, editor. PLoS One [Internet]. 2014;9:e98520. Available from: https://dx.plos.org/10.1371/journal.pone.0098520.

16. Bandmann O, Weiss KH, Kaler SG. Wilson's disease and other neurological copper disor-ders. Lancet Neurol [Internet] Elsevier Ltd. 2015;14:103–13. Available from: https://doi. org/10.1016/S1474-4422(14)70190-5.

17. Walshe JM. Cause of death in Wilson disease. Mov Disord. 2007;22:2216–20.

18. Prashanth LK. Wilson's disease: diagnostic errors and clinical implications. J Neurol Neurosurg Psychiatry [Internet]. 2004;75:907–9. Available from: http://jnnp.bmj.com/cgi/ doi/10.1136/jnnp.2003.026310.

19. Scheiber IF, Brůha R, Dušek P. Pathogenesis of Wilson disease. Handb Clin Neurol. 2017;142:43–55.

20. Scheiber I, Dringen R, Mercer JFB. Copper: effects of deficiency and overload. Met Ions Life Sci [Internet]. 2013; 359–87. Available from: http://link.springer. com/10.1007/978-94-007-7500-8_11

21. Ala A, Walker AP, Ashkan K, Dooley JS, Schilsky ML. Wilson's disease. Lancet [Internet]. 2007;369:397–408. Available from: https://linkinghub.elsevier.com/retrieve/pii/ S0140673607601962.

22. Ferenci P, Roberts EA. Defining Wilson disease phenotypes: from the patient to the bench and back again. Gastroenterology. 2012;142:692–6.

23. Schilsky ML. Wilson disease: diagnosis, treatment, and follow-up. Clin Liver Dis [Internet]. Elsevier Inc. 2017;21:755–67. Available from: https://doi.org/10.1016/j.cld.2017.06.011.

24. Huster D, Khne A, Bhattacharjee A, Raines L, Jantsch V, Noe J, et al. Diverse functional prop-erties of Wilson disease ATP7B variants. Gastroenterology [Internet]. 2012;142:947–956.e5. Available from: https://doi.org/10.1053/j.gastro.2011.12.048.

25. Das SK, Ray K. Wilson's disease: an update. Nat Clin Pract Neurol. 2006;2:482–93.

26. Boga S, Ala A, Schilsky ML. Hepatic features of Wilson disease [Internet]. 1st ed. Handb Clin Neurol. 2017. Available from: https://doi.org/10.1016/B978-0-444-63625-6.00009-4.

27. Członkowska A, Litwin T, Chabik G. Wilson disease: neurologic features. Handb Clin Neurol. 2017;142:101–19.

28. Lorincz MT. Neurologic Wilson's disease. Ann N Y Acad Sci [Internet]. 2010;1184:173–87. Available from: http://doi.wiley.com/10.1111/j.1749-6632.2009.05109.x.

29. Svetel M, Kozić D, Stefanova E, Semnic R, Dragašević N, Kostič VS. Dystonia in Wilson's disease. Mov Disord. 2001;16:719–23.
30. Stremmel W, Meyerrose KW, Niederau C, Hefter H, Kreuzpaintner G, Strohmeyer G. Wilson disease: clinical presentation, treatment, and survival. Ann Intern Med. 1991;115:720–6.
31. Mahajan R, Zachariah U. Wing-beating tremor. N Engl J Med [Internet]. 2014;371:e1. Available from: http://www.nejm.org/doi/10.1056/NEJMicm1312190
32. Walshe JM, Yealland M. Wilson's disease: the problem of delayed diagnosis. J Neurol Neurosurg Psychiatry. 1992;55:692–6.
33. Litwin T, Dusek P, Szafrański T, Dzieżyc K, Członkowska A, Rybakowski JK. Psychiatric manifestations in Wilson's disease: possibilities and difficulties for treatment. Ther Adv Psychopharmacol. 2018;8:199–211.
34. Biswas S, Paul N, Das SK. Nonmotor manifestations of Wilson's disease [Internet]. 1st ed. Int Rev Neurobiol. 2017. Available from: https://doi.org/10.1016/bs.irn.2017.04.010
35. Goel S, Sahay P, Maharana PK, Titiyal JS. Ocular manifestations of Wilson's disease. BMJ Case Rep. 2019;12:1–2.
36. Dusek P, Litwin T, Czlonkowska A. Wilson disease and other neurodegenerations with metal accumulations. Neurol Clin [Internet]. 2015;33:175–204. Available from: https://doi.org/10.1016/j.ncl.2014.09.006.
37. Liu M, Cohen EJ, Brewer GJ, Laibson PR. Kayser-Fleischer ring as the presenting sign of Wilson disease. Am J Ophthalmol [Internet]. 2002;133:832–4. Available from: https://linking-hub.elsevier.com/retrieve/pii/S0002939402014083.
38. Langwińska-Wośko E, Litwin T, Dzieżyc K, Członkowska A. The sunflower cataract in Wilson's disease: pathognomonic sign or rare finding? Acta Neurol Belg. 2016;116:325–8.
39. Klingele TG, Newman SA, Burde RM. Accommodation defect in Wilson's disease. Am J Ophthalmol [Internet]. 1980;90:22–4. Available from: https://doi.org/10.1016/S0002-9394(14)75072-X.
40. Lennox G, Jones R. Gaze distractibility in Wilson's disease. Ann Neurol. 1989;25:415–7.
41. Leśniak M, Członkowska A, Seniów J. Abnormal antisaccades and smooth pursuit eye movements in patients with Wilson's disease. Mov Disord. 2008;23:2067–73.
42. Ingster-Moati I, Bui Quoc E, Pless M, Djomby R, Orssaud C, Guichard JP, et al. Ocular motility and Wilson's disease: a study on 34 patients. J Neurol Neurosurg Psychiatry. 2007;78:1199–201.
43. Shaikh A, Ghasia F. Advances in translational neuroscience of eye movement disorders. New York: Springer; 2019.
44. Wong A. An update on opsoclonus. Curr Opin Neurol. 2007;20:25–31.
45. Sahu JK, Prasad K. The opsoclonus–myoclonus syndrome. Two cases to illustrate the typical clinical features. Case No 1. Pract Neurol. 2011;10:160–6.
46. Klaas JP, Ahlskog JE, Pittock SJ, Matsumoto JY, Aksamit AJ, Bartleson JD, et al. Adult-onset opsoclonus-myoclonus syndrome. Arch Neurol. 2012;69:1598–607.
47. Członkowska A, Tarnacka B, Möller JC, Leinweber B, Bandmann O, Woimant F, et al. Unified Wilson's disease rating scale - a proposal for the neurological scoring of Wilson's disease patients. Neurol Neurochir Pol. 2007;41:1–12.
48. Aggarwal A, Aggarwal N, Nagral A, Jankharia G, Bhatt M. A novel global assessment scale for Wilson's disease (GAS for WD). Mov Disord. 2009;24:509–18.
49. Volpert HM, Pfeiffenberger J, Gröner JB, Stremmel W, Gotthardt DN, Schäfer M, et al. Comparative assessment of clinical rating scales in Wilson's disease. BMC Neurol. 2017;17:1–9.
50. Midena E, Frizziero L, Parrozzani R. Eye signs of Wilson disease [Internet]. Clin Transl Perspect. WILSON Dis. 2019. Available from: https://doi.org/10.1016/B978-0-12-810532-0.00020-3
51. Youn J, Kim JS, Kim HT, Lee JY, Lee PH, Ki CS, et al. Characteristics of neurological Wilson's disease without Kayser-Fleischer ring. J Neurol Sci [Internet]. 2012;323:183–6. Available from: https://doi.org/10.1016/j.jns.2012.09.013.

52. Fenu M, Liggi M, Demelia E, Sorbello O, Civolani A, Demelia L. Kayser–Fleischer ring in Wilson's disease: a cohort study. Eur J Int Med [Internet]. 2012;23:e150–6. Available from: https://linkinghub.elsevier.com/retrieve/pii/S0953620512000921.
53. de Bem RS, Muzzillo DA, Deguti MM, Barbosa ER, Werneck LC, Teive HAG. Wilson's disease in southern Brazil: a 40-year follow-up study. Clinics [Internet]. 2011;66:411–6. Available from: http://www.scielo.br/scielo.php?script=sci_arttext&pid=S1807-59322011000300008&lng=en&nrm=iso&tlng=en.
54. Folhoffer A, Ferenci P, Csak T, Horvath A, Hegedus D, Firneisz G, et al. Novel mutations of the ATP7B gene among 109 Hungarian patients with Wilson's disease. Eur J Gastroenterol Hepatol. 2007;19:105–11.
55. Jacobs DA, Markowitz CE, Liebeskind DS, Galetta SL. The "double panda sign" in Wilson's disease. Neurology. 2003;61:969.
56. Sinha S, Taly AB, Ravishankar S, Prashanth LK, Venugopal KS, Arunodaya GR, et al. Wilson's disease: cranial MRI observations and clinical correlation. Neuroradiology. 2006;48:613–21
57. Hitoshi S, Iwata M, Yoshikawa K. Mid-brain pathology of Wilson's disease: MRI analysis of three cases. J Neurol Neurosurg Psychiatry. 1991;54:624–6.
58. Brewer GJ. Wilson's disease: a clinician's guide to recognition, diagnosis, and management [Internet]. Society. Boston: Springer US; 2001. Available from: http://link.springer.com/10.1007/978-1-4615-1645-3.
59. Ferenci P. Whom and how to screen for Wilson disease. Expert Rev Gastroenterol Hepatol. 2014;8:513–20.
60. Yang X, Tang XP, Zhang YH, Luo KZ, Jiang YF, Luo HY, et al. Prospective evaluation of the diagnostic accuracy of hepatic copper content, as determined using the entire core of a liver biopsy sample. Hepatology. 2015;62:1731–41.
61. Roberts EA, Schilsky ML. Diagnosis and treatment of Wilson disease: an update. Hepatology. 2008;47:2089–111.
62. Chang IJ, Hahn SH. The genetics of Wilson disease [Internet]. 1st ed. Handb Clin Neurol. 2017. Available from: https://doi.org/10.1016/B978-0-444-63625-6.00003-3
63. Ferenci P, Caca K, Loudianos G, Mieli-Vergani G, Tanner S, Sternlieb I, et al. Diagnosis and phenotypic classification of Wilson disease. Liver Int. 2003;23:139–42.
64. Nicastro E, Ranucci G, Vajro P, Vegnente A, Iorio R. Re-evaluation of the diagnostic criteria for Wilson disease in children with mild liver disease. Hepatology. 2010;52:1948–56.
65. Ryan A, Nevitt SJ, Tuohy O, Cook P. Biomarkers for diagnosis of Wilson's disease. Cochrane Database Syst Rev. 2019;2019:CD012267.
66. Aggarwal A, Bhatt M. Advances in treatment of Wilson disease. Tremor Other Hyperkinet Mov. 2018;8:1–13.
67. Członkowska A, Litwin T. Wilson disease – currently used anticopper therapy. Handb Clin Neurol. 2017;142:181–91.
68. Aggarwal A, Bhatt M. The pragmatic treatment of Wilson's disease. Mov Disord Clin Pract. 2014;1:14–23.

X-Linked Adrenoleukodystrophy: Addisonian Crisis in a Patient with Spastic Paraparesis-Ataxia Syndrome

27

Philippe A. Salles and Hubert H. Fernandez

Patient Vignette

A 28-year-old man with a 5-year history of progressive spastic paraparesis of unknown etiology, with comorbid sphincter and sexual dysfunction, was brought to the emergency department (ED) because of a 3-day history of marked exacerbation of spasticity in his lower limbs, followed by two syncopal episodes, emesis, vegetative symptoms, and finally psychomotor agitation. At the ED he was noted to be agitated and confused. He had no fever, but his vital signs were remarkable for hypotension and tachycardia. Brain CT and CSF analysis were unremarkable. His clinical picture progressed with persistent hypotension, hypoglycemia, hyponatremia, hyperkalemia, and a low cortisol level. Suprarenal insufficiency was confirmed, and he was started on steroid replacement, along with correction of hypoglycemia and electrolyte imbalance. While his mentation slowly improved, his spasticity with severe spasms persisted. Neurological and general evaluation during admission was remarkable for hyperpigmented skin and gums, frontotemporal alopecia (Fig. 27.1), cognitive slowness, spastic paraparesis-dystonic syndrome, and mild ataxia with

Supplementary Information The online version of this chapter (https://doi.org/10.1007/978-3-030-75898-1_27) contains supplementary material, which is available to authorized users.

P. A. Salles
Department of Neuroscience, Clínica Dávila, Santiago, Chile

CETRAM, Santiago, Chile

Center for Neurological Restoration, Neurological Institute, Cleveland Clinic, Cleveland, OH, USA

H. H. Fernandez (✉)
Center for Neurological Restoration, Neurological Institute, Cleveland Clinic, Cleveland, OH, USA
e-mail: fernanh@ccf.org

© Springer Nature Switzerland AG 2022
S. J. Frucht (ed.), *Movement Disorder Emergencies*, Current Clinical Neurology, https://doi.org/10.1007/978-3-030-75898-1_27

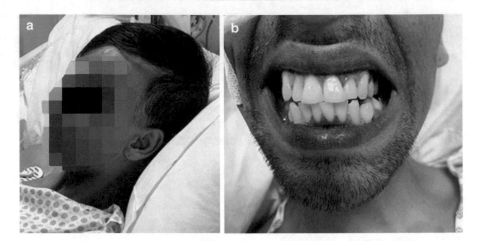

Fig. 27.1 Androgenic pattern of alopecia (**a**) and hyperpigmented skin and gums (**b**)

hypermetric saccades, mild dysmetria, dysdiadochokinesia, and dyssynergia, with generalized hyperreflexia and bilateral Babinski signs. His MRI showed signal changes in parieto-occipital deep white matter and splenium of the corpus callosum (Fig. 27.2). Based on the clinical and radiological characteristics, along with elevated very long-chain fatty acid (VLCFA) levels, X-linked adrenoleukodystrophy was confirmed.

Introduction

X-linked adrenoleukodystrophy (ALD) is both the most common inborn error of metabolism of peroxisomal beta-oxidation and the most frequent monogenetically inherited demyelinating disorder [1]. In the United States, the estimated overall minimum frequency is about 1:21,000 for hemizygote men and 1:14,000 for heterozygote women [2]. Now that newborn screening has been implemented in some parts of the world, the true prevalence could be even higher [3]. It is an X-linked hereditary disease caused by pathogenic variants in the ATP-binding cassette, subfamily D, member 1 (*ABCD1*) gene, located on chromosome Xq28, that codes for the peroxisomal half-transporter of CoA-activated very long-chain fatty acids (VLCFA), responsible for the transportation of VLCFA into the peroxisome [4, 5]. Deficiency of the enzyme very long-chain acyl CoA synthetase (ligase) results in accumulation of endogenous and exogenous saturated VLCFA (fatty acyl chain length of ≥ 22 carbons), particularly tetracosanoic (C24:0) and hexacosanoic acid (C26:0), mainly in the nervous system, the adrenal cortex, and the Leydig cells in the testes [4, 6].

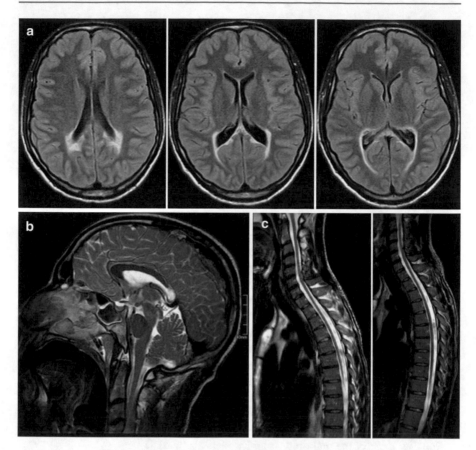

Fig. 27.2 Brain MRI, axial FLAIR with symmetric bilateral posterior peri-atrial white matter and splenium hyperintensities (**a, b**). Cervical-thoracic spine atrophy (**c**)

There is no genotype-phenotype correlation, and there is often marked intrafamilial variability. Clinically, ALD can present with a wide spectrum of neurological and endocrine manifestations. Six main phenotypes among men hemizygotes have been reported. The more prevalent phenotypes are adrenomyeloneuropathy (AMN) and the cerebral form of ALD with a childhood, adolescent, and adult age of presentation. Less frequent phenotypes include pure Addison's disease, spinocerebellar ataxia, and asymptomatic subtypes [1]. Heterozygous women develop an AMN phenotype with a later onset and somewhat milder presentation.

⚷ X-linked adrenoleukodystrophy is the most common inherited peroxisomal disorder, caused by mutations in the ABCD1 gene, resulting in the accumulation of VLCFA mainly in the nervous and endocrine systems. There is no genotype-phenotype correlation. It may present with adrenal insufficiency, progressive brain demyelination, or myelopathy, in different combinations.

Pathophysiology

ABCD1 is widely expressed in many different tissues, and VLCFA levels are highly elevated in almost all tissues. The exact mechanism by which VLCFA are toxic to cells and why cells of the adrenal cortex, testes, and the peripheral and central nervous system are especially vulnerable remains to be resolved [7]. An explanation for the demyelination in the cerebral ALD subtype could be the myelin sheath instability from VLCFA excess in the lipid membrane. High levels of VLCFA could also be cytotoxic to oligodendrocytes and microglia contributing to the demyelination process [8]. Cerebral inflammation is mediated by oxidative stress, activation of macrophages, microglial apoptosis, and endothelial dysfunction, which ultimately damages the blood–brain barrier [9].

Griffin et al. have typed the cells in the perivascular cuffs [10]. Fifty-nine percent were T cells, 24% B cells, and 11% monocytes/macrophages. Fifty-eight percent of the T cells were T4, and 27% T8, while 15% could not be classified. This pattern was similar to that found in the CNS during a cellular immune response, which suggested that an aspect of injury in ALD is likely immunologically mediated [10, 11]. In AMN cases, the current pathogenic hypotheses suggest that impaired mitochondrial function, subsequent oxidative stress, and energy depletion contribute to a noninflammatory dying-back axonopathy of the spinal cord that involves the descending corticospinal tracts in the thoracic and lumbosacral regions and ascending posterior columns in the cervical region [4]. The mechanism of adrenal gland injury in ALD is not well understood. VLCFA are known to accumulate in the zona fasciculata and reticularis of the adrenal cortex, and the chronic accumulation of VLCFA is thought to lead to cytotoxic effects and ultimately apoptosis with atrophy of the adrenal cortex [12].

See Fig. 27.3 for the pathophysiological aspects of ALD.

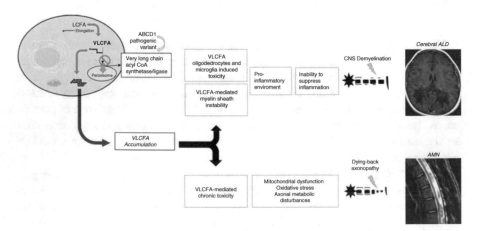

Fig. 27.3 Pathophysiological aspects of ALD. LCFA long-chain fatty acids, VLCFA very long-chain fatty acids, ALD adrenoleukodystrophy, AMN adrenomyeloneuropathy. (Adapted from [4])

Clinical Presentations

Neuropsychiatric Manifestations

ALD has been defined as a disorder with many different phenotypes (Table 27.1). In addition, presenting phenotypes may not be static, and their clinical state may change over time. Patients with ALD are classically asymptomatic at birth [7]. AMN, the combination of myelopathy and peripheral neuropathy, has a near 100% lifetime penetrance. Virtually all men and up to 80% of heterozygous women develop myelopathy [13]. Consequently, there is a high risk for children and adult asymptomatic patients to develop neurological deficits, and for AMN men to develop cerebral demyelination [14]. Although myelopathy may present during adolescence, it typically develops between 20 and 40 years of age. The earliest

Table 27.1 Phenotypes associated with *ABCD1* pathological variants

Phenotype	Relative frequency	AAO (yr)	Adrenal insufficiency	Neuropsychiatric manifestations	RNM pattern	Progression
Childhood cerebral ALD	31–35%	2–10	Usual (79%)	Behavioral and cognitive changes, school difficulties, visual disturbances, hearing loss, spastic gait, and seizures	1 and 5[a]	Rapid (total disability in 2–4 years)
Adolescent cerebral ALD	4–7%	11–21	Usual (62%)	Symptoms resemble those of the childhood cerebral form	2 and 4[a]	Slower than childhood
Adult cerebral ALD	2–5%	>21	Usual (>50%)	Initial symptoms include dementia and psychiatric disturbances; sometimes focal deficits	3[a]	Similar than adolescent
Pure AMN	20–30%	28 ± 9	Usual (>70%)	Mainly involves the spinal cord and presents with slowly progressive stiffness and weakness of legs, impaired vibration sense (neuropathy), sphincter disturbances, and impotence	Spine atrophy	Slowly progressive over decades
Cerebral ALD-AMN	20–23%	–	Usual	Approximately 40% of AMN present with combined cerebral involvement	Mixed	Variable

(continued)

Table 27.1 (continued)

Phenotype	Relative frequency	AAO (yr)	Adrenal insufficiency	Neuropsychiatric manifestations	RNM pattern	Progression
Spinocerebellar	1–2%	20–71	Usual (75%)	Cerebellar ataxia, gait and speech disturbance, pyramidal signs, and autonomic failure	MCP, C, and IC[b]	Slow
Pure Addison's disease	10–20%	>2	Rule (100%)	Age dependent (up to 50% in childhood); these patients are at high risk of eventually developing AMN	Normal	Variable
Asymptomatic		<4 (rare >40)	Uninvolved	Absence of symptoms despite high levels of VLCFA and/or *ABCD1* variant demonstrated; diminished with age (pre-symptomatic stage)	Normal	–
Female carriers	50% >40 years	30–40	Rare (<1%)	Milder clinical symptoms; mainly spastic paraparesis (<1% develop cerebral ALD)	Spine atrophy	Slower than men AMN

AAO age at onset, *ALD* adrenoleukodystrophy, *AMN* adrenomyeloneuropathy, *MCP* middle cerebellar peduncle, *C* cerebellum, *IC* internal capsule

Table references: [1, 9, 33, 34, 35, 36]

[a]Pattern 1, parieto-occipital white matter; pattern 2, frontal white matter; pattern 3, corticospinal tract; pattern 4, cerebellar white matter; pattern 5, concomitant parieto-occipital and frontal white matter

[b]Hyperintensity over bilateral middle cerebellar peduncles, cerebellar white matter, and internal capsule

symptoms are usually urge incontinence, followed by a gradually progressive gait disorder due to spastic paraparesis and sensory ataxia. An axonal peripheral sensorimotor neuropathy is present on electrophysiological testing, but this is frequently overlooked because of the coexisting myelopathy. The age of onset and rate of progression of AMN symptoms are highly variable [7]. In a prospective cohort of men with AMN, Huffnagel et al. determined a median time from onset of myelopathy to the use of a walking aid of 13 years (95% CI 9.1–16.9 years) [15]. Patients with pure AMN, with normal brain MRI, have a better prognosis compared with other phenotypes. Their neuropsychological profile is typically normal except for mild deficits in psychomotor speed and visual memory [16].

According to van Geel et al. after a mean follow-up period of 10 ± 5 years, 19% of adult patients with AMN without symptoms of cerebral involvement developed cerebral ALD, with a mean survival of 2.3 ± 1.9 years after the first manifestation of cerebral disease [14]. Studies have shown that more than 80% of women heterozygous carriers develop a milder AMN phenotype than men, usually after the age of 40. According to some recent reports, AMN can occur in women in their 20s [17]. Signs of dementia, behavioral or visual disturbances, occur in 1–3% of heterozygous women and adrenal insufficiency in only 1% [18]. A prospective cohort study in 42 men with ALD and 32 controls demonstrated that the spinal cord cross-sectional area of patients is smaller compared to healthy controls and correlates with severity of myelopathy as measured by the expanded disability status scale, severity scoring system for progressive myelopathy, and vibration sense scores [19].

There are several reports of ALD presenting as pure familial spastic paraparesis [20], in some cases presenting with an autosomal dominant pedigree [21], or recessive pattern in others [22]. Urinary and bowel symptoms are common in men with AMN and in *ABCD1* variant female carriers. According to Hofereiter et al., in a case series of 19 males with AMN and 29 female carriers, overactive bladder symptoms were reported in 100% of males and 86% of females. Moderate to severe bowel dysfunction was noted in 21% and 10% of males and females, respectively [23]. In a retrospective chart review based on 39 ALD adult patients (28 female carriers), Gomery et al. reported urinary symptoms in 64% of men and 68% of women and bowel symptoms in 44% of men and 64% of women. The most common symptoms included urinary urgency (28% of males, 50% of females), urinary incontinence (41% of males, 57% of females), and constipation (36% of males, 39% of females), as well as urinary frequency and urinary hesitancy in males (both 38%) [24]. Although the precise mechanism is still unclear, severe autonomic dysfunction has also been reported, characterized by orthostatic hypotension, sexual dysfunction [25], and autonomic neuropathy [26].

According to Chen et al., among unrelated Taiwanese patients with adult-onset cerebellar ataxia, ALD accounts for 0.85% (1/118) of the patients with molecularly unassigned hereditary ataxia and 0.34% (1/296) of the patients with sporadic ataxia with autonomic dysfunction. In this cohort, white matter hyperintensities in the corticospinal tracts and in the cerebellar hemispheres were strongly associated with ALD rather than other ataxias [27]. Cerebral demyelination is estimated to occur in about 40% of male ALD patients before the age of 18 years but is well documented to occur also in adulthood [14].

The symptoms associated with cerebral ALD depend on the site of the initial lesions. In children and adolescent boys, the first symptoms are usually cognitive deficits, hyperactive behavior, emotional lability, and decline in school performance [1]. These symptoms are frequently initially attributed to attention deficit hyperactivity disorder, which can delay the diagnosis of ALD. When lesions progress, pyramidal tract signs, central visual impairment, apraxia, astereognosis, auditory impairment, and sometimes seizures occur [1, 28]. Demyelination involving the visual tracts occurs typically months to years after the diagnosis of childhood cerebral ALD, manifesting as progressive visual loss followed by optic atrophy. In a report of 15 childhood cerebral ALD patients, there were strabismus in 10 cases, pale optic discs in 7 cases, macular pigmentary changes in 3, optic nerve hypoplasia in 1, and cataracts in 1 [29]. A pathological examination revealed accumulation of bi-leaflet inclusions in optic nerve macrophages, retinal neurons, and macrophages [30].

An atypical spontaneous "arrested" clinical course of cerebral ALD has been described, without evidence of imaging, neurological, or neuropsychological deterioration for many years after the initial symptoms [5, 31]. All three patients reported by Korenke et al. showed typical first symptoms and neuroimaging alterations of cerebral ALD between 7 and 11 years, with a subsequent arrest of neurologic deterioration for 5 to 12 years; none developed impaired visual or auditory function. This stable clinical course was supported by serial neuroimaging studies, with gadolinium enhancement observed only in the first MRI examination of one of these patients [31]. Some authors warned that it may still reactivate many years later [7].

In adult cerebral ALD, initial symptoms are often psychiatric, especially if the lesions are located in the frontal lobes, and can resemble depression, mania, or psychosis [13]. A review by Rosebush et al. found that 19 of 34 cases (56%) were reported to have psychiatric symptomatology. However, a detailed psychiatric assessment was provided only in 13, and the earliest reported symptom was a change in behavior or personality. Twelve of those 13 patients had symptoms of mania, including disinhibition, emotional lability, increased spending, hypersexuality, and perseveration. In addition, five of these patients were also psychotic. Unfortunately, many of the patients were treatment-resistant and appeared to have an aggressive course [32].

See Fig. 27.4 for the clinical spectrum and natural history of ALD.

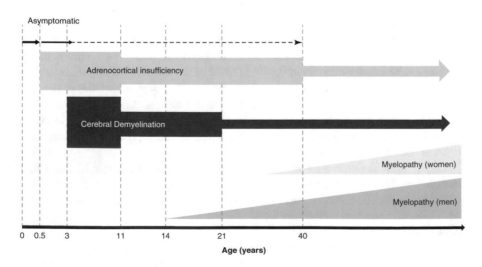

Fig. 27.4 Clinical spectrum and natural history of ALD

Endocrine Dysfunction

X-linked ALD is the most frequent genetic cause of Addison's disease [37]. However, in regions where neonatal screening has not been established, there is a high prevalence of unrecognized adrenocortical insufficiency in *ABCD1* pathological variant children carriers [38]. Primary adrenal insufficiency is characterized by high levels of adrenocorticotropic hormone (ACTH) and low cortisol level. The lifetime prevalence of adrenal insufficiency in ALD is about 80%. The cumulative probability of adrenal insufficiency is highest at the age of 10 years (46.8%) and remains prominent until 40 years of age (an additional 28.6%), decreasing substantially thereafter (an additional 5.6%) [39]. The incidence of adrenal insufficiency varies according to phenotype (see Table 27.1). According to van Geel et al. in a retrospective analysis in 35 of 70 patients with AMN, adrenocortical insufficiency was diagnosed before ALD, and in 33 patients dysfunction was diagnosed after ALD [14]. Sato et al. in a case report have shown that the demand for cortisol is extremely high in advanced adult-onset cerebral ALD. Even with mild infection, because cortisol secretion is limited in these patients, the risk of relative adrenal insufficiency despite normal serum cortisol levels warrants proactive administration of steroids when hyponatremia or hypoglycemia develops [40].

Patients with chronic adrenal insufficiency often have fatigue, anorexia, nausea, vomiting, loss of appetite, poor weight gain or weight loss, and abdominal symptoms. In an acute adrenal crisis, patients may present with hypotension, hypoglycemia, altered mental status, vomiting, and syncope, in addition to chronic symptoms. Salt wasting (hyponatremia and hyperkalemia) is less common with ALD, but patients are described to have impaired aldosterone response to ACTH stimulation and require mineralocorticoid replacement. Hyponatremia may also be present with severe cortisol deficiency, as there may be water retention due to a lack of cortisol inhibition of vasopressin secretion [36]. Corresponding with the relative sparing of the zona glomerulosa from VLCFA accumulation, mineralocorticoid function typically is less affected than glucocorticoid function [12].

Hypogonadism is noticed most frequently after neurologic or adrenal symptoms, but testicular dysfunction has been reported before the appearance of neurologic or adrenal symptoms. In a retrospective report of 26 men with ALD, 46% reported decreased libido and 58% had erectile dysfunction [41]. A prospective controlled study of 49 men with AMN revealed an 82% incidence of testicular dysfunction (elevated gonadotropins or low testosterone/luteinizing hormone ratio), and 54% with erectile dysfunction [42].

Adrenal insufficiency may be absent at the time of ALD diagnosis. In suspected cases, monitoring adrenal function is extremely important in order to secure the diagnosis and prevent Addisonian crisis.

Dermatologic Signs

Early-onset androgenetic alopecia despite hypogonadism and a diffuse reduction in scalp hair and the eyelashes are the main patterns of alopecia described in these patients [43]. Increased skin pigmentation may also be observed as a result of elevations of melanocyte-stimulating hormone, a byproduct of ACTH production. Common areas to note hyperpigmentation include palmar creases, axillae, genitalia, areolae, scars, gums, and the posterior helix of the ear [36]. After adrenarche, loss of pubic and axillary hair due to accumulation of VLCFA in the zona reticularis of the adrenal cortex and consequent poor androgen production may also be noted [36].

Radiologic Findings

Frequently, CT scan shows a symmetric hypodensity bilateral in parieto-occipital white matter with involvement of the splenium of the corpus callosum and enhancement seen along the anterior edge of hypodensity. MRI demonstrates T2/FLAIR hyperintense signal in the same areas as that on CT scan with hypo-intense signal on T1. There is no evidence of restricted diffusion or blooming on susceptibility-weighted images. Histopathologically, in brain lesions of cerebral ALD cases, three distinct zones of white matter involvement are seen. The inner zone is represented by scarring, while the intermediate inflammatory zone is represented by perivascular inflammatory cells and demyelination. Finally, a zone of ongoing demyelination is situated at the periphery, where myelin is breaking down in the absence of inflammation [44]. These areas are also observed in contrast MRI images, where the intermediate zone shows contrast enhancement in the "leading edge" due to ongoing inflammation [45].

Different radiological patterns have been recognized among patients with cerebral ALD: pattern 1, white matter in the parieto-occipital lobe or splenium of corpus callosum; pattern 2, white matter in the frontal lobe or genu of corpus callosum; pattern 3, primary involvement of frontopontine or corticospinal projection fibers without affecting the periventricular white matter; pattern 4, primary involvement of cerebellar white matter; and pattern 5, combined but separate initial involvement of frontal and parieto-occipital white matter. Whereas 80% of patients under 10 years of age presented with pattern 1, the overall frequency of this pattern was somewhat less common in older patients. For the group as whole, 137 (66%) patients presented with pattern 1, 32 (15.5%) with pattern 2, 24 (12%) with pattern 3, 2 (1%) with pattern 4, and 5 (2.5%) with pattern 5. The pattern 1 and 5 groups were on average the youngest, whereas patterns 2 and 4 presented mostly during adolescence, and pattern 3 during adulthood. Progression rates for patterns 1 and 2 were relatively rapid and similar, whereas progression in pattern 3 patients was slow. The progression in pattern 5 patients was extremely rapid [33].

Loes et al. proposed a 34-point brain MRI severity score for cerebral ALD, derived from location and extent of involvement, and the presence of focal and/or global atrophy [46]. This scale is used as a disease progression monitoring tool, with a score <4 considered very early stage, a score 4–8 representing early stage, a score 9–13 representing late stage, and a score of >13 representing advanced disease [47]. Its combination with the radiological pattern, presence of contrast enhancement, and age helped predict progression of lesions [47, 48]. Currently the "Loes scale" is the main radiological criteria used to determine viability for hematopoietic stem cell transplantation in cerebral ALD, with a score ≤ 8 points showing a higher likelihood of benefiting from this treatment [48].

In the pure form of AMN, imaging is dominated by spinal cord atrophy primarily affecting the thoracic cord [28, 49]. Imaging of the brain is either normal or demonstrates only minor abnormalities in the pyramidal tracts traversing the brainstem and internal capsules [28]. On the other hand, patients with AMN may have signs of concealed "arrested" cerebral ALD on MRI, which can help point to a diagnosis of AMN [5]. Liberato et al. described the brain MRI findings in 47 boys with asymptomatic ALD. They reported that 28/47 cases showed brain lesions. Among these cases, 22 had contrast enhancement [50].

Diagnosis

According to a case series reported by van Geel et al., the mean delay in diagnosis of all cases, from the time of onset of symptoms, was almost 10 years; delay was 17 years in adults with initial symptoms of adrenocortical insufficiency [51]. However, this reality is expected to change, because since 2006 a newborn screening test for ALD, using liquid chromatography-tandem mass spectroscopy (LC-MS/MS) measurement of C26:0-lysophosphatidylcholine (C26:0-LPC) in dried blood spot, has been available and already implemented in some regions [3]. This strategy allows pre-symptomatic identification of patients with ALD, close monitoring, and early intervention with hematopoietic stem cell transplantation and adrenal hormone therapy, thereby avoiding the devastating consequences of cerebral ALD and Addisonian crisis, respectively [52].

Usually, when the diagnosis of ALD is suspected based on clinical characteristics and/or brain imaging, plasma VLCFA levels are determined. VLCFA are elevated in almost all male ALD cases irrespective of age, disease duration, metabolic status, or clinical symptoms [53]. Most laboratories measure the concentration of total hexacosanoic acid (C26:0) in dried blood spots, the most frequently used parameter, and its ratio to tetracosanoic (C24:0) and docosanoic (C22:0) acids [11, 54]. The latter remains basically unchanged in plasma samples of ALD [53] (Table 27.2).

Table 27.2 Normal and abnormal plasma levels of VLCFA

VLCFA	C26:0	C24:0/C22:0	C26:0/C22:0
ALD (males)	1.3 ± 0.45 µg/mL	1.71 ± 0.23 µg/mL	0.07 ± 0.03 µg/mL
Female carriers[a]	0.68 ± 0.29 µg/mL	1.3 ± 0.19 µg/mL	0.04 ± 0.02 µg/mL
Normal controls	0.23 ± 0.09 µg/mL	0.84 ± 0.10 µg/mL	0.01 ± 0.004 µg/mL

[a]Elevated in ~80%. Modified from [55]

If ALD is suspected in a woman, the testing strategy should additionally include mutation analysis of the *ABCD1* gene for the correct identification of heterozygous ALD females, because 15% of women with ALD have normal plasma VLCFA levels [9]. Family screening follows the same recommendations [28]. Plasma VLCFA levels strongly depend on dietary intake of VLCFA, for example, by the consumption of peanuts. Thus, blood leucocytes provide an alternative for confirmation of the diagnosis. Following the development of the whole blood spot LC-MS/MS, it has been shown that the C26:0-LPC assay accurately diagnoses males with ALD, and notably offers an accurate diagnostic test for women with ALD, with a reported sensitivity of 100% in 49 females and 126 controls [56].

VLCFA are similarly increased in other peroxisomal disorders such as the Zellweger syndrome spectrum or single enzyme defects of peroxisomal beta-oxidation (acyl-CoA oxidase deficiency and D-bifunctional protein deficiency). Hence mild atypical or late-onset variants of these diseases must be considered in the differential diagnosis, although other peroxisomal disorders can usually be excluded by measuring phytanic acid and plasmalogen levels [53].

In addition to the identification of female carriers and confirmation of the diagnosis in male patients, analysis of *ABCD1* gene variants is also valuable to characterize ALD kindreds and for prenatal diagnosis [53]. To date, more than 849 non-recurrent *ABCD1* mutations have been described, of which 46% are missense mutations [57]. The reported de novo mutation rate ranges from 5% to as high as 19% [58]. As an X-linked inherited disorder, all daughters of an affected male are obligate carriers, whereas his sons can never be affected. When a woman carries the gene for ALD, there is a 50% probability for each pregnancy that the gene is transmitted to a son or daughter. The frequency of de novo mutations in the index case is estimated to be around 4%, which indicates that the *ABCD1* mutation occurred in the germ line. There is evidence of gonadal or gonosomal mosaicism in less than 1% of patients, which means an increased risk of an additional affected offspring. On occasions when no mutations can be detected by DNA sequence analysis, methods such as quantitative polymerase chain reaction, multiple ligation-dependent probe amplification, or Southern blot analysis have been used for recognition of large deletions, duplications, or chromosomal rearrangements [53]. Other tests should include serum ACTH and baseline cortisol levels (24-hour urine cortisol and A.M. and P.M. serum levels). If either is abnormal, an ACTH stimulation test should be performed to evaluate adrenal reserve. The adrenocortical insufficiency in ALD can be life-threatening if not treated, and all patients with ALD should have a regular reassessment of adrenocortical function if the initial results are normal. Routine adrenal testing every 4 to 6 months until 10 years of age, annual testing thereafter until 40 years of age, and solely on-demand testing in case endocrine symptoms manifest from age 41 years onward are recommended [39]. See Fig. 27.5 for a general guide to the diagnosis of X-ALD patients and their management.

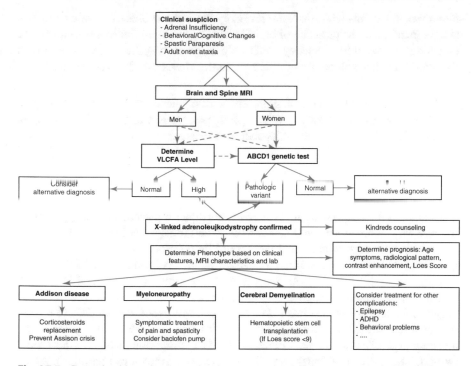

Fig. 27.5 General guide to the diagnosis of symptomatic X-ALD patients and their management

Differential Diagnosis

In children with cerebral ALD, the main differential diagnoses are other childhood-onset leukodystrophies. The mnemonic "**LACK P**roper **M**yelin" may help clinicians to remember the main differential diagnoses among demyelinating leukodystrophies in the childhood (**L**, Leigh's disease; **A**, Alexander's disease and adrenoleukodystrophy; **C**, Canavan's disease; **K**, Krabbe's disease; **P**, Pelizaeus-Merzbacher disease; **M**, metachromatic leukodystrophy) [59]. Remarkably, as mentioned, VLCFA are also increased in other peroxisomal disorders, such as Zellweger syndrome, neonatal adrenoleukodystrophy, and infantile Refsum disease, but these disorders have a different clinical presentation and are rarely confused with ALD [11].

Adults with cerebral ALD should be differentiated from other demyelinating diseases, such as multiple sclerosis, but other adult-onset leukoencephalopathies should also be considered. The spinocerebellar form of ALD could mimic sporadic ataxias such as multiple system atrophy or adult-onset hereditary ataxias. Moreover, AMN could also present with ataxic features. Therefore, ALD should also be considered in the differential of ataxias. However, the most important differential diagnoses in patients with AMN are probably the many causes of spastic paraparesis. As mentioned, the presence of brain MRI abnormalities, family history, and the evidence of adrenal insufficiency could help in suspecting the diagnosis, although the diagnosis must still be considered even in the absence of these elements.

Adult ALD patients may present with atypical phenotypes, such as pure spastic paraparesis mimicking familial spastic paraparesis, or ataxia-dysautonomia syndrome mimicking other neurodegenerative diseases.

Treatment

Currently used therapies for ALD include hormone replacement therapy, dietary therapy with Lorenzo's oil, and hematopoietic cell transplantation.

Patients with adrenal abnormalities should be referred to an endocrinologist, as glucocorticoid and mineralocorticoid treatment should be monitored. Glucocorticoid therapy must be initiated in all patients with confirmed adrenal insufficiency. A recent clinical practice guideline on the treatment of primary adrenal insufficiency suggests the use of hydrocortisone (15–25 mg) or cortisone acetate (20–35 mg) in two or three divided oral doses per day. The highest dose should be given in the morning at awakening, the next either in the early afternoon (2 hours after lunch; two-dose regimen) or at lunch, and in the afternoon (three-dose regimen). As an alternative, prednisolone (3–5 mg/d), administered orally once or twice daily, is suggested. In patients with severe adrenal insufficiency symptoms or adrenal crisis, immediate therapy with intravenous hydrocortisone at an appropriate stress dose prior to the availability of the results of diagnostic tests is recommended [60]. Initiation of mineralocorticoid replacement therapy has been suggested only after clinical and/or biochemical evidence of mineralocorticoid deficiency [12].

Lorenzo's oil is a formula of unsaturated fatty acids (glycerol trioleate C18:1 and glyceryl trierucate C22:1 in a 4:1 ratio); this formula may inhibit elongation of saturated fatty acids [1, 61]. Lorenzo's oil combined with a VLCFA-poor diet has been shown to be helpful in normalizing plasma levels of VLCFA [61]. This combined therapy failed to arrest disease progression of AMN and pre-symptomatic patients in an open trial [62]. In an open single-arm trial of asymptomatic ALD patients with normal brain MRI, Moser et al., using Lorenzo's oil combined with a moderate fat restriction diet, showed a reduced risk of developing MRI abnormalities and an association between the development of MRI abnormalities and a plasma C26:0 levels [63]. Other studies of untreated boys reported similar conversion rates as those reported on Lorenzo's oil. There is no consistent evidence of disease-modifying effects of Lorenzo's oil in AMN, nor a role in reducing the risk of brain lesions in cerebral ALD. A group of experts recommend that "the use of Lorenzo's oil should only be undertaken by centers that have the ability to provide monitoring with MRI, nutritional guidance, and the ability to measure VLCFA and other essential fatty acids. Other centers consider the efficacy of Lorenzo's oil unproven and do not recommend its use" [57].

Allogeneic hematopoietic stem cell transplantation (HSCT) is the only therapeutic approach that can potentially arrest the neuroinflammatory demyelinating cerebral process of X-ALD in boys, particularly if the procedure is performed when patients have no neuropsychiatric compromise and limited extension of demyelinating lesions on brain MRI. After the transplantation procedure, demyelinating lesions may extend for 12 months to 18 months, and then their progression arrests. This interval is likely caused by the slow substitution of brain microglia with bone marrow-derived cells. Similar benefits of allogeneic HSCT have been demonstrated in adults with cerebral ALD. In already symptomatic patients, unfortunately, this procedure has not been shown to be effective in stopping the demyelinating process. More importantly, it can accelerate neurologic deterioration. Furthermore, allogeneic HSCT is associated with risks of graft-versus-host disease and prolonged immune deficiency, particularly in adults, and not all ALD patients have donors despite the availability of cord blood [64].

In practice, for the children up to 12 years of age, HSCT is mainly reserved for patients who present first with Addison's disease or who are identified during genetic counseling, and in whom repeated brain MRI can detect the appearance of the beginning signs of cerebral demyelination. For adults, most transplanted patients were patients who initially had AMN and in whom repeated brain MRI detected early signs of cerebral demyelination.

Increased muscle tone is often severe and difficult to treat. Aggressive treatment is essential, since it causes pain, which in turn aggravates spasticity as well as dystonia in a vicious feedback circle that not only causes suffering but seriously lowers the quality of life of both the patient and his family. Symptomatic treatment is primarily the approach to spasticity, dystonia, and other complications in patients with ALD. Intrathecal baclofen seems to be effective for boys with the cerebral form of ALD with spasticity-dystonia who have not responded adequately to oral medication. It also can be considered as an early option in such cases in the hopes of preventing further complications [65]. Other therapeutic approaches remain under investigation.

⚷ High VLCFA level is the standard biomarker for diagnosis in males, although less reliable in females. Genetic testing is available. Early hematopoietic stem cell transplantation can arrest brain demyelination/inflammation. However, there is no known cure for adrenomyeloneuropathy. Treatment is focused on hormone replacement and symptomatic treatment of spasticity.

References

1. Berger J, Gärtner J. X-linked adrenoleukodystrophy: clinical, biochemical and pathogenetic aspects. Biochim Biophys Acta, Mol Cell Res. 1763;2006:1721–32.
2. Bezman L, Moser AB, Raymond GV, Piero Rinaldo, Watkins PA, Smith KD, et al. Adrenoleukodystrophy: incidence, new mutation rate, and results of extended family screening. Ann Neurol [Internet]. 2001;49:512–7. Available from: http://doi.wiley.com/10.1002/ana.101.

3. Vogel BH, Bradley SE, Adams DJ, D'Aco K, Erbe RW, Fong C, et al. Newborn screening for X-linked adrenoleukodystrophy in New York State: diagnostic protocol, surveillance protocol and treatment guidelines. Mol Genet Metab [Internet]. 2015;114:599–603. Available from: https://doi.org/10.1016/j.ymgme.2015.02.002.

4. Berger J, Forss-Petter S, Eichler FS. Pathophysiology of X-linked adrenoleukodystrophy. Biochimie [Internet]. 2014;98:135–42. Available from: https://doi.org/10.1016/j.biochi.2013.11.023.

5. Lin JE, Armour EA, Heshmati A, Umandap C, Couto JJ, Iglesias AD, et al. Pearls & Oy-sters: adolescent-onset adrenomyeloneuropathy and arrested cerebral adrenoleukodystrophy. Neurology. 2019;93:81–4.

6. Wang A.-G. X-Linked Adrenoleukodystrophy, in: A.-G. Wang (Ed.), Emergency Neuro-Ophthalmology: Rapid Case Demonstrations, Springer Singapore, Singapore, 2018: pp. 137–141. https://doi.org/10.1007/978-981-10-7668-8.

7. Engelen M, Kemp S, Poll-The BT. X-linked adrenoleukodystrophy: pathogenesis and treatment. Curr Neurol Neurosci Rep. 2014;14:1–8.

8. Paláu-Hernández S, Rodriguez-Leyva I, Shiguetomi-Medina JM. Late onset adrenoleukodystrophy: a review related clinical case report. eNeurologicalSci [Internet]. Elsevier; 2019;14:62–7. Available from: https://doi.org/10.1016/j.ensci.2019.01.007.

9. Moser HW, Mahmood A, Raymond GV. X-linked adrenoleukodystrophy. Nat Clin Pract Neurol. 2007;3:140–51.

10. Griffin DE, Moser HW, Mendoza Q, Moench TR, O'Toole S, Moser AB. Identification of the inflammatory cells in the central nervous system of patients with adrenoleukodystrophy. Ann Neurol. 1985;18:660–4.

11. Moser HW, Krieger K. Adrenoleukodystrophy: phenotype, genetics, pathogenesis and therapy* dedicated to the memory of Peter Moser. Brain. 1997;120:1485–508.

12. Zhu J, Eichler F, Biffi A, Duncan CN, Williams DA, Majzoub JA. The changing face of adrenoleukodystrophy. Endocr Rev [Internet]. 2020;1–29. Available from: https://academic.oup.com/edrv/advance-article/doi/10.1210/endrev/bnaa013/5828725.

13. Kemp S, Huffnagel IC, Linthorst GE, Wanders RJ, Engelen M. Adrenoleukodystrophy - Neuroendocrine pathogenesis and redefinition of natural history. Nat Rev Endocrinol [Internet]. 2016;12:606–15. Available from: https://doi.org/10.1038/nrendo.2016.90.

14. Van Geel BM, Bezman L, Loes DJ, Moser HW, Raymond GV. Evolution of phenotypes in adult male patients with X-linked adrenoleukodystrophy. Ann Neurol. 2001;49:186–94.

15. Huffnagel IC, Van Ballegoij WJC, Van Geel BM, Vos JMBW, Kemp S, Engelen M. Progression of myelopathy in males with adrenoleukodystrophy: towards clinical trial readiness. Brain. 2019;142:334–43.

16. Edwin D, Speedie LJ, Kohler W, Naidu S, Kruse B, Moser HW. Cognitive and brain magnetic resonance imaging findings in adrenomyeloneuropathy. Ann Neurol. 1996;40:675–8.

17. Azar C, Nadjar Y. First report of young women presenting with severe form of adrenomyeloneuropathy. J Neurol Sci [Internet]. 2019;405:79. Available from: https://linkinghub.elsevier.com/retrieve/pii/S0022510X19321860.

18. Moser HW, Moser AB, Naidu S, Bergin A. Clinical aspects of adrenoleukodystrophy and adrenomyeloneuropathy. Dev Neurosci [Internet]. 1991;13:254–61. Available from: https://www.karger.com/Article/FullText/112170.

19. Van de Stadt SIW, Van Ballegoij JWC, Labounek R, Huffnagel IC, Kemp S, Nestrasil I, et al. Spinal cord atrophy as a measure of severity of myelopathy in adrenoleukodystrophy., J. Inherit. Metab. Dis. 2020;43:852–60. https://doi.org/10.1002/jimd.12226.

20. Maris T, Androulidakis EJ, Tzagournissakis M, Papavassiliou S, Moser H, Plaitakis A. X-linked adrenoleukodystrophy presenting as neurologically pure familial spastic paraparesis. Neurology. 1995;45:1101–4.

21. Shaw-Smith CJ, Lewis SJG, Reid E. X-linked adrenoleukodystrophy presenting as autosomal dominant pure hereditary spastic paraparesis. J Neurol Neurosurg Psychiatry. 2004;75:686–8.

22. Zhan Z Xiong, Liao X Xin, Du J, Luo Y Ying, Hu Z Ting, Wang J Ling, et al. Exome sequencing released a case of X-linked adrenoleukodystrophy mimicking recessive hereditary

spastic paraplegia. Eur J Med Genet [Internet]. 2013;56:375–8. Available from: https://doi. org/10.1016/j.ejmg.2013.04.008.
23. Hofereiter J, Smith MD, Seth J, Tudor KI, Fox Z, Emmanuel A, et al. Bladder and bowel dysfunction is common in both men and women with mutation of the ABCD1 gene for X-linked adrenoleukodystrophy. JIMD Rep [Internet]. 2015;77–83. Available from: http://link.springer. com/10.1007/8904_2015_414.
24. Gomery P, Corre C, Eichler F. Urinary and Bowel symptoms in adult patient with adrenoleukodystrophy. Neurology. 2018;90:464.
25. Zhang Y, Guo D, Tang Y. Autonomic dysfunction in a patient with X-linked adrenoleukodystrophy. Int J Neurosci [Internet]. 2018;128:783–4. Available from: https://doi.org/10.108 0/00207454.2017.1405953.
26. Schulte-Mattler W, Lindner A, Zierz S. Autonomic neuropathy in a patient with adrenomyeloneuropathy. Eur J Med Res. 1996;1:559–61.
27. Chen YH, Lee YC, Tsai YS, Guo YC, Hsiao CT, Tsai PC, et al. Unmasking adrenoleukodystrophy in a cohort of cerebellar ataxia. PLoS One. 2017;12:1–14.
28. Engelen M, Kemp S, De Visser M, Van Geel BM, Wanders RJA, Aubourg P, et al. X-linked adrenoleukodystrophy (X-ALD): clinical presentation and guidelines for diagnosis, follow-up and management. Orphanet J Rare Dis. 2012;7:1–14.
29. Traboulsi EI, Maumenee IH. Ophthalmologic manifestations of X-linked childhood adrenoleulcodystrophy. Ophthalmology. 1987;94:47–52.
30. Brown FR, Moser HW, Cohen SMZ, Green WR, de la Cruz ZC, Luckenbach MW, et al. Ocular histopathologic studies of neonatal and childhood adrenoleukodystrophy. Am J Ophthalmol. 1983;95:82–96.
31. Korenke GC, Pouwels PJW, Frahm J, Hunneman DH, Stoeckler S, Krasemann E, et al. Arrested cerebral adrenoleukodystrophy: a clinical and proton magnetic resonance spectroscopy study in three patients. Pediatr Neurol. 1996;15:103–7.
32. Rosebush PI, Garside S, Levinson AJ, Mazurek MF. The neuropsychiatry of adult-onset adrenoleukodystrophy. J Neuropsychiatry Clin Neurosci [Internet]. 1999;11:315–27. Available from: http://psychiatryonline.org/doi/abs/10.1176/jnp.11.3.315.
33. Loes DJ, Fatemi A, Melhem ER, Gupte N, Bezman L, Moser HW, et al. Analysis of MRI patterns aids prediction of progression in X-linked adrenoleukodystrophy. Neurology. 2003;61:369–74.
34. Au LWC, Chan AYY, Mok VCT. Teaching NeuroImages: X-linked adrenoleukodystrophy: spinocerebellar variant. Neurology. 2019;93:E731–2.
35. Ogaki K, Koga S, Aoki N, Lin W, Suzuki K, Ross OA, et al. Adult-onset cerebello-brainstem dominant form of X-linked adrenoleukodystrophy presenting as multiple system atrophy: case report and literature review. Neuropathology [Internet]. 2016;36:64–76. Available from: http:// doi.wiley.com/10.1111/neup.12230.
36. Burtman E, Regelmann MO. Endocrine dysfunction in X-linked adrenoleukodystrophy. Endocrinol Metab Clin North Am [Internet]. 2016;45:295–309. Available from: https://doi. org/10.1016/j.ecl.2016.01.003.
37. Aubourg P, Chaussain JL. Adrenoleukodystrophy: The most frequent genetic cause of Addison's disease. Horm Res. 2003;59:104–5.
38. Dubey P, Raymond GV, Moser AB, Kharkar S, Bezman LMH. Adrenal insufficiency in asymptomatic long-chain fatty acid screening. J Pediatr. 2005;146:528–32.
39. Huffnagel IC, Laheji FK, Aziz-Bose R, Tritos NA, Marino R, Linthorst GE, et al. The natural history of adrenal insufficiency in X-linked adrenoleukodystrophy: an international collaboration. J Clin Endocrinol Metab. 2019;104:118–26.
40. Sato T, Umehara T, Nakahara A, Oka H. Relative adrenal insufficiency in adult-onset cerebral X-linked adrenoleukodystrophy. Neurol Clin Pract [Internet]. 2017;7:398–400. Available from: http://cp.neurology.org/lookup/doi/10.1212/CPJ.0000000000000310.
41. Assies J, Gooren LJG, Van Geel B, Barth PG. Signs of testicular insufficiency in adrenomyeloneuropathy and neurologically asymptomatic X-linked adrenoleukodystrophy: a

retrospective study. Int J Androl [Internet]. 1997;20:315–21. Available from: http://doi.wiley. com/10.1046/j.1365-2605.1997.00066.x.

42. Brennemann W, Köhler W, Zierz S, Klingmüller D. Testicular dysfunction in adrenomyeloneuropathy. Eur J Endocrinol. 1997;137:34–9.

43. König A, Happle R, Tchitcherina E, Schaefer JR, Sokolowski P, Köhler W, et al. An X-linked gene involved in androgenetic alopecia: a lesson to be learned from adrenoleukodystrophy. Dermatology. 2000;200:213–8.

44. Schaumburg H, Poewers J, Raine C, Suzuki K, Richardson E. Adrenoleukodystrophy a clinical and pathological study of 17 cases. Arch Neurol. 1975;32:577–91.

45. Eichler F, Mahmood A, Loes D, Bezman L, Lin D, Moser HW, et al. Magnetic resonance imaging detection of lesion progression in adult patients with X-linked adrenoleukodystrophy. Arch Neurol. 2007;64:659–64.

46. Loes DJ, Hite S, Moser H, Stillman AE, Shapiro E, Lockman L, et al. Adrenoleukodystrophy: a scoring method for brain MR observations. Am J Neuroradiol. 1994;15:1761–6.

47. Turk BR, Moser AB, Fatemi A. Therapeutic strategies in adrenoleukodystrophy. Wien Med Wochenschr. 2017;167:219–26.

48. Bladowska J, Kulej D, Biel A, Zimny A, Kałwak K, Owoc-Lempach J, et al. The role of MR imaging in the assessment of clinical outcomes in children with x-linked adrenoleukodystrophy after allogeneic haematopoietic stem cell transplantation. Polish J Radiol. 2015;80:181–90.

49. Resende LL, de Paiva ARB, Kok F, Leite C da C, Lucato LT. Adult leukodystrophies: a step-by-step diagnostic approach. Radiographics. 2019;39:153–68.

50. Liberato AP, Mallack EJ, Aziz-Bose R, Hayden D, Lauer A, Caruso PA, et al. MRI brain lesions in asymptomatic boys with X-linked adrenoleukodystrophy. Neurology. 2019;92:e1698–708.

51. van Geel BM, Assies J, Haverkort EB, Barth PG, Wanders RJA, Schutgens RBH, et al. Delay in diagnosis of X-linked adrenoleukodystrophy. Clin Neurol Neurosurg. 1993;95:115–20.

52. Turk BR, Theda C, Fatemi A, Moser AB. X-linked adrenoleukodystrophy: pathology, pathophysiology, diagnostic testing, newborn screening, and therapies. Int J Dev Neurosci [Internet]. 2019. Available from: https://doi.org/10.1016/j.ijdevneu.2019.11.002.

53. Wiesinger C, Eichler FS, Berger J. The genetic landscape of X-linked adrenoleukodystrophy: inheritance, mutations, modifier genes, and diagnosis. Appl Clin Genet. 2015;8:109–21.

54. Hubbard WC, Moser AB, Liu AC, Jones RO, Steinberg SJ, Lorey F, et al. Newborn screening for X-linked adrenoleukodystrophy (X-ALD): validation of a combined liquid chromatography-tandem mass spectrometric (LC-MS/MS) method. Mol Genet Metab [Internet]. 2009;97:212–20. Available from: https://doi.org/10.1016/j.ymgme.2009.03.010.

55. Steinberg S, Jones R, Tiffany C, Moser A. Investigational methods for peroxisomal disorders. Curr Protoc Hum Genet. 2008;58(1):17.6.1–17.6.23.

56. Huffnagel IC, van de Beek MC, Showers AL, Orsini JJ, Klouwer FCC, Dijkstra IME, et al. Comparison of C26:0-carnitine and C26:0-lysophosphatidylcholine as diagnostic markers in dried blood spots from newborns and patients with adrenoleukodystrophy. Mol Genet Metab [Internet]. 2017;122:209–15. Available from: https://doi.org/10.1016/j.ymgme.2017.10.012.

57. Engelen M, Salzman R, Bonnamain V, Kemp S. The ALD mutation database [Internet]. 2019. Available from: https://adrenoleukodystrophy.info/mutations-biochemistry/mutation-statistics.

58. Horn MA, Retterstøl L, Abdelnoor M, Skjeldal OH, Tallaksen CME. Adrenoleukodystrophy in Norway: high rate of De Novo mutations and age-dependent penetrance. Pediatr Neurol [Internet]. 2013;48:212–9. Available from: https://linkinghub.elsevier.com/retrieve/pii/S0887899412006789.

59. Myelin LP. Pediatric radiology originals Dysmyelinating leukodystrophies: "LACK Proper Myelin". Pediatr Radiol. 1991:477–82.

60. Bornstein SR, Allolio B, Arlt W, Barthel A, Don-Wauchope A, Hammer GD, et al. Diagnosis and treatment of primary adrenal insufficiency: an endocrine society clinical practice guideline. J Clin Endocrinol Metab. 2016;101:364–89.

61. Moser HW, Moser AB, Hollandsworth K, Brereton NH, Raymond G V. "Lorenzo's Oil" therapy for X-linked adrenoleukodystrophy: rationale and current assessment of efficacy. J

Mol Neurosci [Internet]. 2007;33:105–13. Available from: http://link.springer.com/10.1007/s12031-007-0041-4.

62. Aubourg P, Adamsbaum C, Lavallard-Rousseau M-C, Rocchiccioli F, Cartier N, Jambaque I, et al. A two-year trial of Oleic and Erucic Acids ("Lorenzo's Oil") as treatment for adrenomyeloneuropathy. N Engl J Med [Internet]. 1993;329:745–52. Available from: http://www.nejm.org/doi/pdf/10.1056/NEJM199309303291401.

63. Moser HW, Raymond GV, Lu S-E, Muenz LR, Moser AB, Xu J, et al. Follow-up of 89 asymptomatic patients with adrenoleukodystrophy treated with Lorenzo's Oil. Arch Neurol [Internet]. 2005;62:1073. Available from: http://archneur.jamanetwork.com/article.aspx?doi=10.1001/archneur.62.7.1073.

64. Cartier N, Aubourg P. Hematopoietic stem cell transplantation and hematopoietic stem cell gene therapy in X-linked adrenoleukodystrophy. Brain Pathol. 2010;20:857–62.

65. Hjartarson HT, Ehrstedt C, Tedroff K. Intrathecal baclofen treatment an option in X-linked adrenoleukodystrophy. Eur J Paediatr Neurol [Internet]. 2018;22:178–81. Available from: https://doi.org/10.1016/j.ejpn.2017.09.003.

Whipple's Disease

28

Eoin Mulroy, John Lynch, and Timothy Lynch

Patient Vignettes

Patient 1

A 55-year-old man developed right facial twitching without other neurological signs. Hemifacial spasm was diagnosed. Carbamazepine (600 mg daily) and baclofen (60 mg daily) produced no benefit. Five months later, he complained of somnolence, blurred vision, and poor balance. One month later, the facial twitching spread to his neck and tongue, persisting with sleep. He developed dysarthria and complained of poor memory, change in personality, malaise, intermittent fevers, increased sweating, impotence, and inability to ejaculate. One year after the onset of facial twitching, orientation, memory, and language were normal. He was inter-mittently inattentive and had marked dysarthria due to rhythmic lingual retraction and masticatory myorhythmia coinciding with rhythmic contraction of the right side of the face, neck, and chest and right arm. The contractions spread irregularly to the left side of the face, chest, and left arm and leg. Vertical gaze was limited but

Supplementary Information The online version of this chapter (https://doi.org/10.1007/978-3-030-75898-1_28) contains supplementary material, which is available to authorized users.

E. Mulroy (✉)
Dublin Neurological Institute at the Mater Misericordiae University Hospital, Dublin, Ireland

Department of Clinical and Movement Neurosciences, UCL Queen Square Institute of Neurology, London, UK
e-mail: e.mulroy@ucl.ac.uk

J. Lynch (Deceased)

T. Lynch
Department of Neurology, Dublin Neurological Institute at the Mater Misericordiae University Hospital, Dublin, Ireland

© Springer Nature Switzerland AG 2022
S. J. Frucht (ed.), *Movement Disorder Emergencies*, Current Clinical Neurology,
https://doi.org/10.1007/978-3-030-75898-1_28

improved with the oculocephalic maneuver. Saccades were slow in all directions. Pendular vergence oscillations of the right more than of the left eye (frequency = 1 Hz) were synchronous with the masticatory and skeletal myorhythmia (i.e., oculofacial-skeletal myorhythmia [OFSM]). Electromyographic analysis revealed 400-msec bursts of bilateral rhythmic activity. This activity originated at the level of cranial nerve VII, and spread rostrally to involve the muscles of the mastication, and caudally to involve muscles of the neck, arms, and legs. Muscle tone, strength, sensation, deep tendon reflexes, plantar responses, and postural stability were normal. Gait was mildly ataxic.

Serum chemistries; complete blood count (CBC); serum venereal disease research laboratory (VDRL) test result; serum Lyme titer; thyroid function test (TFT) results; antinuclear antibody (ANA) titer; human immunodeficiency virus (HIV) test result; vitamin B12 (B12); folate; CSF cell count, protein, and glucose levels; and electroencephalogram (EEG) were normal. Brain magnetic resonance imaging (MRI) with gadolinium revealed a left frontal periventricular punctate hyperintensity. Technetium-99m hexamethylpropyleneamine oxime (99m Tc = HMPAO) single-photon emission computed tomography (SPECT) revealed decreased activity in the right cerebellar hemisphere. A duodenal biopsy specimen obtained 12 months after the onset of facial twitching was initially normal (periodic acid Schiff [PAS] stain negative, electron microscopy [EM] not performed). After 1 month, a repeat biopsy with Crosby capsule revealed foamy macrophages stained positive with PAS and silver stains and negatively with acid-fast stain. PAS and Grocott methenamine silver stains demonstrated intracytoplasmic granular rod-shaped structures consistent with Whipple's bacillus. Probable CNS WD was diagnosed.

Trimethoprim-sulfamethoxazole (TPM-SMX) (1 double-strength [DS] tablet twice a day) resulted in improvement in malaise and the ocular component of the myorhythmia. When diarrhea developed, TPM-SMX was discontinued, and intravenous ceftriaxone (2 gm daily) resulted in resolution of the diarrhea and sweating, decrement in the myorhythmia, and increase in alertness. After 1 month, he was switched to receive doxycycline monohydrate (200 mg twice a day), with worsening of hemifacial spasms, malaise, and lethargy over the ensuing 9 months. Ceftriaxone (2 gm/day) was resumed, with improvement in hemifacial spasms, malaise, and lethargy over the ensuing 3 months. After 2 years of follow-up, he was taking TPM-SMX (1 DS tablet twice a day). He still had right facial twitching, complaints of poor memory, increased sweating, impotence, and inability to ejaculate. There was moderate improvement in limb myorhythmia, malaise, and vertical gaze.

Patient 2

A 47-year-old woman developed severe progressive insomnia unresponsive to medication, a 10-lb weight loss, double vision, fever, and submandibular lymph node enlargement. Past history was notable for arthritis. No diarrhea, steatorrhea, or other gastrointestinal symptoms were reported. She noted spontaneous rhythmic right eye movement while looking in the mirror. On examination, vertical and horizontal saccades were slow, with diminished abduction of the left eye. Downgaze was full; upgaze was mildly limited. There were spontaneous convergent nystagmoid movements in the right eye unaccompanied by miosis. These movements increased with downward moving optokinetic stimuli.

Over the ensuing 8 months, a progressive ophthalmoparesis resulted in complete loss of voluntary eye movements except for adduction of the right eye. She developed short-term memory loss, depressive symptoms, difficulty swallowing, blurred vision, intermittent hypersomnolence, and increased postural instability. On reexamination, she was intermittently unrousable, with hypomimia and severe dysarthria. Pendular vergence oscillations of both eyes synchronous with the masticatory myorhythmia (oculomasticatory myorhythmia [OMM]) were present. There was mild hypertonia, and normal strength and sensation. Deep tendon reflexes were brisk. Gait was slow, with shuffling, difficulty turning, and postural instability. Levodopa-carbidopa and prednisolone (20 mg daily) were trialled without benefit.

Serum chemistries, CBC, serum Lyme titers, coagulation screen results, ANA titer, B12 and folate levels, TFT results, serum protein electrophoresis, and VDRL and HIV test results were normal. EEG revealed a generalized mildly slow background. CSF analyses revealed protein levels of 50 to 55 mg/dl with a normal glucose concentration, and 0 to 70 PAS-negative mononuclear cells. Brain computed tomography (CT) scans appeared normal, and MRI revealed an Arnold-Chiari type 1 malformation with no brainstem compression. Specimens obtained at two duodenal biopsies indicated mild chronic nonspecific duodenitis. No PAS staining or other changes consistent with WD were detected. EM was not performed, but polymerase chain reaction (PCR) on gut biopsy samples was positive, even though PAS staining was negative. CNS WD was diagnosed based on clinical findings (i.e., OMM). Intravenous ceftriaxone (2 gm daily) for 6 months resulted in complete resolution of OMM and improvement in the supranuclear gaze palsy and malaise. After switching to TPM-SMX (1 DS tablet twice a day), the supranuclear gaze palsy, lethargy, and malaise recurred. After years of follow-up, she was restricted to a wheelchair and fed by gastrostomy tube.

Introduction

First described by George Hoyt Whipple in 1907 [1], Whipple's disease is a chronic, treatable multisystemic infectious disease caused by the gram-positive actinomycete, *Tropheryma whipplei*. Over a century has elapsed since its first recognition, yet Whipple's disease remains a somewhat enigmatic diagnostic challenge. In the central nervous system in particular, Whipple's disease (WD) can mimic almost any other neurologic condition. Diagnosis of WD remains complicated and laborious. Equally, because of a variety of factors, most notably its penchant for the intracellular milieu and slow replication rate, treatment is far from straightforward, requiring prolonged courses of antibiotics, the choice of which is generally informed by limited clinical experience rather than controlled trial evidence. In this chapter, we review the diagnostic conundrum that is Whipple's disease of the central nervous system, touch on the immunopathologic defects which promote transition from asymptomatic carriage to a disease state, highlight red flags which should make clinicians suspect the diagnosis, and conclude with insights from previous treatment trials.

O━━━➤   Whipple's is a particular challenge: difficult to diagnose, pleomorphic in its presentations, and requiring prolonged treatment.

Tropheryma whipplei

Previously considered a rare organism, more recent studies have shown that *T. whipplei* is in fact a common commensal bacterium. This bacilliform bacterium is found ubiquitously in the environment, with highest prevalence in sewage and wastewaters [2]. Transmission likely occurs through the fecal-oral route, and it is likely that most individuals are exposed to the bacterium at some point in their lifetime. Nearly a century would elapse between the original description by Whipple and the eventual identification of the causative bacillus. Sequencing of PCR-amplified bacterial 16s ribosomal RNA from infected tissue, followed by sequencing of other parts of its genome, confirmed the bacillus as a GC-rich gram-positive actinomycete [3–6]. The determination of specific nucleotide sequences within the *T. whipplei* genome also allowed the development of sensitive and specific PCR tools which are now critical in diagnosing both systemic and CNS forms of the disorder [7–9]. The bacterium is predominantly found intracellularly in macrophages and monocytes of affected tissues, though it can also persist extracellularly [10]. Histologically, it generally appears as multiple periodic acid-Schiff (PAS) positive, diastase-resistant inclusions in macrophage cytoplasm [11]. Examination by electron microscopy demonstrates that the areas of intense PAS staining are packed with bacilli, some degenerated.

Epidemiology

Classic Whipple's disease is predominantly a disorder of middle-aged Caucasian men (outnumbering women 8:1), though this is less obvious in the cases reported with predominant CNS manifestations [12]. Farmers and those in regular contact with soil or animals also have a much higher incidence of Whipple's disease [11]; close contact with affected individuals and squalid sanitary conditions also increase the risk [12–14]. Seroprevalence for *T. whipplei* is over 70% in the general population, though most individuals clear the infection. Asymptomatic gastrointestinal carriage is also not uncommon, ranging from 1.5% to 7% in the general population to 12% to 25% in sewage treatment workers [2, 13, 15, 16]. Despite high seroprevalence and asymptomatic carriage rates, Whipple's disease itself remains exceedingly rare, with estimated incidence of less than 1 per 1,000,000 population per year [11]. Such great discrepancy between high levels of exposure/asymptomatic carriage and the tiny number of people that develop disease suggests a strong role for host factors in pathogenesis of disease. In this regard, genetic factors, particularly relating to host cell-mediated immune responses, appear to play a critical role in conferring a lifetime susceptibility to Whipple's disease [17].

Pathophysiology and Immunopathology

The immunopathogenesis of Whipple's disease remains incompletely understood. At its core, it is accepted that dysfunctional macrophage and monocyte function resulting in impaired clearance of the bacterium are at play [18–20]. Such impairments are probably majorly genetically determined, with rare familial cases, disease predominance in Caucasians, specific HLA associations (HLA DRB1*13 and DQB1*06) known to impair antigen presentation, and polymorphisms in certain cytokine genes polarizing immune responses toward T-helper 2 (TH2) activity being associated with the disease [21, 22]. Furthermore, some patients are prone to recurrent relapses with different strains of *T. whipplei* [23]. Moreover, acquired immune deficits have also been recognized as a risk factor for WD. Patients with HIV may be at increased risk [24, 25], as may those receiving the increasingly common biologic therapies for systemic inflammatory disorders [26, 27].

Under normal circumstances, exposure to *T. whipplei* results in a swift and robust immune response resulting in clearance of the organism, or at the very least, asymptomatic carriage. In patients developing WD, however, this response is muted, either due to inherently defective monocyte function or through dysfunctional priming of *T. whipplei*-specific T cells by dendritic cells in the gut, perhaps from inadequate IL-12 production [20, 28]. This failure to clear the organism sets the scene for persistent bacterial replication within gut monocytes and spread to cause systemic disease. In the case of central nervous system disease, entry might be achieved through passage of infected monocytes across the blood-brain barrier [29].

Numerous defective immune responses have been noted in patients with WD. These include impairments of fusion of *T. whipplei* containing phagosomes with lysosomes [30], low serum concentrations of interleukin-12 (which likely inhibits the generation of TH1-helper cells), and overexpression of IL-10 [31–33]. Additionally, there appears to be a significant role for IL-16 in the immunopathogenesis of WD. *T. whipplei* itself stimulates the release of IL-16 from macrophages, which induces macrophage apoptosis and impairs phagosome-lysosome fusion [34, 35]; interestingly, IL-16 levels and apoptotic markers correlate with disease severity and decrease to normal upon successful treatment [30, 36]. *T. whipplei* has been shown to replicate in macrophages and monocytes deactivated with IL-16, while anti-IL-16 antibodies inhibit *T. whipplei* replication [34].

Clinical Presentations of Whipple's Disease

The clinical manifestations of Whipple's disease are insidious in onset, slowly progressive, and, for the most part, highly nonspecific. This often leads to significant delays in diagnosis. Classic Whipple's disease generally begins with a period of intermittent, migratory large joint seronegative arthralgia or arthritis, which generally spans a number of years prior to the development of other symptoms [27]. Predilection for large joints is often seen, with knees, wrists, and ankles affected more often than shoulders or hips [37]. Generally, the ensuing symptoms are gastrointestinal in nature, consisting of weight loss, diarrhea, and steatorrhea. This may be accompanied by intermittent fever and lymphadenopathy. Cardiac involvement is common and may comprise valvular dysfunction, coronary arterial damage, culture-negative endocarditis as well as myocarditis and pericarditis [38–40]. Rarer disease manifestations include increased skin pigmentation, subcutaneous nodules, and bone marrow involvement [41, 42]. Various ocular manifestations of Whipple's disease have been described including uveitis, vitritis, retinitis, keratitis, and optic neuritis [11, 43], which may cause diagnostic confusion with other eye-involving multisystem masqueraders including syphilis and vasculitides.

Neurological Manifestations of Whipple's Disease

Neurological involvement occurs in 10% to 40% of patients with Whipple's disease [44]. In the vast majority of cases, this occurs as a late feature of systemic Whipple's disease, less commonly as a CNS relapse in patients with previously treated systemic Whipple's disease treated, and in exceptional cases as isolated CNS Whipple's disease [44]. Spinal cord and peripheral nerve involvement are also reported [45, 46]. Asymptomatic CNS infection may occur, and even in the absence of neurological symptoms, up to 50% of patients with Whipple's disease are found to have CNS infection by PCR analysis of the CSF [47]. Presenting clinical symptoms are protean. A progressive encephalopathy manifesting as dementia, confusion, apathy, and somnolence is probably the most common neurological sign [44]. Supranuclear ophthalmoplegia, psychiatric symptoms, myoclonus, and gait ataxia are also suggestive [43, 48]. Seizures can occur, as can focal neurological signs resulting from focal mass lesions or strokes secondary to Whipple endocarditis. Hypothalamic dysfunction with secondary hormonal imbalance is common.

Two clinical signs, namely, oculomasticatory myorhythmia (OMM) and oculofacial-skeletal myorhythmia (OFSM), are highly specific for Whipple's disease, especially in the presence of supranuclear gaze palsy [49–51]. Present in about 20% of patients with CNS WD, OMM involves pendular vergence oscillations of the eyes synchronous with rhythmic myoclonic contractions of the masticatory muscles, while OFSM additionally involves contraction of the skeletal musculature;

both are classically thought of as pathognomonic of CNS Whipple's disease [43, 50, 52]. Pendular vergence oscillations are characterized by continuous smooth, rhythmic convergent eye movements with a frequency of 1 Hz varying from 10 to 25 degrees of amplitude per eye, but never diverging beyond the primary position. The oscillations continue throughout sleep and may be subtle and asymmetric. Convergence and divergence are at the same speed and are not accompanied by miosis or accommodation. The anatomical basis for this apparently unique movement disorder is not known but may originate from the upper brainstem. Though myorhythmia as an entity can occur in a number of other conditions, including brainstem and thalamic strokes or structural lesions, its oculomasticatory and oculofacial-skeletal variants do appear to be pathognomonic for WD [53].

O━━┱   Pendular vergence nystagmus, oculomasticatory myorhythmia, and oculofacial-skeletal myorhythmia are unusual but pathognomonic findings in Whipple's disease.

Radiologic Findings

Neuroimaging findings in CNS Whipple's disease are equally as diverse as the clinical manifestations. Importantly, even in the presence of florid clinical signs, brain imaging can be normal [54, 55]. For unknown reasons, there is a predilection for involvement of the diencephalon, and CNS Whipple's is an important differential diagnosis of abnormalities in the brainstem, hypothalamus, and thalamus [54]. Indeed, T2-signal hyperintensity involving these regions either symmetrically or asymmetrically, occasionally extending into the adjacent medial temporal lobes, is the most commonly observed abnormality [54]. Mild-to-moderate cerebral atrophy is thought to be present in about half of cases [54]. Focal or multifocal mass lesions, which tend to show little if any enhancement, may also be seen and may mimic CNS neoplasms [56–58]. Less frequently, leptomeningeal enhancement, stroke-like lesions, or spinal cord involvement may be observed [45, 59]. Signal hyperintensity in the corticospinal tracts on T2-weighted imaging is not uncommon.

Investigations and Diagnosis

Most cases of Whipple's disease are diagnosed based on gut biopsy findings. As most patients with suspected CNS Whipple's disease will have concurrent systemic involvement, this approach to diagnosis generally proceeds in parallel with confirmation of CNS involvement and sampling other clinically involved sites. The cerebrospinal fluid is the medium of choice on which to confirm CNS Whipple's disease, though brain biopsy is occasionally required if systemic involvement is absent, clinical suspicion is high, and CSF studies are unrevealing. Given that CNS involvement is described in around 50% of cases, sometimes without clinical correlate, CSF sampling is recommended in all cases as this will influence treatment decisions [39, 40]. The general laboratory workup of patients with CNS Whipple's disease frequently reveals steatorrhea, impaired xylose absorption, anemia, and hypoalbuminemia, reflecting gut dysfunction (though this will be absent in isolated CNS disease). The hallmark of disease is the finding of *T. whipplei*-infected macrophages which stain positive with PAS and are diastase resistant. Immunohistochemical stains using specific antibodies against *T. whipplei* increase diagnostic sensitivity and may be positive in the absence of PAS-positive staining [60]. Though PCR amplification of *T. whipplei* DNA from stool and saliva is often positive in cases of Whipple's disease, given that asymptomatic gut carriage of *T. whipplei* can occur, a positive gut PCR alone is not diagnostic, and diagnosis always requires a second method of confirmation. The same is not true for sterile sites such as the CSF. Serum *T. whipplei* antibody titers are paradoxically low in patients with WD, rendering this a useless test in this setting.

Cerebrospinal fluid cell count and protein are, more often than not, normal. A moderate pleocytosis and CSF protein elevation may however be observed [43, 55]. PAS staining of the CSF has an equally low yield (positive in about a third of cases). *T. whipplei* PCR on the other hand is highly sensitive (>90%) [55]. Electron microscopy can be used to visualize *T. whipplei* in infected tissues, though it is only available in specialist laboratories and does not form part of routine clinical workup in this condition [39].

Treatment

Prior to its first successful treatment with antibiotics in 1952 [61], Whipple's disease was a universally fatal affliction. For decades thereafter, choices of antibiotic regimes remained poorly informed, and indeed it was only after sequencing of the organism's genome and successful culture of *T. whipplei* in the early 2000s (allowing in vitro testing of antibiotic sensitivity) that its antibiotic susceptibility was defined. Tetracycline was the treatment of choice for many years, until the recognition of alarmingly high relapse rates (especially CNS relapses) with this therapy alone [62]. For this reason, induction therapy with 2 weeks of parenteral high-dose penicillin, third-generation cephalosporins, or carbapenems (antibiotics which achieve high CNS concentrations) is often advocated [11]. Maintenance therapy should generally continue for at least 1 year. Trimethoprim-sulfamethoxazole was previously considered the optimal maintenance strategy following induction; however, evidence now suggests that this may not be the case. Indeed trimethoprim has no action against *T. whipplei*, as the bacterium lacks the gene coding for dihydrofolate reductase, the target of trimethoprim [63]. Recent in vitro studies have also suggested that up to a quarter of *T. whipplei* strains may be resistant to sulfonamides in vitro [64]. Moreover, acquired sulfamethoxazole resistance due to *folP* mutations (the gene encoding dihydropteroate synthase, the target of sulfonamides) has been described [65].

Recent evidence suggests that a combination of oral doxycycline and hydroxychloroquine for 12 months might be a more effective treatment option [23]. This combination is the only one proven to be bactericidal in vitro and has been successfully used in two patients with CNS relapses in whom co-trimoxazole was ineffective [65, 66]. After 12 months of dual therapy, long-term (possibly lifelong) oral doxycycline is advocated by some authors, in order to prevent late relapses or reinfection in susceptible patients [55, 67].

Whipple's disease, whether systemic or localized, should be regarded as a chronic disease prone to relapse. As such, patients should undergo lifelong follow-up in order to identify both relapses and complications of treatment early and institute appropriate management without delay [39, 68, 69]. Most cases of CNS relapse occur late (beyond 2 years), and it is important to recognize that relapses can occur at sites distant from the originally affected organ. After completion of treatment for CNS WD, performing *T. whipplei* PCR on CSF is currently the preferred method for confirming treatment efficacy and eradication of the bacterium from the central nervous system. The most common complication arising from treatment of Whipple's disease is the development of a nonspecific inflammatory syndrome termed IRIS (immune reconstitution inflammatory syndrome) [70]. This complication occurs almost exclusively in patients receiving immunosuppressive therapy (generally following misdiagnosis of their condition as a cryptogenic inflammatory arthritis) prior to starting antibiotics [70, 71]. IRIS may manifest as prolonged fever along with other signs and symptoms of systemic inflammation, e.g., arthritis, orbitopathy, and gut perforation, after initiation of treatment. It occurs in approximately 10% of patients but can have a rapid and fatal course. It generally responds promptly to the addition of oral corticosteroids, which may be life-saving [39].

See Table 28.1 for modified guidelines for diagnostic screening, biopsy, and treatment of CNS Whipple's disease.

Table 28.1 Modified guidelines for diagnostic screening, biopsy, and treatment of CNS Whipple's disease [43]

Definite CNS Whipple's disease

Must have any one of the following three criteria:
1. Oculomasticatory myorhythmia or oculofacial-skeletal myorhythmia and/or pendular vergence nystagmus
2. Positive brain tissue biopsy
3. Positive PCR analysis of cerebrospinal fluid
4. Autopsy-confirmed diagnosis

Probable CNS Whipple's disease
1. Suggestive neurological symptoms and signs (cognitive decline, personality change, supranuclear gaze palsy, etc.)

And

Positive PCR analysis of duodenal tissue

Or

PAS-positive macrophages in duodenal biopsy

+/− Supportive imaging

Possible CNS Whipple's disease

Must have any one of four systemic symptoms, not due to another known etiology:
1. Fever of unknown etiology
2. Gastrointestinal symptoms (steatorrhea, abdominal distension, or pain)
3. Chronic migratory arthralgias or polyarthralgias
4. Unexplained lymphadenopathy, night sweats, or malaise

And

Must have any one of four neurological signs, not due to another known etiology:
1. Supranuclear vertical gaze palsy
2. Rhythmic myoclonus
3. Dementia with psychiatric symptoms
4. Hypothalamic manifestations

Suggested diagnostic sequence

Clinical presentation suggestive (but not pathognomonic) of Whipple's disease (cognitive dysfunction, personality change, weight loss, diarrhea, arthralgia)

Proceed to:
1. Detailed neurological examination: including evaluation for rhythmic myoclonus, supranuclear gaze palsy, pendular vergence nystagmus, cerebellar ataxia
2. Laboratory investigations: hypoalbuminemia, steatorrhea, anemia
3. Neuroimaging: MRI brain with gadolinium including diffusion-weighted imaging

Suggestive clinical +/− biochemical and radiological features

->Proceed to confirm diagnosis:
1. Small bowel biopsy: PAS staining of small intestinal mucosal cells and PCR of gut biopsy sample
2. Cerebrospinal fluid examination including PCR for *T. whipplei*
3. If discreet lesion on imaging, proceed to stereotactic biopsy to outrule neoplasm, and confirm diagnosis (if CSF PCR is negative or if patient fails to respond to appropriate antibiotic therapy)
4. Sampling of any other clinically involved sites

Diagnosis confirmed

1st line
1. Hydroxychloroquine 200 mg TDS *and* doxycycline 200 mg/day for 12 months
   Followed by
2. Doxycycline 200 mg/day lifelong

2nd line
1. Intravenous meropenem 1g TDS for 14 days or ceftriaxone 2g OD for 14 days
   Followed by
2. Trimethoprim-sulfamethoxazole 960 mg twice daily by mouth for 12 months

Conclusion

Whipple's disease is a rare infectious disorder that may first be recognized by a neurologist or movement disorder clinician. As a treatable condition, like Wilson's disease, it is important to maintain a high index of suspicion.

Acknowledgments Dr. John Lynch died at a young age in 2019. He contributed hugely to the care of patients in the West of Ireland and to the education of a generation of medical and nursing students in Ireland. We all miss John's enthusiasm, expertise, and infectious laugh. It was always an absolute pleasure to work on this chapter with John over the years. As a colleague said, "we lost one of the good ones."

References

1. Whipple GH. A hitherto undescribed disease characterized anatomically by deposits of fat and fatty acids in the intestinal and mesenteric lymphatic tissues. Bull Johns Hopkins Hosp 1907.
2. Schöniger-Hekele M, Petermann D, Weber B, Müller C. Tropheryma whipplei in the environment: survey of sewage plant influxes and sewage plant workers. Appl Environ Microbiol. 2007;73(6):2033–5. https://doi.org/10.1128/AEM.02335-06.
3. Bentley SD, Maiwald M, Murphy LD, Pallen MJ, Yeats CA, Dover LG, et al. Sequencing and analysis of the genome of the Whipple's disease bacterium Tropheryma whipplei. Lancet. 2003;361(9358):637–44. https://doi.org/10.1016/S0140-6736(03)12597-4.
4. Raoult D, Ogata H, Audic S, Robert C, Suhre K, Drancourt M, et al. Tropheryma whipplei Twist: a human pathogenic actinobacteria with a reduced genome. Genome Res. 2003;13(8):1800–9. https://doi.org/10.1101/gr.1474603.
5. Relman DA, Schmidt TM, Macdermott RP, Falkow S. Identification of the uncultured Bacillus of Whipple's disease. N Engl J Med. 1992;327(5):293–301. https://doi.org/10.1056/NEJM199207303270501.
6. Wilson KH, Frothingham R, Wilson JAP, Blitchington R. Phylogeny of the Whipple's-disease-associated bacterium. Lancet. 1991;338(8765):474–5. https://doi.org/10.1016/0140-6736(91)90545-Z.
7. Lynch T, Odel J, Fredericks DN, Louis ED, Forman S, Rotterdam H, et al. Polymerase chain reaction-based detection of Tropheryma whippelii in central nervous system whipple's disease. Ann Neurol. 1997;42(1):120–4. https://doi.org/10.1002/ana.410420120.
8. Von Herbay A, Ditton HJ, Maiwald M. Diagnostic application of a polymerase chain reaction assay for the Whipple's disease bacterium to intestinal biopsies. Gastroenterology. 1996;110(6):1735–43. https://doi.org/10.1053/gast.1996.v110.pm8964398.
9. von Herbay A, Ditton H, Schuhmacher F, Maiwald M. Whipple's disease: staging and monitoring by cytology and polymerase chain reaction analysis of cerebrospinal fluid. Gastroenterology. 1997;113(2):434–41. https://doi.org/10.1053/gast.1997.v113.pm9247461.
10. Fredricks DN, Relman DA. Localization of Tropheryma whippelii rRNA in tissues from patients with Whipple's disease. J Infect Dis. 2001;183(8):1229–37. https://doi.org/10.1086/319684.
11. Schneider T, Moos V, Loddenkemper C, Marth T, Fenollar F, Raoult D. Whipple's disease: new aspects of pathogenesis and treatment. Lancet Infect Dis. 2008;8(3):179–90. https://doi.org/10.1016/S1473-3099(08)70042-2.
12. Dobbins W. Whipple's disease. Springfield: Charles C Thomas; 1987.
13. Fenollar F, Puéchal X, Raoult D. Whipple's disease. N Engl J Med. 2007;356(1):55–66. https://doi.org/10.1056/NEJMra062477.

14. Keita AK, Brouqui P, Badiaga S, Benkouiten S, Ratmanov P, Raoult D, et al. Tropheryma whipplei prevalence strongly suggests human transmission in homeless shelters. Int J Infect Dis. 2013;17(1):e67–8. https://doi.org/10.1016/j.ijid.2012.05.1033.
15. Fenollar F, Laouira S, Lepidi H, Rolain J, Raoult D. Value of Tropheryma whipplei quantitative polymerase chain reaction assay for the diagnosis of Whipple disease: usefulness of saliva and stool specimens for first-line screening. Clin Infect Dis. 2008;47(5):659–67. https://doi.org/10.1086/590559.
16. Fenollar F, Trani M, Davoust B, Salle B, Birg M, Rolain J, et al. Prevalence of asymptomatic Tropheryma whipplei carriage among humans and nonhuman primates. J Infect Dis. 2008;197(6):880–7. https://doi.org/10.1086/528693.
17. Lagier JC, Fenollar F, Lepidi H, Raoult D. Evidence of lifetime susceptibility to Tropheryma whipplei in patients with Whipple's disease. J Antimicrob Chemother. 2011;66(5):1188–9. https://doi.org/10.1093/jac/dkr032.
18. Bai JC, Sen L, Diez R, Niveloni S, Mauriño EC, Estevez ME, et al. Impaired monocyte function in patients successfully treated for Whipple's disease. Acta Gastroenterol Latinoam. 1996;26(2):85–9.
19. Desnues B, Ihrig M, Raoult D, Mege JL. Whipple's disease: a macrophage disease. Clin Vaccine Immunol. 2006;13(2):170–8. https://doi.org/10.1128/CVI.13.2.170-178.2006.
20. Marth T, Kleen N, Stallmach A, Ring S, Aziz S, Schmidt C, et al. Dysregulated peripheral and mucosal Th1/Th2 response in Whipple's disease. Gastroenterology. 2002;123(5):1468–77. https://doi.org/10.1053/gast.2002.36583.
21. Biagi F, Badulli C, Feurle GE, Müller C, Moos V, Schneider T, et al. Cytokine genetic profile in Whipple's disease. Eur J Clini Microbiol Infect Dis. 2012;31(11):3145–50. https://doi.org/10.1007/s10096-012-1677-8.
22. Martinetti M, Biagi F, Badulli C, Feurle GE, Müller C, Moos V, et al. The HLA Alleles DRB1*13 and DQB1*06 are associated to Whipple's disease. Gastroenterology. 2009;136(7):2289–94. https://doi.org/10.1053/j.gastro.2009.01.051.
23. Lagier J-C, Fenollar F, Lepidi H, Giorgi R, Million M, Raoult D. Treatment of classic Whipple's disease: from in vitro results to clinical outcome. J Antimicrob Chemother. 2014;69(1):219–27. https://doi.org/10.1093/jac/dkt310.
24. Lozupone C, Cota-Gomez A, Palmer BE, Linderman DJ, Charlson ES, Sodergren E, et al. Widespread colonization of the lung by Tropheryma whipplei in HIV infection. Am J Respir Crit Care Med. 2013;187(10):1110–7. https://doi.org/10.1164/rccm.201211-2145OC.
25. Stein A, Doutchi M, Fenollar F, Raoult D. Tropheryma whipplei pneumonia in a patient with HIV-2 infection. Am J Respir Crit Care Med. 2013;188(8):1036–7. https://doi.org/10.1164/rccm.201304-0692LE.
26. Gaddy JR, Khan ZZ, Chaser B, Scofield RH. Whipple's disease diagnosis following the use of TNF-α blockade. Rheumatology (Oxford). 2012;51(5):946. https://doi.org/10.1093/rheumatology/ker387.
27. Mahnel R, Kalt A, Ring S, Stallmach A, Strober W, Marth T. Immunosuppressive therapy in Whipple's disease patients is associated with the appearance of gastrointestinal manifestations. Am J Gastroenterol. 2005;100(5):1167–73. https://doi.org/10.1111/j.1572-0241.2005.40128.x.
28. Moos V, Schmidt C, Geelhaar A, Kunkel D, Allers K, Schinnerling K, et al. Impaired immune functions of monocytes and macrophages in Whipple's disease. Gastroenterology. 2010;138(1):210–20. https://doi.org/10.1053/j.gastro.2009.07.066.
29. Raoult D, Lepidi H, Harle JR. Tropheryma whipplei circulating in blood monocytes. N Engl J Med. 2001;345(7):548. https://doi.org/10.1056/NEJM200108163450716.
30. Ghigo E, Capo C, Aurouze M, Tung CH, Gorvel JP, Raoult D, et al. Survival of Tropheryma whipplei, the agent of whipple's disease, requires phagosome acidification. Infect Immun. 2002;70(3):1501–6. https://doi.org/10.1128/IAI.70.3.1501-1506.2002.

31. Desnues B, Lepidi H, Raoult D, Mege J. Whipple disease: intestinal infiltrating cells exhibit a transcriptional pattern of M2/alternatively activated macrophages. J Infect Dis. 2005;192(9):1642–6. https://doi.org/10.1086/491745.

32. Kalt A, Schneider T, Ring S, Hoffmann J, Zeitz M, Stallmach A, et al. Decreased levels of interleukin-12p40 in the serum of patients with Whipple's disease. Int J Color Dis. 2006;21(2):114–20. https://doi.org/10.1007/s00384-005-0778-6.

33. Marth T, Neurath M, Cuccherini BA, Strober W. Defects of monocyte interleukin 12 production and humoral immunity in Whipple's disease. Gastroenterology. 1997;113(2):442–8. https://doi.org/10.1053/gast.1997.v113.pm9247462.

34. Desnues B, Raoult D, Mege J-L. IL-16 is critical for Tropheryma whipplei replication in Whipple's disease. J Immunol. 2005;175(7):4575–82. https://doi.org/10.4049/jimmunol.175.7.4575.

35. Ghigo E, Barry AO, Pretat L, Al Moussawi K, Desnues B, Capo C, et al. IL-16 promotes T whipplei replication by inhibiting phagosome conversion and modulating macrophage activation. PLoS One. 2010;5(10):e13561. https://doi.org/10.1371/journal.pone.0013561.

36. Benoit M, Fenollar F, Raoult D, Mege JL. Increased levels of circulating IL-16 and apoptosis markers are related to the activity of Whipple's disease. PLoS One. 2007;2(6):e494. https://doi.org/10.1371/journal.pone.0000494.

37. Puéchal X. Whipple's arthritis. Joint Bone Spine. 2016;83(6):631–5. https://doi.org/10.1016/j.jbspin.2016.07.001.

38. James TN. On the wide spectrum of abnormalities in the coronary arteries of Whipple's disease. Coron Artery Dis. 2001;12(2):115–25. https://doi.org/10.1097/00019501-200103000-00005.

39. Marth T, Moos V, Müller C, Biagi F, Schneider T. Tropheryma whipplei infection and Whipple's disease. Lancet Infect Dis. 2016;16(3):e13–22. https://doi.org/10.1016/S1473-3099(15)00537-X.

40. Marth T, Raoult D. Whipple's disease. Lancet. 2003;361(9353):239–46. https://doi.org/10.1016/S0140-6736(03)12274-X.

41. Tarroch X, Vives P, Salas A, Moré J. Subcutaneous nodules in whipple's disease. J Cutan Pathol. 2001;28(7):368–70. https://doi.org/10.1034/j.1600-0560.2001.280706.x.

42. Walter R, Bachmann SP, Schaffner A, Rüegg R, Schoedon G. Bone marrow involvement in Whipple's disease: rarely reported, but really rare? Br J Haematol. 2001;112(3):677–9. https://doi.org/10.1046/j.1365-2141.2001.02648.x.

43. Louis ED, Lynch T, Kaufmann P, Fahn S, Odel J. Diagnostic guidelines in central nervous system Whipple's disease. Ann Neurol. 1996;40(4):561–8. https://doi.org/10.1002/ana.410400404.

44. Gerard A, Sarrot-Reynauld F, Liozon E, Cathebras P, Besson G, Robin C, et al. Neurologic presentation of Whipple disease: report of 12 cases and review of the literature. Medicine (Baltimore). 2002;81(6):443–57. https://doi.org/10.1097/00005792-200211000-00005.

45. Messori A, Di Bella P, Polonara G, Logullo F, Pauri P, Haghighipour R, et al. An unusual spinal presentation of Whipple disease. AJNR Am J Neuroradiol. 2001;22(5):1004–8.

46. Rusina R, Keller O, Síma R, Zámečník J. Peripheral neuropathy in Whipples disease: a case report. Cesk Patol. 2012;48(2):97–9.

47. von Herbay A, Otto HF, Stolte M, Borchard F, Kirchner T, Ditton H-J, et al. Epidemiology of Whipple's disease in Germany: analysis of 110 patients diagnosed in 1965–95. Scand J Gastroenterol. 1997;32(1):52–7. https://doi.org/10.3109/00365529709025063.

48. Matthews BR, Jones LK, Saad DA, Aksamit AJ, Josephs KA. Cerebellar ataxia and central nervous system whipple disease. Arch Neurol. 2005;62(4):618–20. https://doi.org/10.1001/archneur.62.4.618.

49. Mulroy E, Lynch T. Whipple's disease. In: Encyclopedia of the neurological sciences. Philadelphia: Elsevier; 2014. https://doi.org/10.1016/B978-0-12-385157-4.00367-5.

50. Schwartz MA, Selhorst JB, Ochs AL, Beck RW, Campbell WW, Harris JK, et al. Oculomasticatory myorhythmia: a unique movement disorder occurring in Whipple's disease. Ann Neurol. 1986;20(6):677–83. https://doi.org/10.1002/ana.410200605.

51. Simpson DA, Wishnow R, Gargulinski RB, Pawlak AM. Oculofacial-skeletal myorhythmia in central nervous system Whipple's disease: additional case and review of the literature. Mov Disord. 1995;10(2):195–200. https://doi.org/10.1002/mds.870100210.

52. Lynch T, Fahn S, Louis ED, Odel JG. Oculofacial-skeletal myorhythmia in Whipple's disease. Mov Disord. 1997;12(4):625–6.

53. Baizabal-Carvallo JF, Cardoso F, Jankovic J. Myorhythmia: phenomenology, etiology, and treatment. Mov Disord. 2015;30(2):171–9. https://doi.org/10.1002/mds.26093.

54. Black DF, Aksamit AJ, Morris JM. MR imaging of central nervous system Whipple disease: a 15-year review. Am J Neuroradiol. 2010;31(8):1493–7. https://doi.org/10.3174/ajnr.A2089.

55. Compain C, Sacre K, Puéchal X, Klein I, Vital-Durand D, Houeto J-L, et al. Central nervous system involvement in Whipple disease: clinical study of 18 patients and long-term follow-up. Medicine (Baltimore). 2013;92(6):324–30. https://doi.org/10.1097/MD.0000000000000010.

56. Frazier JL, Quinones-Hinojosa A. Isolated Whipple disease of the brain resembling a tumour. Acta Neurochir. 2009;151(2):173–5. https://doi.org/10.1007/s00701-008-0180-6.

57. Löhr M, Stenzel W, Plum G, Gross WP, Deckert M, Klug N. Whipple disease confined to the central nervous system presenting as a solitary frontal tumor: case report. J Neurosurg. 2004;101(2):336–9. https://doi.org/10.3171/jns.2004.101.2.0336.

58. Wroe SJ, Pires M, Harding B, Youl BD, Shorvon S. Whipple's disease confined to the CNS presenting with multiple intracerebral mass lesions. J Neurol Neurosurg Psychiatry. 1991;54(11):989–92. https://doi.org/10.1136/jnnp.54.11.989.

59. Schröter A, Brinkhoff J, Günthner-Lengsfeld T, Suerbaum S, Reiners K, Messmann H, et al. Whipple's disease presenting as an isolated lesion of the cervical spinal cord. Eur J Neurol. 2005;12(4):276–9. https://doi.org/10.1111/j.1468-1331.2004.01035.x.

60. Baisden BL, Lepidi H, Raoult D, Argani P, Yardley JH, Dumler JS. Diagnosis of Whipple disease by immunohistochemical analysis: a sensitive and specific method for the detection of Tropheryma whipplei (the Whipple bacillus) in paraffin-embedded tissue. Am J Clin Pathol. 2002;118(5):742–8. https://doi.org/10.1309/8YGR-FE7L-39LL-L37C.

61. Paulley JW. A case of Whipple's disease (intestinal lipodystrophy). Gastroenterology. 1952;22(1):128–33. https://doi.org/10.1016/S0016-5085(19)36367-X.

62. Keinath RD, Merrell DE, Vlietstra R, Dobbins WO. Antibiotic treatment and relapse in Whipple's disease. Gastroenterology. 1985;88(6):1867–73. https://doi.org/10.1016/0016-5085(85)90012-5.

63. Boulos A, Rolain JM, Mallet MN, Raoult D. Molecular evaluation of antibiotic susceptibility of Tropheryma whipplei in axenic medium. J Antimicrob Chemother. 2005;55(2):178–81. https://doi.org/10.1093/jac/dkh524.

64. Fenollar F, Perreal C, Raoult D. Tropheryma whipplei natural resistance to trimethoprim and sulphonamides in vitro. Int J Antimicrob Agents. 2014;43(4):388–90. https://doi.org/10.1016/j.ijantimicag.2014.01.015.

65. Fenollar F, Rolain J-M, Alric L, Papo T, Chauveheid M-P, van de Beek D, et al. Resistance to trimethoprim/sulfamethoxazole and Tropheryma whipplei. Int J Antimicrob Agents. 2009;34(3):255–9. https://doi.org/10.1016/j.ijantimicag.2009.02.014.

66. Feurle GE, Moos V, Schneider T, Fenollar F, Raoult D. The combination of chloroquine and minocycline, a therapeutic option in cerebrospinal infection of Whipple's disease refractory to treatment with ceftriaxone, meropenem and co-trimoxazole. J Antimicrob Chemother. 2012;67(5):1295–6. https://doi.org/10.1093/jac/dks008.

67. Fenollar F, Lagier J-C, Raoult D. Tropheryma whipplei and Whipple's disease. J Infect. 2014;69(2):103–12. https://doi.org/10.1016/j.jinf.2014.05.008.

68. Lagier J-C, Fenollar F, Lepidi H, Raoult D. Failure and relapse after treatment with trimethoprim/sulfamethoxazole in classic Whipple's disease. J Antimicrob Chemother. 2010;65(9):2005–12. https://doi.org/10.1093/jac/dkq263.

69. Ramzan NN, Loftus E, Burgart LJ, Rooney M, Batts KP, Wiesner RH, et al. Diagnosis and monitoring of Whipple disease by polymerase chain reaction. Ann Intern Med. 1997;126(7):520–7. https://doi.org/10.7326/0003-4819-126-7-199704010-00004.
70. Feurle GE, Moos V, Schinnerling K, Geelhaar A, Allers K, Biagi F, et al. The immune reconstitution inflammatory syndrome in Whipple disease. Ann Intern Med. 2010;153(11):710. https://doi.org/10.7326/0003-4819-153-11-201012070-00004.
71. Biagi F, Trotta L, Di Stefano M, Balduzzi D, Marchese A, Vattiato C, et al. Previous immunosuppressive therapy is a risk factor for immune reconstitution inflammatory syndrome in Whipple's disease. Digest Liver Dis. 2012;44(10):880–2. https://doi.org/10.1016/j.dld.2012.05.008.

Part V

Practical Risks in the Clinic:
Pitfalls in Management

Emergencies in Huntington's Disease

29

Laura Buyan Dent and Kathleen M. Shannon

Patient Vignettes

Patient 1

A 53-year-old man with a 4-year history of symptomatic Huntington's disease lived alone and was independent in activities of daily living, including balancing his checkbook, shopping, cooking, and cleaning. He followed up regularly with his neurologist and was not currently taking medications. His daughter contacted the neurologist alarmed by a significant change in behavior. She had visited her father at his apartment the prior evening, and he was argumentative and violent without provocation. He turned over chairs and the kitchen table, made threatening remarks to her, and even gesticulated as if he were going to hit her. She became fearful for her safety and called the police. While waiting for them to arrive, her father proceeded to straighten up his apartment, so that no evidence of a disturbance was present when the police arrived. When interviewed by the police, he appeared calm and cooperative, and his daughter decided not to press charges. He agreed to further evaluation by neurology and psychiatry in the emergency room. When directly questioned, he admitted to episodes of impulsive anger, and to feelings that his family was trying to harm him, or to "take his money and put him away." Upon admission to the hospital, olanzapine was initiated and marked improvement in these feelings occurred. Follow-up care with visiting nurse services and support for his daughter allowed him to return home to independent living.

L. Buyan Dent (✉) · K. M. Shannon
Department of Neurology, University of Wisconsin School of Medicine and Public Health, Madison, WI, USA
e-mail: dent@neurology.wisc.edu

© Springer Nature Switzerland AG 2022
S. J. Frucht (ed.), *Movement Disorder Emergencies*, Current Clinical Neurology,
https://doi.org/10.1007/978-3-030-75898-1_29

Patient 2

A 55-year-old right-handed man was diagnosed with HD with DNA testing showing 45 CAG repeats. He developed mild to moderate choreiform movements that were attenuated by risperidone. He was mildly depressed but not agitated. He had cognitive impairment, was very impulsive, and lacked awareness of his physical deficits. Subsequently, he had frequent falls. Approximately 5 years after diagnosis, he fell and sustained a right humeral fracture. Due to the HD-related cognitive difficulties, he was unable to follow the treatment recommendations and developed brachial plexus and radial nerve injury resulting in a flail right limb. He continued to fall on a regular basis. Three years later, he was found down at his skilled nursing facility. Emergency room evaluation revealed a large subdural hematoma with signs of impending herniation. The family opted for nonsurgical treatment and he passed away 3 days later.

Patient 3

A 51-year-old woman with a 10-year history of HD, with choreiform movements controlled by aripiprazole, moderately impaired cognition, and depression, lived with her husband who provided assistance with all activities of daily living. At her last clinic visit, her husband reported some mild worsening of chorea and memory impairment as expected, as well as issues indicating he was likely experiencing caregiver burnout. He contacted the clinic a month later and reported significantly worsening chorea, new episodes of confusion, and lethargy. He denied any signs of infection and was convinced she was now at a terminal stage of HD. She was requesting to use the bathroom frequently and focused on urinary and bowel issues. He was advised to take her to the emergency room, where she was found to be febrile and aspiration pneumonia was suspected. Further evaluation of abnormal liver function tests revealed that she had cholecystitis with perforation and abscess formation. She was treated medically and surgically. When seen in follow-up 6 months later, she was back to her baseline.

Introduction

Huntington's disease (HD) is a neurodegenerative disease caused by an autosomal dominant inherited abnormal expansion in the huntingtin gene on chromosome 4. Although observed for centuries, George Huntington's seminal description in 1872 led to better recognition of this disease. After a worldwide collaboration of scientists and physicians, in 1993 the gene defect causing HD was identified. This dominantly inherited CAG trinucleotide repeat expansion results in the production of abnormal huntingtin protein. The mutant huntingtin protein causes neuronal dysfunction and death via a cascade of various cellular mechanisms. These include toxicity of mutant protein, transcriptional dysregulation, abnormal neuronal aggregation, changes in axonal transport, synaptic dysfunction, excitotoxicity, and mitochondrial dysfunction [1]. At a macroscopic level, pathological changes are seen in both cortical and subcortical striatal regions at early phases of the disease. As the disease progresses, obvious changes are noted including global cerebral atrophy and preferential atrophy of the caudate nucleus and other basal ganglia structures [2].

Clinically HD is characterized by cognitive, psychiatric, and movement abnormalities. Worldwide prevalence varies greatly. The disease prevalence is 10.6–13.7 individuals per 100,000 in Western populations, 1–7 per million prevalence in Asian populations, and lower rates in African populations. This likely occurs due to differences in CAG repeat length in the mutant huntingtin gene, with longer repeat lengths found in populations with higher prevalence [2–4]. Symptom onset is often in the fourth to fifth decades, but onset across the lifespan even in infancy or old age has been observed [5–7]. As knowledge regarding HD evolves and as advances in genetic testing occur, nomenclature regarding the phases of the disease has changed. Following a period of clinical normalcy, patients progress through a 10- to 20-year period of gradual decline that is not clinically perceptible but can be demonstrated using sensitive experimental measures of brain volume, motor function, cognition, and psychiatric function. Subtle but definite motor, behavioral, and cognitive signs emerge from this transitional or pre-manifest period and include clumsiness, mild chorea, difficulty with complex cognitive tasks, and affective or personality changes. Although predominantly behavioral or cognitive presentations of HD are well recognized leading to calls to broaden the definition of manifest illness, current criteria for clinically manifest disease are anchored in the presence of a clinically typical motor syndrome [8–11].

The motor signs and symptoms change in appearance across the spectrum of disease progression. Chorea may be very subtle at first, increases over the course of the illness, and often plateaus in mid-stage disease. Chorea severity may actually decline in later-stage disease. However, with disease progression, rigidity, bradykinesia, and dystonia assume increasing importance, and in many patients these movement disorders come to predominate [12]. The motor picture in end-stage disease includes severe dysarthria and dysphagia, very slow and poorly coordinated movement, severe postural abnormality even when seated, and inability to stand or walk [12].

The cognitive disorder reflects subcortical pathology, with deficits in attention and concentration, processing speed, multitasking, planning and organization, problem-solving, and visuoperceptual abnormalities [13, 14]. Cognitive changes lead to loss of work and driving and contribute to loss of function and poor quality of life in HD. The cognitive disorder progresses to a global dementia in late-stage disease [15]. It is well recognized that HD patients have decreased awareness of many aspects of their clinical state.

⌘━━━ Patients with early HD are often unaware of their chorea, and may not be aware that anything is wrong.

Behavioral and psychiatric changes include abnormal affect (especially depression), personality change, irritability or aggression, anxiety, apathy, and rarely psychosis [16]. Behavioral changes may begin very early in the illness, often before clinically manifest motor changes. Unlike the motor and cognitive changes in HD, behavioral changes do not progress in a linear fashion. Thus, aberrant behaviors can arise suddenly and unexpectedly and may respond to drugs or other therapies [17, 18]. When HD begins before the age of 21 (juvenile HD which is relatively rare), the motor phenotype is characterized by bradykinesia, rigidity, dystonia, myoclonus, and often seizures [7]. Eventually every patient with HD requires 24-hour supervision and assistance with all daily tasks. For many, this level of care is possible only in an institutional setting. Disease duration at death averages about 17 years [2, 19–21].

🔑 HD is unique in movement disorders: a disorder that is 100% penetrant, with disinhibition and cognitive impairment, and certain incapacity.

Emergencies in HD

Given its chronic progressive nature, there is little published literature into the types of emergencies encountered in HD care. In one study of 3612 hospitalizations in HD patients, 22% were related to respiratory illness, 10% to urinary tract infection or sepsis, and 6% to trauma. Twenty-one percent were related to psychiatric diagnoses [22]. Death certificate studies in HD reveal that important causes of death are pneumonia and choking, nutritional deficiency, chronic skin ulcers and debility, and mental disorders including suicide [23–25]. These studies suggest that emergencies in HD generally result from (1) complications of the movement disorder, or (2) psychiatric and behavioral changes or sequelae of their management.

Psychiatric Emergencies in HD

Psychiatric symptoms are nearly universal in HD and span the spectrum from personality changes through affective disorders and psychosis [17, 26, 27]. Psychiatric syndromes precipitate about 20% of acute HD hospitalizations. Dementia and affective disturbances are the most frequent psychiatric causes of hospitalization but are rarely associated with in-hospital mortality [22]. Depression occurs commonly in HD. First-degree relatives of HD patients report that sadness and depression are among the earliest symptoms of the disorder [28]. A study in HD subjects in the Huntington Study Group database showed nearly half of all subject endorsed anxiety or depression and 25% had low self-esteem. Patients in early stages were more likely to endorse symptoms of sadness and depression than were patients in later stages of the illness [29].

George Huntington himself observed a connection between HD and suicide, writing "(t)he tendency to insanity, and sometimes that form of insanity which leads to suicide, is marked" [30]. An increase in suicidality in HD patients compared to the general population is widely accepted, though estimates of the magnitude of this increase vary [26, 31–36]. Suicidal ideation and suicide have been reported in clinically manifest disease, pre-manifest gene carriers, and even family members not known to carry the mutation [31]. In a large study of the Huntington Study Group dataset, including 4171 subjects (1483 "at risk" and 2688 with clinically manifest HD), suicidal ideation was endorsed by 17.5% of these subjects and was "moderate" or "severe with intent and plan" in about 10% of subjects. This study identified two critical periods of increased risk: at the time of development of soft neurological signs early in the "zone of onset" of clinical signs and later when clinical signs begin to impair occupational or financial functions. A cross-sectional study of 2835 HD subjects in the Huntington Study Group database found 10% had a prior suicide attempt [29]. Large studies suggest suicide is the cause of death in 0.1–14% of HD cases [31, 37, 38]. Continued surveillance for depressed mood and suicidal ideation is critical if suicide is to be prevented. HD families should be counseled to recognize suicidality, to remove potential means of suicide from the home, and when and how to handle acute suicidality [26, 34–36].

Other psychiatric syndromes that result in a significant number of HD hospitalizations include dementia-related symptoms (7% of admissions) and psychotic symptoms (4% of admissions). Admissions also occur for ethanol and substance abuse, anxiety and personality disorders, medication toxicity, and others [22]. There are no published high-quality controlled clinical trials of any therapy for psychiatric disorders in HD. An evidence-based review suggested that amitriptyline and mirtazapine were possibly useful for the treatment of depression, that risperidone was possibly useful for psychosis, and that haloperidol, olanzapine, propranolol, and buspirone were possibly useful for behavioral disorders [39]. Currently, HD-related psychiatric symptoms are treated by usual psychiatric standard of care clinical principles [26, 36].

Since dopamine-blocking agents are used to help reduce chorea, neuroleptic malignant syndrome may occur. Neuroleptic malignant syndrome (NMS) was first described in 1960. It is a dramatic iatrogenic disorder resulting from the use of drugs with dopamine receptor-blocking activity. Diagnostic criteria for NMS include hyperthermia, autonomic instability, rigidity, altered consciousness, elevated creatine kinase, and leukocytosis [40]. Onset of symptoms is often within 1 week of initiation or escalation of dose of the causative agent. Once the offending agent has been discontinued, recovery can be slow and complications are common. These include aspiration, rhabdomyolysis, or renal failure. Most often reported with first-generation antipsychotics, NMS has been reported with second-generation antipsychotics and with other agents that block dopamine receptors, including antiemetics. Young and middle-aged men seem to have a higher risk of NMS. Among patients treated with these agents, the incidence of NMS is low (about 0.2%) [41]. Isolated cases of NMS in HD have been reported. Implicated drugs included tetrabenazine [42, 43] and aripiprazole [44]. There is no reliable evidence base for treatment of NMS in HD. Prudence dictates discontinuation of the offending dopamine receptor-blocking agent, or dose reduction as appropriate. Further management should be guided by the usual principles of NMS care in a psychiatric population.

Trauma

Trauma accounts for about 5% of HD hospital admissions and is associated with 2% in-hospital mortality and high likelihood of discharge to a long-term care facility [22]. Falls are a significant cause of injuries in HD. Studies reveal high rates of falls with greater than 75% of people reporting falling on a regular basis during the course of the disease. As the disease progresses, the frequency of falling increases, often with numerous falls per day [45, 46]. HD causes a complex gait disorder that includes progressive slowing, shortening of stride length, and reduced cadence with increased double-support time and base of support. There is significant and progressively increasing variability in all these measures as well [46, 47]. Impulsivity and poor judgment contribute to fall risk, and HD falls are associated with poorer motor function, more aggression, and worse cognition [45, 46]. The most important sequelae of trauma in HD are intracranial injuries and fractures, but open wounds, dislocations, and crushing wounds also occur.

Intracranial injuries prompt nearly half of acute hospitalizations for HD [22]. Many of these admissions were likely for subdural hematoma (SDH). SDH forms when blood accumulates in the potential space between the arachnoid membranes and dura mater due to tearing of the veins that carry blood from the cortical surface to the dural sinuses or by rupture of small cortical arteries [48, 49]. Acute SDH usually presents within a few days of a significant head injury, while chronic SDH generally presents more than 3 weeks from the ictus and tends to be associated with more minor head injury. Age, male gender, alcoholism, cerebral atrophy, and use of anticoagulants are risk factors for SDH.

Cerebral atrophy coupled with a tendency to fall in HD predisposes these patients to the development of SDH (Fig. 29.1). In one center, nearly 7% of 58 cases of subdural hematoma surgeries occurred in patients with HD. About 2.5% of their chronic

Fig. 29.1 CT brain scan in a patient with late-stage HD and multiple falls. There is a chronic subdural hematoma over the right side of the brain with mass effect and midline shift. This hematoma required multiple surgeries and was ultimately fatal

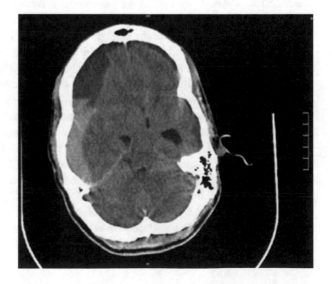

HD population developed SDH [24, 50]. SDH may leave a patient with substantial disability or may be fatal. It typically occurs in a moderately affected HD patient who is still walking without assistance but with significant postural instability and typically presents in a chronic state. Of the four HD subjects with SDH in the afore-mentioned study, age ranged from 44 to 62 years, and disease duration ranged from 3 to 11 years. None had major head trauma, though three had one or more minor head traumas 2–3 months prior to SDH. In one case the diagnosis was incidental. Symptoms in the other three cases included headaches, gait disturbance, hemipare-sis, anisocoria, and coma. One patient had bilateral hematomas. In all, there was evidence of mass effect with shift. All patients were managed with surgical evacua-tion, although reoperation was required in two of four [50].

The most common acute traumatic injuries in a large hospitalization cohort were hip fracture (25%) and limb or other fractures (25%). Soft tissue trauma, crushing injuries, and open wounds were also reported [22]. It is important to note that HD patients often are poorly aware of their physical deficits [2, 51] including pain, so families and physicians must be alert to changes that might reflect the patient having sustained a traumatic injury. Falls in HD can be predicted by performance on mea-sures of gait and balance, such as the Berg Balance Scale, Timed Up and Go test, and the Tinetti Mobility Test [46, 52–54]. Fall prevention is critical in HD and requires judicious use of physical therapy. Walkers and other aids often prove dif-ficult to use by HD patients. A gait belt may be useful to the caregiver. A patient with repeated falls should be encouraged to wear a safety helmet. Passive restraints are often the easy solution to the falling patient, but this approach exposes the patient to the risk of injury or death. Restraint-related deaths in the general popula-tion tends to occur in nursing homes and are associated with cognitive impairment, impulsivity, and involuntary movements, suggesting HD patients may be at particu-lar risk [55]. While restraint-related injury and even death are reported in the HD literature [20], the frequency of these events is unknown. Given these factors, restraints should be avoided in HD patients in favor of other measures to reduce falls.

Pneumonia and Aspiration Pneumonitis

Pneumonia and aspiration pneumonitis are complications of HD, together account-ing for almost 20% of hospitalizations and 42% of deaths in HD [22, 24, 25]. The in-hospital mortality of respiratory disease in HD is about 7%, and more than half of the survivors who had previously lived at home enter institutional care after dis-charge [22]. The importance of respiratory disease in HD relates to the prominence of dysphagia in the illness. While there are no published data on the prevalence of dysphagia by illness stage or on progression of dysphagia, the literature is clear that dysphagia is universal in middle- to late-stage HD. Descriptive series suggest dys-phagia in HD reflects both hyperkinetic (chorea, repetitive swallow, inability to stop respirations) and hypokinetic (mandibular rigidity, slow lingual movements, cough-ing, and choking) features. The combination of hyperkinetic and hypokinetic motor abnormalities, cognitive decline, and behavioral changes causes complex disorders of eating and feeding with abnormalities occurring in almost every aspect of eating and swallowing [56, 57].

Pneumonia and pneumonitis may require intravenous antibiotics and respiratory therapy. The development of this illness should also prompt a speech therapy assessment for swallowing and often requires a formal swallowing study. It is thought that aspiration risk can be reduced by supervised or assisted feeding and by swallowing therapy, but there is a scant evidence base to support these contentions [56]. Pneumonia risk coupled with malnutrition in late-stage disease prompts the consideration of percutaneous feeding tube insertion for most patients in later-stage HD. Published indications for a feeding tube include weight loss greater than 10% over 1 month, dehydration, repeated aspiration, and severe dysphagia [58]. The frequency of feeding tube uptake in the HD community is unknown, but it is far from universal, and there are many factors to consider before making a decision including the patient's expressed wishes regarding artificial feeding.

In addition to the risk of aspiration pneumonitis, there is a risk of asphyxiation from acute choking. The combination of a healthy appetite, impulsivity, cognitive impairment, and deranged swallowing can precipitate an acute choking emergency. Attention to the size and consistency of food and supervised or assisted feeding reduce the risk of this calamity. Caregivers are advised to seek training in acute first aid including an approach to choking.

HD patients are at risk for aspiration, particularly with certain foods (e.g., hot dogs).

HD does not preclude an individual from developing "usual" or "common" medical and surgical conditions. The cognitive and psychiatric manifestations of HD can make the detection of common medical problems difficult. People with HD may not exhibit or be able to report symptoms in a manner that healthcare workers are accustomed. Often when people with HD become ill with common illnesses, their baseline HD symptoms become exacerbated or unmasked. The usual course of disease progression is gradual over years with some acceleration in the pace at more advanced "terminal" stages. If a patient presents with sudden (days to weeks) worsening of baseline symptoms, one has to be alert for other underlying medical conditions or illnesses. Of additional importance is inclusion of healthcare providers that are familiar with the individual. Of course, as HD symptoms progress, quality of life worsens, and people with advanced HD need the benefits of palliative care interventions; however to do so prematurely has obvious ethical implications.

Conclusion

The triad of cognitive decline, psychiatric issues, and choreiform movements alerts one to possible HD. Although great strides have occurred in understanding this disease, especially at a molecular level, it remains an incurable disease, but not without hope. New molecular biological techniques and therapies are undergoing clinical trials in humans at the time of this publication [59, 60]. Although these treatments hopefully will alter the course of this disease by slowing progression or halting progression, individuals with HD will remain at risk of neurologic and medical emergencies. Healthcare workers need to remain alert to identifying signs of acute psychiatric decline, trauma-induced injuries, and acute medical and/or surgical issues that may be difficult to uncover in someone with HD.

References

1. Saudou F. The biology of Huntington. Neuron. 2016;89:910–26.
2. McColgan P, Tabrizi SJ. Huntington's disease: a clinical review. Eur J Neurol. 2018;25:24–34.
3. Rawlins MD, Wexler NS, Wexler AR, Tabrizi SJ, Douglas I, Evans SJ, et al. The prevalence of Huntington's disease. Neuroepidemiology. 2016;46(2):144–53.
4. Harper PS. The epidemiology of Huntington's disease. Hum Genet. 1992;89:365–76.
5. James CM, Houlihan GD, Snell RG, Cheadle JP, Harper PS. Late-onset Huntington's disease: a clinical and molecular study. Age Ageing. 1994;23:445–8.
6. Nance MA, Mathias-Hagen V, Breningstall G, Wick MJ, McGlennen RC. Analysis of a very large trinucleotide repeat in a patient with juvenile Huntington's disease. Neurology. 1999;52:392–4.
7. Nance MA, Myers RH. Juvenile onset Huntington's disease–clinical and research perspectives. Ment Retard Dev Disabil Res Rev. 2001;7:153–7.
8. Ross CA, Reilmann R, Cardoso F, McCusker EA, Testa CM, Stout JC, et al. Movement Disorder Society Task Force viewpoint: Huntington's disease diagnostic categories. Mov Disord Clin Pract. 2019;6(7):541–6.
9. Paulsen JS, Langbehn DR, Stout JC, Aylward E, Ross CA, Nance M, Predict-HD Investigators and Coordinators of the Huntington Study Group, et al. Detection of Huntington's disease decades before diagnosis: the Predict-HD study. J Neurol Neurosurg Psychiatry. 2008;79(8):874–80.
10. Duff K, Paulsen JS, Beglinger LJ, Langbehn DR, Stout JC. Psychiatric symptoms in Huntington's disease before diagnosis: the Predict-HD study. Biol Psychiatry. 2007;62:1341–6.
11. Biglan KM, Ross CA, Langbehn DR, Aylward EH, Stout JC, Queller S, PREDICT-HD Investigators of the Huntington Study Group, et al. Motor abnormalities in premanifest persons with Huntington's disease: the PREDICT-HD study. Mov Disord. 2009;24(12):1763–72.
12. Penney JB Jr, Young AB, Shoulson I, Starosta-Rubenstein S, Snodgrass SR, Sanchez-Ramos J, et al. Huntington's disease in Venezuela: 7 years of follow-up on symptomatic and asymptomatic individuals. Mov Disord. 1990;5(2):93–9.
13. Peavy GM, Jacobson MW, Goldstein JL, Hamilton JM, Kane A, Gamst AC, et al. Cognitive and functional decline in Huntington's disease: dementia criteria revisited. Mov Disord. 2010;25(9):1163–9.
14. Ho AK, Sahakian BJ, Brown RG, Barker RA, Hodges JR, Ané MN, NEST-HD Consortium, et al. Profile of cognitive progression in early Huntington's disease. Neurology. 2003;61(12):1702–6.
15. Paulsen JS, Conybeare RA. Cognitive changes in Huntington's disease. Adv Neurol. 2005;96:209–25.
16. Anderson KE, Marshall FJ. Behavioral symptoms associated with Huntington's disease. Adv Neurol. 2005;96:197–208.
17. Paulsen JS, Ready RE, Hamilton JM, Mega MS, Cummings JL. Neuropsychiatric aspects of Huntington's disease. J Neurol Neurosurg Psychiatry. 2001;71:310–4.
18. Zappacosta B, Monza D, Meoni C, Austoni L, Soliveri P, Gellera C, et al. Psychiatric symptoms do not correlate with cognitive decline, motor symptoms, or CAG repeat length in Huntington's disease. Arch Neurol. 1996;53(6):493–7.

19. Wheelock VL, Tempkin T, Marder K, Nance M, Myers RH, Zhao H, Huntington Study Group, et al. Predictors of nursing home placement in Huntington disease. Neurology. 2003;60(6):998–1001.
20. Nance MA, Sanders G. Characteristics of individuals with Huntington disease in long-term care. Mov Disord. 1996;11:542–8.
21. Walker FO. Huntington's disease. Lancet. 2007;369:218–28.
22. Dubinsky RM. No going home for hospitalized Huntington's disease patients. Mov Disord. 2005;20:1316–22.
23. Lanska DJ, Lanska MJ, Lavine L, Schoenberg BS. Conditions associated with Huntington's disease at death. A case-control study. Arch Neurol. 1988;45:878–80.
24. Sorensen SA, Fenger K. Causes of death in patients with Huntington's disease and in unaffected first-degree relatives. J Med Genet. 1992;29:911–4.
25. Rodrigues FB, Abreu D, Damásio J, Goncalves N, Correia-Guedes L, Coelho M, Ferreira JJ, REGISTRY Investigators of the European Huntington's Disease Network. Survival, mortality, causes and places of death in a European Huntington's disease prospective cohort. Mov Disord Clin Pract. 2017;4(5):737–42.
26. Galts CPC, Bettio LEB, Jewett DC, Yang CC, Brocardo PS, Rodrigues ALS, et al. Depression in neurodegenerative diseases: common mechanisms and current treatment options. Neurosci Biobehav Rev. 2019;102:56–84.
27. Testa CM, Jankovic J. Huntington disease: a quarter century of progress since the gene discovery. J Neurol Sci. 2019;396:52–68.
28. Kirkwood SC, Su JL, Conneally P, Foroud T. Progression of symptoms in the early and middle stages of Huntington disease. Arch Neurol. 2001;58:273–8.
29. Paulsen JS, Nehl C, Hoth KF, Kanz JE, Benjamin M, Conybeare R, et al. Depression and stages of Huntington's disease. J Neuropsychiatry Clin Neurosci. 2005;17(4):496–502.
30. Huntington G. On chorea. Med Surg Rep. 1872;26:317–21.
31. Di Maio L, Squitieri F, Napolitano G, Campanella G, Trofatter JA, Conneally PM. Suicide risk in Huntington's disease. J Med Genet. 1993;30:293–5.
32. Paulsen JS, Hoth KF, Nehl C, Stierman L. Critical periods of suicide risk in Huntington's disease. Am J Psychiatry. 2005;162:725–31.
33. Fiedorowicz JG, Mills JA, Ruggle A, Langbehn D, Paulsen JS. Suicidal behavior in prodromal Huntington disease. Neurodegener Dis. 2011;8(6):483–90. Epub 2011 Jun 9.
34. McGarry A, McDermott MP, Kieburtz K, Fung WLA, McCusker E, Peng J, Huntington Study Group 2CARE Investigators and Coordinators, et al. Risk factors for suicidality in Huntington disease: an analysis of the 2CARE clinical trial. Neurology. 2019;92(14):e1643–51.
35. Honrath P, Dogan I, Wudarczyk O, Görlich KS, Votinov M, Werner CJ, Enroll-HD Investigators, et al. Risk factors of suicidal ideation in Huntington's disease: literature review and data from Enroll-HD. J Neurol. 2018;265(11):2548–61.
36. Kachian ZR, Cohen-Zimerman S, Bega D, Gordon B, Grafman J. Suicidal ideation and behavior in Huntington's disease: systematic review and recommendations. J Affect Disord. 2019;250:319–29.
37. Farrer LA. Suicide and attempted suicide in Huntington disease: implications for preclinical testing of persons at risk. Am J Med Genet. 1986;24:305–11.
38. Schoenfeld M, Myers RH, Cupples LA, Berkman B, Sax DS, Clark E. Increased rate of suicide among patients with Huntington's disease. J Neurol Neurosurg Psychiatry. 1984;47:1283–7.
39. Bonelli RM, Wenning GK. Pharmacological management of Huntington's disease: an evidence-based review. Curr Pharm Des. 2006;12:2701–20.
40. Levenson JL. Neuroleptic malignant syndrome. Am J Psychiatry. 1985;142:1137–45.
41. Robottom BJ, Weiner WJ, Factor SA. Movement disorders emergencies part 1: hypokinetic disorders. Arch Neurol. 2011;68:567–72.
42. Burke RE, Fahn S, Mayeux R, Weinberg H, Louis K, Willner JH. Neuroleptic malignant syndrome caused by dopamine-depleting drugs in a patient with Huntington disease. Neurology. 1981;31:1022–5.

43. Ossemann M, Sindic CJ, Laterre C. Tetrabenazine as a cause of neuroleptic malignant syndrome. Mov Disord. 1996;11:95.
44. Gahr M, Orth M, Abler B. Neuroleptic malignant syndrome with aripiprazole in Huntington's disease. Mov Disord. 2010;25:2475–6.
45. Grimbergen YA, Knol MJ, Bloem BR, Kremer BP, Roos RA, Munneke M. Falls and gait disturbances in Huntington's disease. Mov Disord. 2008;23:970–6.
46. Vuong K, Canning CG, Menant JC, Loy CT. Gait, balance, and falls in Huntington disease. Handb Clin Neurol. 2018;159:251–60.
47. Rao AK, Muratori L, Louis ED, Moskowitz CB, Marder KS. Spectrum of gait impairments in presymptomatic and symptomatic Huntington's disease. Mov Disord. 2008;23:1100–7.
48. Gennarelli TA, Thibault LE. Biomechanics of acute subdural hematoma. J Trauma. 1982;22:680–6.
49. Maxeiner H, Wolff M. Pure subdural hematomas: a postmortem analysis of their form and bleeding points. Neurosurgery. 2002;50:503–8. discussion 508–509.
50. Pechlivanis I, Andrich J, Scholz M, Harders A, Saft C, Schmieder K. Chronic subdural haematoma in patients with Huntington's disease. Br J Neurosurg. 2006;20:327–9.
51. Hoth KF, Paulsen JS, Moser DJ, Tranel D, Clark LA, Bechara A. Patients with Huntington's disease have impaired awareness of cognitive, emotional, and functional abilities. J Clin Exp Neuropsychol. 2007;29:365–76.
52. Busse ME, Wiles CM, Rosser AE. Mobility and falls in people with Huntington's disease. J Neurol Neurosurg Psychiatry. 2009;80:88–90.
53. Kloos AD, Kegelmeyer DA, Young GS, Kostyk SK. Fall risk assessment using the Tinetti mobility test in individuals with Huntington's disease. Mov Disord. 2010;25:2838–44.
54. Rao AK, Muratori L, Louis ED, Moskowitz CB, Marder KS. Clinical measurement of mobility and balance impairments in Huntington's disease: validity and responsiveness. Gait Posture. 2009;29:433–6.
55. Miles SH. Restraints and sudden death. J Am Geriatr Soc. 1993;41:1013.
56. Kagel MC, Leopold NA. Dysphagia in Huntington's disease: a 16-year retrospective. Dysphagia. 1992;7:106–14.
57. Heemskerk AW, Roos RA. Dysphagia in Huntington's disease: a review. Dysphagia. 2010;26:62–6.
58. Moskowitz CB, Marder K. Palliative care for people with late-stage Huntington's disease. Neurol Clin. 2001;19:849–65.
59. Tabrizi SJ, Leavitt BR, Landwehrmeyer GB, Wild EJ, Saft C, Barker RA, Phase 1–2a IONIS-HTTRx Study Site Teams, et al. Targeting huntingtin expression in patients with Huntington's disease. N Engl J Med. 2019;380(24):2307–16.
60. Wild EJ, Tabrizi SJ. One decade ago, one decade ahead in Huntington's disease. Mov Disord. 2019;34:1434–9.

Genetics and Genetic Counseling-Related Issues

30

Martha A. Nance

Patient Vignettes

Patient 1

A 32-year-old woman presented to clinic with her partner, also 32 years old. She reported that she was 12 weeks' pregnant, with a pregnancy that was desired. Her partner had recently informed her that he was at risk for Huntington's disease, as his mother and uncle had died of the disorder. They had not previously discussed his family history, and he had never been evaluated by a neurologist. The woman requested that he be tested urgently and, if his test showed that he carried the genetic abnormality that causes Huntington's disease, that she be offered a prenatal test to determine whether the fetus carried the abnormal gene.

The couple met with the social worker and genetic counselor to discuss their options. The woman expressed the desire to continue the pregnancy if she could be assured that "her baby" would not have HD. She was not sure what she would do if "it" tested positive for the gene, but felt that she might terminate the pregnancy. The at-risk partner discussed his fears about the possibility of a diagnosis of HD, and also indicated that he was not interested in predictive testing or a neurologic exam. After discussion with the woman's obstetrician, chorionic villus sampling was performed, with testing for the huntingtin gene (HTT). This decision was based on current practices related to maternal rights for fetal testing. The test showed that the fetus did not carry the mutation that causes Huntington's disease, a CAG repeat expansion.

M. A. Nance (✉)
Struthers Parkinson's Center, Golden Valley, MN, USA
e-mail: martha.nance@parknicollet.com

© Springer Nature Switzerland AG 2022
S. J. Frucht (ed.), *Movement Disorder Emergencies*, Current Clinical Neurology,
https://doi.org/10.1007/978-3-030-75898-1_30

Patient 2

A 65-year-old man with Parkinson's disease called his neurologist confused and upset. He, his sister, and cousin were affected with Parkinson's disease, diagnosed by movement disorders experts. His cousin, aware of the diagnoses in other family members, had undergone direct-to-consumer testing "for Parkinson's disease," which was negative. Genetic testing on the 65-year-old patient at the time of his diagnosis, using a "Parkinson's gene testing panel" available through the company that our clinic prefers to use, tested 20 different genes all of which were normal. However, the patient's sister also underwent testing for Parkinson's disease through her neurologist in another state; her test panel only included seven genes, but she was found to have a mutation in the glucocerebrosidase A (GBA) gene, which she was told was the cause of her Parkinson's disease. She was also told that her children could also potentially inherit another disease, called Gaucher disease. Multiple family members in multiple generations were confused, angry at the patient's sister, and angry at the doctors and the direct-to-consumer company for failing to detect the gene mutation in the sister.

Test reports were obtained from the sister and cousin, and the neurologist met with the family by video during the patient's appointment. The underlying problem was that different laboratory panels test different genes using different methods. The direct-to-consumer test looked for a single specific mutation in GBA, which was not the mutation present in this family. The 20-gene panel evaluated genes associated with Parkinson's disease, but GBA was not among them. The discrepancy between the test panels was explained to the patient and his family members, and he and his cousin underwent GBA testing through the laboratory that performed the sister's test. His test was positive, but his cousin's was negative, illustrating that the etiology of Parkinson's disease is complex and that nongenetic "phenocopies" may occur even in families where there is an identified genetic cause of Parkinson's disease. Some GBA mutations that are associated with Parkinson's disease are also associated with the recessive condition, Gaucher disease, in children who receive an abnormal gene from both parents. The children of the patient and his sister and other siblings were encouraged to ask for a referral to a genetic counselor, to consider testing for the family's GBA mutation, which might clarify their risk for both Parkinson's disease and also Gaucher disease in future generations.

Introduction

In the ideal outpatient clinic, diagnoses (including genetic ones) are provided by caring and knowledgeable physicians with an abundance of time, complemented by easy access to educational materials, support staff, and a treatment plan to address the newly diagnosed condition. The subspecialties of medical genetics/genomics and genetic counseling developed in response to the unique diagnostic and management issues that accompany genetic disorders. Genetics specialists can help the neurologist to avoid crises related to the genetic aspects of neurogenetic disorders and to help alleviate them if they arise. However, the busy neurologist may not have detailed knowledge of a particular genetic condition, or may not have immediate access to a genetics specialist, and so may encounter a neurogenetic emergency. We describe below some problematic situations that can arise related to genetic testing and neurogenetic disorders and suggest strategies to prevent or manage them.

There are four clinically distinct situations in which genetic testing might be offered: for diagnostic confirmation, predictive testing, prenatal or preimplantation testing, and carrier testing. Superficially, diagnostic genetic testing is a familiar concept for the neurologist. However, after a genetic diagnosis is made in an affected individual, additional requests for information or additional types of testing may quickly ensue, with which the neurologist is less familiar. The patient might request prenatal (or preimplantation) genetic testing for a current or future pregnancy; and siblings, children, or other relatives might want to consider carrier testing (for a recessively inherited condition) or pre-symptomatic or predictive testing (usually in the context of a dominantly inherited condition). While other clinicians will certainly be involved in the decision to perform prenatal or preimplantation testing, the neurologist may be asked to perform predictive or carrier testing, or at least to direct family members to where it can be performed. The lack of guidance or provision of incorrect information to families at this point can have adverse effects that resonate over generations.

Psychosocial Emergencies Following a Diagnostic Gene Test

By definition, a genetic disorder is inborn and permanent. If a person is not the first in the family to be diagnosed with a neurogenetic condition, then the diagnosis may confirm the parent or patient's worst fear, a fear that may have been smoldering for years or generations. On the other hand, if the diagnosis is new to the family, the patient may experience, in addition to grief for their own situation, guilt for having "brought the disease" into the family. There is also a potential for the diagnosis of a genetic condition to bring to light such issues as unknown adoption, nonpaternity, and incest, with obvious potential impact on family relationships. Family members may demand immediate testing to clarify their risk status. In addition, many neurogenetic movement disorders—Parkinson's disease, Huntington's disease, and some of the hereditary ataxias and dystonias—can have cognitive and behavioral effects that impact a patient's ability to cope with or fully understand a genetic diagnosis and its broader implications for others in the family.

The risk of adverse psychological events following the diagnosis of a neurogenetic condition varies depending on the condition. Suicidal ideation occurs in up to 23.5% of people with "possible" (soft signs suggesting) Huntington's disease, and over 15% of those in Stage I or Stage II of the disease, before declining later in the disease, suggesting that individuals at and around the time of diagnosis are particularly susceptible to suicidality [1]. Suicide has been reported in patients with myoclonus-dystonia syndrome, and also following deep brain stimulation surgery for dystonia [2, 3]. In one review, suicide attempts occurred in 7/45 patients with

Wilson's disease [4]. Suicidal thinking was present in 11% of a convenience sample of outpatients with Parkinson's disease [5]. Although suicide has not been reported, depression occurs in about 25% of patients with spinocerebellar ataxia and 50% of patients with hereditary spastic paraplegia [6, 7]. Although depression is common in Tourette syndrome, suicide appears to be uncommon, and suicide has only rarely been reported in patients with essential tremor or any of the hereditary ataxia syndromes. Whether people with suicidality, depression, or psychosis are more sensitive at the time of a diagnosis, with or without genetic confirmation, and whether genetic diagnosis is likely to trigger a less-than-lethal level of depression, is generally not known.

Huntington's disease presents a unique situation in neurogenetics, in which all individuals with the disease have the same mutation at the same location in the same gene (with the minor exception of HD "look-alikes" such as Huntington's disease-like 2 (HDL-2), dentatorubral-pallidoluysian (DRPLA), and spinocerebellar ataxia type 17 (SCA17)). Because of this, a relatively inexpensive targeted analysis of the CAG repeat expansion in the huntingtin gene is available, and counseling regarding the relationship between the presence of the gene mutation and the development of the disease is relatively straightforward. The situation becomes more complex for the hereditary ataxias, dystonias, and spastic paraplegias, where mutations in several different genes can lead to a similar phenotype, mutations in the same gene can lead to different phenotypes, and multiple different mutations in the same gene can occur, which may or may not be detected using any given assay [8]. The potential for uncertainty or unexpected results following genetic testing is thus greater in these conditions and may create discomfort or distrust between patient, family, and clinician.

For Parkinson's disease, the situation is even more complex, as demonstrated in the Patient 2 vignette. Mutations in multiple different genes have been shown to be associated with Parkinson's disease. Nongenetic phenocopies can occur (people from a "Parkinson's family" who have Parkinson's disease but do not carry the family gene mutation). Gene test panels vary widely as to which genes and which mutations they include, and, as we will discuss later, reduced penetrance for many of the identifiable mutations complicates the discussion with at-risk but clinically unaffected individuals. There is also the possibility that individuals may carry mutations in more than one Parkinson's gene. The role of genetic testing in Parkinson's disease has recently been reviewed [9]. Finally, in this rapidly evolving area of neurogenetics, as more people are undergoing genetic testing, more sequence variants are identified in Parkinson's disease genes that have uncertain significance, because they have not been seen or reported in the medical literature before. These "variants of uncertain significance" (VUSes) are the genetic equivalent of the "unidentified bright objects" seen frequently on brain MRI scans, which neurologists learn to interpret with a heavy dose of clinical context [10]. Some genetic testing laboratories report VUSes, and others do not. Failure of the clinician to discuss VUSes described in a test report, or overestimation of their relevance, is common and may lead to confusion and misunderstanding, with consequences for the patient and other family members [11].

Requests for "Emergency" Diagnostic Testing

While a diagnostic gene test can provide a definitive confirmation of a patient's diagnosis, other than in a child with an acute metabolic crisis due to an inborn error of metabolism, it is rarely an emergency to obtain this confirmation. In some cases, a clinical diagnosis might be allowed to trump a negative or inconclusive genetic test result. Unfortunately, both patients and doctors can overestimate the information content of a diagnostic/confirmatory gene test, which can create an unnecessary sense of urgency around its use. The following two cases illustrate this point.

Patient 3

A 40-year-old woman asks for an urgent evaluation. She is performing poorly in the workplace, with increasing clumsiness over the last 3–4 years, ataxia, and a change in speech. Coworkers are accusing her of being intoxicated at work. Her deceased mother and grandfather had similar symptoms, and her brother has "hereditary ataxia." She would like an ataxia gene test, so that she can apply for disability before she gets fired from her job, which seems imminent. Examination shows dysarthria, gait spasticity and ataxia, limb ataxia, slow eye movements, and hyporeflexia. No additional information can be obtained about the other family members; she is estranged from her brother.

This patient should be given a working clinical diagnosis of hereditary ataxia, with further evaluation to include MR imaging (primarily to rule out other treatable potential causes of ataxia and spasticity, such as multiple sclerosis) and an attempt to access the brother's gene test results. If the brother in fact came to a specific genetic diagnosis, for instance, spinocerebellar ataxia type 2 (SCA2), then the patient's working diagnosis can be amended to SCA2 pending a focused test of that particular gene. If the brother never came to a specific genetic diagnosis, or if his records are truly inaccessible, then the patient will need a more expensive "ataxia genetic panel." It is important to note that the patient's disability is due to the progressive and severe nature of the neurological findings, not to the specific genetic diagnosis. Even if the patient's gene test is normal and the family diagnosis remains uncertain, she is still disabled due to a progressive neurodegenerative disease process.

Patient 4

A 35-year-old man is admitted to the psychiatric crisis unit for the third time in 2 years. He lives on the street in his town in the summer but makes his way south in the winter. He only comes to medical attention in a crisis situation, and little additional medical or family history has been available. This time, however, a family member appears at his bedside and says that the patient's father and brother both have Huntington's disease. The psychiatry resident orders a stat HD gene test and a neurology consult.

Rather than a stat gene test, this patient needs a thorough medical history and neurologic exam. He may also benefit from formal neuropsychological testing. If he has obvious chorea and/or cognitive decline from his prior employment as an architect, then the working diagnosis of HD is evident, and the gene test is not an emergency. If the exam shows subtle changes that could be consistent with HD, then a nonurgent test to rule that condition in or out is reasonable. If he has no movement disorder, has been on the streets since his early 20s, has never worked more than temporary jobs, and was diagnosed 15 years ago with paranoid schizophrenia, then the clinical diagnosis of HD is not evident, and any genetic testing would be considered "predictive" and should only be done if and when the patient requests it. No matter what the results of the gene test are, or whether it is performed or not, the patient needs urgent and ongoing psychiatric care. The gene test can be performed at a time when the patient is not in the midst of a psychiatric crisis and is more able to understand the implications of the results.

A final comment should be made about the potential impact of diagnostic genetic testing on employment. The Genetic Information Nondiscrimination Act (GINA) prevents discrimination in employment or insurance because of gene test results [12]. This will be discussed in the next section, as it is relevant to individuals undergoing carrier testing or pre-symptomatic testing, and is not relevant to diagnostic genetic testing in a patient who already has a diagnosis or neurologic symptoms of a disease.

Psychosocial Complications of Predictive Testing

Guidelines written over 25 years ago (shortly after the identification of the HD gene) recommended a course of genetic counseling, psychological assessment, and neurologic examination prior to the completion of a predictive gene test [13]. The purpose of these guidelines was to protect patients requesting predictive testing from experiencing adverse psychological and social consequences of testing for an incurable disease, which would not be offset by any therapeutic strategies to delay or prevent the disease. These guidelines are still referred to today as a model for pre-symptomatic genetic testing of other adult-onset neurogenetic disorders [14]. A worldwide survey of over 4500 individuals tested at "predictive testing centers" showed that the risk of catastrophic events (defined as suicide, suicide attempt, psychiatric hospitalization) after predictive testing was less than 1% [15]. It is not known whether the outcomes are different for patients who undergo predictive testing in a less rigorously supported situation, such as through their primary care physician, neurologist, or psychiatrist without the added benefits of genetic counseling and psychosocial assessment and support.

It is also not known whether a more abbreviated testing protocol could be used for other neurogenetic movement disorders. Given that the genetic complexity and heterogeneity of other groups of movement disorders (ataxias, dystonias, spastic paraplegias, parkinsonian syndromes) are greater than HD, it seems safest to make use of genetics specialists if a patient requests predictive testing, carrier testing, or genetic risk factor assessment for virtually any movement disorder. Knowing that the primary risks of predictive testing are psychosocial, the clinician may also wish to involve a social worker or psychologist, if they plan to provide predictive testing for patients. Recent studies have pointed out the importance of support for tested patients, in particular the possibility of psychological stress if the test result precipitates changes in family dynamics or contradicts what the patient thought the outcome would be [16]. As genetic testing for Parkinson's disease becomes more widespread, requests for predictive genetic testing will undoubtedly ensue. The neurologist is strongly advised to refer such patients to a genetic counselor for an in-depth discussion of the possibility of nongenetic PD occurring in patients who test negative, as well as the likelihood of reduced penetrance for the most common "dominant" PD genes, such as LRRK2 and GBA, and the potential psychosocial consequences of early knowledge of genetic status [9].

Next-generation sequencing opens up the possibility of predictive testing for neurodegenerative disorders even in the absence of a family history or a known genetic diagnosis. Goldman et al. used a "modified Huntington's disease genetic testing protocol" that included pre- and post-test genetic counseling, neurologic and psychological evaluations in a pilot study of 24 individuals evaluated through next-generation sequencing (including patients without a specific known family diagnosis), and found this procedure to be safe and generally well-received [17].

O━━━▶ Genetic testing for Huntington's disease should **never** be ordered without careful pre- and post-test counseling and psychological care.

A situation occasionally arises in which a third party inappropriately requests an urgent predictive gene test to be performed. For instance, an employer may wish to know whether an employee carries a gene that will cause incoordination or cognitive/behavioral impairment. This is the situation in which GINA provides important protections, by preventing an employer (with more than 15 employees) from requiring genetic testing, or asking about results of a previously performed test. This legislation also prevents health insurers from requiring a gene test or providing coverage differently because of the results of a gene test [12]. Importantly, GINA does not provide protection to tested individuals in relation to other kinds of insurance, such as life, long-term care, disability, or homeowner's insurance.

Occasionally, a young adult whose parent is at risk for a dominantly inherited condition requests predictive testing. In this situation, a positive test result for the patient means that the parent, who did not request testing and may not want to know their genetic status, must also carry the abnormal gene (the same applies to an identical twin). Although we have made the decision to proceed with testing in these cases after counseling and consultation with our institutional ethics committee, adverse consequences of this kind of decision have been observed [18].

We have been involved in situations where a party in a custody dispute demands testing of a parent at risk for HD to determine that person's future ability to work or to care for the child. In this situation, we have tried to make clear to all the distinction between a diagnostic test in a person who is having symptoms of HD (in which case the neurologic exam or cognitive tests identify an impairment), the gene test that confirms the clinical diagnosis, and a test to determine whether an asymptomatic person carries a gene for a condition that may not manifest until years later. Predictive testing in the United States leans strongly on the ethical principle of autonomy, the right of the testing individual to choose whether to be tested free of coercion, with a clear understanding of the medical benefits, which may be zero, and the psychosocial risks [19]. An analogous discussion has been applied to the idea of testing children at risk for adult-onset diseases before they have the cognitive, emotional, and legal ability to make decisions for themselves. There may be specific individuals or situations in which predictive genetic testing of a minor is reasonable, for instance, an emancipated minor [20]. Finally, there is concern that the use of direct-to-consumer tests by minors could lead to deleterious psychosocial effects [21].

The potential for genetic discrimination, such as loss of insurance, related to predictive testing of asymptomatic individuals for conditions such as HD has been discussed for years [22]—there are few detailed case reports of actual events [23]. One study showed that family history of HD, rather than the gene test itself, presented a greater risk for events perceived as examples of discrimination and that the events more commonly related to insurance, family, and social situations, and less often to work, healthcare, or public situations [24]. Finally, there is an upcoming potential problem of confidentiality as we move into the era of open access to electronic medical records [25]. The neurologist who treats patients with genetic neurologic disorders should be sensitive to the potential social impact of the diagnosis, genetic risk status, or gene test results—obtained at any point in the patient's life—on self-image and on their standing within the family, workplace, and community.

Prenatal Testing

Prenatal tests for neurogenetic conditions are sometimes requested urgently or emergently, because of time pressure related to the pregnancy. The best strategy to avoid these situations is detailed and repeated proactive communication with the patient and family. The day that the patient is given a diagnosis of DYT1 dystonia or SCA3 ataxia may not be the best day to have a detailed discussion about reproductive and testing options, but the conversation needs to occur and may need to occur more than once for full understanding. Printed materials from disease-specific lay organizations can be helpful, and for the patient of child-bearing potential, referral to a genetic counselor for a detailed discussion is appropriate. A surprising amount of genetic misinformation and misunderstanding still exists, and sometimes having multiple family members present (or in the COVID era, logged in by video) for a genetics discussion can help to avoid the misunderstandings that can emerge as one family member talks to another, who talks to another. A recent study shows that individuals at risk for hereditary ataxia are more interested in preimplantation genetic diagnosis than in prenatal testing. Preimplantation genetic diagnosis requires in vitro fertilization, followed by testing of an individual cell from the embryo and implantation of an embryo documented to be free of the tested gene mutation, an invasive process and procedure that must be discussed in detail and planned prior to pregnancy [26].

Many of the genetic movement disorders have a long, slow course, and a patient's children who were once teenagers may end up providing care and support for their affected parent. Those young adults may begin to have questions about their own at-risk status and the possibility of predictive or prenatal testing and should be encouraged to seek out accurate information.

A pregnant patient requesting emergency predictive or prenatal testing should always be referred to a genetic counselor, who can work with the neurologist and obstetrician to make appropriate decisions about the patient, the pregnancy, and the role of genetic testing. The only "therapy" to offer following a positive gene test result is termination of the pregnancy, which may not be acceptable to the patient. Current practice in the United States permits pregnant women to request genetic testing of a fetus "to prepare" (for instance, for a child with Down syndrome or some other childhood-onset condition), and it is difficult to justify permitting testing for some genetic conditions but not others, meaning that it is ethically permissible to test a pregnant woman even if she does not intend to terminate the pregnancy. Outcomes of continued pregnancies following a positive test result, and recommendations for those managing these patients have been discussed [27].

Family Crises Related to a Genetic Diagnosis

The unit of care in genetics is the family, and so genetic medicine, by its very nature, has the potential to create or become enmeshed in conflicts between a particular individual and others in their family. We have seen challenging situations particularly in the Huntington's disease clinic. In (more than) one case, the family brought the patient to the clinic under false pretenses for evaluation and diagnosis of a condition the patient was unaware of or did not think they had [28]. Conversely, another at risk patient may attribute decades of anxiety and depression to manifest effects of HD, even in the absence of motor or cognitive effects [29]. It can be very difficult to attend to the needs and desires of both the patient and the family when they are in opposition. In the pre-symptomatic patient, there is no medical benefit to be gained by testing, no matter how many family members request the test on behalf of the patient—the patient's autonomy should prevail. However, in a symptomatic patient, it may be important for medical, legal, and psychosocial reasons to establish a clear diagnosis. Treatment of symptoms, however, can often proceed with or without a specific genetic diagnosis.

The clinician must also be sensitive to the emotional challenges faced by family caregivers related to the patient, such as siblings and children, and to the special burden faced by a spouse simultaneously caring for an affected adult and an affected child. We recall a 14-year-old daughter who was called upon by her father to come to her mother's appointment, in case the mother needed assistance with menstrual hygiene in a public restroom. When at age 16 the daughter refused to be so involved with her mother's care, urgent nursing home placement became necessary.

Another crisis situation can arise when families are misinformed or have misunderstandings about the genetic aspects of their disease. Based on observations within their kindred, or misinformation provided decades ago, families may still believe that their disease skips generations, affects only males or females, never affects the second-born child, or is nongenetic. Correcting these misimpressions is important but may cause ripples through the family [30]. Once again, referral to a genetic counselor, who may be able to take extra time, schedule family conferences, and use visual aids to illustrate various genetic principles, can be very helpful to the busy clinician. Disease-specific lay organizations often have printed or online materials about the genetic aspects of their disease(s). Finally, the online resource, GeneReviews® (www.ncbi.nlm.nih.gov/books/NBK1116/), provides excellent, current, and detailed information for the clinician about the genetic and clinical aspects and approaches to genetic testing for many neurogenetic conditions [31].

Conclusion

By understanding the unique aspects of genetic medicine, and making use of genetics specialists such as genetic counselors, the neurologist should avoid most emergencies related to genetic testing for neurogenetic disorders. Most of the crises that do arise are of a psychosocial nature, so enlisting the support of social workers, nurse case managers, psychologists, or psychiatrists can help the neurologist to defuse the crises that do arise.

References

1. Paulsen JS, Hoth KF, Nehl C, Stierman L. Critical periods of suicide risk in Huntington's disease. Am J Psychiatry. 2005;162:725–31.
2. Foncke EM, Schuurman PR, Speelman JD. Suicide after deep brain stimulation of the internal globus pallidus for dystonia. Neurology. 2006;66:142–3.
3. Misbahuddin A, Placzek M, Lennox G, Taanman JW, Warner TT. Myoclonus-dystonia syndrome with severe depression is caused by an exon-skipping mutation in the epsilon-sarcoglycan gene. Mov Disord. 2007;22:1173–5.
4. Oder W, Grimm G, Kollegger H, Ferenci P, Schneider B, Deecke L. Neurological and neuropsychiatric spectrum of Wilson's disease: a prospective study of 45 cases. J Neurol. 1991;238:281–7.
5. Nazem S, Siderowf AD, Duda JE, Brown GK, Ten Have T, Stern MB, et al. Suicidal and death ideation in Parkinson's disease. Mov Disord. 2008;23:1573–9.
6. Lo RY, Figueroa KP, Pulst SM, Perlman S, Wilmot G, Gomez C, et al. Depression and clinical progression in spinocerebellar ataxias. Parkinsonism Relat Disord. 2016;22:87–92.
7. Vahter L, Braschinsky M, Hladre S, Gross-Paju K. The prevalence of depression in hereditary spastic paraplegia. Clin Rehabil. 2009;23:857–61.

8. Witek N, Hawkins J, Hall D. Genetic ataxias: update on classification and diagnostic approaches. Curr Neurol Neurosci Rep. 2021;21(3):13.
9. Cook L, Schulze J, Naito A, Alcalay RN. The role of genetic testing for Parkinson's disease. Curr Neurol Neurosci Rep. 2021;21(4):17.
10. Di Fonzo A, Monfrini E, Erro R. Genetics of movement disorders and the practicing clinician; who and what to test for? Curr Neurol Neurosci Rep. 2018;18(7):37.
11. Macklin SK, Jackson JL, Atwal PS, Hines SL. Physician interpretation of variants of uncertain significance. Familial Cancer. 2019;18(1):121–6.
12. Clifton JM, VanBeuge SS, Mladenka C, Wosnik KK. The Genetic Information Nondiscrimination Act 2008: what clinicians should understand. J Am Acad Nurse Pract. 2010;22:246–9.
13. Anonymous. Guidelines for the molecular genetics predictive test in Huntington's disease: International Huntington Association (IHA) and the World Federation of Neurology (WFN) Research Group on Huntington's Chorea. Neurology. 1994;44:1533–6.
14. Grandis M, Obici L, Luigetti M, Briani C, Benedicenti F, Bisogni G, et al. Recommendations for pre-symptomatic genetic testing for hereditary transthyretin amyloidosis in the era of effective therapy: a multicenter Italian consensus. Orphanet J Rare Dis. 2020;15(1):348.
15. Almqvist EW, Bloch M, Brinkman R, Craufurd D, Hayden MR. A worldwide assessment of the frequency of suicide, suicide attempts, or psychiatric hospitalization after predictive testing for Huntington disease. Am J Hum Genet. 1999;64:1293–304.
16. Forrest Keenan K, McKee L, Miedzybrodzka Z. Help or hindrance: young people's experiences of predictive testing for Huntington's disease. Clin Genet. 2015;87(6):563–9.
17. Goldman J, Xie S, Green D, Naini A, Mansukhani MM, Marder K. Predictive testing for neurodegenerative diseases in the age of next-generation sequencing. J Genet Couns. 2020;30(2):553–62.
18. Bonnard A, Herson A, Gargiulo M, Durr A. Reverse presymptomatic testing for Huntington disease: double disclosure when 25% at-risk children reveal the genetic status to their parent. Eur J Hum Genet. 2019;27(1):22–7.
19. Lilani A. Ethical issues and policy analysis for genetic testing: Huntington's disease as a paradigm for diseases with a late onset. Hum Reprod Genet Ethics. 2005;11:28–34.
20. Borry P, Stultiens L, Nus H, Cassiman JJ, Direickx K. Presymptomatic and predictive genetic testing in minors: a systematic review of guidelines and position papers. Clin Genet. 2006;70:374–81.
21. Borry P, Howard HC, Senecal K, Avard D. Health-related direct-to-consumer genetic testing: a review of companies' policies with regard to genetic testing in minors. Familial Cancer. 2010;9:51–9.
22. Oster E, Dorsey ER, Bausch J, Shinaman A, Kayson E, Oakes D, et al. Fear of health insurance loss among individuals at risk for Huntington disease. Am J Med Genet A. 2008;146A:2070–7.
23. Kitzman R. Views of discrimination among individuals confronting genetic disease. J Genet Couns. 2010;19:68–83.
24. Bombard Y, Veenstra G, Friedman JM, Creighton S, Currie L, Paulsen JS, et al. Perceptions of genetic discrimination among people at risk for Huntington's disease: a cross-sectional survey. BMJ. 2009;338:b2175.
25. Black KJ, Barton SK, Perlmutter JS. Presymptomatic testing and confidentiality in the age of the electronic medical record. J Neuropsychiatry Clin Neurosci. 2021;33(1):80–3.
26. Cahn S, Rosen A, Wilmot G. Spinocerebellar ataxia patient perceptions regarding reproductive options. Mov Disord Clin Pract. 2019;7(1):37–44.
27. Wadrup F, Holden S, MacLeod R, Miedzybrodzka Z, Németh AH, Owens S, UK Huntington's Disease Predictive Testing Consortium, et al. A case-note review of continued pregnancies found to be at a high risk of Huntington's disease: considerations for clinical practice. Eur J Hum Genet. 2019;27(8):1215–24.

28. Hoth KF, Paulsen JS, Moser DJ, Tranel D, Clark LA, Bechara A. Patients with Huntington's disease have impaired awareness of cognitive, emotional, and functional abilities. J Clin Exp Neuropsychol. 2007;29:365–76.
29. Browner CH, Preloran HM. Neurogenetic diagnoses. New York: Routledge; 2010. p. 37–48.
30. Stuttgen K, Bollinger J, McCague A, Dvoskin R, Mathews D. Family communication patterns and challenges of Huntington's disease risk, the decision to pursue presymptomatic testing, and test results. J Huntingtons Dis. 2020;9(3).265–74.
31. GeneReviews® website. www.ncbi.nlm.nih.gov/books/NBK1116/. Accessed 28 March 2021.

Driving in Parkinson's Disease

31

Ergun Y. Uc

Patient Vignettes

Patient 1

A 58-year-old man with Parkinson's disease (PD) for 3 years, working full time, has an intermittent resting tremor in the left hand with no balance or gait problems. He is on ropinirole 5 mg TID. He is concerned about excessive daytime sleepiness during driving. He did well on road testing and had very mild executive dysfunction and slight decrease in visual contrast sensitivity. After decreasing his ropinirole dose, his sleepiness improved. He continues to drive without problems but avoids nighttime driving and congested roads.

Patient 2

A 78-year-old woman with postural-instability-gait-disorder (PIGD) parkinsonism of 8-year duration responded modestly to levodopa. While driving she had several near-misses despite restricting her driving to favorable weather and road conditions. Mental status evaluation revealed executive, visuospatial, and memory impairment consistent with mild-moderate dementia. Her visual contrast sensitivity and useful field of view were markedly impaired. In the driving simulator, she showed increased swerving and slow reaction to hazards with resultant crashes. Road test was deemed unsafe to undertake and she was recommended to cease driving.

E. Y. Uc (✉)
Department of Neurology, Division of Movement Disorders and Parkinson's Foundation
Center of Excellence, University of Iowa Carver College of Medicine, Iowa City, IA, USA
e-mail: ergun-uc@uiowa.edu

© Springer Nature Switzerland AG 2022
S. J. Frucht (ed.), *Movement Disorder Emergencies*, Current Clinical Neurology,
https://doi.org/10.1007/978-3-030-75898-1_31

Patient 3

A 63-year-old woman with PD for 8 years experienced wearing off and excessive daytime sleepiness on carbidopa/levodopa 25/100, 1 tablet QID, and pramipexole 1.5 mg TID. She had multi-domain mild cognitive impairment with moderate decrease in visual contrast sensitivity and useful field of view. She committed more safety errors on the road than healthy drivers and completely missed a hazard in a foggy environment in the driving simulator with a resultant crash. After gradual withdrawal of pramipexole and increase of carbidopa/levodopa, her sleepiness resolved and her driving improved. Due to moderate disease severity and presence of MCI, annual road tests were recommended. Her disease continued to progress with increased mobility and cognitive impairment, and she ceased driving 3 years later after a near-miss.

Introduction

In addition to the characteristic motor dysfunction, PD also impairs cognition, vision, and alertness [1–3], resulting in decreased driving safety [4–7]. Drivers with PD perform worse on driving simulator [8–13] and road tests [4–6] compared to their healthy peers. Their driving problems worsen with multitasking [14–16] or under conditions of low visibility [8]. They also may be at increased risk for crashes. Although driving simulation studies [6, 8, 10] and retrospective surveys [17, 18] have demonstrated increased crash rates in drivers with PD, this has not yet been confirmed by community-based, prospective, controlled studies [19]. Drivers with PD use more compensation strategies and cease driving earlier than their healthy peers, which could partially explain the lack of increased crash rates in PD [19]. Periodic multidisciplinary evaluations in close cooperation with the patient, caregivers, and state authorities are needed to asses driving fitness and to offer alternative transportation methods in appropriate cases [7, 20]. Research on driver rehabilitation in PD is in progress, but there are no clear proven methods [21]. The role of automation ranging from collision mitigation technologies in newer vehicles to fully autonomous vehicles requires further investigation [7].

The Scope of the Problem

Driving is an important activity of daily living and is essential for mobility and independence for many individuals. With increased longevity, the number of elderly drivers is rising, which will be accompanied by an increase of drivers with neurological diseases of aging such as dementia, stroke, and PD. One of the most important concerns in drivers with PD is the potential for increased risk for crashes. While there has been some decrease in the number of fatalities in recent years [22], motor vehicle crashes are a major public health problem with about 42,000 fatalities and a financial cost of ~$231 billion in 2000 [23]. Indeed, driving simulation studies have shown increased crash rates in PD [8, 10], and retrospective surveys have suggested increased crashes in drivers with PD [17, 18]. However, increased real-life crash risk in drivers with PD has not been confirmed by community-based prospective controlled studies or epidemiological research so far [6, 19, 24, 25]. Another potential unfavorable driving outcome in drivers with PD is loss of vehicular mobility (driving cessation) as shown on cross-sectional, retrospective and prospective surveys [6, 17–19, 26–28].

The goal in counseling drivers with PD is to prevent crashes while preserving mobility and independence. The methods for assessing driver safety and requirements for reporting in potentially impaired persons vary across the world [25] and among states within the USA [29]; no clear guidelines have been established for PD [30]. Medical diagnosis or a clinician's assessment alone are not accurate enough to determine driving competence in patients with cognitive impairment [31, 32]. While a proportion of drivers with PD use compensatory strategies such as reduction of driving exposure, avoidance of difficult driving conditions (inclement weather, darkness, rush hour, difficult maneuvers) suggesting some insight into their limitations [19], both patients [33–35] and their neurologists [33] have been shown to overestimate the patient's driving ability.

The Framework to Start Driving

Driving performance is determined by factors related to the driver (e.g., age; medical condition; cognitive, visual, motor, behavioral dysfunction; decreased alertness; substance abuse; etc.), environment (e.g., weather, road conditions), vehicle (e.g., maintenance, presence of warning or safety devices), presence of distractions, and their interactions [36].

Michon proposed a hierarchical model of cognitive control of driving with concurrent activity at three levels: (1) strategic, (2) tactical/maneuvering, and (3) operational/vehicle control. The decisions to drive during inclement weather or route selection (e.g., freeways vs. urban streets) are examples of strategic behavior which affect driving performance and safety on a time scale of minutes to days. Adjusting speed and car following distance, choice of lane, and decision to overtake according to road rules and conditions are examples of tactical behaviors and affect driving on a time scale of 5–60 seconds. Maintaining lane position with ongoing steering adjustments, keeping a safe distance to the car in front from moment to moment, and reacting to hazards represent operational behaviors, which affect driving on the time scale of 0.5–5 seconds [2].

At an operational level, driver actions can be analyzed using an information processing model (Fig. 31.1): (1) perception and attention to stimulus (e.g., visual and auditory inputs) and interpretation of the road situation; (2) planning a reaction to the stimulus based on relevant previous experience in similar situations; (3) execution of selected plan (e.g., by applying the accelerator, brake, or steering controls); and (4) monitoring the outcome of the behavior with subsequent self-correction [2]. The driver's response to the stimulus (e.g., a hazard such as an illegal

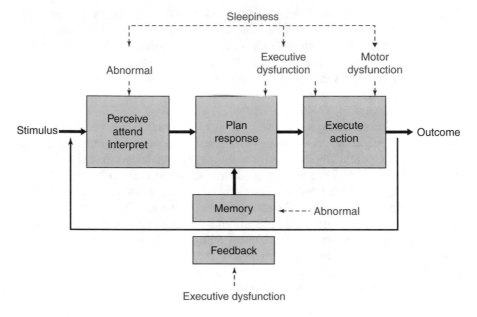

Fig. 31.1 Information processing model for driver error in PD. (Reprinted by permission from Springer Nature: Uc and Rizzo [2], Copyright 2008)

intersection incursion by another vehicle) is either safe (able to stop) or unsafe (e.g., crash) as a result of errors at one or more of these stages [2].

Neural Substrates of Driving

Driving engages the parieto-occipital cortices, cerebellum, and cortical regions associated with perception and motor control, as shown by fMRI studies during simulation [37] or positron emission tomography (PET) scanning after a road drive [38]. Alcohol degrades driving performance and decreases activation in these areas [39]. Even a simple auditory-verbal distraction such as listening to sentences produces a significant deterioration in vehicle control during straight driving and is associated with increased activation in temporal regions at the expense of decreased activation of parietal regions. This suggests that language comprehension performed concurrently with driving draws mental resources (spatial processing by the parietal lobe) away from the primary task and produces deterioration in driving performance [40]. During more complex driving tasks, especially when making left-hand turns at busy intersections compared to more simple driving tasks, a widely distributed brain network was identified. During distracted driving using an auditory task, brain activation shifted dramatically from the posterior, visual, and spatial areas to the prefrontal cortex, suggesting that activation in the posterior brain important for visual attention and alertness was reduced to recruit other brain regions to perform a secondary, cognitive task [41] and to monitor for errors during increased demand [42]. EEG studies suggest an impaired resistance to distractor interference and a reduced inhibition of prepotent responses in older drivers, most pronounced when the processing of task-relevant and task-irrelevant stimuli engages the same mental resources [43]. Alcohol amplifies the negative effects of distraction on brain activation and driving performance [44, 45].

PD pathology involves many regions in the brain, leading to cognitive, visual, and motor impairments that can interfere with driving performance at different levels [2, 3]. For example, decreased decision-making ability/executive dysfunction due to frontostriatal dysfunction can lead to poor strategic and tactical choices such as driving under challenging conditions and making risky maneuvers. Impairments in attention, visual perception, memory, executive functions, motor speed, and self-monitoring can lead to driver errors at operational levels with unsafe responses to sudden hazards [37]. One could expect that negative consequences of distraction would be worse in patients with neurodegenerative disease such as PD.

Driving Research in PD

Due to the complexity of the task of driving and PD, multiple complimentary assessment methods in comparison to a control group need to be studied longitudinally to determine the predictors of driving safety and outcomes. Off-road batteries usually combine questionnaires on general health, mood and sleep, quality of life, driving history, and habits with performance-based measures of cognition, vision, and motor function. As real-life crashes are rare events, driving performance in a simulator and a road test in an instrumented vehicle are used as intermediate steps to uncover relationships between cognitive, visual, motor impairments, and driving outcomes. While most driving experience consists of uneventful long stretches, there are interspersed segments with multitasking. Some of the secondary tasks are required as part of driving (e.g., following a new route to reach a destination, paying attention to landmarks and traffic signs, listening to radio for weather updates), and others may be discretionary (e.g., speaking on a cell phone, talking to a passenger, eating). The secondary tasks can have a degrading effect on driver safety and performance, especially in drivers with cognitive dysfunction.

Off-Road Evaluation

Demographics
The patients in reported studies of driving in PD are usually in their mid-60s or 70s and predominantly male, with mild-moderate disease severity, living in the community (e.g., Uc et al. [5]). The male predominance among drivers in the PD group may reflect that men are at higher risk for PD [18] and that women in this age group have not traditionally been the main driver in the family, or might have more

readily relinquished their driving privileges once they developed PD [15]. Of note, gender has not been found to be a predictor of driving performance in PD [46] consistent with our results when we adjusted for driving outcomes for gender [4, 5, 8, 14–16, 19].

Assessments of Cognition, Vision, and Motor Function and Indices of Parkinsonism Sleep and Psychiatric Problems

Although individual tests may differ between batteries used by various research teams, they attempt to probe different aspects of visual perception, cognition (e.g., executive functions, attention, and memory), motor function, mood, and sleep. As driving is a primarily visual task, these batteries are rich in visual tests and may cover all aspects of visual function from the retinal to the cortical level. Drivers with PD in most studies had mild-moderate parkinsonism and performed worse compared to controls in most visual and cognitive abilities, albeit usually showing mild deficits [4, 5, 19, 34, 47–53].

Effect of Sleep-Related Impairments

Ever since Frucht et al. [54] observed that PD patients taking the dopamine agonist ropinirole or pramipexole may experience "sleep attacks" leading to car crashes, excessive daytime sleepiness (EDS) or "sleep attacks" have been reported with all dopaminergic medications used to treat PD [55]. About 33% (range 16–74%) of patients with PD suffer from EDS; the estimates for "sleep attacks" are 1–14%, with 1–4% experiencing them during driving [56]. EDS increases significantly over time and is associated with several clinical variables, including dopaminergic therapy whose influence is dose-dependent [57]. The mechanisms of sleepiness and sleep attacks in PD might include a complex drug-disease interaction with degeneration in sleep centers in the brain, and side effects of dopaminergic medications, particularly direct dopamine agonists [56].

Sleep attacks remain a significant concern for PD patients treated with dopamine agonists.

Several studies using self-report measures such as the Epworth Sleepiness Scale (ESS; cutoff score 7–10) found a relationship between EDS and driving performance in PD; real sleep attacks without any prior sleepiness were rare [17, 58–62]. In particular, use of ergot dopamine agonists (e.g., bromocriptine, cabergoline, and pergolide) has been associated with crashes and sleepiness [58], but these are either off the market or not in widespread use anymore in the USA. Furthermore, the ESS does not correlate well with a more objective measure of sleepiness [55]. Empirical studies using experimental performance measures for driving and physiological measures of sleep while driving are needed to describe the characteristics of sleep-related driving problems and predictors of poor outcomes due to wakefulness disorders in PD [61]. There are active research projects using EEG and other electrophysiological techniques to assess drowsiness during driving [63–70].

Effect of PD Treatment

Road testing in drivers with PD has usually been done when the patients are in the "on" state due to ethical (subject protection) and practical (normally subjects would not start driving without treatment effect) concerns. Thus, there are no data on driving performance comparing "on" and "off" states of PD patients on the road. However, this can be potentially tested in the safe environment of a driving simulator. No significant correlations of dopaminergic medication dosage (levodopa equivalent dose per day (LEDD)) could be found with empirical driving performance [4, 5, 12, 14–16, 34]. We found that higher LEDD at baseline predicts earlier driving cessation [19], probably as a surrogate measure of disease severity. Higher LEDD was also found to be associated with a history of major crashes in PD [71]. There are limited data comparing the effect of dopaminergic medication class (levodopa vs. direct agonists) on driving. Uc et al. (2007) classified PD drivers as being on levodopa, dopamine agonist, levodopa and dopamine agonist, or other/no treatment and made formal comparisons among these groups. There was no effect of medication group status on safety errors or performance on the route following task.

Standardized Road Tests

The main outcome measures of these road tests were pass/fail (or safe/unsafe) ratings by driving experts as categorical measures, and at-fault error counts (Table 31.1) or driver ratings as continuous performance measures. Failure rates up to 62% in community testing of drivers with PD have been reported [72]. A systematic review of past controlled studies found that 30–56% of PD drivers failed the road test, whereas only 0–24% controls failed across studies [21]. A meta-analysis found that the odds of on-the-road test failure in drivers with PD was 6.16 times higher than controls (95% confidence interval [CI] 3.79–10.03) and that overall driving ratings were significantly worse for the PD group [6]. Analyses were done to determine the cognitive, visual, and motor predictors of pass/fail ratings or error counts. Below are some specific examples.

Cross-Sectional Studies

Heikkila et al. showed that PD patients and their neurologists overestimate their driving ability [33]. The driving abilities of PD patients were estimated by a neurologist and by a psychologist using tests and an interview, by a driving instructor

Table 31.1 Driving safety errors in PD

General classification
Total errors
Serious/critical errors
Errors during multitasking
Location
Stop signs
Traffic signals
Roundabouts
Maneuver
Turns
Lane changing
Merging
Parking
Vehicle control
Lane observance
Speed control
Blind spot errors

Classification, locations, maneuvers observed to be worse than controls

on the basis of a driving test, and by the patients themselves using a global scale. Patients with PD performed worse than controls both on neuropsychological tests and road test. The driving instructor found 35% of PD drivers unsafe, while none of the patients were rated unsafe by themselves or the neurologist. There was a significant correlation between the driving instructors scores and the psychologist's estimates, but not with the neurologist's estimates. Drivers with PD committed significantly more at-fault errors, especially in urban conditions. Slower information processing correlated with more driving errors in the PD group [33].

🔑 Neurologists routinely overestimate PD patients' ability to drive.

Grace et al. found impaired driving performance in both mild Alzheimer's disease and PD vs. controls [73]. While drivers with AD were more impaired on the road than PD, drivers with PD experienced more difficulty in maneuvers requiring head turning. Driving performance in PD was related to disease stage; impairments in visuospatial abilities, executive functions, and memory; and axial rigidity and postural instability, but not to the UPDRS motor total score [73]. Wood et al. found higher fail rates in PD compared to controls [34]. Drivers with PD also made significantly more errors than the control group during maneuvers that involved changing lanes and lane keeping, monitoring their blind spot, reversing, car parking, and traffic light-controlled intersections [34]. The driving instructor had to intervene to avoid an incident significantly more often for drivers with PD than for controls [34]. Impairments in dexterity, contrast sensitivity, and executive functions predicted failure on the road test within the PD group in the study [51].

Devos et al. (2007) rated ~1/4 of their PD driver sample as unfit to drive, which was predicted accurately using a model with the following variables: disease duration, contrast sensitivity, Clinical Dementia Rating, and motor part of the Unified PD Rating Scale [35]. This model was validated in a second cohort [74].

Adding driving simulator performance to the model increased the accuracy further [35]. In these cohorts, 65% of PD drivers passed and 35% failed the on-road driving evaluation [49]. The failing group performed worse on all on-road items and on all motor, visual, and cognitive tests compared to the passing group. When adjusted for age and gender, poor performance on lateral positioning at low speed, speed adaptations at high speed, and left turning maneuvers were the key road skills that determined the pass/fail decision. Measures of visual scanning, motor severity, PD subtype, visual acuity, executive functions, and divided attention were independent predictors of pass/fail decisions [49]. Classen et al. found that ~40% of PD and ~20% of controls failed a road test, predicted by the Useful Field of View (UFOV) test, and developed cutoff points for UFOV [75, 76]. While objective tests and scales are important to understand and predict driving performance in PD, information provided by caregivers is invaluable as the caregiver impressions explained 56% of variability in road test scores, whereas PD scales and motor tests only explained 30% of the variability [77].

Longitudinal Studies

Uc et al. tested drivers with PD and healthy controls in a longitudinal cohort study: participants drove a standardized route in an instrumented vehicle and were invited to return 2 years later [4, 5]. A professional driving expert reviewed drive data and videos to score safety errors. At baseline, drivers with PD performed worse on visual, cognitive, and motor tests and committed more road safety errors compared to controls. Interestingly ~1/4 of the PD group drove as good as controls at baseline [5]. Lane violations were the most common error category, and group differences in some error categories became insignificant after results were adjusted for demographics and familiarity with the local driving environment. Within the PD group, older age and worse performance on tests of visual acuity, contrast sensitivity, attention, visuospatial abilities, visual memory, and general cognition predicted error counts. Measures of visual processing speed and attention (UFOV test) and far visual acuity were jointly predictive of error counts in a multivariate model [5]. An alternative model using CFT-COPY (another strong univariate predictor) resulted in slightly smaller but still significant R-squared value. The advantage of CFT-COPY is that it is a paper-pencil test, which is in public domain and is quick to administer [5].

A smaller proportion of drivers with PD compared to controls in the Uc et al. study [5] returned for repeat testing (42.8% vs. 62.7%; $p < 0.01$) as seen in Fig. 31.2 [4]. At baseline, returnees with PD had made fewer errors than non-returnees with PD and performed similar to control returnees [4]. Baseline global cognitive performance of returnees with PD was better than that of non-returnees with PD but worse than for control returnees. Despite dropout of the more impaired drivers within the PD cohort, returning drivers with PD, who drove like controls without PD at baseline, showed greater cognitive decline and many more driving safety errors than controls after 2 years (~40% vs. 10%; $p < 0.001$) [4]. Driving error count increase in the returnees with PD was predicted by greater error count and worse visual acuity at baseline, and by greater interval worsening of global cognition,

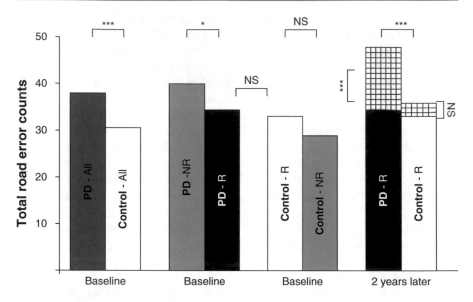

Fig. 31.2 Total error counts (medians) at baseline and after 2-year follow-up. At baseline, the PD group performed worse compared to controls. The baseline counts of PD returnees (PD-R) were lower (better) than PD non-returnees (PD-NR), and similar to control returnees (control-R). There were no significant differences between control-returnees and control non-returnees (control-NR). Two years later, PD-R have much higher error counts than control-R. The increase in error counts in PD-R (median = 13.5) was highly significant, whereas the control-R had only a minor nonsignificant increase in error counts (median = 3.0). NS, nonsignificant. (Reprinted with permission from Uc et al. [4])

Unified PD Rating Scale activities of daily living score, executive functions, visual processing speed, and attention [4]. The returning PD drivers were probably at a compensated state in terms of driving safety at baseline despite their poorer cognition at the time, but their driving also decompensated over 2 years ago. This study clearly shows that even the "cream of the crop" drivers can deteriorate over relatively a short time and justifies periodic monitoring of driving abilities (e.g., once a year).

Effects of Multitasking on Driving in PD

Uc et al. compared multitasking abilities of drivers with PD and controls by administering tasks on navigation (route following) [16], visual search [14], and mental arithmetic (to simulate auditory-verbal distraction) [15]. Drivers with PD took longer to finish the route-following task [16]. Higher proportions of PD drivers made incorrect turns, got lost, or committed at-fault safety errors [16]. Within the PD group, the navigational and safety errors were predicted by poor performance on cognitive and visual tests, but not by the severity of motor dysfunction [16]. During the same drive, drivers were asked to report sightings of specific landmarks and traffic signs along a four-lane commercial strip to assess the ability for visual search and recognition of roadside targets [14]. The drivers with PD identified significantly fewer landmarks and traffic signs, and they committed more at-fault safety errors during the task than control subjects, even after adjusting for baseline errors. Within the PD group, the most important predictors of landmark and traffic sign identification rate were performance on visual speed of processing and attention and visuospatial abilities. Trail Making Test (B-A), a measure of cognitive flexibility independent of motor function, was the only independent predictor of at-fault safety errors in drivers with PD [14]. In another experiment in this cohort of PD patients and controls, the effects of auditory-verbal distraction on driving performance in PD were assessed using the Paced Auditory Serial Addition Task (PASAT) [15]. Despite driving slower, drivers with PD were more affected by the distracter task with increased safety errors. Decreased performance on tests of cognitive flexibility, verbal memory, postural control, and increased daytime sleepiness predicted worsening of driving performance due to distraction within the PD group [15].

Driving Simulation

Although actual road testing provides richer and more balanced visual, tactile, vibratory, and vestibular cues to the driver for the control of the vehicle [2], the road conditions vary between subjects, and some maneuvers may be unsafe to test. On the other hand, driving simulators replicate the experimental conditions for each subject and enable administration of challenging tasks in a safe environment with complete experimental control [78]. Driving simulators may vary widely in their technical characteristics (e.g., motion base vs. fixed base, interactivity, resolution, and field of view). Validation of individual simulators and driving scenarios is needed to derive meaningful conclusions from their administration. Another important concern about simulators is "simulator sickness" (similar to motion sickness), also known as simulator adaptation syndrome, in a proportion of drivers due to visual vestibular mismatch, which can reduce performance or preclude simulation altogether [79]. Most studies in the following section were performed on medium-high fidelity simulators with a fixed motion base.

Drivers with PD are able to tolerate simulated driving similarly to elderly healthy drivers [8]. Simulator studies in drivers with PD showed impaired steering accuracy, slower driving reaction times, and missing red lights [80, 81]; impaired lane keeping and increased crashes [8, 10], especially rear-end collisions [80]; and crashes at intersections under low visibility conditions [8]. In these studies, PD driver performance was associated with cognitive and visual dysfunction as well as severity of parkinsonism, especially for reaction times in tasks where speed of response was critical (e.g., reaction to sudden hazard such as an illegal intersection incursion by another vehicle) [8]. While increased incidence of crashes could not be shown in prospective cohort studies (possibly due to attrition of at-risk drivers or methodological issues such as small sample sizes or short follow-up) [6, 19], a meta-analysis found the odds of crashes 2.63 (95% CI 1.64–4.22) times higher for people with PD compared to controls in driving simulator experiments [6], showing the value of simulator studies for outcomes that cannot be safely or feasibly tested in real-life road tests or prospective epidemiological studies.

Drivers with PD have difficulty generating internal cues from memory and rely on external cues such as warnings and signs for better driving performance due to attentional and executive dysfunction, akin to usefulness of visual cues to overcome freezing. Concurrent, distracting auditory-verbal or motor tasks take a larger toll on vehicle control and reaction to hazards in drivers with PD compared to controls, although they tend to drive slower and perform worse on the secondary tasks. The impact of these secondary tasks on drivers with PD is associated with increased severity of their executive and attentional dysfunction.

Increased levels of cognitive demands may affect drivers with PD worse as also shown in the road tests [14–16]. In a sign recall task in a simulator, the performance of PD drivers was initially similar to controls when the instructions were direct but dropped below controls when drivers were required to apply the instructions from working memory [82]. Mental flexibility and the updating of information in working memory are key executive functions that can affect driving. Using neuropsychological tests to evaluate updating (via the n-back task), flexibility (via the plus-minus task), and information processing speed (via the Stroop test), their equivalent tasks in a driving simulator (recalling road signs for the updating task, indicating the shape or color of road signs according to roadside for the flexibility task, braking at the same time as the car ahead for the information processing speed task), updating deficits both on neuropsychological testing and driving were found in PD compared to controls. There were no significant differences between groups in tasks measuring flexibility or information processing speed. Trail Making Test (B-A) was strongly predictive of PD drivers' simulator task updating score [13]. A 2-year cohort study in PD and control drivers using both neuropsychological and driving simulator tasks revealed a significant decline in executive functions in PD compared to controls, especially in shift cost, associated with modifications in their driving habits over time [47].

Psychological factors such as emotion recognition and impulse control can also be significant contributors to driving safety: compared to controls, drivers with neurodegenerative diseases such as Alzheimer's disease, frontotemporal dementia, dementia with Lewy bodies, and Huntington's disease showed significantly worse emotion recognition, particularly of anger, disgust, fear, and sadness [83]. Patients took significantly more risks in the driving simulator rides, which was associated with poor recognition of fear [83]. In addition to severity of parkinsonism and cognitive impairment, presence and severity of impulse control disorders as measured by QUIP (Questionnaire for Impulsive-Compulsive Disorders in PD) was also predictive of crashes in patients with PD [71].

Real-Life Driving Outcomes

Real-life driving outcomes can be studied using retrospective or prospective self-report questionnaires and state records. Naturalistic driving studies where the driver's car is outfitted with special sensors and cameras for long-term observation can add an objective component to these observations; however, their use is limited by feasibility and funding concerns.

Driving History and Habits

Questionnaires (e.g., Driving Habits Questionnaire [19]) are used to collect self-report information on driving exposure (e.g., miles/week, days/week), driving history (crashes and citations), perceptions and judgments on own impairments and driving ability, and use of compensatory strategies (e.g., no driving at night, in snow). The driving history can be verified by using state records. Caregiver perspective can also give valuable insights on driving ability and deficiency awareness of the patient [77].

There are no well-established epidemiologic data on crash risk in PD. However, a retrospective, cross-sectional questionnaire study from a movement disorders center found that 20% of PD patients had stopped driving [18]. The frequency of crashes in subjects with more severe PD (Hoehn and Yahr stage III and higher) was fivefold higher than controls, whereas patients with mild PD (HY I) reported almost twice as many crashes as the controls. An MMSE score of 23 or less was associated with a threefold increased crash rate [18].

A large mail and phone survey from Germany [17] revealed that ~80% of the PD patients held a driving license and ~60% of them were still actively driving. Of the patients holding a driving license, 15% had been involved in and 11% had caused at least one accident during the past 5 years. The risk of crashes significantly increased for patients who felt moderately impaired by PD, had an increased ESS score, and had reported "sleep attacks" while driving. Female gender, more severe parkinsonism and sleepiness, higher age, and longer disease duration were associated with driving cessation [17]. In a cross-sectional study among PD patients, Cubo et al. [26] found that, compared to current drivers, the ex-drivers were significantly older, had longer disease duration, had more overall cognitive dysfunction, and had greater motor impairment, as measured by the Clinical Impression of Severity Index, HY stage, and the SCOPA (Scales for Outcomes in Parkinson's disease) motor scale and difficulty in activities of daily life. Aging and ADL impairment were the principal clinical predictors that differentiated drivers from ex-drivers [26].

Review of the records of drivers with PD referred to the Scottish Driving Assessment Service over a 15-year period revealed that 66% were able to continue driving with about half receiving recommendations for vehicle modifications [28]. Ability to drive was predicted by the severity of parkinsonism, reaction time, presence of significant comorbidities, and poor score on road testing [28]. Our longitudinal prospective cohort study of 106 drivers with PD and 130 elderly control drivers [19] showed that 40.6% of PD drivers ceased driving compared to 16.9% of control drivers with an estimated HR (95% CI) of 7.09 (3.66, 13.75) for PD, adjusted for age, gender, education, and driving exposure at baseline. This is consistent with prior retrospective reports, where PD was found to be a major factor in driving cessation, but not a significant factor in crashes [27, 84]. The Kaplan-Meier plot (Fig. 31.3) shows the probability of still driving (or inversely, the risk of driving

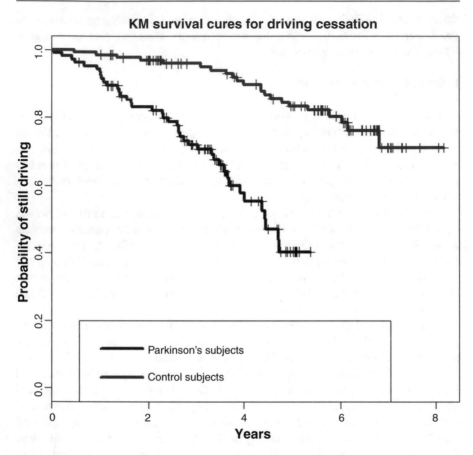

Fig. 31.3 Kaplan-Meier curves for driving cessation (logrank test χ $\chi^2 = 37.53^2 = 37.53$, p-value < 0.0001) between subjects with Parkinson's disease and elderly control subjects. (Reprinted with permission from Uc et al. [19])

cessation) at any particular time point during the follow-up and allows visual comparison between groups for between-group comparisons over time [19]. For example, the cumulative incidence (95% CI) of driving cessation at 2 years after baseline was 17.6% (11.5%, 26.5%) for PD and 3.1% (1.2%, 8.1%) for controls [19]. Significant individual risk factors for driving cessation within PD included older age, decreased driving exposure, poorer ratings of driving ability by self and others, higher number of road errors and past crashes, increased use of compensation strategies, poorer performances in most measures of vision, and higher severity of parkinsonism. A multivariate analysis of risk factors in PD showed a preference to be driven by others, higher UFOV total score, higher UPDRS-ADL score, and higher daily levodopa equivalent as the most important risk factors for driving cessation [84]. Among driving simulator measures at baseline, crash occurrence was not predictive of driving cessation, but high standard deviation of lane position predicted future driving cessation [85]. There was no statistically significant difference between groups on crashes; however the study had limited power to detect differences in crashes due to the small number of crashes that occurred. Of note, our results in PD are similar to observations in Alzheimer's disease (AD) by other researchers where driving cessation was the main outcome without showing increased crashes [32]. The likely reasons for these findings may include attrition of potentially unsafe drivers with AD or PD before a potential crash or restricted driving and strategic compensation [19]. Our results were consistent with a recent meta-analysis: self-reported real-life crash involvement did not differ between people with PD and healthy controls (odds ratio = 0.84, 95% CI 0.57–1.23, $p = 0.38$) [6].

In a naturalistic driving study, electronic devices were installed in the vehicles of drivers with PD and controls for 2 weeks, and driving data were matched with aerial maps, weather and daylight archives, and trip logs to examine driving context [86]. Compared to controls, the PD group drove significantly less overall (number of trips, distance, duration), and proportionately less at night and on days with bad weather suggesting more restricted driving practices [86], congruent with lower ratings of driving comfort and abilities as in self-reports [19]. However, they drove significantly faster (and over the speed limit) on highways and freeways, and 19% reported driving problems over the 2 weeks [86], suggesting that they may not necessarily drive more cautiously or safely at operational or tactical levels despite taking compensatory measures at strategic levels.

Driver Rehabilitation

Driving rehabilitation strategies include training underlying abilities (e.g., motor function, information processing speed, or executive functions) or focusing on driving skills [21]. The literature on driving rehabilitation in PD is limited. Driving simulator training exposes drivers to different driving situations in dynamic and realistic conditions, aiming to improve the impaired driving skills, or lead to strategies that compensate for impaired driving skills [7]. Simulator training programs use driving scenarios that can be tailored to the needs of the drivers and increase in difficulty to continue challenging the drivers throughout the training sessions. Immediate feedback can be provided through video replay functions so that the drivers can actively participate in identifying their challenges and provide solutions to overcome these challenges [7]. A potential issue of simulator training is the simulator adaptation syndrome (SAS, similar to motion sickness) due to mismatch between the simulator's visual cues of movement and the subject's kinesthetic and vestibular cues of being stationary [7]. As an example from neurology, an intense simulator training program led to significant improvements within the simulator and was associated with passing an official driving assessment in stroke survivors [87]. However, there was no difference in driving cessation in these stroke patients between the simulator training and control groups at 5 years [87].

There are several preliminary studies on simulator training in PD. In the first pilot study by our group [88], drivers with PD completed training sessions in a driving simulator that mimicked multiple intersections of varying visibility and traffic load where an incurring vehicle posed a crash risk. After training, participants had fewer crashes and responded faster to the incurring vehicle. However, it is not clear whether these improvements are the result of an actual training effect or rather familiarity with the simulated environment and scenarios. In a follow-up study, four drivers with PD who performed poorly on an on-road driving test completed sessions using the same scenarios reported before [88] as well as various scenarios on decision-making, hazard perception, and response behavior [89]. All participants improved their performance on the simulator tasks after training. In addition, the majority of participants completed the on-road driving test with fewer errors [89]. In another pilot study, drivers with PD completed 10 hours of simulator training, individually customized according to their pre-training performance on specific on-road driving skills [90]. After training, participants performed better on tests of cognition and visual scanning, as well on a driving test, including passing the road test after having failed before the simulator training [90].

With population aging, the advances in autonomous vehicle technology using Adaptive Driver Assistance Systems (ADAS) offers promise for maintaining or improving safe transportation, mobility, and quality of life [7]. The effect of low-level ADAS on intersection behavior, speed, and headway control in a pilot study showed that elderly healthy drivers gained more confidence using ADAS after several training sessions [91]. In speed and headway control experiments, automated warnings improved adherence to speed limit and safe following of the lead vehicle in both PD and control groups. However, removing ADAS after short-term exposure led to deterioration of performance in all speed measures in the PD group [92]. More research is needed on the effect of ADAS in maintaining safe vehicular independence in the elderly and in patients with PD [7].

Policy Issues

There are currently no uniform legal criteria to guide individuals with PD and healthcare professionals on fitness to drive [7]. A consensus statement by an expert panel involving the National Highway Traffic Safety Administration and the American Occupational Therapy Association provided general recommendations on fitness-to-drive decision-making according to PD disease severity [93] using a similar decision process as advocated in an evidence-based review on driving in PD [20]. As in Fig. 31.4 [20], individuals with low severity of parkinsonism and minimal non-motor/cognitive risk factors are usually deemed fit to drive [93]. A comprehensive baseline driving evaluation is recommended to establish baseline fitness to drive with annual follow-up driving evaluations. Cessation of driving is recommended for patients with advanced parkinsonism and multiple risk factors. This advice should be conveyed to the driver, and reporting to the driving license agencies should be considered according to the local jurisdiction. Continued consultation on

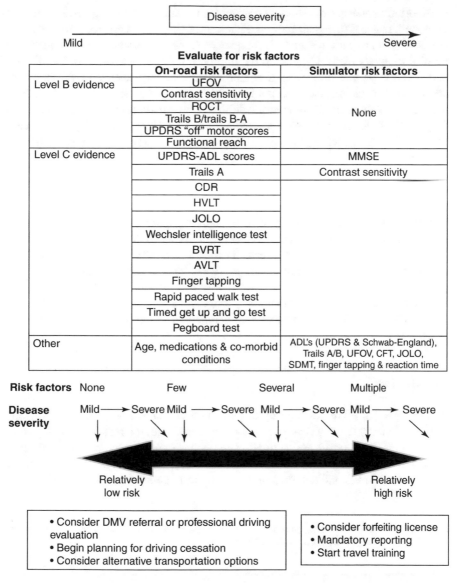

Fig. 31.4 Approach to driving fitness in PD and levels of evidence for various assessment tools. The lower part of the figure shows the interaction of PD motor severity with presence of visual and cognitive risk factors. For example, a patient with mild motor severity would be at increased risk for unsafe driving if he/she has multiple visual and cognitive risk factors. AVLT, Auditory Verbal Learning Test; BVRT, Benton Visual Retention Task; CDR, Clinical Dementia Rating Scale; ROCT, Rey-Osterrieth Complex Figure Test; HVLT, Hopkins Verbal Learning Test; JOLO, Judgment of Line Orientation; SDMT, Symbol Digit Modalities Test; UFOV, Useful Field of View. (Reprinted with permission from Crizzle et al. [20])

transportation alternatives should be provided to patient and caregiver. For drivers with moderate parkinsonism and some non-motor risk factors, the recommendations are less certain, and research is in progress. Each patient should undergo a multidisciplinary evaluation due to the highly individualized nature of the disease and variable progression using a comprehensive battery testing motor function, cognition, and vision and incorporating other non-motor aspects such as sleep, mood, and autonomic dysfunction. Additional information can be obtained from recent driving record and insights provided by the patient and family into driving safety concerns or changes in driver habits (e.g., compensation strategies to lower risk).

Reporting requirements for medically impaired drivers are not uniform across the USA and across the world. Healthcare providers should familiarize themselves with local rules and regulations on reporting of medically impaired drivers. The American Academy of Neurology (AAN) "supports optional reporting of individuals with medical conditions that may impact one's ability to drive safety, especially in cases where public safety has already been compromised, or it is clear that the person no longer has the skills needed to drive safely," and advocates immunity for physicians "both for reporting and not reporting a patient's condition when such action is taken in good faith, when the patient is reasonably informed of his or her driving risks, and when such actions are documented by the physician in good faith" [68, 94].

Conclusion

Driving is impaired in the majority of patients with PD and progressively worsens resulting in early driving cessation and potentially increased risk of crashes. While general guidelines on fitness to drive have been proposed, each patient should be evaluated individually with periodic follow-up [7]. Research on rehabilitation of driving skills in PD and automation of driving to maintain vehicular mobility is in progress [7].

Acknowledgments EYU is supported by NIH R01 grant NS044930 and VA Merit Review grants 1 I01 RX000170 and 1 I01 RX002987-01A1.

References

1. Uc EY, Rizzo M, Anderson SW, Qian S, Rodnitzky RL, Dawson JD. Visual dysfunction in Parkinson disease without dementia. Neurology. 2005;65:1907–13.
2. Uc EY, Rizzo M. Driving and neurodegenerative diseases. Curr Neurol Neurosci Rep. 2008;8:377–83.
3. Zhang Q, Aldridge GM, Narayanan NS, Anderson SW, Uc EY. Approach to cognitive impairment in Parkinson's disease. Neurotherapeutics. 2020;17(4):1495–510.
4. Uc EY, Rizzo M, O'Shea AMJ, Anderson SW, Dawson JD. Longitudinal decline of driving safety in Parkinson disease. Neurology. 2017;89:1951–8.

5. Uc EY, Rizzo M, Johnson AM, Dastrup E, Anderson SW, Dawson JD. Road safety in drivers with Parkinson disease. Neurology. 2009;73:2112–9.
6. Thompson T, Poulter D, Miles C, Solmi M, Veronese N, Carvalho AF, et al. Driving impairment and crash risk in Parkinson disease: a systematic review and meta-analysis. Neurology. 2018;91:e906–16.
7. Ranchet M, Devos H, Uc EY. Driving in Parkinson disease. Clin Geriatr Med. 2020;36:141–8.
8. Uc EY, Rizzo M, Anderson SW, Dastrup E, Sparks JD, Dawson JD. Driving under low-contrast visibility conditions in Parkinson disease. Neurology. 2009;73:1103–10.
9. Madeley P, Hulley JL, Wildgust H, Mindham RH. Parkinson's disease and driving ability. J Neurol Neurosurg Psychiatry. 1990;53:580–2.
10. Zesiewicz TA, Cimino CR, Malek AR, Gardner N, Leaverton PL, Dunne PB, et al. Driving safety in Parkinson's disease. Neurology. 2002;59:1787–8.
11. Stolwyk RJ, Triggs TJ, Charlton JL, Iansek R, Bradshaw JL. Impact of internal versus external cueing on driving performance in people with Parkinson's disease. Mov Disord. 2005;20:846–57.
12. Stolwyk RJ, Triggs TJ, Charlton JL, Moss S, Iansek R, Bradshaw JL. Effect of a concurrent task on driving performance in people with Parkinson's disease. Mov Disord. 2006;21:2096–100.
13. Ranchet M, Paire-Ficout L, Marin-Lamellet C, Laurent B, Broussolle E. Impaired updating ability in drivers with Parkinson's disease. J Neurol Neurosurg Psychiatry. 2011;82:218–23.
14. Uc EY, Rizzo M, Anderson SW, Sparks J, Rodnitzky RL, Dawson JD. Impaired visual search in drivers with Parkinson's disease. Ann Neurol. 2006;60:407–13.
15. Uc EY, Rizzo M, Anderson SW, Sparks JD, Rodnitzky RL, Dawson JD. Driving with distraction in Parkinson disease. Neurology. 2006;67:1774–80.
16. Uc EY, Rizzo M, Anderson SW, Sparks JD, Rodnitzky RL, Dawson JD. Impaired navigation in drivers with Parkinson's disease. Brain. 2007;130:2433–40.
17. Meindorfner C, Korner Y, Moller JC, Stiasny-Kolster K, Oertel WH, Kruger HP. Driving in Parkinson's disease: mobility, accidents, and sudden onset of sleep at the wheel. Mov Disord. 2005;20:832–42.
18. Dubinsky RM, Gray C, Husted D, Busenbark K, Vetere-Overfield B, Wiltfong D, et al. Driving in Parkinson's disease. Neurology. 1991;41:517–20.
19. Uc EY, Rizzo M, Johnson AM, Emerson JL, Liu D, Mills ED, et al. Real-life driving outcomes in Parkinson disease. Neurology. 2011;76:1894–902.
20. Crizzle AM, Classen S, Uc EY. Parkinson disease and driving: an evidence-based review. Neurology. 2012;79:2067–74.
21. Devos H, Ranchet M, Akinwuntan AE, Uc EY. Establishing an evidence-base framework for driving rehabilitation in Parkinson's disease: a systematic review of on-road driving studies. NeuroRehabilitation. 2015;37:35–52.
22. National Center for Statistics and Analysis. Preview of motor vehicle traffic fatalities in 2019 (Research Note. Report No. DOT HS 813 021). National Highway Traffic Safety Administration. October 2020 [online]. Available at: https://crashstats.nhtsa.dot.gov/Api/Public/ViewPublication/813021. Accessed December 6.
23. Shafi S, Parks J, Gentilello L. Cost benefits of reduction in motor vehicle injuries with a nationwide speed limit of 65 miles per hour (mph). J Trauma. 2008;65:1122–5.
24. Homann CN, Suppan K, Homann B, Crevenna R, Ivanic G, Ruzicka E. Driving in Parkinson's disease – a health hazard? J Neurol. 2003;250:1439–46.
25. Klimkeit EI, Bradshaw JL, Charlton J, Stolwyk R, Georgiou-Karistianis N. Driving ability in Parkinson's disease: current status of research. Neurosci Biobehav Rev. 2009;33:223–31.
26. Cubo E, Martinez Martin P, Gonzalez M, Bergareche A, Campos V, Fernández JM, et al. What contributes to driving ability in Parkinson's disease. Disabil Rehabil. 2010;32:374–8.
27. Lafont S, Laumon B, Helmer C, Dartigues JF, Fabrigoule C. Driving cessation and self-reported car crashes in older drivers: the impact of cognitive impairment and dementia in a population-based study. J Geriatr Psychiatry Neurol. 2008;21:171–82.
28. Singh R, Pentland B, Hunter J, Provan F. Parkinson's disease and driving ability. J Neurol Neurosurg Psychiatry. 2007;78:363–6.

29. Wang CC, Carr DB, Older DP. Older driver safety: a report from the older drivers project. J Am Geriatr Soc. 2004;52:143–9.
30. AAMVA. Driver fitness medical guidelines. DOT HS 811 210. Washington, DC: National Highway Traffic Safety Administration. US Department of Transportation; 2009.
31. Ott BR, Anthony D, Papandonatos GD, D'Abreu A, Burock J, Curtin A, et al. Clinician assessment of the driving competence of patients with dementia. J Am Geriatr Soc. 2005;53:829–33.
32. Ott BR, Heindel WC, Papandonatos GD, Festa EK, Davis JD, Daiello LA, et al. A longitudinal study of drivers with Alzheimer disease. Neurology. 2008;70:1171–8.
33. Heikkila VM, Turkka J, Korpelainen J, Kallanranta T, Summala H. Decreased driving ability in people with Parkinson's disease. J Neurol Neurosurg Psychiatry. 1998;64:325–30.
34. Wood JM, Worringham C, Kerr G, Mallon K, Silburn P. Quantitative assessment of driving performance in Parkinson's disease. J Neurol Neurosurg Psychiatry. 2005;76:176–80.
35. Devos H, Vandenberghe W, Nieuwboer A, Tant M, Baten G, De Weerdt W. Predictors of fitness to drive in people with Parkinson disease. Neurology. 2007;69:1434–41.
36. Galski T, Bruno RL, Ehle HT. Driving after cerebral damage: a model with implications for evaluation. Am J Occup Ther. 1992;46:324–32.
37. Spiers HJ, Maguire EA. Neural substrates of driving behaviour. NeuroImage. 2007;36:245–55.
38. Jeong M, Tashiro M, Singh LN, Yamaguchi K, Horikawa E, Miyake M, et al. Functional brain mapping of actual car-driving using [18F]FDG-PET. Ann Nucl Med. 2006;20:623–8.
39. Meda SA, Calhoun VD, Astur RS, Turner BM, Ruopp K, Pearlson GD. Alcohol dose effects on brain circuits during simulated driving: an fMRI study. Hum Brain Mapp. 2009;30:1257–70.
40. Just MA, Keller TA, Cynkar J. A decrease in brain activation associated with driving when listening to someone speak. Brain Res. 2008;1205:70–80.
41. Schweizer TA, Kan K, Hung Y, Tam F, Naglie G, Graham SJ. Brain activity during driving with distraction: an immersive fMRI study. Front Hum Neurosci. 2013;7:53.
42. Choi MH, Kim HS, Yoon HJ, Lee JC, Baek JH, Choi JS, et al. Increase in brain activation due to sub-tasks during driving: fMRI study using new MR-compatible driving simulator. J Physiol Anthropol. 2017;36:11.
43. Karthaus M, Wascher E, Getzmann S. Effects of visual and acoustic distraction on driving behavior and EEG in young and older car drivers: a driving simulation study. Front Aging Neurosci. 2018;10:420.
44. Allen AJ, Meda SA, Skudlarski P, Calhoun VD, Astur R, Ruopp KC, et al. Effects of alcohol on performance on a distraction task during simulated driving. Alcohol Clin Exp Res. 2009;33:617–25.
45. Calhoun VD, Pearlson GD. A selective review of simulated driving studies: combining naturalistic and hybrid paradigms, analysis approaches, and future directions. NeuroImage. 2012;59:25–35.
46. Crizzle AM, Classen S, Lanford D, Malaty IA, Okun MS, Wagle Shukla A, et al. Driving performance and behaviors: a comparison of gender differences in Parkinson's disease. Traffic Inj Prev. 2013;14:340–5.
47. Ranchet M, Broussolle E, Paire-Ficout L. Longitudinal executive changes in drivers with Parkinson's disease: study using neuropsychological and driving simulator tasks. Eur Neurol. 2016;76:143–50.
48. Classen S, Holmes JD, Alvarez L, Loew K, Mulvagh A, Rienas K, et al. Clinical assessments as predictors of primary on-road outcomes in Parkinson's disease. OTJR (Thorofare N J). 2015;35:213–20.
49. Devos H, Vandenberghe W, Tant M, Akinwuntan AE, De Weerdt W, Nieuwboer A, et al. Driving and off-road impairments underlying failure on road testing in Parkinson's disease. Mov Disord. 2013;28:1949–56.
50. Ranchet M, Broussolle E, Poisson A, Paire-Ficout L. Relationships between cognitive functions and driving behavior in Parkinson's disease. Eur Neurol. 2012;68:98–107.
51. Worringham CJ, Wood JM, Kerr GK, Silburn PA. Predictors of driving assessment outcome in Parkinson's disease. Mov Disord. 2006;21:230–5.

52. Stolwyk RJ, Charlton JL, Triggs TJ, Iansek R, Bradshaw JL. Neuropsychological function and driving ability in people with Parkinson's disease. J Clin Exp Neuropsychol. 2006;28:898–913.
53. Heikkila VM, Kallanranta T. Evaluation of the driving ability in disabled persons: a practitioners' view. Disabil Rehabil. 2005;27:1029–36.
54. Frucht S, Rogers JD, Greene PE, Gordon MF, Fahn S. Falling asleep at the wheel: motor vehicle mishaps in persons taking pramipexole and ropinirole. Neurology. 1999;52:1908–10.
55. Comella CL. Daytime sleepiness, agonist therapy, and driving in Parkinson disease. JAMA. 2002;287:509–11.
56. De Cock VC, Vidailhet M, Arnulf I. Sleep disturbances in patients with parkinsonism. Nat Clin Pract Neurol. 2008;4:254–66.
57. Amara AW, Chahine LM, Caspell-Garcia C, Long JD, Coffey C, Högl B, et al. Longitudinal assessment of excessive daytime sleepiness in early Parkinson's disease. J Neurol Neurosurg Psychiatry. 2017;88:653–62.
58. Ueno T, Kon T, Haga R, Nishijima H, Tomiyama M. Motor vehicle accidents in Parkinson's disease: a questionnaire study. Acta Neurol Scand. 2018;137:218–23.
59. Ghorayeb I, Loundou A, Auquier P, Dauvilliers Y, Bioulac B, Tison F. A nationwide survey of excessive daytime sleepiness in Parkinson's disease in France. Mov Disord. 2007;22:1567–72.
60. Amick MM, D'Abreu A, Moro-de-Casillas ML, Chou KL, Ott BR. Excessive daytime sleepiness and on-road driving performance in patients with Parkinson's disease. J Neurol Sci. 2007;252:13–5.
61. Moller JC, Stiasny K, Hargutt V, Cassel W, Tietze H, Peter JH, et al. Evaluation of sleep and driving performance in six patients with Parkinson's disease reporting sudden onset of sleep under dopaminergic medication: a pilot study. Mov Disord. 2002;17:474–81.
62. Hobson DE, Lang AE, Martin WR, Razmy A, Rivest J, Fleming J. Excessive daytime sleepiness and sudden-onset sleep in Parkinson disease: a survey by the Canadian Movement Disorders Group. JAMA. 2002;287:455–63.
63. Perrier J, Jongen S, Vuurman E, Bocca ML, Ramaekers JG, Vermeeren A. Driving performance and EEG fluctuations during on-the-road driving following sleep deprivation. Biol Psychol. 2016;121:1–11.
64. Duma GM, Mento G, Manari T, Martinelli M, Tressoldi P. Driving with intuition: a preregistered study about the EEG anticipation of simulated random car accidents. PLoS One. 2017;12:e0170370.
65. Nguyen T, Ahn S, Jang H, Jun SC, Kim JG. Utilization of a combined EEG/NIRS system to predict driver drowsiness. Sci Rep. 2017;7:43933.
66. Taeho H, Miyoung K, Seunghyeok H, Kwang SP. Driver drowsiness detection using the in-ear EEG. Annu Int Conf IEEE Eng Med Biol Soc. 2016;2016:4646–9.
67. Barua S, Ahmed MU, Begum S. Classifying drivers' cognitive load using EEG signals. Stud Health Technol Inform. 2017;237:99–106.
68. Yang L, Ma R, Zhang HM, Guan W, Jiang S. Driving behavior recognition using EEG data from a simulated car-following experiment. Accid Anal Prev. 2018;116:30–40.
69. Protzak J, Gramann K. Investigating established EEG parameter during real-world driving. Front Psychol. 2018;9:2289.
70. Yang L, Guan W, Ma R, Li X. Comparison among driving state prediction models for car-following condition based on EEG and driving features. Accid Anal Prev. 2019;133:105296.
71. Ando R, Iwaki H, Tsujii T, Nagai M, Nishikawa N, Yabe H, et al. The clinical findings useful for driving safety advice for Parkinson's disease patients. Intern Med. 2018;57:1977–82.
72. Lloyd K, Gaunt D, Haunton V, Skelly R, Mann H, Ben-Shlomo Y, et al. Driving in Parkinson's disease: a retrospective study of driving and mobility assessments. Age Ageing. 2020;49:1097–101.
73. Grace J, Amick MM, D'Abreu A, Festa EK, Heindel WC, Ott BR. Neuropsychological deficits associated with driving performance in Parkinson's and Alzheimer's disease. J Int Neuropsychol Soc. 2005;11:766–75.

74. Devos H, Vandenberghe W, Nieuwboer A, Tant M, De Weerdt W, Dawson JD, et al. Validation of a screening battery to predict driving fitness in people with Parkinson's disease. Mov Disord. 2013;28:671–4.
75. Classen S, McCarthy DP, Shechtman O, et al. Useful field of view as a reliable screening measure of driving performance in people with Parkinson's disease: results of a pilot study. Traffic Inj Prev. 2009;10:593–8.
76. Classen S, Brumback B, Crawford K, Jenniex S. Visual attention cut points for driver fitness in Parkinson's disease. OTJR (Thorofare N J). 2019;39:257–65.
77. Cordell R, Lee HC, Granger A, Vieira B, Lee AH. Driving assessment in Parkinson's disease--a novel predictor of performance? Mov Disord. 2008;23:1217–22.
78. Uc EY, Rizzo M, Anderson SW, Shi Q, Dawson JD. Unsafe rear-end collision avoidance in Alzheimer's disease. J Neurol Sci. 2006;251:35–43.
79. Uc EY, Rizzo M. Driving in Alzheimer's disease, Parkinson's disease, and stroke. In: Fisher DL, Rizzo M, Caird J, Lee JD, editors. Handbook of driving simulation for engineering, medicine, and psychology. Boca Raton: CRC Press, Taylor & Francis Group; 2011.
80. Uc EY, Rizzo M, Liu D, Anderson SW, Dawson JD. Increased rear-end collisions in drivers with Parkinson's disease. Mov Disord. 2009;24:S315.
81. Lings S, Dupont E. Driving with Parkinson's disease. A controlled laboratory investigation. Acta Neurol Scand. 1992;86:33–9.
82. Vardaki S, Devos H, Beratis I, Yannis G, Papageorgiou SG. Exploring the association between working memory and driving performance in Parkinson's disease. Traffic Inj Prev. 2016;17:359–66.
83. van den Berg NS, Reesink FE, de Haan EHF, Kremer HPH, Spikman JM, Huitema RB. Emotion recognition and traffic-related risk-taking behavior in patients with neurodegenerative diseases. J Int Neuropsychol Soc. 2021;27:136–45.
84. Campbell MK, Bush TL, Hale WE. Medical conditions associated with driving cessation in community-dwelling, ambulatory elders. J Gerontol. 1993;48:S230–4.
85. Uc E, Rizzo M, Anderson S, Dawson J. Simulated driving in low visibility predicts real world driving outcomes in Parkinson's disease. Neurology. 2016;86:S19.004.
86. Crizzle AM, Myers AM. Examination of naturalistic driving practices in drivers with Parkinson's disease compared to age and gender-matched controls. Accid Anal Prev. 2013;50:724–31.
87. Akinwuntan AE, De Weerdt W, Feys H, Pauwels J, Baten G, Arno P, et al. Effect of simulator training on driving after stroke: a randomized controlled trial. Neurology. 2005;65:843–50.
88. Dawson JD, Rizzo M, Anderson SW, Dastrup E, Uc EY. Collision avoidance training using a driving simulator in drivers with Parkinson's disease: a pilot study. Proc Int Driv Symp Hum Factors Driv Assess Train Veh Des. 2009;2009:154–60.
89. Uc E, Rizzo M, Anderson S, Lawrence J, Dawson J. Driver rehabilitation in Parkinson's disease using a driving simulator: a pilot study. Proc Int Driv Symp Hum Factors Driv Assess Train Veh Des. 2011;2011:248–54.
90. Devos H, Morgan JC, Onyeamaechi A, Bogle CA, Holton K, Kruse J, et al. Use of a driving simulator to improve on-road driving performance and cognition in persons with Parkinson's disease: a pilot study. Aust Occup Ther J. 2016;63:408–14.
91. Dotzauer M, Caljouw SR, de Waard D, Brouwer WH. Intersection assistance: a safe solution for older drivers? Accid Anal Prev. 2013;59:522–8.
92. Dotzauer M, Caljouw SR, De Waard D, Brouwer WH. Longer-term effects of ADAS use on speed and headway control in drivers diagnosed with Parkinson's disease. Traffic Inj Prev. 2015;16:10–6.
93. Classen S, National Highway Traffic Safety Administration, American Occupational Therapy Association. Consensus statements on driving in people with Parkinson's disease. Occup Ther Health Care. 2014;28:140–7.
94. Bacon D, Fisher RS, Morris JC, Rizzo M, Spanaki MV. American Academy of Neurology position statement on physician reporting of medical conditions that may affect driving competence. Neurology. 2007;68:1174–7.

Suicide Risk in Parkinson's Disease

32

Valerie Voon

Patient Vignette

A 48-year-old man was evaluated in a movement disorders center for consideration of deep brain stimulation for advanced Parkinson's disease (PD). He developed symptoms of PD at the age of 39 and had received treatment with levodopa and dopamine agonists for 8 years. His current problems included marked motor fluctuations requiring him to take levodopa every 2 hours and moderately severe peak-dose dyskinesias. Neuropsychological testing revealed no cognitive impairment. As part of his preoperative evaluation, psychiatric evaluation revealed an underlying mild to moderate depression and mild anxiety. Social support was limited, as he lived alone with one sibling located in the area. He was currently retired on medical disability.

He underwent successful implantation of bilateral subthalamic deep brain stimulators without incident. Postoperative course was uneventful, and there was substantial improvement in his motor performance, with reduction in his levodopa by 60%. Despite this improvement, his depression worsened postoperatively, and close evaluation by his psychiatrist revealed mild suicidal ideation, with some thoughts of a plan. He was admitted to the psychiatry service, and a course of antidepressants was begun. Psychotherapy and supportive counselling were also engaged. His depression improved, and he was ultimately discharged home. One year later, his depression remains well controlled.

V. Voon (✉)
Department of Psychiatry, University of Cambridge, Addenbrooke's Hospital, Cambridge, UK
e-mail: vv247@cam.ac.uk

© Springer Nature Switzerland AG 2022
S. J. Frucht (ed.), *Movement Disorder Emergencies*, Current Clinical Neurology,
https://doi.org/10.1007/978-3-030-75898-1_32

Introduction

Parkinson's disease (PD) is characterized by a range of disease- or medication-related neuropsychiatric symptoms including depression, apathy, psychosis, anxiety, and cognitive and behavioral changes. Recent studies suggest the rates of completed suicides in PD to be greater than the general population [1]. Suicidal ideation appears to be common in PD. Suicide is a major but possibly preventable public health issue identified by the World Health Organization as one of the top ten causes of death. Suicide is multifactorial and is associated in the general population with depression, gender, age, marital status, comorbid physical illness, and previous suicide attempts [2]. In this chapter, the studies on suicidal behaviors in PD are reviewed and categorized into suicidal ideation and completed suicides.

Suicidal Ideation

Suicidal ideation is common in PD, reported across multiple studies between 12% and 30% of PD patients [3–7]. Suicidal ideation is most commonly associated with depression, reported in almost all studies. Other mental health symptoms such as psychosis, anxiety, impulse control disorders, and hopelessness have also been reported to be elevated [4]. Demographic factors such as lower age and PD-related factors such as lower age of PD onset, greater motor complications, more non-motor symptoms, and greater perceived disability are also associated with suicidal ideation [4, 5]. Suicidal ideation was increased in early-onset PD ($N = 577$) relative to late-onset PD ($N = 2973$) (22% vs. 13%) with ideation associated with depression, dyskinesias, nonsmoking, lower education, and higher non-motor symptoms [8].

Completed Suicides

An early study suggested completed suicides may be lower than the general population although multiple more recent studies have challenged this observation. Using the US National Centre of Health Statistics mortality database from 144,364 patients with PD, 122 (0.08%) had committed suicide, a rate 10 times lower than that of the general population (0.8%) [9]. The PD patients with completed suicides had higher rates of depression compared to PD patients who died from other causes, again emphasizing the role of depression. In a smaller study using the Ontario provincial coroner's records with prescription records as a marker of illness from 1354 elderly patients who had died by suicide, suicide was not more or less likely to occur with PD (odds ratio on multivariate analysis: 1.11) as compared to other medical disorders such as congestive heart failure, chronic lung disease, and seizures (odds ratio: 1.30–2.41) and psychiatric disorders (odds ratio: 2.60–3.94) [10]. Similarly, in a large Finnish database study of 555 hospital-treated patients above the age of 50 who had completed suicide, only 1.6% of all subjects were PD patients [11]. Previous suicide attempts in PD patients were common, occurring in 44% of cases as compared to other patients in 9.9%. Other associated characteristics included being male, recent diagnosis, living in a rural area and multiple somatic illnesses. However, multiple subsequent studies across differing countries show elevated rates with the standardized mortality ratio in PD in South Korea at 1.99 [12]; in Serbia [4] and the United Kingdom [13], the rate is five times higher than expected rates, and in the Netherlands an odds ratio of PD in those committing suicide via poisoning was 2.9 [14]. In a nationwide retrospective Danish cohort study from 1980 to 2016, the adjusted incidence rate ratio was elevated at 2.4 [15]. In a population-based cohort study using Taiwan's National Health Insurance and Taiwan Death Registry, the risk of suicide was elevated in PD ($N = 35,891$) (hazards ratio 2.1) relative to controls ($N = 143,557$) [16]. Suicides in PD were associated with younger age, urban dwelling, higher psychiatric rates, and often use of high lethality methods (jumping). The differences in rates may be related to cross-cultural differences in suicidal behavior, although multiple large-scale studies across multiple countries suggest elevated completed suicide rates relative to the general population. Taken together, suicidal ideation in PD is common, and completed suicides appear to be higher than the general population, although influenced by country.

Deep Brain Stimulation and Suicidal Outcomes

STN DBS appears to be associated with higher suicide outcomes in retrospective case-control studies but not in prospective randomized controlled trials. In a large international multicenter study reported in 2008 involving 55 centers, completed suicides occurred in 0.45% (24/5311) and attempted suicides in 0.9% (48/5311) [17]. Suicides occurring in the first postoperative year (0.26%) (263/100,000/year) were higher than the World Health Organization Standardized Mortality Ratio for suicide, age- and gender-matched (SMR: 12.63–15.64; $P < 0.001$), and remained elevated to the fourth postoperative year (0.04%) (38/100,000/year) (SMR: 1.81–2.31; $P < 0.05$) (Fig. 32.1). The excess number of deaths was 13 for the first postoperative year. Seventy-five percent of events occurred within the first 17 postoperative months. Postoperative mortality in the first year following STN DBS from other causes (e.g., hemorrhage, infection) has been reported at 0.41%. Thus, postoperative suicidal outcomes represent the highest risk for mortality following STN DBS.

A large single-center study of STN DBS patients, reported 10 years later in 2018, reported completed (0.75%, 4/543) and attempted (4.11%, 22/543) suicide rates [18]. The authors emphasize that the rate in the first (1/543), second, and third years were higher than the expected standardized mortality ratio. Those with ideation or

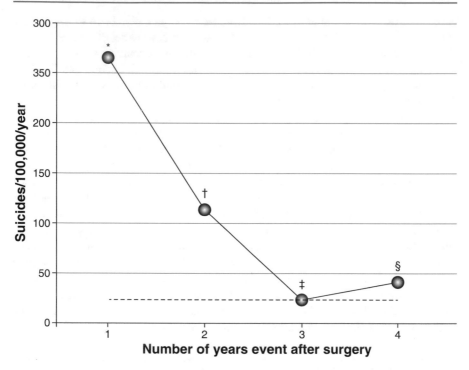

Fig. 32.1 Comparison of the suicide rate per postoperative year following subthalamic stimulation for advanced Parkinson's disease with the baseline suicide rate (printed with permission from Brain). *$P < 0.001$, weighted SMR = 12.64–15.64; †$P < 0.001$, weighted SMR = 5.13–6.91; ‡$P >$ 0.05, weighted SMR = 0.91–1.16; §$P < 0.05$, weighted SMR = 1.81–2.31. The observed postoperative STN DBS suicide rates per 100,000/year (*solid line*) and the lowest (*gray dotted line*) and highest (*black dotted line*) age-, gender-, and country-adjusted WHO expected suicide rates per 100,000/year are reported. (Reprinted from Voon et al. [17], with permission from Oxford University Press)

attempting suicide after STN DBS showed greater psychotic symptoms, family psychiatric history, psychiatric medication use, and higher frontal and depression scores.

In contrast, a randomized DBS and medical control trial, Phase 1 with DBS ($N = 121$) versus 6 months of best medical therapy ($N = 134$) reported no suicidal behaviors with similar rates of new-onset suicidal ideation (1.9% and 0.9%) [19]. The Phase 2 trial randomized to STN ($N = 147$) or GPi ($N = 152$) showed similar rates of suicidal ideation (1.5% and 0.7%). In an open-label STN DBS randomized medication-controlled trial with early motor complications, over the 2-year period, 2/124 STN DBS and 1/127 died by suicide [20]. In subsequent meta-analyses of STN DBS patients involving four cross-sectional, four cohort, and two randomized controlled trials and two case-control trial studies, STN DBS had a higher odds ratio but was not significantly higher relative to PD controls (OR = 2.84, $P = 0.18$) [21]. However, suicidal ideation and/or behaviors were significantly higher than the general population (lnSMR = 3.83, $P < 0.001$). Another meta-analysis including 18 studies showed the pooled rate of suicidal ideation was 4%, suicidal attempts 1%, and suicides 1% [22]. These conflicting results between retrospective clinical cohorts and prospective randomized trials are likely related to differences in comparator groups (medically treated PD versus general population), sample size, and duration of follow-up. Clinical trials will also more frequently follow up, inquire, and treat neuropsychiatric symptomatology with more careful follow-up relative to general clinical populations. Given the rare nature of suicides, smaller studies should be cautiously interpreted and may be influenced by reporting bias. The rate of suicide attempts in this PD clinical cohort may also be underreported or represent a greater proportion of successful attempts. The rates of completed suicides may also change over time given increased awareness of the issue and changes in preoperative and postoperative practices.

The rate of suicide is commonly elevated following any life-altering surgery. For instance, the suicide rate following epilepsy surgery is 1% or 31 times higher than the general population [23]. The baseline rate of suicide in epilepsy is eight times higher than the general population [24]. The study of associated behaviors allows us to address potentially modifiable risk factors. In a study of 200 STN DBS PD patients, 1/200 (1%) had completed and 4/200 (2%) had attempted suicides [25]. Suicidal behaviors were associated with postoperative depression and impaired impulse regulation in this study. Similarly, the multicenter study compared 27 attempted suicides and 9 completed suicides with 70 STN DBS controls selected from the patients who underwent surgery immediately prior to and immediately following the identified case at the same center [17]. Postoperative depression ($P < 0.001$), being single ($P = 0.007$), and a history of impulse control disorders or compulsive medication use ($P = 0.005$) were independent associated factors accounting for 51% of the variance of attempted suicide risk. Other associated factors included being younger, younger PD onset, and previous suicide attempt ($P < 0.05$). A trend was observed associated with greater changes in dopaminergic medications ($P = 0.05$). Overall, postoperative depression was the primary factor associated with both attempted and completed suicides after stringent correction for multiple comparisons. See Table 32.1 for a summary of factors associated with STN DBS for PD.

Postoperative depression following STN DBS has been associated with significant decreases in dopaminergic medications [26], a prior history of depression [27], and significant psychosocial postoperative changes [28] and has also been linked to serotonergic modulation in an animal model [29]. Possible effects of STN stimulation, dopaminergic medications, and the interaction between the two may also play a role in impulsivity.

Table 32.1 Summary of factors associated with attempted suicides following STN DBS for Parkinson's disease

	Probably associated (P < 0.01)	Possibly associated (P < 0.05)	Not associated (P > 0.05)	Unknown
Preoperative individual factors	Hx of impulse control disorders or compulsive medication use	Previous attempt Younger age Younger Parkinson's disease onset	Gender Preoperative cognitive status	Family history of suicide
Postoperative state	Postoperative depression[a] Postoperative apathy		Motor efficacy Stimulation parameters Postoperative cognitive changes	Interaction of stimulation with impulse control
Medication		Percent LEDD decrease**		Dopaminergic withdrawal state
Psychosocial factors	Single		Country-specific suicide rates	Expectations identity changes Relationship changes Supports other stressors

[a]Postoperative depression remains significant following Bonferroni correction. Reprinted from Voon et al. [17], with permission from Oxford University Press
**$P = 0.05$

Conclusion

Suicidal ideation is common in PD. Although completed suicides were once suggested to occur much less frequently than expected, large-scale studies across multiple countries suggests an elevated risk relative to the general population. Country-specific or cultural factors may play a modifying role. Suicidal behaviors in PD demonstrate a clear and consistent association with depression, thus highlighting the necessity to screen for and treat depressive symptoms along with actively screening for suicidal ideation in depressed patients. Other potential associated factors for suicide attempts include psychosis, impulse control disorders, younger age, and anxiety disorders. The early postoperative state following STN DBS poses an increased risk of suicide relative to the general population although whether this is elevated relative to matched medicated controls is less clear. Since suicidal behaviors are preventable and modifiable, careful assessment and education is indicated.

Suicidal behaviors correlate with depression in PD patients, and the early post-operative period following bilateral STN DBS is a period of increased risk.

Preoperative assessment should include a psychosocial assessment focusing on potential risk factors for suicide attempts, including being single and a previous history of impulse control disorders. Other possible factors include being younger, younger age of PD onset, and a history of previous attempts. Patients at higher risk should be counselled preoperatively along with family involvement and active postoperative follow-up. Preoperative psychoeducation should warn of the rare but possible risks with the goal of highlighting that these postoperative neuropsychiatric symptoms are treatable if recognized and adequately followed. Preoperative psychotropic medications should be maintained to avoid withdrawal states. Dopaminergic medication titration should be instituted with care to avoid the dopaminergic withdrawal state given its possible association with suicidal behaviors and potential liability with postoperative depression.

Patients and their caregivers should be questioned on neuropsychiatric behaviors and suicidal ideation in the postoperative period, particularly in the first 3 years after surgery. Patients with suicidal ideation or attempts should be referred to a psychiatrist. Issues of safety should be considered if a suicide attempt occurs, including the need for certification, hospitalization, and observation. The index of suspicion for postoperative depression should be high and those with depression carefully monitored and treated. The etiology of any postoperative depressive or apathy symptoms should be considered and may require resumption of the dopaminergic medication if related to the withdrawal state, or possibly resumption of a dopamine agonist or of other preoperative medications that may have been inadvertently discontinued such as benzodiazepines or antidepressants. A time-limited confusional state may require careful observation or possibly a low dose of an atypical neuroleptic. Hypomania can be managed with observation, if time limited and mild, or may require changes in dopaminergic medications or stimulation parameters. Psychosocial issues should be addressed including changes in relationships or identity and may require referrals for counselling or support.

Suicidal outcomes in PD represent a potentially modifiable form of mortality. Further studies to address modifiable risk factors would be useful for clinical management.

References

1. Shepard MD, Perepezko K, Broen MPG, Hinkle JT, Butala A, Mills KA, et al. Suicide in Parkinson's disease. J Neurol Neurosurg Psychiatry. 2019;90(7):822–9. https://doi.org/10.1136/jnnp-2018-319815.
2. Kessler RC, Borges G, Walters EE. Prevalence of and risk factors for lifetime suicide attempts in the National Comorbidity Survey. Arch Gen Psychiatry. 1999;56(7):617–26. Retrieved from http://www.ncbi.nlm.nih.gov/entrez/query.fcgi?cmd=Retrieve&db=PubMed&dopt=Citation&list_uids=10401507.
3. Belvisi D, Berardelli I, Ferrazzano G, Costanzo M, Corigliano V, Fabbrini G, et al. The clinical correlates of suicidal ideation in Parkinson's disease. Parkinsonism Relat Disord. 2019;63:54–9. https://doi.org/10.1016/j.parkreldis.2019.02.047.
4. Kostic VS, Pekmezovic T, Tomic A, Jecmenica-Lukic M, Stojkovic T, Spica V, et al. Suicide and suicidal ideation in Parkinson's disease. J Neurol Sci. 2010;289(1–2):40–3. https://doi.org/10.1016/j.jns.2009.08.016.

5. Kummer A, Cardoso F, Teixeira AL. Suicidal ideation in Parkinson's disease. CNS Spectr. 2009;14(8):431–6. Retrieved from http://www.ncbi.nlm.nih.gov/entrez/query.fcgi?cmd=Retr ieve&db=PubMed&dopt=Citation&list_uids=19890237.

6. Nazem S, Siderowf AD, Duda JE, Brown GK, Ten Have T, Stern MB, et al. Suicidal and death ideation in Parkinson's disease. Mov Disord. 2008;23(11):1573–9. https://doi.org/10.1002/ mds.22130.

7. Ozdilek B, Gultekin BK. Suicidal behavior among Turkish patients with Parkinson's disease. Neuropsychiatr Dis Treat. 2014;10:541–5. https://doi.org/10.2147/ndt.S60450.

8. Ou R, Wei Q, Hou Y, Zhang L, Liu K, Kong X, et al. Suicidal ideation in early-onset Parkinson's disease. J Neurol. 2021;268(5):1876–84. https://doi.org/10.1007/s00415-020-10333-4.

9. Myslobodsky M, Lalonde FM, Hicks L. Are patients with Parkinson's disease suicidal? J Geriatr Psychiatry Neurol. 2001;14(3):120–4. Retrieved from http://www.ncbi.nlm.nih.gov/ entrez/query.fcgi?cmd=Retrieve&db=PubMed&dopt=Citation&list_uids=11563434.

10. Juurlink DN, Herrmann N, Szalai JP, Kopp A, Redelmeier DA. Medical illness and the risk of suicide in the elderly. Arch Intern Med. 2004;164(11):1179–84. https://doi.org/10.1001/ archinte.164.11.1179.

11. Mainio A, Karvonen K, Hakko H, Sarkioja T, Rasanen P. Parkinson's disease and suicide: a profile of suicide victims with Parkinson's disease in a population-based study during the years 1988-2002 in Northern Finland. Int J Geriatr Psychiatry. 2009;24(9):916–20. https://doi. org/10.1002/gps.2194.

12. Lee T, Lee HB, Ahn MH, Kim J, Kim MS, Chung SJ, et al. Increased suicide risk and clinical correlates of suicide among patients with Parkinson's disease. Parkinsonism Relat Disord. 2016;32:102–7. https://doi.org/10.1016/j.parkreldis.2016.09.006.

13. Roberts SE, John A, Kandalama U, Williams JG, Lyons RA, Lloyd K. Suicide following acute admissions for physical illnesses across England and Wales. Psychol Med. 2018;48(4):578–91. https://doi.org/10.1017/s0033291717001787.

14. Eliasen A, Dalhoff KP, Horwitz H. Neurological diseases and risk of suicide attempt: a case-control study. J Neurol. 2018;265(6):1303–9. https://doi.org/10.1007/s00415-018-8837-4.

15. Erlangsen A, Stenager E, Conwell Y, Andersen PK, Hawton K, Benros ME, et al. Association between neurological disorders and death by suicide in Denmark. JAMA. 2020;323(5):444–54. https://doi.org/10.1001/jama.2019.21834.

16. Chen YY, Yu S, Hu YH, Li CY, Artaud F, Carcaillon-Bentata L, et al. Risk of suicide among patients with Parkinson disease. JAMA Psychiat. 2021;78(3):293–301. https://doi.org/10.1001/ jamapsychiatry.2020.4001.

17. Voon V, Krack P, Lang AE, Lozano AM, Dujardin K, Schupbach M, et al. A multicentre study on suicide outcomes following subthalamic stimulation for Parkinson's disease. Brain. 2008;131(Pt 10):2720–8. https://doi.org/10.1093/brain/awn214.

18. Giannini G, Francois M, Lhommée E, Polosan M, Schmitt E, Fraix V, et al. Suicide and suicide attempts after subthalamic nucleus stimulation in Parkinson disease. Neurology. 2019;93(1):e97–e105. https://doi.org/10.1212/wnl.0000000000007665.

19. Weintraub D, Duda JE, Carlson K, Luo P, Sagher O, Stern M, et al. Suicide ideation and behaviours after STN and GPi DBS surgery for Parkinson's disease: results from a randomised, controlled trial. J Neurol Neurosurg Psychiatry. 2013;84(10):1113–8. https://doi.org/10.1136/ jnnp-2012-304396.

20. Lhommée E, Wojtecki L, Czernecki V, Witt K, Maier F, Tonder L, et al. Behavioural outcomes of subthalamic stimulation and medical therapy versus medical therapy alone for Parkinson's disease with early motor complications (EARLYSTIM trial): secondary analysis of an open-label randomised trial. Lancet Neurol. 2018;17(3):223–31. https://doi.org/10.1016/ s1474-4422(18)30035-8.

21. Du J, Liu X, Zhou X, Wang H, Zhou W, Jiang J, et al. Parkinson's disease-related risk of suicide and effect of deep brain stimulation: meta-analysis. Parkinsons Dis. 2020;2020:8091963. https://doi.org/10.1155/2020/8091963.

22. Xu Y, Yang B, Zhou C, Gu M, Long J, Wang F, et al. Suicide and suicide attempts after sub-thalamic nucleus stimulation in Parkinson's disease: a systematic review and meta-analysis. Neurol Sci. 2021;42(1):267–74. https://doi.org/10.1007/s10072-020-04555-7.
23. Pompili M, Girardi P, Tatarelli G, Angeletti G, Tatarelli R. Suicide after surgical treatment in patients with epilepsy: a meta-analytic investigation. Psychol Rep. 2006;98(2):323–38. Retrieved from http://www.ncbi.nlm.nih.gov/entrez/query.fcgi?cmd=Retrieve&db=PubMed&dopt=Citation&list_uids=16796084.
24. Pompili M, Girardi P, Ruberto A, Tatarelli R. Suicide in the epilepsies: a meta-analytic investigation of 29 cohorts. Epilepsy Behav. 2005;7(2):305–10. https://doi.org/10.1016/j.yebeh.2005.05.010.
25. Soulas T, Gurruchaga JM, Palfi S, Cesaro P, Nguyen JP, Fenelon G. Attempted and completed suicides after subthalamic nucleus stimulation for Parkinson's disease. J Neurol Neurosurg Psychiatry. 2008;79(8):952–4. https://doi.org/10.1136/jnnp.2007.130583.
26. Thobois S, Ardouin C, Lhommee E, Klinger H, Lagrange C, Xie J, et al. Non-motor dopamine withdrawal syndrome after surgery for Parkinson's disease: predictors and underlying meso-limbic denervation. Brain. 2010;133(Pt 4):1111–27. https://doi.org/10.1093/brain/awq032.
27. Berney A, Vingerhoets F, Perrin A, Guex P, Villemure JG, Burkhard PR, et al. Effect on mood of subthalamic DBS for Parkinson's disease: a consecutive series of 24 patients. Neurology. 2020;59(9):1427–9. Retrieved from http://www.ncbi.nlm.nih.gov/entrez/query.fcgi?cmd=Retrieve&db=PubMed&dopt=Citation&list_uids=12427897.
28. Schupbach M, Gargiulo M, Welter ML, Mallet L, Behar C, Houeto JL, et al. Neurosurgery in Parkinson disease: a distressed mind in a repaired body? Neurology. 2006;66(12):1811–6. https://doi.org/10.1212/01.wnl.0000234880.51322.16.
29. Temel Y, Boothman LJ, Blokland A, Magill PJ, Steinbusch HW, Visser-Vandewalle V, et al. Inhibition of 5-HT neuron activity and induction of depressive-like behavior by high-frequency stimulation of the subthalamic nucleus. Proc Natl Acad Sci U S A. 2007;104(43):17087–92. https://doi.org/10.1073/pnas.0704144104.

Index